Human Gametes and Preimplantation Embryos

David K. Gardner • Denny Sakkas
Emre Seli • Dagan Wells
Editors

Human Gametes and Preimplantation Embryos

Assessment and Diagnosis

Springer

Editors
David K. Gardner, DPhil
Department of Zoology
University of Melbourne
Melbourne, VIC, Australia

Emre Seli, MD
Department of Obstetrics, Gynecology
and Reproductive Sciences
Yale School of Medicine
New Haven, CT, USA

Denny Sakkas, PhD
Boston IVF
Waltham, MA, USA

Dagan Wells, PhD, FRCPath
Nuffield Department of
Obstetrics and Gynaecology
University of Oxford
Oxford, UK

ISBN 978-1-4614-6650-5 ISBN 978-1-4614-6651-2 (eBook)
DOI 10.1007/978-1-4614-6651-2
Springer New York Heidelberg Dordrecht London

Library of Congress Control Number: 2013936260

Printed on acid-free paper

Springer is part of Springer Science+Business Media (www.springer.com)

Foreword

Human reproduction is very inefficient. Considering the overpopulation of many regions of our world, how can this be true? The simplistic answer is that the reproductive cycle operates about 13 times each year.

In normal reproduction, although greatly influenced by age, on average only about one in five unions of sperm and egg result in a normal neonate. There is abundant evidence that about two-thirds of these failures are due to chromosomal aneuploidy. One can speculate that the remainder are due to mismatches at the molecular level.

Clinical IVF superimposes its own inefficiency on the inefficiency of normal reproduction. On an egg retrieval basis, IVF requires about ten mature eggs for each neonate. To be sure there is some correction by cryopreservation. These considerations point to the great importance for clinical IVF of an ability to identify one or more biomarkers during oogenesis, spermatogenesis, or embryogenesis, which can predict a normal neonate.

David Gardner, Denny Sakkas, Emre Seli, and Dagan Wells, all distinguished workers in this pursuit, from Australia, the United States and the United Kingdom, have gathered an inclusive and brilliant group of investigators whose work has contributed and surely will continue to contribute to this search.

This encyclopedia of amazing and complicated molecular reactions, which must be just right for each of us to exist, is required reading for anyone who wishes to join the pursuit for the magic biomarker. In addition, every reproductive physician and embryologist will surely be better informed by becoming familiar with the contents of this book as it will give insight and understanding of what is being influenced by their efforts.

It needs to be noted that this book concerns the gametes and the embryo and gives no consideration to the role played by the endometrium. This is in keeping with the biblical story of the seed and soil, which has been aptly paraphrased by many, stating that reproductive inefficiency is due to the seed and not the soil. However, there may well be a minority of cases where there is a problem with the soil.

When a unique biomarker or biomarkers can predict a normal neonate and is widely applied in clinical IVF, a change in mindset of the patient and the physician may well be required. The magic biomarkers will accomplish, in the laboratory, what nature has been doing forever by overcoming what we call the inefficiency of human reproduction. Both patient and staff must understand and be prepared that there may be retrieval cycles that will be characterized by no transfers, especially among patients in the latter 30s and beyond.

However, there is a real compensating possibility that we will understand how to harvest enough eggs to minimize or eliminate the inefficiency of reproduction enhanced by retrieval from a single menstrual cycle. This book should be in the library and minds of every IVF program around the world.

Howard W. Jones, Jr., MD
Professor Emeritus
Eastern Virginia Medical School
Norfolk, VA, USA
Johns Hopkins University School of Medicine
Baltimore, MD, USA

Preface

The plight of infertile couples has been greatly alleviated over the past three decades. Assisted Reproductive Technologies have facilitated the birth of over five million children and counting. Such a wonderful outcome has only been made possible through the tireless work of numerous physicians, nurses, and scientists all around the world. Advances in ovarian stimulation, and laboratory conditions and procedures, have facilitated greater success rates and safer outcomes. Concomitantly, high-order multiple gestations, once a common complication, are now being retired to the archives of human IVF. Nonetheless, the incidence of twins remains high in several communities, culminating in IVF being responsible for a disproportionate percentage of multiple births. The once elusive goal of routine single embryo transfer is finally becoming a reality in some countries. However, in order for single embryo transfer to become the standard of care for all, it is imperative that accurate, rapid, and economical methods of quantifying embryo viability are developed to ensure that the most viable euploid embryo is selected for transfer. Ideally, such tests would be noninvasive, lessening the risks to the embryo and reducing costs and workload in the embryology laboratory.

It was with the goal of single embryo transfer for all patients that we set out to review the established and developing methods for embryo selection, outline promising new technologies, and speculate about the future of embryo selection. The scope of this project covers the analysis of embryo morphological characteristics, both as static observations (conventional scoring) or with time as a continuous variable (morphokinetics), the capability of novel genetic screening approaches for the analysis of embryo ploidy and gene defects, and finally the analysis of both proteome and metabolome of gametes and embryos. The rapid advancement in several technologies described in this book will not only ensure that we are able to obtain highly valuable and novel insights into events during the first week of human life, but will facilitate the creation of assays to identify the most suitable embryo for transfer (and cryopreservation).

It has been our privilege to have worked with the many distinguished contributors for this volume. We dedicate this book to the millions of infertile couples worldwide. It is our collective goal in the IVF community to make their journey to parenthood short in duration and successful.

Melbourne, VIC, Australia — David K. Gardner, DPhil
Waltham, MA, USA — Denny Sakkas, PhD
New Haven, CT, USA — Emre Seli, MD
Oxford, UK — Dagan Wells, PhD, FRCPath

Contents

Contributors

Ashok Agarwal, PhD Clinical Andrology Laboratory and Reproductive Tissue Bank, Glickman Urological and Kidney Institute, Cleveland, OH, USA

Center for Reproductive Medicine, Cleveland Clinic, Cleveland, OH, USA

R. John Aitken, PhD, ScD Discipline of Biological Sciences, Faculty of Science and IT, University of Newcastle, NSW, Australia

Juan G. Alvarez, MD, PhD Department of Male Infertility, Centro ANDROGEN, La Coruña, Spain

Baris Ata, MD, MCT Department of Obstetrics and Gynecology, Uludag University Hospital, Bursa, Republic of Turkey

Mark A. Baker, PhD Discipline of Biological Sciences, Faculty of Science and IT, University of Newcastle, Callaghan, NSW, Australia

Basak Balaban, BSc Assisted Reproduction Unit, American Hospital of Istanbul, Istanbul, Turkey

Can Bruce, PhD Department of Molecular Biochemistry and Biophysics, W. M. Keck Foundation Biotechnology Resource Laboratory, Yale School of Medicine, New Haven, CT, USA

María Cruz, PhD IVI Alicante, Alicante, Spain

Joy Delhanty, PhD Fetal and Maternal Medicine, Institute for Women's Health, University College, London, UK

Elpida Fragouli, PhD Nuffield Department of Obstetrics and Gynaecology, University of Oxford, Oxford, UK

Reprogenetics UK, Oxford, UK

Bhushan K. Gangrade, PhD IVF Laboratory, Center for Reproductive Medicine, Orlando, FL, USA

David K. Gardner, DPhil Department of Zoology, University of Melbourne, Melbourne, VIC, Australia

Tsilya Gerasimova, PhD Department of Obstetrics, Gynecology and Reproductive Sciences, Yale School of Medicine, New Haven, CT, USA

Alan H. Handyside, MA, PhD The Bridge Centre, London Bridge, London, UK

Franchesca D. Houghton, BSc(Hons), DPhil Centre for Human Development, Stem Cells & Regeneration, Faculty of Medicine, University of Southampton, Southampton, UK

Gabor Huszar, MD Sperm Physiology Laboratory, Department of Obstetrics, Gynecology, and Reproductive Sciences, Yale School of Medicine, New Haven, CT, USA

Benedetta Iussig, MSc Clinica Valle Giulia, GENERA Rome, Marostica, Italy

Ubertide Centre for Reproductive Medicine, Rome, Italy

Mandy G. Katz-Jaffe, PhD National Foundation for Fertility Research, Lone Tree, CO, USA

David L. Keefe, MD Department of Obstetrics and Gynecology, New York University School of Medicine, NYU Langone Medical Center, New York, NY, USA

Maria Köster, DVM Department Gynecological Endocrinology and Reproductive Medicine, University of Bonn, Bonn, Germany

Helena Kristiansson, PhD Department of Obstetrics, Gynecology and Reproductive Sciences, Yale School of Medicine, New Haven, CT, USA

Maria D. Lalioti, PhD Department of Obstetrics, Gynecology and Reproductive Sciences, Yale School of Medicine, New Haven, CT, USA

Michelle Lane, PhD Repromed, Dulwich, SA, Australia

Susanna McReynolds, PhD National Foundation for Fertility Research, Lone Tree, CO, USA

Marcos Meseguer, PhD IVF Unit, Clinical Embryology Laboratory, Instituto Valenciano de Infertilidad, Valencia, Spain

Markus Montag, MD IVF Laboratory, Department of Gynecological Endocrinology & Fertility Medicine, University of Heidelberg, Heidelberg, Germany

Manuel Muñoz, MD Instituto Valenciano de Infertilidad, Alicante, Spain

David L. Potter, BSc Department of Zoology, The University of Melbourne, Melbourne, VIC, Australia

Laura Rienzi, MS GENERA Centre for Reproductive Medicine, Rome, Italy

Denny Sakkas, PhD Boston IVF, Waltham, MA, USA

Thomas Schimming, PhD Independent Image Processing IT Professional, Munich, Germany

Emre Seli, MD Department of Obstetrics, Gynecology and Reproductive Sciences, Yale School of Medicine, New Haven, CT, USA

George A. Thouas, BSc, MRepSc, PhD Department of Zoology, The University of Melbourne, Melbourne, VIC, Australia

Nathan R. Treff, PhD Reproductive Medicine Associates of New Jersey, Basking Ridge, NJ, USA

Department of Obstetrics, Gynecology, and Reproductive Sciences, UMDNJ—Robert Wood Johnson Medical School, New Brunswick, NJ, USA

Filippo Ubaldi, MD Clinica Valle Giulia, GENERA Roma, Marostica, Italy

Umbertide Centre for Reproductive Medicine, Rome, Italy

Asli Uyar, PhD Department of Obstetrics and Gynecology, Yale School of Medicine, New Haven, CT, USA

Jonathan Van Blerkom, PhD Department of Molecular, Cellular and Developmental Biology, University of Colorado, Boulder, CO, USA

Leeanda Wilton, PhD Preimplantation Genetics, Melbourne IVF, East Melbourne, VIC, Australia

Dagan Wells, PhD, FRCPath Nuffield Department of Obstetrics and Gynaecology, University of Oxford, Oxford, UK

Institute of Reproductive Sciences, Oxford, UK

1 Current Practices and Regulations for Embryo Transfer Worldwide: Implications on IVF Outcome

Baris Ata and Emre Seli

The birth of Louise Brown opened a new era in reproductive medicine. Following decades of research on animal models and humans, the first successful human in vitro fertilization (IVF) procedure involved the fertilization of a single metaphase two (MII) oocyte collected in a natural cycle [1]. However, soon it was realized that pregnancy and birth rates per treatment cycle could be increased in parallel with the number of oocytes collected [2]. This was achieved by using exogenous gonadotropin administration to overcome the decrease in endogenous follicle stimulating hormone levels in serum, which is responsible for limiting the number of growing antral follicles in the early follicular phase. In this manner, it has been possible to maintain the growth of a larger number of follicles that would otherwise undergo atresia and to collect more MII oocytes to be fertilized [3]. Stimulation protocols were later improved to involve gonadotropin releasing hormone analogues to prevent premature ovulation and even to schedule treatment procedures [4]. Controlled ovarian hyperstimulation (COS) with various combinations of exogenous gonadotropins and GnRH analogues proved to increase the success rate of IVF, and the results achieved by most treatment centers exceed spontaneous conception rates in healthy fertile couples [5].

However, this success was achieved through the simultaneous transfer of multiple embryos in the majority of IVF cycles. Transferring multiple embryos rapidly became the norm and it was not uncommon to transfer five or six embryos at a time. This has led to an "iatrogenic" epidemic of multiple pregnancies. The incidence of multiple pregnancies fluctuated around 30 % of all IVF pregnancies and triplets and higher order multiple pregnancies (HOMP) comprised approximately 5 % of all IVF pregnancies worldwide [6–8]. Compared to spontaneous pregnancies, these figures correspond to almost a 20- and 50-fold increase in the incidence of twins and higher order multiples, respectively [9]. In the United States, while IVF cycles accounted for only 1 % of all births in the year 2006, 18 % of multiple births resulted from IVF, and a striking 48 % of all IVF neonates were the products of multiple gestations, a frequency 15- to 20-fold greater than with spontaneous conceptions [10, 11].

Risks Associated with IVF

Multiple Pregnancy as the Most Common Cause of Morbidity and Mortality Associated with IVF

Multiple pregnancies are associated with serious complications for IVF children. Compared to singletons the neonatal mortality of twins and

B. Ata (✉)
Department of Obstetrics and Gynecology, Uludag University Hospital, Bursa, Republic of Turkey
e-mail: barisata@hotmail.com

E. Seli
Department of Obstetrics, Gynecology and Reproductive Sciences, Yale School of Medicine, New Haven, CT, USA

D.K. Gardner et al. (eds.), *Human Gametes and Preimplantation Embryos: Assessment and Diagnosis*, DOI 10.1007/978-1-4614-6651-2_1,

triplet and HOMPs are increased by 7- and 22-fold, respectively [12]. The mean gestational age of delivery is approximately 35 weeks for twin and 32 weeks for triplet gestations [13]. Consequently, while multiple births constitute only 3 % of all births in the United States, they account for 13 % of preterm births before 37 weeks of gestational age, and 25 % of very low birth weight infants [14]. The higher rate of preterm delivery in neonates from multiple infant pregnancies does not only compromise their chances of survival but also increases their risk of physical handicap. The risks associated with preterm delivery include neurological problems. Cerebral palsy is significantly more frequent in babies born from multiple gestations due to the strong association between premature delivery and cerebral palsy [15]. While the incidence of cerebral palsy is about 2 per 1,000 live births in the general population, it is estimated to increase to 9, 31, and 111 per 1,000 live births in twin, triplet, and quadruplet pregnancies, respectively [16, 17]. Overall, 1 in 5 triplet pregnancies and 1 in 2 quadruplet pregnancies result in at least one child suffering a significant long-term handicap [17].

Maternal Risks Associated with Multiple Pregnancy

Multiple pregnancy increases the risk of serious maternal complications. The risk of pregnancy-induced hypertension and preeclampsia in twins is reported to be five to tenfold higher in multiple pregnancies than in singletons [18]. Similarly, the incidence of gestational diabetes is increased in parallel to the number of fetuses. Compared to singletons, the risk of gestational diabetes is increased twofold in twin pregnancies and more than threefold in triplets [18]. Risk of operative delivery, postpartum hemorrhage, and maternal mortality are all increased in multiple pregnancies [19].

Financial Implications of Multiple Pregnancies Resulting from IVF

On top of the medical complications, multiple pregnancies also cause a significant financial burden on the couple and the society. These complications lead to an increased length and number of hospital stays, and as a consequence, a significant increase in healthcare costs. In fact, neonatal intensive care unit (NICU) admission is ultimately required for 25 % of twins, 75 % of triplets, and nearly all quadruplets, again with the enormous increase in costs associated with lengthy inpatient care [20, 21]. The Board on Health Sciences Policy has estimated that the mean healthcare cost for each preterm infant born in the United States was $51,600 [22]. These costs include prenatal, peripartum, and neonatal care, as well as the costs of increased care and education through the first 5 years of life. Using these values and the data provided by the Society of Assisted Reproductive Technologies (SART), we have estimated the yearly cost of preterm births that result from IVF-associated multiple pregnancies to be $1 billion per year between 2000 and 2006 [23].

Efforts to Limit Multiple Pregnancy

In the early days of human IVF more emphasis was given on achieving a pregnancy, regardless of the number of fetuses. However, advances in IVF procedures and increasing embryo implantation rates over time led to an unprecedented increase in multiple pregnancies. Healthcare professionals and authorities soon realized the burden of IVF multiple pregnancies on the couple and the society. Today the vast majority of practitioners define the aim of IVF as to achieve a healthy singleton live birth at term. Even twin pregnancies are, rightfully, regarded as a complication.

Simply, limiting the number of embryos transferred in an IVF cycle would be expected to solve the problem of multiple pregnancies. Unfortunately, voluntary measures to limit the number of embryos transferred have not been successful in yielding the desired reduction in multiple pregnancies worldwide. Nevertheless, increasing awareness of the complications associated with triplets and HOMPs have led to a decrease in the number of embryos transferred and in the number of triplets and HOMPs. However, twin pregnancies still comprise a substantial proportion of IVF pregnancies. According to the latest reports available twin pregnancies comprised 37 % of all IVF live births in the United States (fresh non-donor egg cycles in 2009) and 19.9 % in Europe (fresh cycles in 2006) [24, 25]. Despite decreasing proportions of triplets and HOMP, the absolute number of IVF multiples are still rising due to the high percentage of twins and ever increasing number of IVF cycles performed annually. The International Committee for Monitoring Assisted Reproductive Technologies estimated that in the year 2003 over 930,000 IVF cycles have been performed worldwide, representing a 10 % increase over the 2002 estimate of 820,000 IVF cycles, and 24.8 % of all pregnancies achieved were twins while 2.0 % was triplets or HOMPs [26].

Current Practices of Embryo Transfer and Clinical Outcomes of IVF Across Continents

Europe

Recognizing the burden of IVF multiples on the society, some European countries were the first to introduce legal limitations on the number of embryos transferred. In 2003, Belgian government decided to reimburse up to six IVF cycles in a lifetime of a woman up to her 43rd birthday in return of limiting the number of embryos transferred in an IVF cycle. According to Belgian legislation, single embryo transfer (SET) is obligatory at the first IVF attempt for all patients younger than 36 years. For the second cycle SET also has to be performed as the first choice, but double embryo transfer (DET) is allowed when only embryos of poor quality are available. From the third cycle on, DET is allowed without restriction. For patients between 36 and 39 years DET can be performed on the first and second occasions. From the third cycle on, replacement of up to three embryos is allowed. For patients older than 39 years, there is no legal limit to the number of transferred embryos. A retrospective analysis evaluating the effect of new regulations on IVF outcome in Belgium revealed that the percentage of SET was increased from 14 to 49 % [27]. Embryo implantation rate did not change significantly; it was 25.9 and 23 % before and after the regulations, respectively. The overall pregnancy rate was maintained (36 % vs. 37 % before and after regulations, respectively). However, twin pregnancies were decreased from 19 to 3 %. The results of the study by Gordts et al. and of another similar study by Van Landuyt et al. demonstrate that elective SET enacted by the Belgian regulations significantly decreased the twin pregnancy rate without a reduction in the overall pregnancy rate [27, 28].

In 2003, Sweden introduced regulations that are similar to those implemented in Belgium. It is noteworthy that IVF clinics in Sweden had already voluntarily decreased the number of embryos transferred from 3 to 2 since 1993. This rare example of successful voluntary limitation had already almost completely eliminated triplets and HOMPs in Sweden. The new regulation was aimed to decrease the rate of twin pregnancies which had remained relatively high. Elective SET was recommended for the first two treatment cycles in women aged less than 36 years, provided that the woman had at least two good quality embryos. DET was allowed in other cases. By the year 2004, the proportion of SET was increased to 67.4 % from 30.6 % in 2002. While the live birth rate per transfer remained stable (26.8 % in 2002 and 25 % in 2004), the multiple birth rate was dramatically decreased from 19.4 to 5.7 % [29].

According to the latest report of the European IVF Monitoring Consortium (EIM), in the year 2006, a single embryo was transferred in 69.9 and 49.2 % of all IVF/ICSI cycles in Sweden and Belgium resulting in twin delivery rates of 5.7 % and 13.2 %, respectively [29]. Among the 27 countries reporting to EIM, Norway and Finland outstand as the only other countries where SETs comprised approximately 50 % of all IVF/ICSI cycles in the same year. Despite the absence of strict legal restrictions a single embryo was transferred in 54.7 and 48 % of IVF/ICSI cycles in Finland and Norway, respectively. These four countries and Iceland were the only European countries which reported a twin delivery rate of less than 15 % coupled with a triplet delivery rate of less than 1 % in the same year. At the other end of the spectrum, in eight countries (8/27, 29.6 %) three or more embryos were transferred in more than 50 % of IVF/ICSI cycles. Twin delivery rates ranged between 16.7 and 30 % while triplets ranged between 0 and 14 % in these countries [25].

Despite the successful examples set by Belgium and Sweden, most European countries do not have strict legal limitations on the number of embryos transferred. Those with regulations liberally limit the number of embryos transferred with three embryos per cycle, some depending on patient age or rank of treatment cycle. Notably, since 2009 Turkey has made SET mandatory for the first two transfer cycles in women less than 35 years of age, and no more than two embryos are allowed regardless of cycle rank, female age, or government reimbursement status. Unfortunately national data has not been available at the time of writing this chapter so we are unable to comment on the effects of these limitations on treatment outcome.

North America

On the other side of the Atlantic Ocean, Quebec province in Canada has taken the lead in limiting the number of embryos transferred by law in return of government reimbursement for IVF. Quebec law states that only one embryo should be transferred in either a fresh or frozen IVF cycle. However, the physicians are given the option of transferring two embryos to women less than 36 years and up to three embryos (no more than two blastocysts) to women aged 37 years or older, provided that they can justify the rationale for transferring more than one embryo. In return, Quebec government reimburses up to three IVF cycles with conventional COS or up to six IVF cycles with mild stimulation. The law came into effect as of 5th of August 2010. Bissonnette et al. have reported that the proportion of elective SET rose to 50 % from 1.6 % in the province within 3 months after the law [30]. Although the overall clinical pregnancy rate fell to 31.6 % from 42.8 %, almost half of all women under 40 years of age had at least one embryo cryopreserved following the fresh IVF cycle. The average number of embryos cryopreserved per patient was 3.4, which can be reasonably expected to balance the cumulative pregnancy rate. Importantly, multiple pregnancy rate was decreased to 3.7 % from 25.6 %. The clinical pregnancy (32 %) and the relatively low twin pregnancy (13 %) rates achieved in women who received elective DET attest to the fact that clinicians have judiciously used the option of transferring an additional embryo across the province. Furthermore, there were no triplet pregnancies at all. It seems that Quebec will be providing better access to reproductive care to its residents using the funds saved by cutting the costs of multiple pregnancies. Other Canadian provinces are expected to implement similar legislations and reimbursement programs soon.

In the United States, however, the situation is very different than Canada; there are no legal limitations on the number of embryos transferred in an IVF cycle. In the United States a single embryo was transferred in only 13.5 % of IVF cycles using fresh non-donor eggs or embryos in 2009 [24]. In 34.9 % of IVF cycles using fresh non-donor eggs or embryos 3 or more embryos were transferred; 3.7 % of women received five or more embryos. This has resulted in 30 % rate of multiple infant deliveries, relatively 50 % higher than the European rate at 20.8 % [24, 25]. It is important to note that while the US data is for the year 2009, the European figure belongs to 2006. However, the rate of multiple infant delivery in the United States was similar at 30.7 % in 2006.

The higher multiple delivery rates in the United States than Europe and Quebec is most likely due to different reimbursement policies. Out of pocket IVF cost is the highest in the United States than anywhere else in the world [31]. Moreover, in the majority of states IVF is not covered by insurance carriers. It is very likely that the financial pressure on both patients and physicians in the United States lead to transferring more embryos as they try to maximize the chances of achieving a pregnancy with the least number of attempts. In fact, embryo transfer practice seems to differ between states with or without insurance coverage for IVF. Martin and colleagues compared IVF outcomes between states with (where insurance carriers were required to cover at least one IVF cycle for a couple) and without a mandate for IVF coverage [32]. The average number of embryos transferred (2.6 vs. 2.2) and the multiple birth rates (32 % vs. 29.4 %) were both significantly lower in states with a mandate.

South America

There are no legal limitations on the number of embryos transferred in South American Countries. However, more than 90 % of all South American IVF centers are registered with Latin America Network of Assisted Reproduction (RED) [33]. Clinics are required to follow RED norms in order to be accredited by the network. According to the guidelines published in 2007, RED requires that the rate of multiple pregnancies is less than 30 % of clinical pregnancies defined as ongoing pregnancy beyond 12th gestational week, and that the rate of triplet pregnancies does not exceed 1 %. HOMPs are not acceptable. In order to achieve this goal RED recommends limiting the number of embryos transferred according to female age and number of previous treatment cycles and no more than two embryos should be transferred in about 60 % of all IVF cycles. RED states that these recommendations will be revised to decrease the suggested number of embryos to be transferred. It should be noted that RED accreditation is voluntary and an unaccredited center can continue to operate as long as it complies with legal requirements in its home country.

According to the annual RED report covering the year 2009, 27,174 fresh IVF/ICSI cycles were started. The average number of embryos transferred was 2.4. This resulted in 7,500 (27.6 %) clinical pregnancies. While twin pregnancies comprised 19.5 % of all clinical pregnancies, the rate of triplet and HOMP was 2 %. Despite the absence of legal limitations, South American figures seem closer to European figures than the US figures. However, compared to Quebec and European countries with legal limitations rate of multiples is still high in Latin American countries and there seems to be room for improvement.

Asia

In Japan, the number of embryos transferred is not regulated by law. However, government reimbursement is only provided when IVF is performed by a center that is registered with the Japanese Society of Obstetrics and Gynecology (JSOG). Starting in 2008, JSOG has recommended that one embryo is transferred, with a maximum of two embryos for those over 35-years-old or who have failed IVF treatments more than once [34]. Accordingly, 59.9 % of all fresh IVF cycles resulted in SET and 35.6 % in DET. Resultantly the rate of multiple pregnancies was decreased to 7.4 % in 2008 from 11 % in 2007 [34]. The rate of SET cycles in Japan is higher than the rates in Quebec, Belgium, Norway, and Finland, only surpassed by Sweden. However, the rate of live birth per transfer was 13.6 % for IVF cycles using fresh embryos, a figure less than that achieved in Quebec, Sweden, Finland, Belgium, and Norway.

In South Korea, while there are no strict legal regulations, the government provides guidelines on the number of embryos transferred. Two and three good quality embryos can be transferred to women under 35 years of age and women aged 35–40 years, respectively. An additional embryo is allowed when the embryo quality is poor. For women older than 40 years of age there is no limit on the number of embryos transferred. Similarly, in China, a maximum of two embryos can be placed to women younger than 35, and a maximum of three embryos to women who are 35 or older.

Australia and New Zealand

Despite the absence of legal regulations for the number of embryos transferred, all IVF clinics are required to be accredited by the Reproductive Technology Accreditation Committee (RTAC).

RTAC Code of Practice requires clinics to provide evidence that they regularly monitor multiple pregnancy rates and take corrective actions that continuously attempt to reduce the incidence of multiple pregnancies in all treatment cycles [35]. RTAC requires IVF clinics to recommend SET for all women under 35, and to ensure that no more than two embryos are transferred to women between 35 and 40 years of age [35].

Consequently, according to the latest report of the Australian Institute of Health and Welfare, there has been a significant increase in the number of SET cycles in Australia and New Zealand [36]. In 2005, the proportion of SET cycles accounted for 48.3 % of embryo transfer cycles and by 2009 this proportion had increased to 69.7 % ($p<0.01$). There was also a significant decline in the proportion of cycles in which three or more embryos were transferred, from 1.9 % in 2005 to 0.7 % in 2009 ($p<0.01$). Despite increasing proportion of SET cycles clinical pregnancy rates remained stable at around 23 % per cycle while the rate of multiple birth deliveries was decreased to 8.2 % in 2009 from 14.1 % in 2005.

Conclusions

Multiple pregnancy is regarded as the most important complication of IVF. With the exception of the rare occurrence of monochorionic twinning following SET, IVF multiples are caused by multiple embryo transfer. Therefore, an SET policy would prevent almost all multiple pregnancies in women undergoing IVF. However, both physicians and patients feel the pressure to achieve a pregnancy with the least treatment attempts. Consequently, despite the obvious trend toward decreasing the number of embryos transferred worldwide, triplets and HOMP still occur and twin pregnancies comprise a substantial proportion of IVF pregnancies.

Reimbursement policies which decrease the out of pocket cost of IVF for the couple together with legal, but reasonable, restrictions on the number of embryos transferred seem to achieve remarkable decrease in multiple pregnancies while maintaining pregnancy rates. This is very well demonstrated by the examples set by Quebec and some European countries. Such reimbursement strategies are expected to decrease financial burden of IVF multiples on the healthcare systems and allow funds to be used for increasing access to IVF by those in need.

The ultimate aim should be to implement a universal SET policy. The major obstacle in achieving this goal is our failure to choose the implantation competent embryo by current methods of embryo assessment. The ideal method to identify an implantation competent embryo among those generated in an IVF cycle should be embryologist and embryo friendly; it should be easy to use, highly sensitive and specific, noninvasive, as well as cost-effective. During the last decade a number of new methods have been introduced to select the best gametes and embryos. However, the quest for optimal method continues. In the following chapters of this book world renowned experts discuss pros and cons of these emerging technologies.

Acknowledgments The authors would like to acknowledge Basak Balaban from the American Hospital, Istanbul, Turkey, Weon Young Son from McGill University Health Centre, Montreal, Quebec, David Mortimer from Oozoa, Vancouver, Canada, David Edgar from Melbourne IVF, Australia, Osamu Okitsu from Miyake Clinic, Japan, Soledad Sepulveda, Grup PRANOR, Peru. We are thankful for their kind help in providing essential information for this chapter.

References

1. Steptoe PC, Edwards RG. Birth after the reimplantation of a human embryo. Lancet. 1978;2(8085):366.
2. Trounson AO, Leeton JF, Wood C, et al. Pregnancies in humans by fertilization in vitro and embryo transfer in the controlled ovulatory cycle. Science. 1981; 212(4495):681–2.
3. Lopata A. Successes and failures in human in vitro fertilization. Nature. 1980;288(5792):642–3.
4. Hughes EG, Fedorkow DM, Daya S, et al. The routine use of gonadotropin-releasing hormone agonists prior to in vitro fertilization and gamete intrafallopian transfer: a meta-analysis of randomized controlled trials. Fertil Steril. 1992;58(5):888–96.
5. Engmann L, Maconochie N, Bekir JS, et al. Cumulative probability of clinical pregnancy and live

birth after a multiple cycle IVF package: a more realistic assessment of overall and age-specific success rates? Br J Obstet Gynaecol. 1999;106(2):165–70.
6. Belgian College of Physicians for Reproductive Medicine. Annual report for activities of medically assisted reproduction, Belgium, version 1.0.2008. 2008. Available from: http://www.belrap.be/Documents/Reports/Global/Report_IVF08_16SEP10.pdf
7. Centers for Disease Control and Prevention, American Society for Reproductive Medicine, Society for Assisted Reproductive Technology. 2006 Assisted reproductive technology success rates: national summary and fertility clinic reports. Atlanta: US Department of Health and Human Services, Centers for Disease Control and Prevention; 2008.
8. Gunby J, Bissonnette F, Librach C, Cowan L. Assisted reproductive technologies (ART) in Canada: 2007 results from the Canadian ART Register. Fertil Steril. 2011;95(2):542–7.e1–10.
9. Adamson D, Baker V. Multiple births from assisted reproductive technologies: a challenge that must be met. Fertil Steril. 2004;81(3):517–22, discussion 526.
10. Sunderam S, Chang J, Flowers L, et al. Assisted reproductive technology surveillance—United States, 2006. Morb Mortal Wkly Rep. 2009;58(SS–5):1–26.
11. Reddy UM, Wapner RJ, Rebar RW, Tasca RJ. Infertility, assisted reproductive technology, and adverse pregnancy outcomes: executive summary of a National Institute of Child Health and Human Development workshop. Obstet Gynecol. 2007;109(4): 967–77.
12. Oleszczuk JJ, Oleszczuk AK, Keith DM, Keith LG. Twin and triplet births: facts, figures, and costs. Female Patient. 2003;28(6):11.
13. Martin JA, Hamilton BE, Sutton PD, et al. Births: final data for 2005. Natl Vital Stat Rep. 2007;56(6): 1–103.
14. Luke B, Martin JA. The rise in multiple births in the United States: who, what, when, where, and why. Clin Obstet Gynecol. 2004;47(1):118–33.
15. Hvidtjorn D, Grove J, Schendel DE, et al. Cerebral palsy among children born after in vitro fertilization: the role of preterm delivery–a population-based, cohort study. Pediatrics. 2006;118(2):475–82.
16. Petterson B, Nelson KB, Watson L, Stanley F. Twins, triplets, and cerebral palsy in births in Western Australia in the 1980s. BMJ. 1993;307(6914):1239–43.
17. Yokoyama Y, Shimizu T, Hayakawa K. Prevalence of cerebral palsy in twins, triplets and quadruplets. Int J Epidemiol. 1995;24(5):943–8.
18. Malone FD, Kaufman GE, Chelmow D, et al. Maternal morbidity associated with triplet pregnancy. Am J Perinatol. 1998;15(1):73–7.
19. The ESHRE Capri Workshop Group. Multiple gestation pregnancy. Hum Reprod. 2000;15(8):1856–64.
20. Chelmow D, Penzias AS, Kaufman G, Cetrulo C. Costs of triplet pregnancy. Am J Obstet Gynecol. 1995;172(2 Pt 1):677–82.
21. Luke B, Bigger HR, Leurgans S, Sietsema D. The cost of prematurity: a case-control study of twins vs singletons. Am J Public Health. 1996;86(6):809–14.
22. Behrman R, Butler A, editors. Board on Health Sciences Policy, Institute of Medicine. Preterm birth: causes, consequences, and prevention. Washington, DC: The National Academies; 2006.
23. Bromer JG, Ata B, Seli M, et al. Preterm deliveries that result from multiple pregnancies associated with assisted reproductive technologies in the USA: a cost analysis. Curr Opin Obstet Gynecol. 2011;23(3): 168–73.
24. Centers for Disease Control and Prevention, American Society for Reproductive Medicine, Society for Assisted Reproductive Technology. 2009 Assisted reproductive technology success rates: national summary and fertility clinic reports. Atlanta: US Department of Health and Human Services, Centers for Disease Control and Prevention; 2011.
25. de Mouzon J, Goossens V, Bhattacharya S, et al. Assisted reproductive technology in Europe, 2006: results generated from European registers by ESHRE. Hum Reprod. 2010;25(8):1851–62.
26. Nygren KG, Sullivan E, Zegers-Hochschild F, et al. International Committee for Monitoring Assisted Reproductive Technology (ICMART) world report: assisted reproductive technology 2003. Fertil Steril. 2011;95(7):2209–22; 2222.e1–17.
27. Gordts S, Campo R, Puttemans P, et al. Belgian legislation and the effect of elective single embryo transfer on IVF outcome. Reprod Biomed Online. 2005;10(4): 436–41.
28. Van Landuyt L, Verheyen G, Tournaye H, et al. New Belgian embryo transfer policy leads to sharp decrease in multiple pregnancy rate. Reprod Biomed Online. 2006;13(6):765–71.
29. Karlstrom PO, Bergh C. Reducing the number of embryos transferred in Sweden-impact on delivery and multiple birth rates. Hum Reprod. 2007;22(8): 2202–7.
30. Bissonnette F, Phillips SJ, Gunby J, et al. Working to eliminate multiple pregnancies: a success story in Quebec. Reprod Biomed Online. 2011;23(4):500–4.
31. Ata B, Seli E. Economics of assisted reproductive technologies. Curr Opin Obstet Gynecol. 2010;22(3): 183–8.
32. Martin JR, Bromer JG, Sakkas D, Patrizio P. Insurance coverage and in vitro fertilization outcomes: a U.S. perspective. Fertil Steril. 2011;95(3):964–9.
33. Red Latinoamericana de Reproduccion Asistida. Registro Latinoamericano de Reproducci6n Asistida, 2009. 2012. Available from: http://www.redlara.com/aa_ingles/quem_somos.asp
34. Japan Society of Obstetrics and Gynecology. ART registry of Japan, 2008. 2009. Available from: http://www.jsog.or.jp/english/
35. Fertility Society of Australia, Reproductive Technology Accreditaion Committee. Code of practice for assisted reproductive technology units. Melbourne: FSA; 2010.
36. Wang YA, Macaldowie A, Hayward I, et al. Assisted reproductive technology in Australia and New Zealand 2009. Australian Institute of Health and Welfare, Assisted Reproduction Series. 2011; No. 15.

Analysis of the Zona Pellucida as an Indicator of Oocyte Developmental Potential

2

Markus Montag, Thomas Schimming, and Maria Köster

In human-assisted reproductive technologies (ART) the search for parameters to assess the quality and developmental potential of human gametes and embryos is of great importance. There is a clear need to gather as much information as possible in order to allow for identification of those gametes or embryos which may finally implant and give birth to a healthy child. Although experience is a key factor in embryology, the overall trend is to replace subjective judgment and decision making with objective devices that assist in the process of gamete and embryo classification. The technology of such a device should rely on physiological properties, it should be easy to use, and should include an automatic user interface which will facilitate acceptance in the daily routine laboratory work. A technique which is available in all embryology laboratories is microscopy. Different microscopic technologies can be used to visualize subcellular structures within cells. One such technology is polarization microscopy.

M. Montag (✉)
IVF Laboratory, Department of Gynecological Endocrinology & Fertility Medicine, University of Heidelberg, Heidelberg, Germany
e-mail: markus.montag@med.uni-heidelberg.de

T. Schimming
Independent Image Processing IT Professional, Munich, Germany

M. Köster
Department Gynecological Endocrinology and Reproductive Medicine, University of Bonn, Bonn, Germany

Historical Background

Polarization microscopy dates back to the nineteenth century. It enables a look on structures which possess birefringence properties and which are otherwise invisible by standard light microscopy [1]. Polarization microscopy implies the use of a polarization filter and a crossed compensator and can only visualize structures which are properly orientated in regard to the polarized light. In the field of cell biology polarization microscopy was initially used to study the architecture of animal cells and in particular microtubule-dependent structures, e.g., the mitotic spindle in living cells [2, 3]. With the introduction of intracytoplasmic sperm injection (ICSI) and the potential risk of damaging the metaphase-II spindle in human oocytes during injection, this technique attracted the interest of some people working in the field of assisted reproduction [4]. However, oocytes and embryos are rather large cells and the time needed to search for the position and orientation of the spindle was too long with the standard polarization microscopy technique.

A new kind of polarization microscope was presented in 1995 [5]. This system was based on computational improvements in order to allow for a real-time image of birefringent structures in large cells and independent of the specimen orientation. As this system was adapted to the need of embryology, it was immediately applied to mammalian oocytes and allowed to visualize the elements within the mammalian oocyte which are

D.K. Gardner et al. (eds.), *Human Gametes and Preimplantation Embryos: Assessment and Diagnosis*,
DOI 10.1007/978-1-4614-6651-2_2,

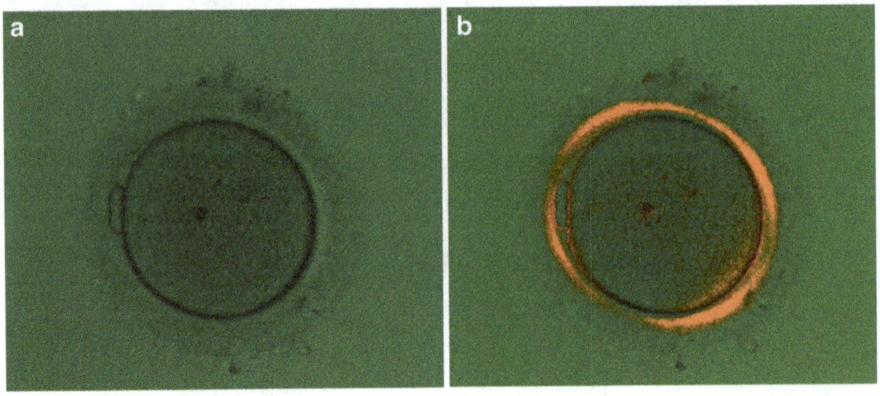

Fig. 2.1 Comparison of normal light microscopic image (**a**) and the corresponding polarization microscopic image (**b**) shown as an overlay picture with the information of the birefringence intensity in the zona pellucida in *red* and the normal light microscopic image in *green*

birefringent: the zona pellucida and the meiotic spindle (Fig. 1) [6, 7].

Polarization microscopy is a noninvasive technique and thus its use in human embryology does not interfere with embryo development as there is no direct intervention other than microscopy and a wavelength which is not different from the one used for standard light microscopy. As this microscopic assessment can be combined with other routine handling steps, there is not much of additional manipulation of oocytes or embryos. Consequently this technique was implemented in several laboratories and resulted in numerous publications which focused on the use of spindle imaging by polarization microscopy in ART. Systematic reviews on the topic of spindle birefringence imaging have been published and may be of value for the interested reader [8–10].

Zona Pellucida Assessment by Polarization Microscopy

Besides the birefringence of the spindle, the presence of a birefringent signal in the zona pellucida of mammalian oocytes has also been described. The first report was on hamster oocytes where polarization microscopy allowed distinguishing three-layers in the zona pellucida, namely an outer layer with low birefringence properties, a middle layer with no birefringence and an inner layer with a very pronounced birefringence [6]. The same properties were confirmed later for the zona pellucida of human oocytes [11]. Despite these early reports, it is still unknown which molecule or which component within the zona pellucida is the main source for its birefringence. The zona pellucida is a paracrystalline network structure composed of the zona proteins (ZP) and embedded glycoproteins and polysaccharides [12]. The zona is formed during the follicular maturation mainly by the oocyte and partly by the granulosa cells [13–16]. All studies on zona imaging do support the hypothesis that the extent of birefringence of the inner zona layer is primarily an indication for the degree of order of the contributing structures within the zona. Therefore zona imaging may reflect the state of cytoplasmic maturity which is reached by a given oocyte during the maturation process.

In contrast to polarization microscopy, conventional light microscopic assessment of the zona pellucida does not serve as a prognostic marker for oocyte assessment. Although a large diameter of the zona pellucida may be problematic for the hatching process and subsequent implantation, other morphological zona characteristics cannot be used as a predictive factor for the success of assisted reproductive treatment [17].

Initial Studies on the Prognostic Value of Zona Birefringence in Human ART

It was found that the birefringence of the inner layer of the zona pellucida showed variations in intensity and in spatial distribution among different oocytes. This opened the field of zona imaging, which means the analysis of the inner cell layer of the zona in regard to the potential of the corresponding oocyte and developing embryo to give a pregnancy. A first retrospective study was presented by Shen and coworkers who evaluated birefringence intensity of the inner zona layer in ART patients. These authors found in ICSI cycles a correlation between conception cycles and zona birefringence in the sense that patients who conceived were more likely to have embryos transferred which were grown from oocytes with a high birefringence of the inner zona layer [18]. Another retrospective study reported a correlation between high zona birefringence and the potential of an embryo to develop to the blastocyst stage [19]. These initial studies stimulated further studies on the potential value of zona birefringence measurement as a prognostic tool in ART.

In a first prospective study a polarization imaging system was used to assess the retardance of the inner zona layer in unfertilized metaphase-II-oocytes [20]. The authors investigated intensity as well as uniformity and classified oocytes subjectively as showing high birefringence or low birefringence. This classification was used as the only criterion to preselect preferentially oocytes derived from the high birefringence group after fertilization for further culture and latter transfer. The resulting implantation, pregnancy, and live birth rates were significantly different between cycles where the transferred embryos were derived from oocytes with high vs. low birefringence. Implantation and pregnancy rates were twofold higher after transfer of exclusively high birefringent cells compared to transfers involving only low birefringent cells. Furthermore, development of embryos derived from high birefringent oocytes on day 3 was superior compared to low birefringent cells. This study was encouraging in view of the potential of zona imaging as a possible prognostic marker for oocyte quality assessment. However, a major drawback was given by the fact that half of the patients presented with oocytes which showed low birefringence and hence a selection was impossible.

Objective Zona Imaging Using Automatic Birefringence Assessment

A major problem of subjective evaluation and selection is that it cannot be considered as robust and reliable. Therefore, further efforts were undertaken to enable an objective zona evaluation while eliminating any subjective user interference. Due to its shape and structure, the zona pellucida is an ideal target for automatic detection and assessment of birefringent characteristics. Two different strategies have been developed and were used for automatic zona imaging. The first approach is based on a software module that calculates a real-time score based on zona intensity and uniformity (Fig. 2) [8]. The underlying algorithm was derived from the results of the subjective zona assessment study reported above and it was validated in a prospective study [8, 20]. This study actually confirmed the results previously obtained by subjective evaluation.

Another approach is based on the detection of the radial orientation of glycoproteins in the inner zona layer [21]. Any disruption or irregularity of the inner zona layer leads to an angular deviation of the radial orientation of the birefringent structures and thus allows identifying a presumably suboptimal oocyte. To date only one study has used the latter approach for a retrospective evaluation of its applicability and to reveal a possible effect on treatment outcome. However, this study failed to show a correlation between zona imaging and improved success rates [22]. At present it is unclear if these conflicting findings are based on the different principle and/or algorithm used by that device or if it is a real contradictionary result.

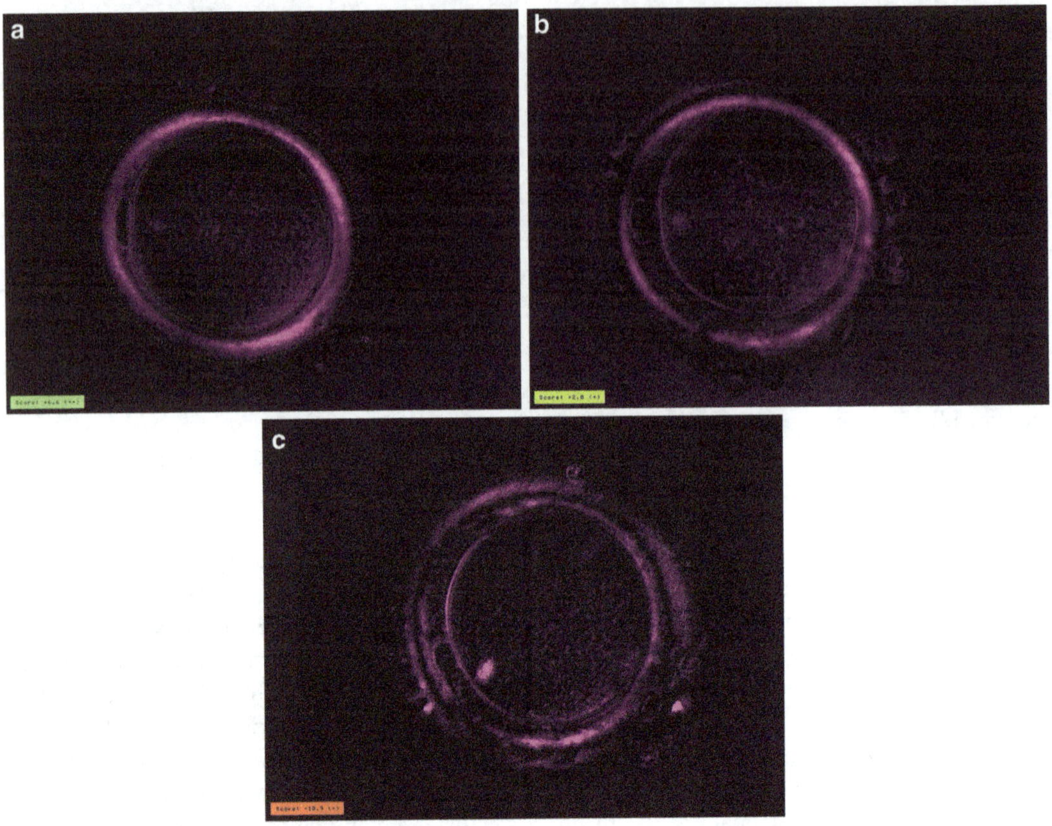

Fig. 2.2 Different patterns of zona pellucida birefringence in human oocytes. A very intense and homogeneous inner zona birefringence gives the highest zona score (**a**). Decreasing intensity (**b**) and a higher variation in the birefringence distribution (**c**) lead to lower zona scores

Automated Zona Imaging in ICSI Cycles

Using the automated zona imaging system presented by Montag & van der Ven, Ebner and colleagues explored in a prospective study the relationship between the birefringence of the inner zona layer and preimplantation development up to the blastocyst stage [8, 23]. They found that when the automatic detection of the birefringence of the inner zona layer in the oocytes failed, the corresponding embryos showed significantly lower compaction rates and blastocyst formation rates, and were significantly less involved in the initiation of a pregnancy. Hence they concluded that automatic zona scoring can be a strong predictor of blastocyst formation. Another study reported a positive correlation between automatically assessed zona pellucida birefringence score and implantation and pregnancy rates [24]. These authors also showed that the miscarriage rate was higher when the transferred embryos were exclusively derived from oocytes with a low zona birefringence score.

However, despite that most of the studies performed with zona imaging do report a benefit in regard to ART success, the underlying physiology of zona imaging is unclear and there is no explanation what distinguishes human oocytes with high birefringence from those with low birefringence. Preliminary data indicate that oocyte competence assessed by polarization microscopy correlates with different expression profiles of certain genes in subpopulations of the cumulus-oophorus complex. Some of these genes are already known to be involved in oocyte-cumulus interaction and in oocyte maturation [25, 26]. A summary of the different studies and their respective outcomes are listed in Table 1.

Table 2.1 Studies applying zona imaging in human-assisted reproduction

References	Study type	Fertilization method	Stage/outcome observed
[18]	Retrospective	ICSI	Unfertilized oocytes/high zona birefringence correlated with conception cycles
[19]	Retrospective	ICSI	Unfertilized oocytes/high zona birefringence was associated with improved embryo development and blastocyst formation rate
[8, 20]	Prospective	ICSI	Unfertilized oocytes/high zona birefringence correlated with embryo development on day 3 and improved implantation and pregnancy rates
[23]	Prospective	ICSI	Unfertilized oocytes/zona imaging correlated with blastocyst formation rate
[24]	Prospective	ICSI	Unfertilized oocytes/high zona birefringence correlated with improved implantation and pregnancy rates and reduced miscarriage rate
[27]	Retrospective	IVF	Fertilized oocytes/no correlation of zona birefringence after IVF with embryo development or clinical results
[31]	Retrospective	IVF+ICSI	Embryos on day 3/no correlation between fresh and frozen-thawed embryos; no correlation of zona birefringence with embryo development or clinical results

Automated Zona Imaging in IVF Cycles

To date only one study applied zona imaging to IVF cycles [27]. These authors found no predictive value of zona imaging in fertilized oocytes. However, they reported a negative correlation between ZPB intensity and the age of female patients as well as a higher zona score in germinal vesicle stage oocytes compared to mature metaphase-II-oocytes. In view of these results one has to note that as soon as the sperm has entered the oocyte, major changes occur in the zona pellucida to prevent further sperms from entering the oocyte. This may also involve alterations of those parts of the zona layer which mediate zona birefringence. Thus zona imaging in IVF cycles deserves further investigations in order to better understand these findings.

Factors Influencing Zona Birefringence

The correlation between oocyte maturity and zona imaging has already been mentioned by several studies [23, 27]. One study investigated the fate of zona birefringence in immature oocytes from stimulated cycles which were matured in vitro to metaphase-II [28]. Overall zona birefringence intensity was higher in immature oocytes compared to mature ones. Although maturation did not change the percentage of oocytes with a good predictive zona birefringence pattern, a positive and prognostic effect of zona birefringence was only noted for oocytes which were already retrieved at the metaphase-II-stage. Similar findings were reported by others [29]. This implies that zona imaging may not be beneficial for classifying cytoplasmic maturity in in vitro matured oocytes.

Only one preliminary study investigated so far the use of polarization microscopy for zona imaging of metaphase-II-oocytes during freezing and thawing [30]. It was shown that the freezing and the thawing process had an influence on the score obtained by zona imaging and that exposure of metaphase-II-oocytes to cryoprotectants has an impact on the zona and in particular on the birefringence of the inner zona layer. Another study assessed the impact of cryopreservation of day-3 embryos on zona imaging [31]. No differences were found between fresh and frozen-thawed embryos, however, in both groups zona imaging was done on day 3 and proper studies on the possible change of zona birefringence intensity during the early phase of embryonic development are still missing, thus making these data difficult to interpret at the moment. One study was undertaken to investigate changes in zona birefringence during the late embryo development from the morula to the hatched blastocyst stage [32]. There was an obvious correlation between zona imaging and zona hardness in embryos at the morula stage vs. the hatched blastocyst stage. Whether these changes are due to physiological alterations

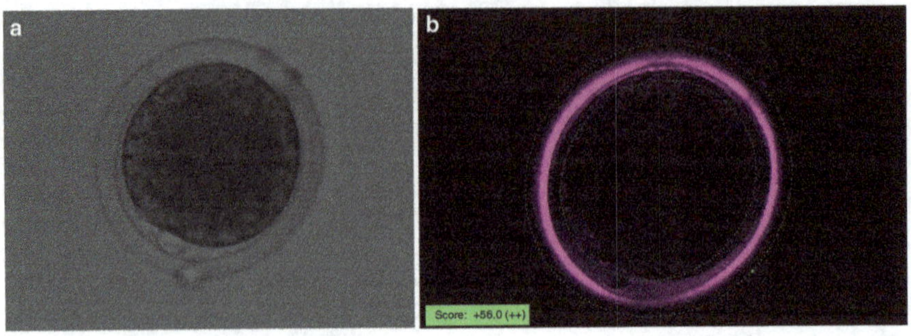

Fig. 2.3 Comparison of normal light microscopic image (**a**) and the corresponding automatic polarization zona image is shown in a bovine oocyte. Note the very intense and uniform birefringence image (**b**) which is typical for bovine oocytes makes a subjective distinction of zona birefringence intensity impossible

of the zona pellucida or simply reflect the effect of zona compression which can be observed prior hatching as reported for mouse embryos is not yet understood [33, 34].

Zona Imaging in Other Species

The use of zona imaging is now entering the veterinarian field. One study applied zona imaging to bovine oocytes which were derived by in vitro maturation from slaughterhouse ovaries (Fig. 3) [35]. After in vitro maturation the zona birefringence intensity parameters were lower in oocytes that reached metaphase-II compared with arrested stages. Also a positive development to blastocyst stage was associated with lower zona birefringence intensity parameters. These results imply that developmentally competent, in vitro matured bovine oocytes exhibit lower zona birefringence intensity parameters and thus birefringence imaging seems to be also suitable technique to predict bovine preimplantation embryo development. However, overall, these findings for in vitro matured bovine oocytes are in contrast to in vivo human-derived oocytes, where high zona birefringence intensity is a positive prognostic marker. If the difference is solely due to the difference in maturation in vitro or in vivo is unclear.

Finally it was shown that—like human and unlike bovine—equine oocytes with a high developmental capacity revealed greater birefringence scores compared with oocytes of lower developmental competence, proving again the benefit of selecting oocytes by zona birefringence imaging [36].

Summary

In summary, assessing oocyte developmental potential by zona pellucida birefringence analysis attracts more and more interest in the human as well as in the veterinarian-assisted reproductive field. Polarization microscope systems can be easily implemented in the routine daily laboratory work allowing for an easy application of the technique as a new prognostic tool. It enables by noninvasive means the visualization of structures which are otherwise inaccessible. According to the data reported so far in observational studies, zona birefringence does help in identifying oocytes with a higher chance to develop to blastocyst and contribute to viable pregnancies. Further studies are welcome to establish the link between the data measured right now and the underlying physiology and follicular background of the corresponding oocytes.

References

1. Brewster D. On the laws of polarisation and double refraction in regularly crystallized bodies. Phil Trans Royal Soc. 1818;108:199–273.
2. Swann MM, Mitchison JM. Refinements in polarized light microscopy. J Exp Biol. 1950;27:226–37.
3. Inoué S. Polarization optical studies of the mitotic spindle. I. The demonstration of spindle fibers in living cells. Chromosoma. 1953;5:487–500.

4. Palermo G, Joris H, Devroey P, Van Steirteghem AC. Pregnancies after intracytoplasmic injection of single spermatozoon into an oocyte. Lancet. 1992;340:17–8.
5. Oldenbourg R, Mei G. New polarized light microscope with precision universal compensator. J Microsc. 1995;180:140–7.
6. Keefe D, Tran P, Pellegrini C, Oldenbourg R. Polarized light microscopy and digital image processing identify a multilaminar structure of the hamster zona pellucida. Hum Reprod. 1997;12:1250–2.
7. Silva CS, Kapura K, Oldenbourg R, Keefe DL. The first polar body does not predict accurately the location of the metaphase II meiotic spindle in mammalian oocytes. Fertil Steril. 1999;71:719–21.
8. Montag M, van der Ven H. Oocyte assessment and embryo viability prediction: birefringence imaging. Reprod Biomed Online. 2008;17:454–60.
9. Petersen C, Oliveira JBA, Mauri AL, Massaro FC, Baruffi RL, Pontes A, et al. Relationship between visualization of meiotic spindle in human oocytes and ICSI outcomes: a meta-analysis. Reprod Biomed Online. 2009;18:235–43.
10. Montag M, Köster M, van der Ven K, van der Ven H. Gamete competence assessment by polarizing optics in assisted reproduction. Hum Reprod Update. 2011;17:654–66.
11. Pelletier C, Keefe DL, Trimarchi JR. Noninvasive polarized light microscopy quantitatively distinguishes the multilaminar structure of the zona pellucida of living human eggs and embryos. Fertil Steril. 2004;81:850–6.
12. Wassarman PM, Jovine L, Litscher ES. Mouse zona pellucida genes and glycoproteins. Cytogenet Genome Res. 2004;105:228–34.
13. Nikas G, Paraschos T, Psychoyos A, Handyside AH. The zona reaction in human oocytes as seen with scanning electron microscopy. Hum Reprod. 1994; 9:2135–8.
14. Sinowatz F, Toepfer-Petersen E, Kolle S, Palma G. Functional morphology of the zona pellucida. Anat Histol Embryol. 2001;30:257–63.
15. Bogner K, Hinsch KD, Nayudu P, Konrad L, Cassara C, Hinsch E. Localization and synthesis of zona pellucida proteins in the marmoset monkey (Callithrix jacchus) ovary. Mol Hum Reprod. 2004;10:481–8.
16. Gook D, Martic M, Borg J, Edgar DH. Identification of zona pellucida proteins during human folliculogenesis. Hum Reprod. 2004;19 Suppl 1:140.
17. Ten J, Mendiola J, Vioque J, de Juan J, Bernabeu R. Donor oocyte dysmorphisms and their influence on fertilization and embryo quality. Reprod Biomed Online. 2007;14:40–8.
18. Shen Y, Stalf T, Mehnert C, Eichenlaub-Ritter U, Tinneberg HR. High magnitude of light retardation by the zona pellucida is associated with conception cycles. Hum Reprod. 2005;20:1596–606.
19. Rama Raju GA, Prakash GJ, Krishna KM, Madan K. Meiotic spindle and zona pellucida characteristics as predictors of embryonic development: a preliminary study using polscope imaging. Reprod Biomed Online. 2007;14:166–74.
20. Montag M, Schimming T, Köster M, Zhou C, Dorn C, Rösing B, et al. Oocyte zona birefringence intensity is associated with embryonic implantation potential in ICSI cycles. Reprod Biomed Online. 2008;16:239–44.
21. Frattarelli JL, Miller KA, Fletcher-Holmes DW, Nagy ZP. The use of quantitative birefringence imaging to assess oocyte competence. Hum Reprod. 2007;22 Suppl 1:i166.
22. Heyndrickxs B, De Gheselle S, Lierman S, Gerris J, De Sutter P. Efficiency of polarized light microscopy as a predictive tool for oocyte quality. Hum Reprod. 2011;25:535–44.
23. Ebner T, Balaban B, Moser M, Shebl O, Urman B, Ata B, et al. Automatic user-independent zona pellucida imaging at the oocyte stage allows for the prediction of preimplantation development. Fertil Steril. 2010;94:913–20.
24. Madaschi C, Aoki T, Aoki T, de Almeida Ferreira Braga DP, de Cássia Sávio Figueira R, Semião Francisco L, et al. Zona pellucida birefringence score and meiotic spindle visualization in relation to embryo development and ICSI outcomes. Reprod Biomed Online. 2009;18:681–6.
25. Van der Ven K, Montag M, Drengner C, Köster M, van der Ven H. Differential gene expression profiles in cells of the corona radiata and outer cumulus oophorus in relation to oocyte competence. Hum Reprod. 2009;24 Suppl 1:i32.
26. Assidi M, Montag M, van der Ven K, Sirard M. Biomarkers of human oocyte developmental competence expressed in cumulus cells before ICSI: a preliminary study. J Assist Reprod Genet. 2011;28:173–88.
27. Cheng J, Huang L, He B, Lu F, Wang X, Wu Z, et al. Quantitative analysis of the intensity of zona pellucida birefringence of oocytes during IVF cycles. Reproduction. 2011;141:779–87.
28. Almeida Ferreira Braga DP, Cassia Savio Figueira R, Queiroz P, Madaschi C, Iaconelli A, Borges E. Zona pellucida birefringence in in vitro and in vivo matured oocytes. Fertil Steril. 2010;94:2050–3.
29. Petersen CG, Vagnini LD, Mauri AL, Massaro FC, Silva LF, Cavagna M, et al. Evaluation of zona pellucida birefringence intensity during in vitro maturation of oocytes from stimulated cycles. Reprod Biol Endocrinol. 2011;9:53.
30. Montag M, Köster M, Rösing R, van der Ven K, van der Ven H. Non-invasive assessment of cryopreserved oocytes through polarized light microscopy. In: Borini A, Coticchio G, editors. Preservation of human oocytes. London: Informa Healthcare; 2009. p. 174–83.
31. Gu YF, Lu CF, Lin G, Lu GX. A comparative analysis of the zona pellucida birefringence of fresh and frozen-thawed human embryos. Reproduction. 2010; 130:121–7.
32. Iwayama H, Hoshi S, Yamashita M. Birefringence parameter available for quantitative analysis of human zona hardness. Zygote. 2011;19:323–9.

33. Montag M, Koll B, van der Ven H. Use of a laser to evaluate zona pellucida hardness at different stages of mouse embryonic development in vitro and in vivo. J Assist Reprod Genet. 2000;17:178–81.
34. Montag M, Koll B, Holmes P, van der Ven H. Significance of the number of embryonic cells and the state of the zona pellucida for hatching of mouse blastocysts in vitro versus in vivo. Biol Reprod. 2000;62:1738–44.
35. Koester M, Mohammadi-Sangcheshmeh A, Montag M, Rings F, Schimming T, Tesfaye D, et al. Evaluation of bovine zona pellucida characteristics in polarized light as a prognostic marker for embryonic developmental potential. Reproduction. 2011;141:779–87.
36. Mohammadi-Sangcheshmeh A, Held E, Tesfaye D, Schellander K, Hoelker M. 160 zona pellucida birefringence correlates with cumulus morphology and glucose-6-phosphate dehydrogenase acti vity of equine oocytes. Reprod Fertil Dev. 2011;24:192.

Morphological Assessment of Oocytes, Pronuclear and Cleavage Stage Embryos

3

Laura Rienzi, Benedetta Iussig, and Filippo Ubaldi

The efficiency of human-assisted reproductive techniques (ART) is still low and most of the embryos transferred fail to implant. As a consequence, the policy of simultaneously replacing multiple embryos has been adopted but unfortunately this practice has led to an undesirable increase in multiple pregnancy rate [1]. The ability to objectively assess gametes and embryos with the most developmental potential is challenging and would also represent a tool for troubleshooting. In fact, it would help reduce the number of embryos transferred without affecting the overall pregnancy rate but lowering, at the same time, multiple gestations. To date, the evaluation of embryo quality relies mainly on morphology and routine inverted microscopic investigations are performed at predetermined checkpoints [2]. A number of different grading systems have been described in the literature but there are some concerns regarding the predictive value of these parameters. Recently, the Alpha Scientists in Reproductive Medicine and the ESHRE Special Group of Embryology stated that an international consensus on oocyte and embryo morphological assessment is needed. In fact, the standardization would help to validate the morphological criteria as end-points in clinical trials and other studies that assess the effect of new technologies and new products, improving the safety and efficacy of IVF treatments [3]. The document produced by the two societies in collaboration will be referred to as the "Consensus document" and will be discussed in this chapter [3].

L. Rienzi (✉)
GENERA Centre for Reproductive Medicine,
Rome, Italy
e-mail: riezi@generaroma.it

B. Iussig • F. Ubaldi
Clinica Valle Giulia, GENERA Rome, Marostica, Italy

Ubertide Centre for Reproductive Medicine, Rome, Italy

Morphological Assessment of Oocytes

Morphological evaluation of oocytes has been superficial, at least in the last few years. In fact the general approach is the postponement of the problem: all the available mature oocytes are inseminated and the selection is done at the preimplantation embryo level. However, since the embryo competence is likely due to oocyte quality, the introduction of earlier evaluations, in conjunction with the well-known cleavage stage embryo assessment, may be fundamental for the improvement of the in vitro fertilization techniques. In fact it could help reducing the number of oocytes inseminated, and thus the number of supernumerary embryos produced. "Good quality" oocytes should be preferred to "bad quality" ones for insemination in order to avoid the production of potentially abnormal embryos. Moreover, when possible, this earlier selection could help in the identification of an appropriate number of oocytes to be used in egg donation programs. Unfortunately, the literature on oocyte morphological assessment and the impact of certain egg

D.K. Gardner et al. (eds.), *Human Gametes and Preimplantation Embryos: Assessment and Diagnosis*,
DOI 10.1007/978-1-4614-6651-2_3, © Springer Science+Business Media New York 2013

features on embryo development and clinical results is still controversial, and this is probably due to the complex picture depicted [2].

Cumulus-Corona-Oocyte Complex Evaluation

Cumulus-corona-oocyte complex (CCOC) assessment generally represents the first-line evaluation in the everyday work of an average IVF laboratory. Cumulus cells surround the oocyte and establish a bidirectional communication that is fundamental for the growth of both the egg and the follicle [4–7]. The innermost layer of the cumulus oophorus is called "corona radiata." The cumulus-corona mass of fully mature oocytes is expected to be highly expanded as a consequence of the secretion of hyaluronic acid that interposes among the cells and separates them conferring to the complex a fluffy appearance [8]. However, in stimulated cycles the CCOC morphology is not strictly connected to the oocyte maturity; this seems to be due to a different sensitivity to the drugs used, with the subsequent lack of synchrony between the expansion of cumulus and the egg maturation process [8–11]. To date there is little evidence of a clear relationship between the aspect of the CCOC and the oocyte/embryo developmental competence [2]. However, given the fundamental metabolic connection between cumulus cells and eggs, the aspect of CCOC should predict the intrinsic quality of gametes and their further developmental potential [12, 13]. Therefore, an appropriate CCOC scoring system should be a tool for troubleshooting. Apart from the different grading systems described so far, recently the Consensus document suggested the use of a simple binary score (0 or 1) to describe "poor" CCOC or "good" CCOC on the basis of cumulus expansion and corona radiation [3, 10, 12–15].

Nuclear Maturity Evaluation

The removal of the cumulus-corona cell mass allows for a more accurate evaluation of oocyte morphology and more importantly nuclear maturity. Nuclear maturity is morphologically defined as the presence of the first polar body (IPB) in the perivitelline space (PS). In this condition the egg is at the resting stage of metaphase II (MII), characterized by the alignment of the homologous chromosomes on the spindle equatorial plate during the second division of meiosis. It is generally recognized that in about 85 % of the cases the retrieved oocytes display the IPB and are classified as MII, whereas 10 % present an intracytoplasmic structure called the "germinal vesicle" (GV), characteristic of the prophase of the first meiotic division. Approximately 5 % of the oocytes have neither visible GV nor IPB extruded: these oocytes are generally classified as metaphase I (MI) [16].

Additional information on oocyte nuclear status can be obtained with the use of polarized light microscopy combined with software for image processing for the noninvasive visualization of the meiotic spindle (MS) and other oocyte birefringent structures. The MS is a microtubular structure involved in chromosome segregation, and thus is crucial in the sequence of events leading to the correct completion of meiosis and fertilization. Parallel-aligned MS microtubules are birefringent and able to shift the plane of polarized light inducing a retardance; these properties enable the system to generate contrast and image the MS structure [17] (Fig. 1a). This technique allows both a qualitative and a quantitive analysis. First of all, MS presence gives more accurate information about the nuclear stage. In particular, some oocytes were found to be clearly immature (at the stage of early telophase I) when observed with the polarized light microscopy. At this stage, there is continuity between the ooplasm and the cytoplasm of the forming IPB and the MS is interposed between the two separating cells (75–90 min). These oocytes would have been classified as "mature" when assessed by routine light microscopy based solely on the presence of the IPB. Moreover, the MS has been found to disappear in late telophase I, reforming only 40–60 min after [18, 19]. However, it must be underlined that other factors can contribute to MS absence. For example, suboptimal culture

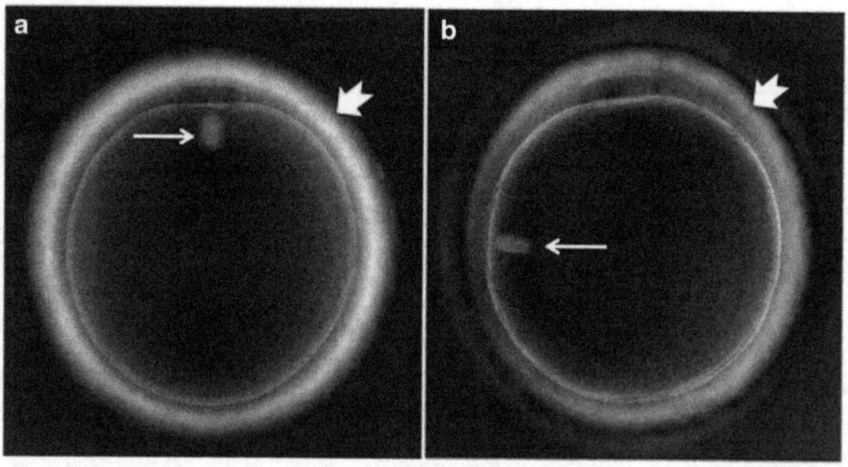

Fig. 3.1 Metaphase II oocytes observed by polarized light microscopy. Meiotic spindles (MS) (*long arrows*) and ZP inner layers (*short arrows*) are clearly visible. (**a**) The MS is aligned under the first polar body (IPB); (**b**) the MS is dislocated and placed at about 90° from the IPB

conditions, such as temperature fluctuations and chemical stress during manipulation, can account for MS disassembly [20–25]. Moreover, the MS may be artifactually not visualized if not correctly orientated during the analysis [26, 27]. Finally, the percentage of oocytes with detectable MS is related to the time elapsed from HCG administration and is higher after ≥38 h post-administration of HCG [28]. This finding may be explained by the fact that more oocytes are still in pro-metaphase II at time intervals closer to HCG administration [19]. Data regarding the correlation between the presence of MS and IVF/ICSI outcomes are controversial. In fact, although MS presence is generally correlated to higher fertilization rates and better embryo development, pregnancy and implantation rates seem not to be significantly affected [29].

Besides its role played in chromosome segregation, the MS is also a key organelle in the creation of the IPB and IIPB. Its position at the very periphery of the cell, attached to the oolemma cortex, is believed to determine the true animal pole and the plane of the first cleavage and thus the PB extrusion site [27, 30]. However, the IPB has been found to be frequently dislocated from the MS location and the manipulation required for cumulus-corona cells removal has been identified as the cause of this artifactual displacement [26, 31, 32] (Fig. 1b). The software associated with polarized light microscopy is able to calculate the deviation degree and it has been found that mechanical stress-induced IPB dislocation superior to 90° correlates with lower fertilization ability [26]. Another possible drawback of IPB displacement is the potential injury of MS during the microinjection procedure. In fact, a displaced IPB may be a false indicator of the real position of MS, which can then be disturbed by an ICSI micropipette [16, 33].

Finally, since the degree of MS birefringence is directly proportional to the molecular organization of the structure and the density of microtubules, it has been postulated that higher spindle retardance may correlate with oocyte competence and better embryo development and clinical results [34–38]. However, the literature on this correlation is still controversial and some authors failed to find any statistical significant correlation between the degree of birefringence and IVF/ICSI outcomes [39]. Instead, there should be a relationship between spindle retardance and maternal age [37, 39]. However, it must be kept in mind that spindle retardance seems to be MS orientation-dependent and probably correlated with the time of investigation, thus its reliability as a new marker of oocyte quality should be questioned [19].

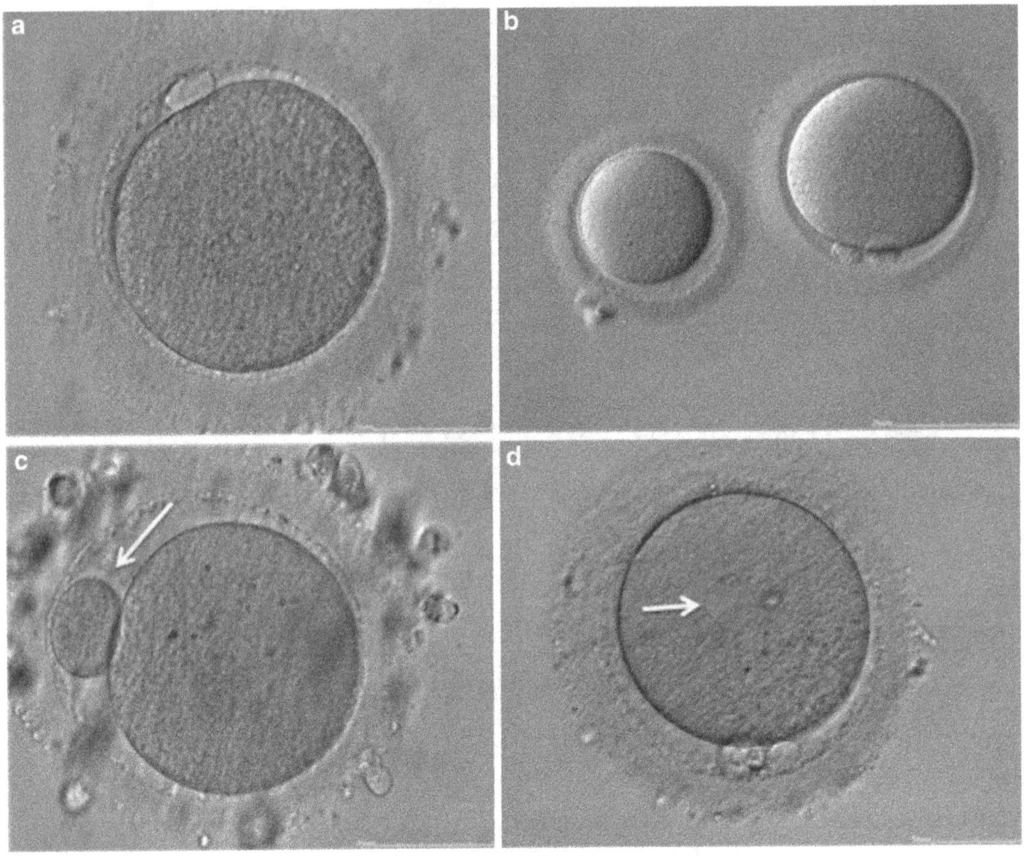

Fig. 3.2 Metaphase II oocytes with different morphological characteristics. (**a**) Normal appearing MII oocyte; (**b**) giant MII oocyte compared to a normal sized MI oocyte; (**c**) MII oocyte with giant IPB (*arrow*); (**d**) MII oocyte presenting SER aggregations (*arrows*)

Metaphase II Oocyte Morphological Evaluation

It has been recognized that oocytes undergo both nuclear and cytoplasmic maturation. This latter comprises the events that prepare the oocyte for activation, fertilization, and further development. Since these processes can be desynchronized, the simple assessment of nuclear maturity is highly unlikely to indicate the proper developmental competence of oocytes [40]. Therefore, a variety of cytoplasmic/extracytoplasmic factors have also been recently taken into account.

The normal morphology of a metaphase II oocyte consists of a spherical structure enclosed by a uniform zona pellucida and a small perivitelline space containing one single unfragmented polar body. The cytoplasm is translucent and moderately granular, with no inclusions [3] (Fig. 2a). However the majority of oocytes present the so-called one or multiple morphological abnormalities that have been investigated in order to find a correlation with the IVF/ICSI outcomes. Although many papers have been written on this subject, a recent systematic review of the literature found out that none of the features investigated so far was unanimously correlated with normal or compromised development and slight deviations should be considered as expression of phenotypic variance [2, 3]. As a consequence, the Alpha and ESHRE Scientists noted that a prolonged evaluation of gametes doesn't necessarily lead to knowledge improvement. Therefore, the costs vs. benefits of a more detailed morphological classification should be considered in order to avoid an excessive stress to the oocytes [3].

The oocyte shape is of biological interest only if exceptionally large (Fig. 2b). In fact the so-called giant oocytes may contain additional set of chromosomes and two distinct MS are present [41, 42]. These oocytes should not be inseminated in order to avoid the risk of aneuploidy [3]. As to the ovoidal shape, some authors found a correlation with abnormal cleavage and delay in in vitro parameters [43].

The Zona Pellucida (ZP) is a trilaminar glycoprotein structure that plays a crucial role in the protection of oocytes and embryos and in the fertilization process. Each ZP layer is characterized by different molecular arrangements and exhibits different birefringence patterns: the inner and the outer layers are constituted respectively by radiant and tangentially oriented filaments and appear birefringent if visualized with the light microscopy (Fig. 1). On the contrary, the middle layer has minimal birefringence, probably caused by a random orientation of the filaments [44]. The darkness, thickness, and the retardance of ZP, in particular those of the inner layer, have been suggested by many authors as new markers of oocyte competence [37, 44–46]. However, literature results are still controversial and the Alpha Scientists in conjunction with the ESHRE Special Interest Group of Embryology stated that, to date, there's no clear evidence of the reliability of ZP characteristics, at least thickness measurement, as markers of oocyte quality [2]. However, it was also noted that there could be patient-specific effects and thus exceptional observations should be performed [3].

The perivitelline space (PS) interposes between the ZP and the oolemma and accomodates the polar bodies. The presence of inclusions is considered anomalous but not sufficient to support any negative correlation with IVF/ICSI outcomes; similarly, contradictory results were obtained regarding the effect of large PVS on further developmental potential [2, 3]. However, an exceptionally large PVS may reflect an overmaturity of the ooplasm and a note should be made [3, 47].

The IPB can appear smooth ("normal" morphology), fragmented, degenerated or large. The evaluation of polar body appearance and consequences on further development has been troublesome. For example, early IPB division and disintegration (prior to 20 h after extrusion) may be a sign of disrupted events in meiosis and decreased development and implantation ability [48–52]. However, fragmented IPB has been associated with the time elapsed from denudation and ICSI and correlated to post-ovulatory aging instead of being considered a proper marker of oocyte quality [53, 54]. Similarly, a degenerated IPB may reflect asynchrony between nuclear and cytoplasmic maturation and be the result of overmaturity of the oocytes but its impact on embryo development has not been clearly demonstrated [2, 54]. It has been concluded that only large IPB (Fig. 2c) should be noted; in fact, large IPB may indicate an inability of the MS to migrate correctly at the very periphery of the cell and thus may account for oocyte aneuploidy [3, 39, 55].

The cytoplasmic texture includes different characteristics such as diffuse or centrally located granularity and presence of inclusions. Among these features, nonhomogeneous cytoplasm is of unknown biological significance whereas the presence of translucent smooth endoplasmic reticulum clusters (SER) is troublesome [3] (Fig. 2d). In fact, it seems that SER aggregation is associated with an abnormal calcium surge and pathway and is correlated with lower chances of successful pregnancy, early fetal demise, and certain fetal anomalies [56–58]. Given the severity of impaired outcomes, it has been strongly recommended not to inseminate this type of oocytes [3]. As to the vacuoles, only large ones (>14 μm) seem to be associated with fertilization failure [3].

Unfortunately, it is clear that these evaluations are not sufficient to select between normal appearing oocytes the one with higher developmental potential. Thus far, later morphological analysis, such as pronuclear and cleavage stage embryo assessment, is still essential in routine clinical applications in order to gain reliable information about embryo implantation fate.

Morphological Assessment of Pronuclear Stage Embryos

During the natural fertilization process, a spermatozoon passes the cellular investments, contacts the zona pellucida, undergoes the acrosomal reaction, and attaches to the oolemma for its subsequent incorporation into the oocyte. A complex intracellular cascade of events, "oocyte activation," is then initiated and comprises the calcium surge, cortical granule release, cytoplasm rearrangement, and the resumption of meiosis. The oocyte completes the second division of meiosis with the split of the chromosomes at the centromeres and the separation of the sister chromatids to the oocyte or a second polar body. In this manner, the egg contributes a haploid number of chromosomes and amount of nuclear DNA. Within a few hours male and female pronuclei are formed: this stage is termed "pronuclear stage." It has been suggested that the morphology of pronuclear stage embryos may be correlated with further development, thus it could be an additional valuable selection criterion for embryo transfer and cryopreservation [31, 59–67].

As to the timing of fertilization assessment, it would be advisable to take into account the different insemination methods used (standard IVF or ICSI): in fact, since ICSI bypasses some time-consuming processes, the ICSI-derived zygotes may be early [68]. Therefore, fertilization check is normally performed 16 h after ICSI and 18 h after standard IVF [3, 69]. The first sign of fertilization is the presence of two pronuclei (PN) in the ooplasm and two polar bodies (PB) extruded in the perivitelline space. Actually, this simple first-line evaluation may be troublesome: in fact, PN appearance can be asynchronous and PBs may have disintegrated before the fertilization check. In these cases, time-lapse recordings should be helpful in the recognition of correctly fertilized oocytes. However, it is likely that better embryos develop from zygotes with shorter intervals between the appearance of the two pronuclei [31].

The PN should be juxtaposed, centrally located, and evenly sized. Male PN appear in the center of the ooplasm while the female PN in the cytoplasmic region near the IIPB. The female PN then moves towards the male PN until the two abut [31]. The lack of correct apposition and localization of the pronuclei in the cytoplasm can be caused by the abnormal function of the sperm-derived centriole and microtubules which are responsible for PN alignment, and this is correlated with poor developmental potential and implantation [60, 62, 66, 70–72]. Therefore, the configuration of widely separated pronuclei is considered severely atypical and zygotes of this kind should not be transferred [3]. Similarly, pronuclear stage embryos with PN of unequal size or fragmented have an increased incidence of chromosomal abnormalities and, if possible, should not be used [3, 72–75]. The failure of PN growth may be the consequence of fertilization with immature sperm cells [76, 77].

Pronuclear orientation relative to the PBs might be an additional feature to relate to embryo development. In fact, the oocyte seems to establish polarity by pronuclear rotation towards the IIPB after fertilization [78]. This alignment is fundamental because the IIPB extrusion site defines the polar axis of the first cleavage division [79]. A misalignment of the PN and PBs has been related to decrease morphologically quality and chromosomal abnormalities of the early embryo [72, 80].

The central point of pronuclear scoring is the evaluation (in terms of number, size, and distribution) of the nucleolar precursor bodies (NPBs) present within the nuclei. NPBs are the precursors of nucleoli, which are the sites of ribosomal gene transcription and are thus essential for protein synthesis. Nucleoli are formed by a dense fibrillar component (DFC) required for rDNA transcription, a fibrillar center (FC), a structural part that acts as storage for inactive transcription factors, and a granular component (GC), which consist in a collection of maturing preribosomes [81, 82]. Nucleoli are first seen in oocytes in antral follicles, where they are completely formed and synthesize rRNA. During the maturation process that leads to ovulation, rRNA synthesis decreases and nucleoli appear small and dissociated, composed only by the FC; they are known as "nucleolar precursor bodies" [83]. At fertilization, the subsequent increase of rRNA synthesis, sees them grow and coalesce to reach their final form at the time of embryonic genome activation [81, 84–87].

A variety of scoring systems have been proposed through the years but the most popular ones are those used by Tesarik and Scott [59–63]. These grading systems are very similar to each other and differ only in the terminology adopted. In both cases, much attention has been paid to the identification of any asynchrony between the two pronuclei (different NPBs' number and/or size and/or distribution). In fact, asynchronous pronuclear stage embryos have slower development, undergo abnormal cleavage more frequently leading to more fragmentation, and result in lower blastocyst and implantation rates [59, 60, 62–66]. Notwithstanding, the prognostic value of pronuclear classification is still controversial and this is probably due to different experimental designs and terminology used [88, 89]. Recently, Alpha Scientists in collaboration with the ESHRE Special Interest Group in Embryology found a consensus suggesting the allocation of NPBs' patterns into only three categories: symmetrical (equal number/size/distribution of NPBs), asymmetrical (other arrangements, including peripherally located PN), and abnormal (pronuclei with 0 or 1 NPBs) [3].

Another level of pronuclear stage embryo assessment relies on the cytoplasmic appearance. Some authors found a positive correlation between the presence of a cytoplasmic halo and day-3 embryo grading, blastocyst rate and implantation rate [59, 90, 91]. The "halo" effect is described as the microtubule-mediated redistribution of organelles, in particular mitochondria, from the cortex to the perinuclear region, the most metabolically active site of the cell [31, 59, 92]. Moreover, it could be an indicator of the rotational effect of the male pronucleus during PN alignment in order to place the centrosome and complete fertilization and subsequent mitotic division [66]. However, to date there's insufficient evidence of a prognostic value of the halo appearance in embryo selection [3].

The prognostic value of pronuclear score alone is still a matter of debate but it seems to be more informative if used in conjunction with the cleavage stage embryo grading [67, 93–95]. Therefore, the combination of these morphological evaluations may lead to the optimization of the selection of embryos for transfer.

Morphological Assessment of Cleavage Stage Embryos

In most of the cases, pronuclear stage embryos divide mitotically (cleavage) into daughter cells, called "blastomeres," without a discernible increase in overall size. Different morphological criteria for cleavage embryo assessment have been described through the years in the literature and a variety of characteristics have been proposed as indicative of embryo viability: early cleavage, cleavage rate, blastomere size, presence of multinucleation, extent of fragmentation, and distribution of fragments [59, 96–117].

Lately, it has been suggested that the embryo's capacity to reach the blastocyst stage could have an additional prognostic value, and an increase in pregnancy and implantation rates has been reported after fresh or cryopreserved blastocyst transfers [118–122]. However, data are still controversial, since some authors found comparable results after cleavage embryo transfers [93, 123, 124]. Moreover, most embryos fail to develop to the blastocyst stage in extended in vitro culture and it's not possible to know how many of these embryos would have implanted if they had been replaced earlier [93, 125].

One of the most critical factors in the evaluation of cleavage stage embryos is the strict timing for the assessment. In fact, this is the only way for a comparative embryo selection [126]. For standardization, it has been agreed to perform the 2- and 3-day evaluation, respectively, at 44 ± 1 and 68 ± 1 h post-insemination. Syngamy and embryo cleavage assessment should be done, respectively, at 23 ± 1 h post-insemination, and 26 ± 1 h after ICSI or 28 ± 1 h after standard IVF [3]. Early cleavage in two daughter cells has been associated with higher development and pregnancy and implantation rates; therefore, it could be used as a valuable additional embryo selection criterion at the discretion of the laboratory [3, 59, 96, 98–101].

The Alpha and ESHRE Scientists agreed that the expected stage of development for a 2- and 3-day embryo is, respectively, 4 cells and 8 cells [3].

Too slow or too fast cleavage embryos have little developmental potential and present a high degree of chromosomal abnormalities [103–106, 117, 127, 128]. For embryos with 2, 4, and 8 cells, the blastomeres should have equal or very similar size. In fact, embryos with uneven sized blastomeres seem to have lower developmental capacity [104, 105, 107]. This impairment may be due to the unequal distribution of proteins, mRNA, mitochondria, and other organelles between the sister cells as well as the disruption of the polarization of certain proteins and gene products within the oocyte [78, 116]. Furthermore, the genetic analysis conducted on unevenly cleaved embryos revealed a higher degree of multinucleation and chromosomal abnormalities [107]. As to the other stages (5, 6, 7 cells), uneven blastomere size may be simply the effect of asynchronous cleavage rather than abnormal cytoplasmic distribution [3, 69].

A central point in the cleavage embryo assessment is the correct identification and differentiation of blastomeres and fragments. These latter indicators are defined as anucleate membrane-bound cytoplasmic structures <45 μm diameter in day-2 embryos and <40 μm diameter in day-3 embryos [3]. The cause of cell fragmentation is unknown and its impact on embryo development uncertain [69]. Fragmentation is considered "mild" when <10 %, moderate if 10–25 %, and severe when >25 % [3]. Mild and moderate fragmentation has not been associated with impaired IVF/ICSI outcomes [107, 115, 129]. Finally, fragment localization has been proposed as a new marker of embryo quality; however, this pattern is difficult to evaluate since these structures are dynamic and may vary or disappear during culture [3, 116].

Another very important morphological parameter in embryo selection is multinucleation, namely the presence of more than one nucleus (micronuclei included) in a single blastomere [3]. The evaluation of multinucleation should be done on day-2 because of the greater cell size and the better optical accessibility that facilitate the analysis [3]. Multinucleation rates vary greatly in the literature [109, 112, 130]. Culture media composition and improper temperature control have been proposed as possible factors that affect multinucleation rate and the underlying mechanisms include (1) karyokinesis in the absence of cytokinesis; (2) partial fragmentation of the nuclei; and (3) defective chromosome migration at the mitotic anaphase [20, 131, 132]. Multinucleation has been linked to chromosomal abnormality as well as to uneven cleavage and cleavage rate and fragmentation degree [107, 108, 112]. It is thus not a surprise that multinucleated embryos have lower developmental potential and lead to an increased risk of abortion [3].

Other morphological features, such as cytoplasmic texture, have been suggested to be related to the embryonic developmental potential. The embryo cytoplasm is considered normal if pale and clear or finely granular in appearance, although the definitive norm has yet to be established. In fact, some authors found increased cytoplasmic granularity and tiny pits in some day-3 embryos and suggested that these could be early signs of cytoplasmic activity correlated to a better development to the morula and blastocyst stages [106, 133–135]. However, a more recent study failed to find any significant correlation between cytoplasmic texture and fertilization rate, embryo quality, and pregnancy, implantation, and miscarriage rates [136]. To date there are insufficient evidences to support the prognostic value of the blastomere's cytoplasmic appearance and more research is required [3]. Similarly, even if early compaction on day 3 is atypical, it is still of unknown biological significance [3].

A great number of scoring systems that include all the features pointed as markers of embryo viability have been proposed [69, 137–140]. However, at present the lack of standardization (in the nomenclature used as well as the number of characteristics considered and the calculated threshold values) is an obstacle for an easy and univocal interpretation of the different results. Therefore, it has been suggested to use simple categories named "good," "fair," and "poor" as related to embryo quality. A "good" cleavage embryo is characterized by mild fragmentation (<10 %), stage-specific cell size, and absence of multinucleation, whereas a "fair" embryo is defined by the presence of moderate fragmentation

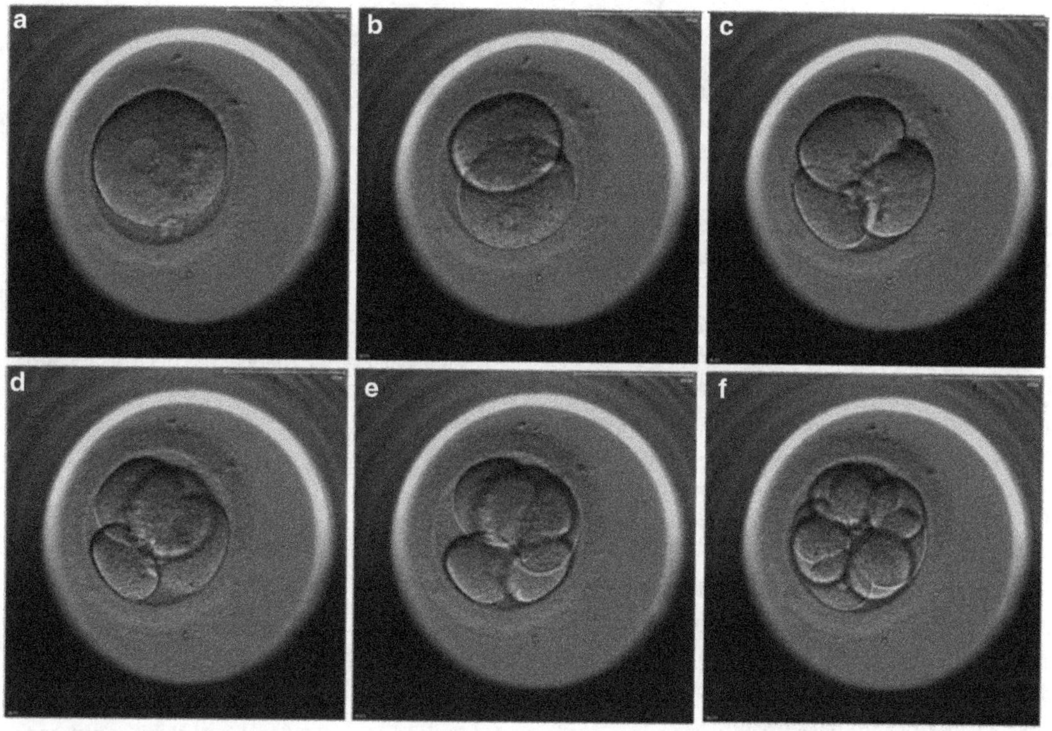

Fig. 3.3 Sequence of events recorded in time-lapse cinematograpy from 2PN formation (**a**) to 2-cell cleavage stage embryo (**b**), 3-cell cleavage stage embryo (**c**), 4-cell cleavage stage embryo (**d**), 5-cell cleavage stage embryo (**e**), and 8-cell cleavage stage embryo (**f**)

(10–25 %), stage-specific cell size for the majority of blastomeres, and no evidence of multinucleation. Finally, a "poor" embryo presents severe fragmentation (>25 %), cell size not stage-specific, and evidence of multinucleation [3].

One major limit relative to classic embryo selection based on morphology is the static evaluation (that means only few observations at specific time points) regardless of the dynamic nature of the human embryo. Continual monitoring by means of time-lapse cinematography leads to a more complete picture of embryo morphological changes and permits a better correlation of morphokinetics with further development and clinical fate (Fig. 3). Indeed, timing of different embryonic developmental events post-insemination has been proposed as an additional criterion in embryo selection [141–143]. Early disappearance of pronuclei, onset of the first cleavage division, and synchrony in the reappearance of the nuclei after the first cleavage have been shown to be correlated to the embryo cleavage status and pregnancy rate [141]. Moreover, blastocyst rate seems to be affected by the duration of the first cleavage division and the time required for the division of 2-cell and 3-cell embryos, respectively [142]. A more recent study revealed that an optimal time range (time window) exists for every early cell division, supporting the hypothesis that viable embryos undergo tightly regulated cellular events [143]. In particular, the time required by a 4-cell embryo to divide into 5 cells (t5), the duration of the period as a 3-cell embryo (s2), and the duration of the second cell cycle (cc2) are strong predictors of the further implantation fate and may be combined with the morphology score in the identification of the embryos with the higher developmental potential [143].

Conclusions

Morphological assessment of gametes and embryos is still the key-point in the everyday work of an IVF laboratory. In fact, it is simple, noninvasive, and cost-effective. The combination of different morphological criteria, from the oocyte to the pronuclear stage and the cleavage embryo, has proven to be predictive for embryo developmental potential, even if the overall efficacy of ART is still low, considering that most of the embryos produced fail to implant. The improving knowledge about gametes and embryo physiology would allow the identification of novel markers of embryo quality to be used as additional selection criteria. The recent "-omics" technology (metabolomics, trascriptomics, and proteomics) is promising in widening the horizon of human-assisted reproduction and will probably be an additional tool for improvement. Furthermore, preimplantation genetic screening may help in the determination of embryonic "health" through the screening of the genetic constitution of the embryo. Unfortunately, even if their promise is powerful, they are still far from routine introduction in the IVF clinic and further investigation is needed to ensure the reliability and sensitivities of these methods.

References

1. Edwards RG, Beard HK. Blastocyst stage transfer: pitfalls and benefits. Hum Reprod. 1999;14:1–6.
2. Rienzi L, Vajta G, Ubaldi F. Predictive value of oocyte morphology in human IVF: a systematic review of the literature. Hum Reprod Update. 2011;17:34–45.
3. Alpha Scientists in Reproductive Medicine and ESHRE Special Interest Group of Embryology. The Istanbul consensus workshop on embryo assessment: proceedings of an expert meeting. Hum Reprod. 2011;26:1270–83.
4. Dong J, Albertini DF, Nishimori K, et al. Growth differentiation factor-9 is required during early ovarian folliculogenesis. Nature. 1996;383:531–5.
5. Albertini DF, Combelles CMH, Benecchi E, et al. Cellular basis for paracrine regulation of ovarian follicle development. Reproduction. 2001;121:647–53.
6. Hutt KJ, Albertini DF. An oocentric view of folliculogenesis and embryogenesis. Reprod Biomed Online. 2007;14:758–64.
7. Gilchrist RB, Lane M, Thompson JG. Oocyte-secreted factors: regulators of cumulus cell function and oocyte quality. Hum Reprod Update. 2008;14: 159–77.
8. Testart J, Frydman R, De Mouzon J, et al. A study of factors affecting the success of human fertilization in vitro. I. Influence of ovarian stimulation upon the number and condition of oocytes collected. Biol Reprod. 1983;28:415–24.
9. Laufer N, Tarlatzis BC, DeCherney AH, et al. Asynchrony between human cumulus-corona cell complex and oocyte maturation after human menopausal gonadotropin treatment for in vitro fertilization. Fertil Steril. 1984;42:366–72.
10. Rattanachaiyanont M, Leader A, Léveillé MC. Lack of correlation between oocyte-corona-cumulus complex morphology and nuclear maturity of oocytes collected in stimulated cycles for intracytoplasmic sperm injection. Fertil Steril. 1999;71:937–40.
11. Bar-Ami S, Gitay-Goren H, Brandes JM. Different morphological and steroidogenic patterns in oocyte/cumulus-corona cell complexes aspirated at in vitro fertilization. Biol Reprod. 1989;41:761–70.
12. Ng ST, Chang TH, Jackson Wu TC. Prediction of the rates of fertilization, cleavage and pregnancy success by cumulus-coronal morphology in an in vitro fertilization program. Fertil Steril. 1999;72:412–7.
13. Lin YC, Chang SY, Lan KC, et al. Human oocyte maturity in vivo determines the outcome of blastocyst development in vitro. J Assist Reprod Genet. 2003;20:506–12.
14. Veeck LL. The human oocyte. In: Veeck LL, editor. An atlas of human gametes and conceptuses. New York: Parthenon Publishing; 1999. p. 19–24.
15. Ebner T, Moser M, Shebl O, et al. Blood clots in the cumulus-oocyte complex predict poor oocyte quality and post-fertilization development. Reprod Biomed Online. 2008;16:801–7.
16. Rienzi L, Ubaldi F. Oocyte retrieval and selection. In: Gardner DK, Weissman A, Howles CM, Shoham Z, editors. Textbook of assisted reproductive technologies. Laboratory and clinical perspectives. 3rd ed. London, UK: Informa Healthcare; 2009. p. 85–101.
17. Oldenbourg R. Polarized light microscopy of spindles. Methods Cell Biol. 1999;61:175–208.
18. Montag M, Schimming T, Van der Ven H. Spindle imaging in human oocytes: the impact of the meiotic cell cycle. Reprod Biomed Online. 2006;12:442–6.
19. Montag M, Köster M, Van der Ven K, et al. Gamete competence assessment by polarizing optics in assisted reproduction. Hum Reprod Update. 2011;17: 654–66.
20. Pickering SJ, Brande PR, Johnson MH, et al. Transient cooling to room temperature can cause irreversible disruption of the meiotic spindle in human oocyte. Fertil Steril. 1990;54:102–8.
21. Almeida PA, Bolton VN. The effect of temperature fluctuations on the cytoskeletal organisation and chromosomal constitution of the human oocyte. Zygote. 1995;3:357–65.
22. Zenzes MT, Bielecki R, Casper RF, et al. Effects of chilling to 0 degrees C on the morphology of meiotic spindles in human metaphase II oocytes. Fertil Steril. 2001;75:769–77.
23. Wang WH, Meng L, Hackett RJ, et al. Limited recovery of meiotic spindles in living human oocytes

after cooling-rewarming observed using polarized light microscopy. Hum Reprod. 2001;16:2374–8.
24. Sun XF, Wang WH, Keefe DL. Overheating is detrimental to meiotic spindles within in vitro matured oocytes. Zygote. 2004;12:65–70.
25. Rienzi L, Martinez F, Ubaldi F, et al. Polscope analysis of meiotic spindle changes in living metaphase II human oocytes during the freezing and thawing procedures. Hum Reprod. 2004;19:655–9.
26. Rienzi L, Ubaldi F, Martinez F, et al. Relationship between meiotic spindle location with regard to the polar body position and oocyte developmental potential after ICSI. Hum Reprod. 2003;18:1289–93.
27. Cooke S, Tyler JPP, Driscoll GL. Meiotic spindle location and identification and its effect on embryonic cleavage plane and early development. Hum Reprod. 2003;18:2397–405.
28. Cohen Y, Malcov M, Schwartz T, et al. Spindle imaging: a new marker for optimal timing of ICSI? Hum Reprod. 2004;19:649–54.
29. Petersen C. Relationship between visualization of meiotic spindle in human oocytes and ICSI outcomes: a meta-analysis. Reprod Biomed Online. 2009;18:235–43.
30. Maro B, Verlhac MH. Polar body formation: new rules for asymmetric divisions. Nat Cell Biol. 2002;4:E281–3.
31. Payne D, Flaherty SP, Barry MF, et al. Preliminary observations on polar body extrusion and pronuclear formation in human oocytes using time-lapse video cinematography. Hum Reprod. 1997;12:532–41.
32. Moon JH, Hyun CS, Lee SW, et al. Visualization of the metaphase II meiotic spindle in living human oocytes using the Polscope enables the prediction of embryonic developmental competence after ICSI. Hum Reprod. 2003;18:817–20.
33. Silva CP, Kommineni K, Oldenbourg R, et al. The first polar body does not predict accurately the location of the metaphase II meiotic spindle in mammalian oocytes. Fertil Steril. 1999;71:719–21.
34. Sato H, Ellis GW, Inoue S. Microtubular origin of meiotic spindle from birifrangence. Demonstration of the applicability of Wiener's equation. J Cell Biol. 1975;67:501–17.
35. Trimarchi JR, Karin RA, Keefe DL. Average spindle retardance observed using the polscope predicts cell number in day 3 embryos. Fertil Steril. 2004;82 Suppl 2:S268.
36. Shen Y, Stalf T, De Santis L, et al. Light retardance by human oocyte spindle is positively related to pronuclear score after ICSI. Reprod Biomed Online. 2006;6:737–51.
37. Raju R, Prakash GJ, Krishna KM, et al. Meiotic spindle and zona pellucida characteristics as predictors of embryonic development: a preliminary study using Polscope imaging. Reprod Biomed Online. 2007;14:166–74.
38. Kilani S, Cooke S, Kan A, et al. Are there non-invasive markers in human oocytes that can predict pregnancy outcome? Reprod Biomed Online. 2009;18:674–80.
39. De Santis L, Cino I, Rabellotti E, et al. Polar body morphology and spindle imaging as predictors of oocyte quality. Reprod Biomed Online. 2005;11: 36–42.
40. Ebner T, Moser M, Tews G. Is oocyte morphology prognostic of embryo developmental potential after ICSI? Reprod Biomed Online. 2006;12:507–12.
41. Rosenbusch B, Schneider M, Glaser B, et al. Cytogenetic analysis of giant oocytes and zygotes to assess their relevance for the development of digynic triploidy. Hum Reprod. 2002;17:2388–93.
42. Balakier H, Bouman D, Sojecki A, et al. Morphological and cytogenetic analysis of human giant oocytes and giant embryos. Hum Reprod. 2002;17:2394–401.
43. Ebner T, Shebl O, Moser M, et al. Developmental fate of ovoid oocytes. Hum Reprod. 2008;23:62–6.
44. Pelletier C, Keefe DL, Trimarchi JR. Noninvasive polarized light microscopy quantitatively distinguishes the multilaminar structure of the zona pellucida of living human eggs and embryos. Fertil Steril. 2004;81:850–6.
45. Shen Y, Mehnert C, Eichenlaub-Ritter U, et al. High magnitude of light retardation by the zona pellucida is associated with conception cycles. Hum Reprod. 2005;20:1596–606.
46. Montag M, Schimming T, Koster M, et al. Oocyte zona birefringence intensity is associated with embryonic implantation potential in ICSI cycles. Reprod Biomed Online. 2008;16:239–44.
47. Xia P. Intracytoplasmic sperm injection: correlation of oocyte grade based on polar body, perivitelline space and cytoplasmic inclusions with fertilization rate and embryo quality. Hum Reprod. 1997;12: 1750–5.
48. Ortiz M, Lucero P, Croxatto H. Post ovulatory aging of human ova: spontaneous division of the first polar body. Gamete Res. 1983;7:269–76.
49. Scott L. The biological basis of non-invasive strategies for selection of human oocytes and embryos. Hum Reprod Update. 2003;9:237–49.
50. Ebner T, Moser M, Yaman C, et al. Elective transfer of embryos selected on the basis of first polar body morphology is associated with increased rates of implantation and pregnancy. Fertil Steril. 1999; 72:599–603.
51. Ebner T, Yaman C, Moser M, et al. Prognostic value of first polar body morphology on fertilization rate and embryo quality in intracytoplasmic sperm injection. Hum Reprod. 2000;15:427–30.
52. Ebner T, Moser M, Sommergruber M, et al. First polar body morphology and blastocyst formation rate in ICSI patients. Hum Reprod. 2002;17:2415–8.
53. Ciotti PM, Notarangelo L, Morselli-Labate AM, et al. First polar body morphology before ICSI is not related to embryo quality or pregnancy rate. Hum Reprod. 2004;19:2334–9.
54. Eichenlaub-Ritter U, Schmiady H, Kentenich H, et al. Recurrent failure in polar body formation and premature chromosome condensation in oocytes

from a human patient: indicators of asynchrony in nuclear and cytoplasmic maturation. Hum Reprod. 1995;10:2343–9.
55. Verlhac MH, Lefebvre C, Guillard P, et al. Asymmetric division in mouse oocytes: with or without Mos. Curr Biol. 2000;10:1303–6.
56. Otsuki J, Okada A, Morimoto K, et al. The relationship between pregnancy outcome and smooth endoplasmic reticulum clusters in MII human oocytes. Hum Reprod. 2004;19:1591–7.
57. Ebner T, Moser M, Shebl O, et al. Prognosis of oocytes showing aggregation of smooth endoplasmic reticulum. Reprod Biomed Online. 2008;16:113–8.
58. Akarsu C, Caglar G, Vikdan K, et al. Smooth endoplasmatic reticulum aggregations in all retrieved oocytes causing recurrent multiple anomalies: case report. Fertil Steril. 2009;92:1496–8.
59. Scott L, Smith S. The successful use of pronuclear embryo transfers the day following oocyte retrieval. Hum Reprod. 1998;13:1003–13.
60. Tesarik J, Greco E. The probability of abnormal preimplantation development can be predicted by a single static observation on pronuclear stage morphology. Hum Reprod. 1999;14:1318–23.
61. Ludwig M, Schopper B, Al-Hasani S, et al. Clinical use of a pronuclear stage score following intracytoplasmic sperm injection: impact on pregnancy rates under the conditions of the German embryo protection law. Hum Reprod. 2000;15:325–9.
62. Tesarik J, Junca AM, Hazout A, et al. Embryos with high implantation potential after intracytoplasmic sperm injection can be recognized by simple, noninvasive examination of pronuclear morphology. Hum Reprod. 2000;15:1396–9.
63. Scott L, Alvero R, Leondires M, et al. The morphology of human pronuclear embryos is positively related to blastocyst development and implantation. Hum Reprod. 2000;15:2394–403.
64. Wittemer C, Bettahar-Lebugle K, Ohl J, et al. Zygote evaluation: an efficient tool for embryo selection. Hum Reprod. 2000;15:2591–7.
65. Balaban B, Urman B, Isiklar A, et al. The effect of pronuclear morphology on embryo quality parameters and blastocyst transfer outcome. Hum Reprod. 2001;16:2357–61.
66. Scott L. Pronuclear scoring as a predictor of embryo development. Reprod Biomed Online. 2003;6:201–14.
67. Scott L, Finn A, O'Learyt T, et al. Morphologic parameters of early cleavage-stage embryos that correlate with fetal development and delivery: prospective and applied data for increased pregnancy rates. Hum Reprod. 2007;22:230–40.
68. Nagy ZP, Janssenswillen C, Janssens R, et al. Timing of oocyte activation, pronucleus formation and cleavage in humans after intracytoplasmic sperm injection (ICSI) with testicular spermatozoa and after ICSI or in-vitro fertilization on sibling oocytes with ejaculated spermatozoa. Hum Reprod. 1998;13:1606–12.
69. Rienzi L, Ubaldi F, Iacobelli M, et al. Significance of morphological attributes of the early embryo. Reprod Biomed Online. 2005;10:669–81.
70. Sathananthan AH, Kola I, Osborne J, et al. Centrioles in the beginning of human development. Proc Natl Acad Sci USA. 1991;88:4806–10.
71. Schatten G. The centrosome and its mode of inheritance: the reduction of the centrosome during gametogenesis and its restoration during fertilization. Dev Biol. 1994;165:299–335.
72. Gianaroli L, Magli MC, Ferraretti AP, et al. Pronuclear morphology and chromosomal abnormalities as scoring criteria for embryo selection. Fertil Steril. 2003;80:341–9.
73. Sadowy S, Tomkin G, Munnè S, et al. Impaired development of zygotes with uneven pronuclear size. Zygote. 1998;63:137–41.
74. Munnè S, Cohen J. Chromosome abnormalities in human embryos. Hum Reprod Update. 1998;4:842–55.
75. Edirisinghe WR, Jemmott R, Smith C, et al. Association of pronuclear Z scores with rates of aneuploidy in in vitro-fertilised embryos. Reprod Fertil Dev. 2005;17:529–34.
76. Ogura A, Matsuda J, Yanagimachi R. Birth of normal young after electrofusion of mouse oocytes with round spermatids. Proc Natl Acad Sci USA. 1994;91:7460–2.
77. Tesarik J, Mendoza C. Spermatid injection into human oocytes. I. Laboratory techniques and special features of zygote development. Hum Reprod. 1996;11:772–9.
78. Edwards RG, Beard HG. Oocyte polarity and cell determination in early mammalian embryos. Mol Hum Reprod. 1997;3:863–905.
79. Gardner RL. Specification of embryonic axes begins before cleavage in normal mouse development. Development. 2001;128:839–47.
80. Garello C, Baker H, Rai J, et al. Pronuclear orientation, polar body placement, and embryo quality after intracytoplasmic sperm injection and in-vitro fertilization: further evidence for polarity in human oocytes? Hum Reprod. 1999;14:2588–95.
81. Goessens G. Nucleolar structure. Int Rev Cytol. 1984;87:107–58.
82. Schwarzacher H, Mosgoeller W. Ribosome biogenesis in man: current views on nucleolar structures and function. Cytogenet Cell Genet. 2000;91:243–52.
83. Crozet N, Kanka J, Motlik J, et al. Nucleolar fine structure and RNA synthesis in bovine oocytes from antral follicles. Gamete Res. 1986;14:65–73.
84. Tesarik J, Kopecny V. Development of human male pronucleus: ultrastructure and timing. Gamete Res. 1989;24:135–49.
85. Tesarik J, Kopecny V. Assembly of the nuclear precursor bodies in human male pronuclei is correlated with an early RNA synthetic activity. Exp Cell Res. 1990;191:153–6.
86. Flechon J, Kopecny V. The nature of the "nucleulus precursor body" in early preimplantation embryos: a

review of fine-structure cytochemical, immunocytochemical and autoradiographic data related to nucleolar function. Zygote. 1998;6:183–91.
87. Hyttel P, Viuff D, Laurincik J, et al. Risk of in-vitro production of cattle and swine embryos: aberrations in chromosome numbers, ribosomal RNA gene activation and perinatal physiology. Hum Reprod. 2000;15 Suppl 5:87–97.
88. Salumets A, Hyden-Granskog C, Suikkari AM, et al. The predictive value of pronuclear morphology of zygotes in the assessment of human embryo quality. Hum Reprod. 2001;16:2177–81.
89. James AN, Hennessy S, Reggio B, et al. The limited importance of pronuclear scoring of human zygotes. Hum Reprod. 2006;21:1599–604.
90. Stalf T, Herrero J, Mehnert C, et al. Influence of polarization effects in ooplasma and pronuclei on embryo quality and implantation in an IVF program. J Assist Reprod Genet. 2002;19:355–62.
91. Ebner T, Moser M, Sommergruber M, et al. Presence, but not type or degree of extension, of a cytoplasmic halo has a significant influence on preimplantation development and implantation behaviour. Hum Reprod. 2003;18:2406–12.
92. Van Blerkom J, Davis P, Alexander S. Differential mitochondrial distribution in human pronuclear embryos leads to disproportionate inheritance between blastomeres: relationship to microtubular organization, ATP content and competence. Hum Reprod. 2000;15:2621–33.
93. Rienzi L, Ubaldi F, Iacobelli M, et al. Day 3 embryo transfer with combined evaluation at the pronuclear and cleavage stages compares favourably with day 5 blastocyst transfer. Hum Reprod. 2002;17:1852–5.
94. Nagy ZP, Dozortsev D, Diamond M, et al. Pronuclear morphology evaluation with subsequent evaluation of embryo morphology significantly increases implantation rates. Fertil Steril. 2003;80:67–74.
95. Weitzman VN, Schnee-Riesz J, Benadiva C, et al. Predictive value of embryo grading for embryos with known outcomes. Fertil Steril. 2010;93:658–62.
96. Shoukir Y, Campana A, Farley T, et al. Early cleavage of in-vitro fertilized human embryos to the 2-cell stage: a novel indicator of embryo quality and viability. Hum Reprod. 1997;12:1531–6.
97. Sakkas D, Shoukir Y, Chardonnens D, et al. Early cleavage of human embryos to the two-cell stage after intacytoplasmic sperm injection as an indicator of embryo viability. Hum Reprod. 1998;13:182–7.
98. Sakkas D, Percival G, D'Arcy Y, et al. Assessment of early cleaving in vitro fertilized human embryos at the 2-cell stage before transfer improves embryo selection. Fertil Steril. 2001;76:1150–6.
99. Salumets A, Hyden-Granskog C, Makinen S, et al. Early cleavage predicts the viability of human embryos in elective single embryo transfer procedures. Hum Reprod. 2003;18:821–5.
100. Neuber E, Rinaudo P, Trimarchi JR, et al. Sequential assessment of individually cultured human embryos as an indicator of subsequent good quality blastocyst development. Hum Reprod. 2003;18:1307–12.
101. Van Montfoort AP, Dumoulin JC, Kester AD, et al. Early cleavage is a valuable addition to existing embryo selection parameters: a study using single embryo transfers. Hum Reprod. 2004;19:2103–8.
102. Guerif E, Le Gouge A, Giraudeau B, et al. Limited value of morphological assessment at day 1 and 2 to predict blastocyst development potential: a prospective study based on 4042 embryos. Hum Reprod. 2007;22:1973–81.
103. Lewin A, Schenker JG, Safran A, et al. Embryo growth rate in vitro as an indicator of embryo quality in IVF cycles. J Assist Reprod Genet. 1994;11:500–3.
104. Giorgetti C, Terriou P, Auquier P, et al. Embryo score to predict implantation after in-vitro fertilization: based on 957 single embryo transfers. Hum Reprod. 1995;10:2427–31.
105. Ziebe S, Petersen K, Lindberg S, et al. Embryo morphology or cleavage stage: how to select the best embryos for transfer after in-vitro fertilization. Hum Reprod. 1997;12:1545–9.
106. Desai NN, Goldstein J, Rowland DY, et al. Morphological evaluation of human embryos and derivation of an embryo quality scoring system specific for day 3 embryos: a preliminary study. Hum Reprod. 2000;15:2190–6.
107. Hardarson T, Hanson C, Sjögren A, et al. Human embryos with unevenly sized blastomeres have lower pregnancy and implantation rates: indications for aneuploidy and multinucleation. Hum Reprod. 2001;16:313–8.
108. Kligman I, Benavida C, Alikani M, et al. The presence of multinucleated blastomeres in human embryos is correlated with chromosomal abnormalities. Hum Reprod. 1996;11:1492–8.
109. Jackson KV, Ginsburg ES, Hornstein MD, et al. Multinucleation in normally fertilized embryos is associated with an accelerated ovulation induction response and lower implantation and pregnancy rates in in vitro fertilization-embryo transfer cycles. Fertil Steril. 1998;70:60–6.
110. Palmstierna M, Murkes D, Csemiczky G, et al. Zona pellucida thickness variation and occurrence of visible mononucleated blastomers in preembryos are associated with a high pregnancy rate in IVF treatment. J Assist Reprod Genet. 1998;15:70–5.
111. Pelinck MJ, De Vos M, Dekens M, et al. Embryos cultured in vitro with multinucleated blastomeres have poor implantation potential in human in-vitro fertilization and intracytoplasmic sperm injection. Hum Reprod. 1998;13:960–3.
112. Van Royen E, Mangelschots K, Vercruyssen M, et al. Multinucleation in cleavage stage embryos. Hum Reprod. 2003;18:1062–9.
113. Staessen C, Camus M, Bollen N, et al. The relationship between embryo quality and the occurrence of multiple pregnancies. Fertil Steril. 1992;57:626–30.
114. Roseboom TJ, Vermeiden JP, Schoute E, et al. The probability of pregnancy after embryo transfer is

affected by the age of the patient, cause of infertility, number of embryos transferred and the average morphology score, as revealed by multiple logistic regression analysis. Hum Reprod. 1995;10:3035–41.
115. Alikani M, Cohen J, Tomkin G, et al. Human embryo fragmentation in vitro and its implications for pregnancy and implantation. Fertil Steril. 1999;71:836–42.
116. Antczak M, Van Blerkom J. Temporal and spatial aspects of fragmentation in early human embryos: possible effects on developmental competence and association with the differential elimination of regulatory proteins from polarized domains. Hum Reprod. 1999;14:429–47.
117. Van Royen E, Mangelschots K, De Neuborg D, et al. Characterization of a top quality embryo, a step towards single-embryo transfer. Hum Reprod. 1999;14:2345–9.
118. Gardner DK, Lane M, Stevens J, et al. Blastocyst score affects implantation and pregnancy outcome: towards a single blastocyst transfer. Fertil Steril. 2000;73:1155–8.
119. Schoolcraft WB, Gardner DK. Blastocyst culture and transfer increases the efficiency of oocyte donation. Fertil Steril. 2000;74:482–6.
120. Langley MT, Marek DM, Gardner DK, et al. Extended embryo culture in human assisted reproduction treatments. Hum Reprod. 2001;16:902–8.
121. Schwarzler P, Zech H, Auer M, et al. Pregnancy outcome after blastocyst transfer as compared to early cleavage stage embryo transfer. Hum Reprod. 2004;19:2097–102.
122. Blake DA, Farquhar CM, Johnson N, et al. Cleavage stage versus blastocyst stage embryo transfer in assisted conception. Cochrane Database Syst Rev. 2007;(17):CD002118.
123. Coskun S, Hollanders J, Al-Hassan S, et al. Day 5 versus day 3 embryo transfer: a controlled randomized trial. Hum Reprod. 2000;15:1947–52.
124. Huisman GJ, Fauser BC, Eijkemans MJ, et al. Implantation rates after in vitro fertilization and transfer of a maximum of two embryos that have undergone three to five days of culture. Fertil Steril. 2000;73:117–22.
125. Alper M, Brinsden P, Fischer R, et al. To blastocyst or not to blastocyst? That is the question. Hum Reprod. 2001;16:617–9.
126. Bavister B. Culture of preimplantation embryos: facts and artefacts. Hum Reprod Update. 1995;1:91–148.
127. Almeida PA, Bolton VN. The relationship between chromosomal abnormality in the human preimplantation embryo and development in vitro. Reprod Fertil Dev. 1996;8:235–41.
128. Magli MC, Gianaroli L, Ferraretti AP, et al. Embryo morphology and development are dependent on the chromosomal complement. Fertil Steril. 2007;87:534–41.
129. Van Royen E, Mangelschots K, De Neuborg D, et al. Calculating the implantation potential of day 3 embryos in women younger than 38 years of age: a new model. Hum Reprod. 2001;16:326–32.
130. Balakier H, Cadesky K. The frequency and developmental capability of human embryos containing multinucleated blastomeres. Hum Reprod. 1997;12:800–4.
131. Winston NJ, Braude PR, Pickering SJ, et al. The incidence of abnormal morphology and nucleocytoplasmic ratios in 2-, 3- and 5-day human preembryos. Hum Reprod. 1991;6:17–24.
132. Munnè S, Cohen J. Unsuitability of multinucleated human blastomeres for preimplantation genetic diagnosis. Hum Reprod. 1993;8:1120–5.
133. Hartshorne G. The embryo. Hum Reprod. 2000;15:31–41.
134. Tesarik J, Kopecny V, Plachot M, et al. Early morphological signs of embryonic genome expression in human preimplantation development as revealed by quantitative electron microscopy. Dev Biol. 1988;128:15–20.
135. Wiemer KE, Garrisi J, Steuerwald N, et al. Beneficial aspects of co-culture with assisted hatching when applied to multiple-failure in-vitro fertilization patients. Hum Reprod. 1996;11:2429–33.
136. Rienzi L, Ubaldi F, Minasi MG, et al. Blastomere cytoplasmic granularity is unrelated to developmental potential of day 3 human embryos. J Assist Reprod Genet. 2003;20:314–7.
137. Veeck LL. Preembryo grading and degree of cytoplasmic fragmentation. In: Veeck LL, editor. An atlas of human gametes and conceptuses. New York: Parthenon publishing; 1999. p. 46–50.
138. Fisch JD, Rodriguez H, Ross R, et al. The Graduated Embryo Score (GES) predicts blastocyst formation and pregnancy rate from cleavage-stage embryos. Hum Reprod. 2001;16:1970–5.
139. Cutting R, Morrol D, Roberts SA, et al. Elective single embryo transfer: guidelines for practice British Fertility Society and Association of Clinical Embryologists. Hum Fertil. 2008;11:131–46.
140. Stensen MH, Tanbo T, Storeng R, et al. Routine morphological scoring systems in assisted reproduction treatment fail to reflect age-related impairment of oocyte and embryo quality. Reprod Biomed Online. 2010;21:118–25.
141. Lemmen JG, Agerholm I, Ziebe S. Kinetic markers of human embryo quality using time-lapse recordings of IVF/ICSI-ferilized oocytes. Reprod Biomed Online. 2008;17:385–91.
142. Wong CC, Loewke KE, Bossert NL, et al. Non-invasive imaging of human embryos before embryonic genome activation predicts development to the blastocyst stage. Nat Biotechnol. 2010;28:1115–21.
143. Meseguer M, Herrero J, Tejera A, et al. The use of morphokinetics as a predictor of embryo implantation. Hum Reprod. 2011;26:2658–71.

Morphological Assessment of Blastocyst Stage Embryos: Types of Grading Systems and Their Reported Outcomes

4

Basak Balaban and David K. Gardner

The benefits of single embryo transfer (SET) to mother and baby are well documented and SET is rapidly becoming the standard of care for several groups of patients, especially those <38 and oocyte donor programs [1]. The advantages of blastocyst transfer have been well argued and growing data supports the move to day 5 transfer as an effective means of moving to SET while the transfer of embryos at the blastocyst stage has been shown to not only increase implantation rates, but decrease pregnancy losses [2–8].

The human embryo, like that of the mouse, can be cultured to the blastocyst stage in a wide variety of culture conditions, and several extensive reviews have been written on this topic [9–12]. It is the view of the authors that the safest and most effective way to culture human embryo until day 5 is with sequential media, whereby the media are renewed after 48 h to ensure the lowest possible accumulation of ammonium in the medium, and to mirror the nutrient gradients present as the embryo progresses through the oviduct to the uterus [13]. Using such media, and employing a reduced oxygen concentration (5 %) together with an appropriate quality control system, it is quite feasible to obtain implantation rates of over 50 % for patients <38 and oocyte donors (both patient groups acting as bench marks for the IVF laboratory).

Given the high implantation potential of human blastocysts, and that when more than one blastocyst is transferred the incidence of twins is typically around 50 %, it is paramount that effective selection criteria are used in order to identify the blastocyst with the best chance of resulting in a pregnancy [5]. Recent studies on the utilization of omics-based technologies in clinical in vitro fertilization (IVF) applications have reported promising results to enhance the noninvasive assessment and predictive detection of implantation potential of single human embryos in vitro [14]. Furthermore, the analysis of the proteome/secretome, together with an increased understanding of the complex relationships regulating the metabolome, have been and will continue to be extremely valuable in the optimization of culture and cryopreservation procedures [15, 16]. However, to date, there are still no routinely applicable techniques or analytical devices available, and the omics-based technologies tend to reside in a few selected research laboratories. Consequently, IVF clinics worldwide continue to select embryos for transfer based on their developmental rate and morphological features as assessed by conventional light microscopy. It is envisaged that new suitable physiological-based tests will be used to augment morphometric analysis.

Consequently, the immediate necessity for an accurate morphological grading system for blastocyst stage embryos predicting the implantation

B. Balaban (✉)
Assisted Reproduction Unit, American Hospital of Istanbul, 34365 Istanbul, Turkey
e-mail: basakb@amerikanhastanesi.org

D.K. Gardner
Department of Zoology, University of Melbourne, Melbourne, VIC, Australia

D.K. Gardner et al. (eds.), *Human Gametes and Preimplantation Embryos: Assessment and Diagnosis*, DOI 10.1007/978-1-4614-6651-2_4, © Springer Science+Business Media New York 2013

potential and the clinical outcome is evident [17]. One of the clear advantages of examining the morphology of a blastocyst is that one can readily see the differentiation of the two cell types, the inner cells mass (ICM) and the trophectoderm (Td). This gives a distinct advantage over the analysis of cleavage stage morphology, as one can already determine whether the true embryonic tissue has formed successfully.

Development of Grading Systems for the Human Blastocyst

One of the first grading systems based on morphological characteristics of blastocysts was published by Docras et al., where morphological characteristics were correlated with clinical outcome data [18–20]. Although established as a grading system as early as 1993, the first study showing the clinical efficacy of it was published in 2000 [19]. Blastocyst classification took into consideration primarily the developmental speed of blastocyst formation; the cavitation and degree of expansion of the blastocoel cavity, and the characteristics of the ICM. The validity of the grading system was confirmed by measuring β-hCG secreted by the individual blastocyst grown on culture cells. Top quality blastocysts defined as Grade I (BG1) were characterized by early cavitation, resulting in the formation of an eccentric and then expanded cavity lined by a distinct ICM region and Td layer. Grade II (BG2) blastocysts exhibited a transitional phase where single or multiple vacuoles were seen, which over subsequent days developed into the typical blastocyst appearance of the Grade I blastocysts. Grade III (BG3) blastocysts were defined as those with several degenerative foci in the ICM, with cells appearing dark and necrotic (Fig. 1).

A subsequent study by Balaban et al. examined the relationship between blastocyst quality defined by the Docras grading system and the results of 350 day 5 or 6 embryo transfers, with subsequent assessment of implantation and clinical pregnancy rates [19]. Cycles were stratified according to the homogeneityoftransferredembryos.Heterogenous cycles were comprised of all blastocysts of the same grade. Transfer cycles involving hatching blastocysts were analyzed separately. Results of the heterogenous and Grade III blastocyst transfer cycles revealed that implantation rate per embryo and the clinical pregnancy and multiple pregnancy rates were significantly decreased only when poor quality blastocysts were transferred. Very high multiple pregnancy rate were observed when the patient received at least one top quality (Grade I), or one moderate quality (Grade II) for transfer, whereas in the group of patients who received only poor quality (Grade III) blastocysts for embryo transfer, significantly less multiple implantations were encountered, despite the fact of significantly more blastocysts being transferred. Results from homogenous cycles showed that the clinical pregnancy, implantation rate, and multiple pregnancy rate were significantly higher when top quality or moderate quality blastocysts were transferred in comparison to poor quality blastocysts. Although the clinical pregnancy, implantation and multiple pregnancy rates were higher when top quality blastocysts were transferred in comparison to moderate quality blastocysts, the results were not statistically different. In cycles where all blastocysts transferred were hatching a 57.7 % clinical pregnancy rate, a 43.9 % implantation rate per embryo, and a 82.1 % multiple pregnancy rate were achieved. In patients who had no hatching blastocysts available for transfer, respective rates were 27.8 %, 19.1 %, and 40.6 % ($P<0.05$ for all).

In conclusion, this study demonstrated that there is a close relationship between the success of blastocyst transfer and morphological appearance, hence quality of the blastocyst. It was of major importance to demonstrate that this grading system could be used to reduce the number of blastocysts to be transferred to prevent multiple pregnancies without compromising the pregnancy rate.

Inclusion of Inner Cell Mass and Trophectorderm Data in the Grading System

With the increase of blastocyst transfer procedures in assisted reproduction centers around the world, the majority of published clinical articles correlating blastocyst morphology with the

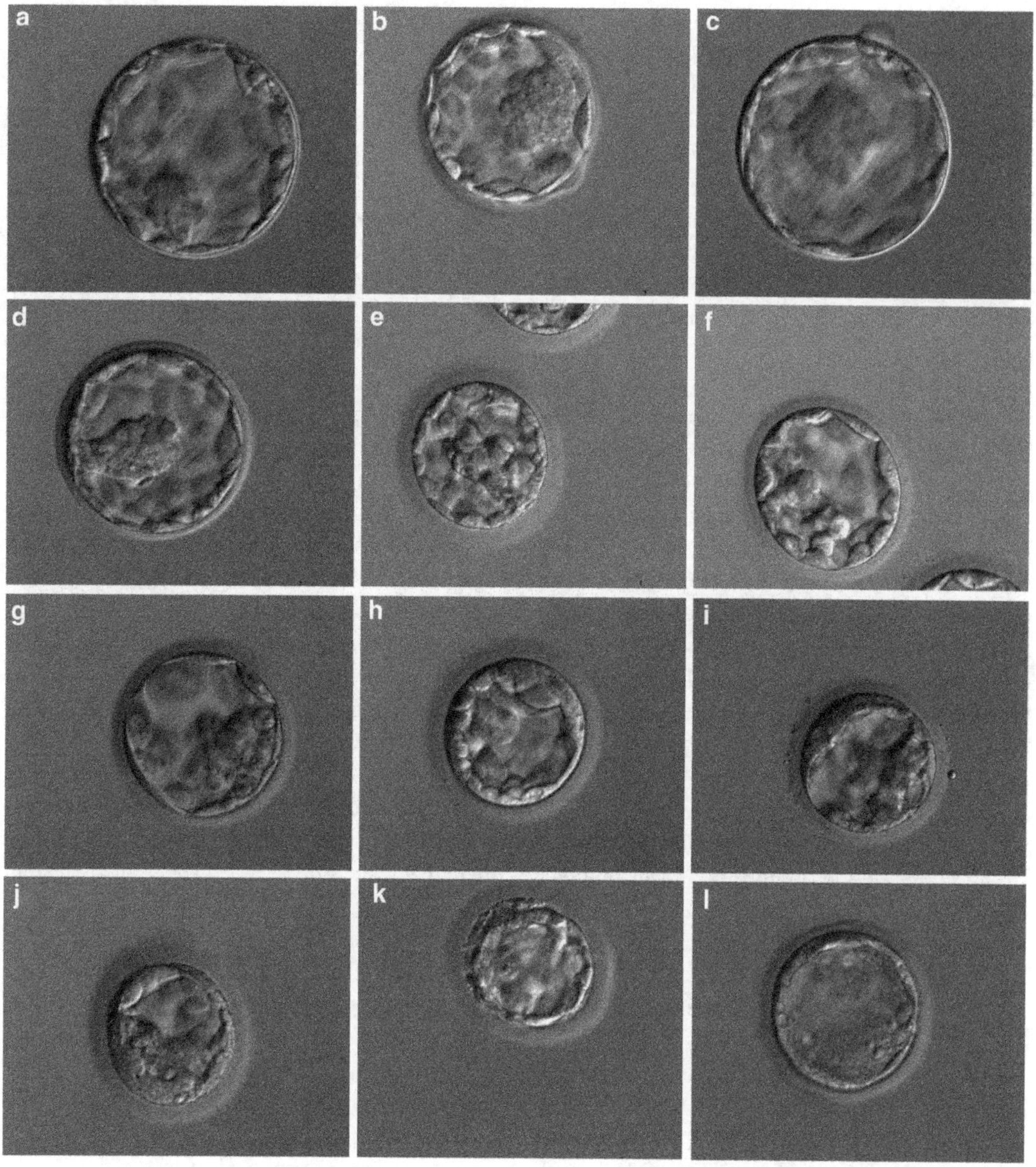

Fig. 4.1 (**a–d**) BG1—top quality blastocysts graded by the Docras scheme [18] (at 117 h post-insemination following ICSI). Blastocysts are fully expanded and there is a distinct ICM and the Td is formed. The diversity of morphologies which reside within each grade is evident, making it difficult to identify the definitive blastocyst for transfer. (**e–h**) BG2—good quality blastocysts graded by the Docras scheme [18] (at 117 h post-insemination following ICSI). Delayed development compared to BG1. (**i–l**) BG3—poor quality blastocysts graded by the Docras scheme [18] (at 117 h post-insemination following ICSI). Blastocysts have several degenerative foci in the ICM with cells appearing dark and necrotic

clinical outcome have used the grading system described by Gardner and Schoolcraft or a modified version based on the same criteria [21]. This advanced grading system took into consideration the morphology of ICM as well as Td cells, in addition to the degree of expansion and developmental rate of the blastocysts. The developmental stages, and the expansion rate of the blastocysts are defined by numbers as follows: 1 (early blastocyst), where the blastocoel is less than half the volume of the embryo; 2 (blastocyst), with blastocoel being greater than half the volume of the embryo; 3 (full blastocyst), with the blastocoel completely filling the embryo; 4 (expanded blastocyst), where the blastocoel volume is larger than originally seen in the early embryo and the zona pellucida starts to thin; 5 (hatching blastocyst), where trophectoderm starts to herniate through the zona pellucida; and 6 (hatched blastocyst), where the blastocyst has completely escaped from the zona pellucida. In the second step of Gardner grading system, an analysis of both the ICM and Td quality is performed for the blastocysts scored as grade 3 or higher. Inner cell mass quality consisted of three independent grades as follows: A, symbolizing a tightly packed ICM with many cells; B, loosely grouped with several cells; or C, very few cells. Trophectoderm quality is also classified by another three grades: A, symbolizing Td with many cells forming a cohesive epithelium; B, few cells forming a loose epithelium; and C, very few large cells (Fig. 2). Therefore, a fully hatched blastocyst with a tightly packed ICM and highly populated and cohesive Td would be graded "6AA."

A study by Gardner and Schoolcraft showed a strong correlation between the clinical outcome (implantation rates, pregnancy and twinning rates) and the morphological scores of blastocysts graded using this system [22]. The study was performed on 107 patients undergoing culture and transfer of two blastocysts, with a patient receiving two top scoring blastocysts (≥3AA) the implantation and pregnancy rates were 70 % and 87 % respectively, with a 61 % twinning rate. When only one top quality blastocysts were available for transfer, the implantation and pregnancy rates were 50 %, and 70 %, with a twinning rate of 50 %. In contrast, when only low-scoring blastocysts (<3AA) were available for transfer, implantation and pregnancy rates were 28 % and 44 %, with a twinning rate of 29 %. This study clearly demonstrated that the ability to transfer one high-scoring blastocyst should lead to pregnancy rate s greater than 60 %, without complication of twins. This initial study was subsequently validated on a much larger sample of 790 patients showing the same relationship between blastocyst score and transfer outcome [23]. The same clinic has also shown that a substantial number of patients can benefit from single blastocyst transfers when the implantation potential of top quality blastocysts is quantitated prior to transfer [24]. This prospective randomized study was performed on 48 women with good prognosis, where the clinical outcome of 23 women who received single blastocyst for transfer was compared with 25 women who received two blastocysts for transfer. The transfer of a single blastocyst resulted in an implantation and ongoing pregnancy rate of 60.9 % with no twins, whereas double embryo transfers resulted in an implantation rate of 56 %, with an ongoing pregnancy rate of 76 %, of which 47.4 % were twin pregnancies. Thus, the clinical efficacy of blastocyst transfer where the degree of expansion and quality of ICM and Td are jointly observed for the selection of a single blastocyst is of critical value for eliminating multiple births while maintaining high pregnancy rates.

Given that these grading systems demonstrate an effective means of morphological identification of blastocysts with high implantation rates, a randomized controlled trial of both systems was performed by Balaban et al. to compare their clinical predictive value side by side [18]. Clinical results of 66 good prognosis patients in each grading system group were compared in the study. Despite the fact that the overall patient characteristics, laboratory outcome, and the number of blastocysts transferred in each study group were similar, clinical pregnancy, implantation, and multiple pregnancy rates were higher when blastocysts were selected for transfer according to Gardner's grading system compared with those of the Dokras system (clinical pregnancy: 66.7 % vs. 53.0 %, not statistically different; implantation rate: 37.6 % vs. 25.0 %, $P<0.01$; multiple pregnancy rate: 38.6 % vs. 17.1 %, $P<0.05$). When the main cohorts were grouped according to the quality of the blastocysts transferred, the Gardner grading system was shown to be a better predictor of pregnancy and implantation outcome, especially when the blastocysts to be transferred are of high quality. In contrast the Dokras grading system was a better predictor of a negative outcome if only poor quality blastocysts are available for transfer.

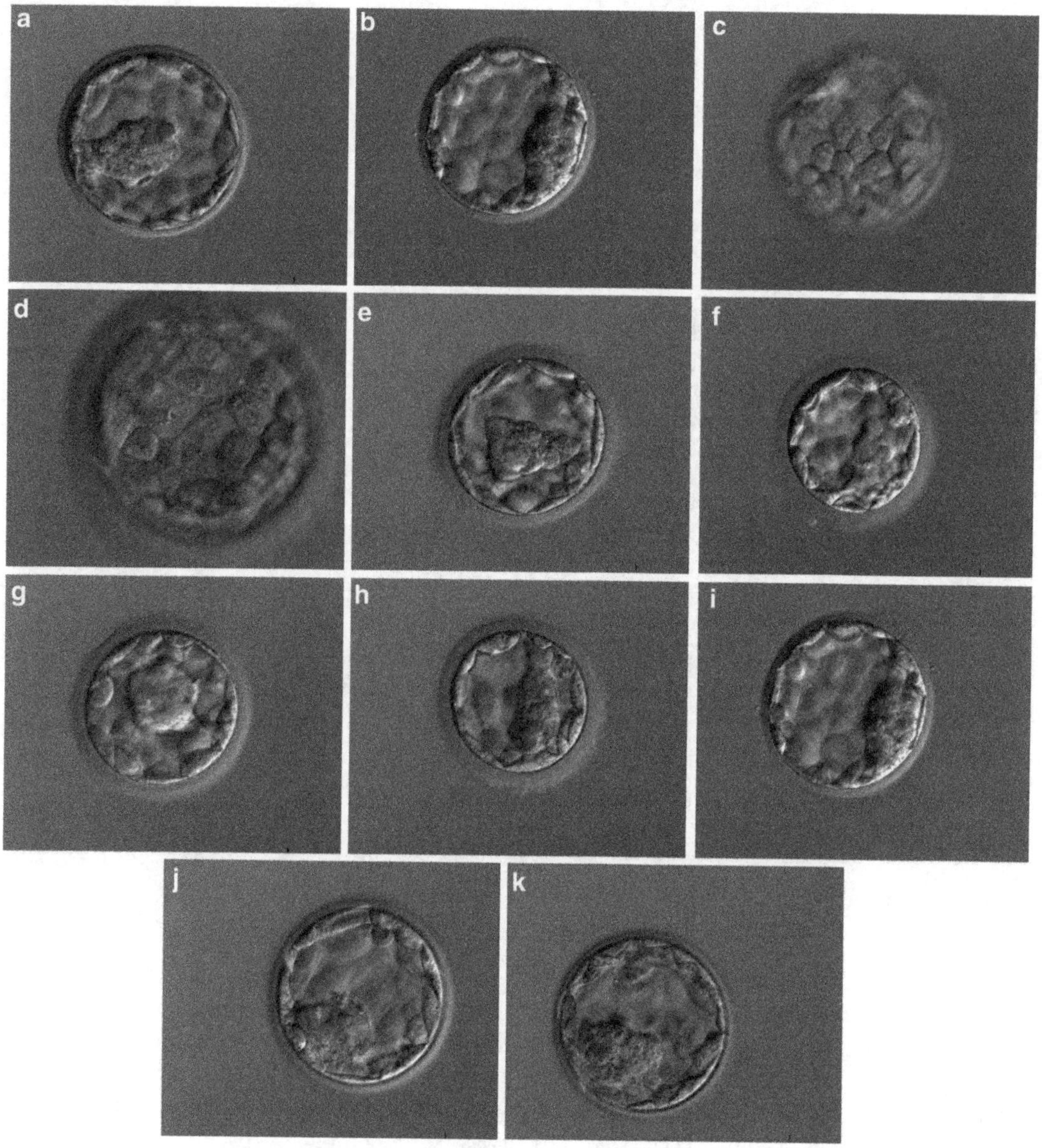

Fig. 4.2 (**a**, **b**) Using the Gardner grading scheme [21] these blastocysts are graded as A for the ICM, which consists of many tightly packed cells. (**c**, **d**) Using the Gardner grading scheme [21] these blastocysts are graded as A for the Td, with many cells forming a cohesive epithelium. (**e–h**) Blastocysts scored as 3AA with the Gardner grading scheme. (**e**) Transferred with delivery of a healthy boy. (**f**) Transferred with delivery of a healthy boy. (**g**) Transferred with delivery of a healthy girl. (**h**) Transferred, not implanted. (**i–l**) Blastocysts scored as 4AA with the Gardner grading scheme: (**i**) Transferred with delivery of a healthy boy. (**j**) Transferred with delivery of a healthy girl. (**k**) Transferred, did not implant. (**l**) Transferred, implanted with a late trimester abortion. (**m**, **n**) Blastocysts scored as 5AA with the Gardner grading scheme: (**m**) Transferred with delivery of a healthy boy. (**n**) Transferred with delivery of a healthy boy. (**o**, **p**) Blastocysts scored as 3CC with the Gardner grading scheme. Both embryos were transferred, but none implanted. (**q**, **r**) Blastocysts scored as 5BB with the Gardner grading scheme. (**q**) Transferred, did not implant. (**r**) Transferred with delivery of a healthy boy. (**s**, **t**) Blastocysts scored as 5BA with the Gardner grading scheme. (**s**) Transferred, did not implant. (**t**) Transferred with delivery of a healthy boy

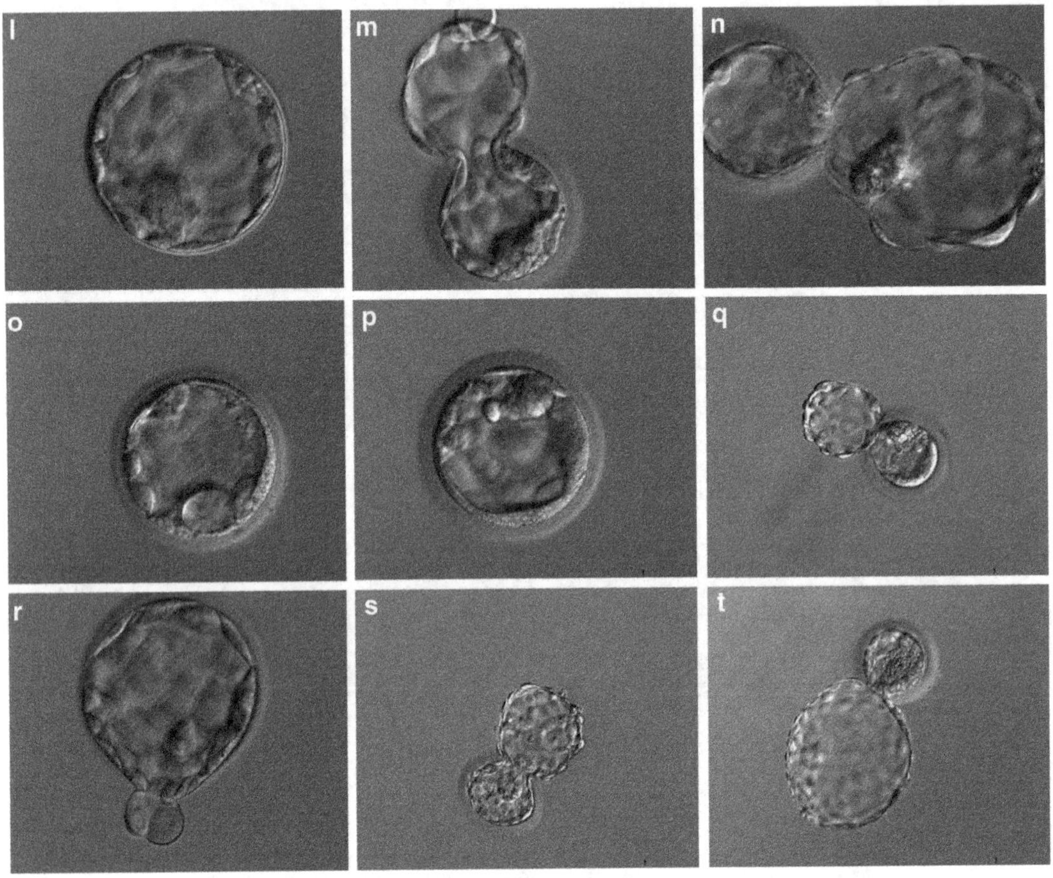

Fig. 4.2 (continued)

Various studies have been published since the introduction of both grading systems, with the aim of identifying the most predictive morphological parameter of the human blastocyst that can be used to determine the highest implantation and pregnancy outcome. The study by Shapiro et al., performed on 93 women, demonstrated that the timing of blastocoel development and grade of expansion are important predictors of implantation potential, with implantation rates of 43 % for embryos transferred to women receiving only expanded blastocysts, compared to 17 % for embryos transferred to women receiving one or more less developed blastocysts [25]. Pregnancy rates were higher for women receiving only expanded blastocysts than for women receiving one or more less developed blastocysts, although the difference was not significant.

Zaninovic et al. subsequently brought up the discussion of whether blastocyst expansion, more so than ICM formation or Td quality, plays the more critical role in reflecting the viability of scored blastocysts [26]. A retrospective analysis was performed on 156 patients who underwent fresh or frozen/thawed day 5 blastocyst transfer. The expansion of blastocysts was graded according to three options—(1) no expansion; (2) slightly expanded; or (3) fully expanded, and ICM and Td quality were also scored, in line with the Gardner grading system. The results revealed that the morphology of the blastocyst, measured with this 3-part grading system for blastocyst expansion significantly correlated with implantation rates, demonstrating an implantation potential that approaches 70 %, even with the transfer of a single 3AA blastocyst. However, when expansion or inner cell mass quality was compared individually, no significant differences in implantation rate were found. In contrast significantly higher implantation rates resulted from transferring blastocysts with a high Td score, above the other parameters. The authors therefore proposed that the Td is the most important individual factor for implantation, as it plays a crucial role in blastocyst attachment, trophoblast development, and subsequent uterine invasion, allowing the ICM direct embryo development after implantation.

Richter et al. went on to examine the predictive value of quantitative measurements of blastocyst morphology (blastocyst diameter, number of trophectoderm cells, and ICM morphology) [27]. Following 174 transfers it was observed that blastocyst diameter and trophectoderm cell numbers were unrelated to implantation rates. The authors showed that expanded blastocysts with ICMs of >4,500 μm^2 implanted at a higher rate than did those with smaller ICMs (55 % vs. 31 %). More expanded blastocysts on day 5 with slightly oval ICM implanted (58 %) compared with those with either rounder ICM (7 %) or more elongated ICMs (33 %). Implantation rates were highest (71 %) for embryos with both optimal ICM size and shape, with pregnancy rates higher for day 5 blastocysts with ICMs of optimally shape, rather than size. Similar findings for the predictive value of ICM quality as a correlate of implantation potential were reported by Marek et al., who determined that the highest clinical pregnancy rate (41.7 %) was obtained following transfer of a blastocyst with a Grade A ICM (grading performed according to Gardner grading system) compared to one with an ICM of Grade B (24.1 %) or C (6.3 %) [28]. The implantation rates for Grade A, B, and C for their ICM were 41.7 %, 24.1 %, and 6.3 % respectively, demonstrating a linear relationship.

More recently, the study by Shapiro et al. utilized a set of 25 objectively measurable criteria including blastocyst diameter, size of the ICM, and trophectoderm cell number, to develop a predictive model of clinical pregnancy in a group of 361 blastocyst transfers [29]. Day 5 blastocyst characteristics such as blastocyst diameter, Td cell count, and ICM size were found to be significantly higher in the group of clinically pregnant women ($n=147$), compared with the nonpregnant group ($n=214$). Of all the parameters, blastocyst diameter was found to be the most significant predictor of clinical pregnancy in the multivariate model.

Rehman et al. proposed another numerical blastocyst morphology grading system they called the blastocyst quality score (BQS) based on the Gardner grading system [30]. The aim of that study was to overcome the limitations of the Gardner grading system associated with the use of alphanumerical label for each combination of degree of expansion, ICM grade, and Td grade. The limitations described were the inability to calculate the mean blastocyst grade for the two or more transferred, or to determine the mean grade of the whole embryo cohort at any given point in time, as well as difficulty in grouping or stratifying embryos statistically. For the BQS, the definition of developmental rate and expansion of a blastocyst was similar to the Gardner grading system (1–6), except that ICM, and Td quality presented by letters in Gardner grading system were converted to numerically values (ICM or Td Grade A = 3, Grade B = 2, and Grade C = 1). Additive and multiplicative combinations were evaluated for the three component numbers that represent expansion, ICM, and Td. So for example, a 4AA blastocyst was given an additive blastocyst score (BQS-A) of 10 (=4 + 3 + 3), or a multiplicative blastocyst score (BQS-M) of 36 (=4 × 3 × 3), with BQS-M showing a greater spread of values in between lower and higher quality blastocysts. Analysis of 1,292 intracytoplasmic sperm injection (ICSI) and 842 standard IVF cycles showed that BQS-M of the transferred embryos had higher analytical power for predicting clinical pregnancy rates than the Gardner score alone. More recently the study by Matsuura et al., demonstrated a positive correlation between BQS and estimated blastocyst cell number, suggesting BQS can be clinically useful to evaluate blastocyst quality and culture systems [31].

It is of no doubt that the best way of understanding the efficacy of a grading system is to correlate it directly with the main endpoint of live birth outcome, instead of only pregnancy and implantation. The first study to analyze the results of 1,117 fresh single day 5 blastocyst transfers and their live birth outcome related to Gardner score was published recently by Ahlstrom et al. [32]. All three parameters: blastocyst expansion, ICM, and Td quality show a significant association with live birth rates. However, once adjusted for known significant confounders, it was shown that trophoectoderm quality was the only statistically significant independent predictor of live birth outcome (37.8 %). Patient and cycle variables were analyzed separately by univariate analysis, and for grade of blastocyst expansion, there was nearly a twofold increase in the odds of live birth for grade 3 blastocysts when compared with lower grades ($P<0.001$). Grade 4 blastocysts had a further decreased chance of live birth when compared with blastocysts of grade 3 ($P<0.01$). When the effect of ICM and Td grades were analyzed, the likelihood of live birth was statistically significantly lower for Grade B ICM blastocysts compared with grade A ICM blastocysts ($P<0.001$), however blastocysts with Grade 3 ICM quality could not be analyzed as the sample size was insufficient. Blastocysts with Grade B trophoectoderm resulted in significantly higher live birth rates compared with grade A ($P<0.0001$), and for Td of Grade C compared with Grade B ($P=0.0176$). This study therefore shows that a 4BA blastocyst has a statistically greater chance of forming a live newborn than a 4AB blastocyst for all female ages, and that a 3BA blastocyst is more likely to than a 4AB.

The methodological weakness of the data described above examining the primary predictive morphological parameter of the human blastocyst, is that of the described studies are retrospective. More prospective randomized trials will be needed to understand the predictive value of different morphological markers of human blastocysts, and perhaps improve the grading system according to updated evidence-based data.

Moving Forward: The Alpha/ESHRE Consensus on Blastocyst Grading

Selecting embryos at different stages for transfer based on their developmental rate and morphological features, as well as the choice of embryo grading scheme applied, makes inter-clinic comparisons extremely difficult. Recently, an expert panel of scientists agreed on a consensus on embryo assessment, basing their criteria on the Gardner grading system [33, 34]. The only changes made to this were the use of numerical references for ICM and Td quality instead of letters representations, similar to the BQS, such that the A,B, and C for ICM and Td were graded as 1, 2, and 3 respectively. The aim of these changes is therefore to use numeric scores to facilitate the entering of individual parameters into electronic database systems, which will ultimately facilitate statistical analysis, especially in multicenter trials. Despite the fact that introduction of this new grading scheme may significantly delay the availability of inter-clinic comparisons when applied over the next few years, it still needs to be further investigated in terms of clinical predictivity by new prospective randomized trials (Fig. 3).

Key Morphological Parameters for Frozen-Thawed Blastocysts

The re-expansion of the blastocoel after thawing of cryopreserved blastocysts had been shown to be the most vital morphological predictor of implantation potential [35, 36]. It has been reported in the literature that independently of the freezing technique used for cryopreserving blastocysts, the re-expansion of the blastocoel as a sign of viability should be expected within 24 h after thawing or warming [37, 38].

One of the first studies examining the effect of post-thaw morphological characteristics of human blastocysts on pregnancy outcome, other than re-expansion, was published by Desai and Goldfarb [39]. The study analyzed 66 thaw and 56 fresh transfer cycles, with clinical pregnancy

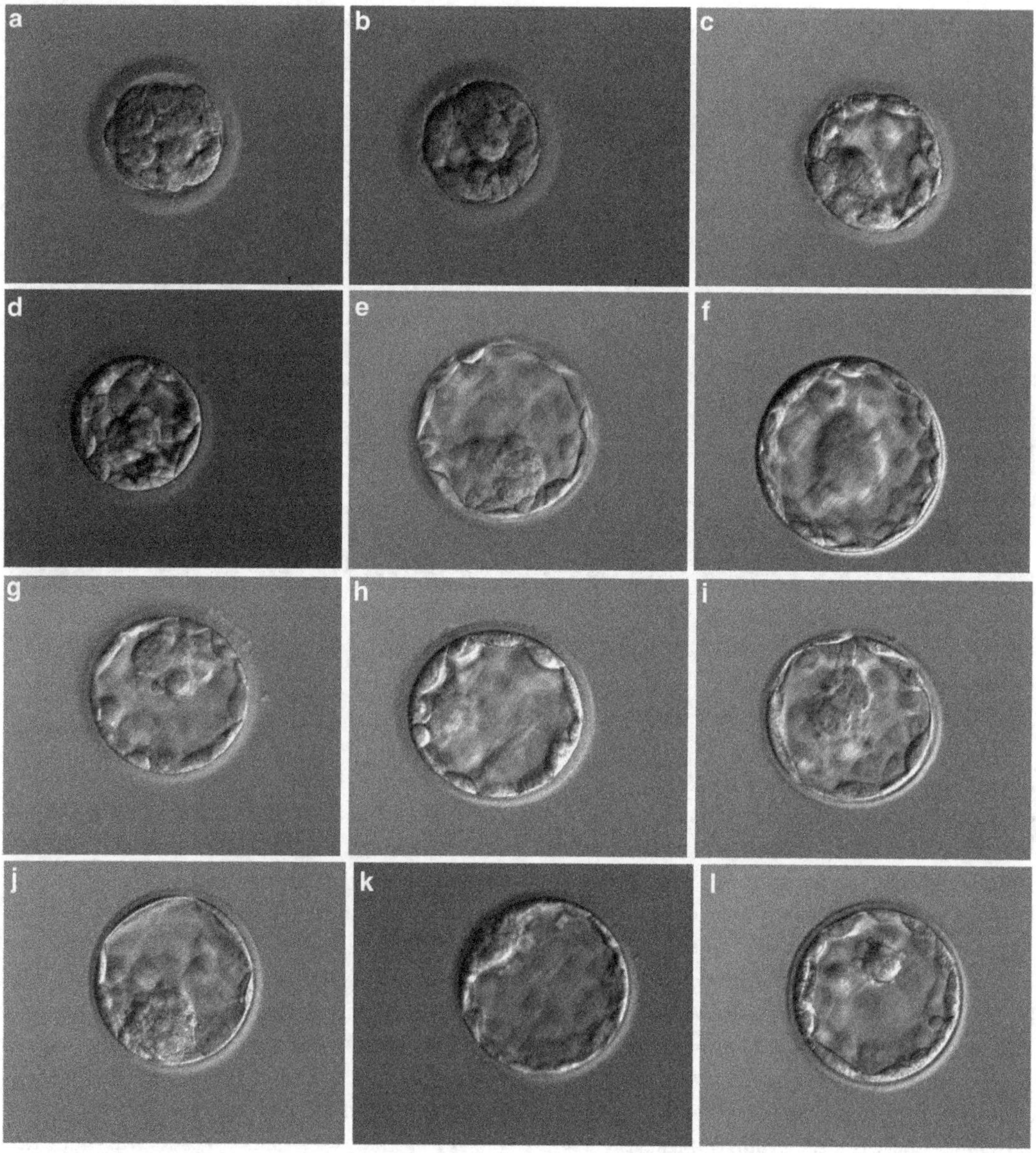

Fig. 4.3 (**a**, **b**) Blastocysts scored as 1 with the Alpha/ESHRE Consensus Grading. (**c**, **d**) Blastocysts scored as 2 with the Alpha/ESHRE Consensus Grading. (**e**, **f**) Blastocysts scored as 3.1.1 with the Alpha/ESHRE Consensus Grading. (**g**, **h**) Blastocysts scored as 3.2.2 with the Alpha/ESHRE Consensus Grading. (**i**, **j**) Blastocysts scored as 3.1.3 with the Alpha/ESHRE Consensus Grading. (**k**, **l**) Blastocysts scored as: (**k**) 3.2.3 with the Alpha/ESHRE Consensus Grading; (**l**) 3.3.1 with the Alpha/ESHRE Consensus Grading. (**m**, **n**) Blastocysts scored as: (**m**) 3.2.2 with the Alpha/ESHRE Consensus Grading; (**n**) 3.3.2 with the Alpha/ESHRE Consensus Grading. (**o**, **p**) Blastocysts scored as 3.3.3 with the Alpha/ESHRE Consensus Grading. (**q**, **r**) Blastocysts scored as 4.1.1 with the Alpha/ESHRE Consensus Grading

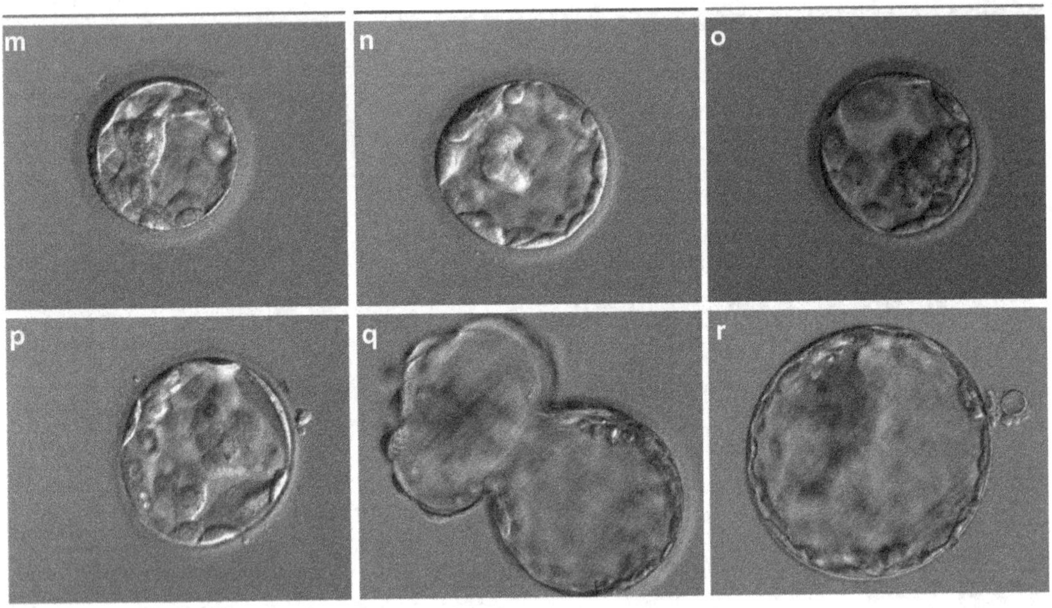

Fig. 4.3 (continued)

of 27 % and a live birth rate of 18 %. The effect of post-thaw morphological characteristics of blastocysts, such as blastocyst developmental stage, ICM, and Td morphology were compared with the clinical pregnancy rate. Post-thaw blastocyst morphology at transfer was found to be an important prognostic factor associated with success. The ability of the blastocyst to re-expand within a few hours (2–4 h after thawing) was found to be a strong indicator of blastocyst viability potential. Although there were no significant differences between the group of blastocysts with different ICM qualities and clinical pregnancy rate, Td grade was proposed to be a vital factor in successful implantation.

Abbeel et al. reported the effect of blastocyst developmental rate and stage on cryosurvival outcome, and further development after thawing [38]. Of the high grade blastocysts frozen (expanded and hatching blastocysts with early cavitation and good quality ICM and Td), morphological recovery immediately after thawing was higher for early blastocysts than for expanded and hatching blastocysts. Conversely, the ongoing survival in subsequent culture was higher for advanced and hatching blastocysts than compared to early blastocysts. The effect of ICM and Td morphology on survival rates was not examined separately, as more than one blastocyst was transferred and the good quality blastocysts were pooled during transfer that were frozen with two different techniques.

Recently, and in agreement with the previous studies, Shu et al. examined the value of fast blastocoel re-expansion in the selection of viable thawed blastocysts for transfer [40]. They observed that the rates of survival and fast blastocoel re-expansion of partially intact blastocyst were significantly reduced compared to fully intact blastocysts. Transfer of blastocysts with a faster re-expanding blastocoel cavity, compared to transfers with more delayed re-expansion, resulted in significantly higher rates of clinical pregnancy (37.1 % vs. 16.8 %) and implantation (26.7 % vs. 11.3 %). What would make an excellent adjunct to morphology and rate of post-thaw expansion is the analysis of embryonic metabolism, which we have previously shown to be beneficial at the cleavage stages after thawing [41].

Key Morphological Parameters for Vitrified Blastocysts

Similar to the findings with slow freezing of human blastocysts, the re-expansion of vitrified and warmed blastocysts play an important role in implantation potential and clinical outcome [42]. Stehlik et al. proposed that during slow freezing, dehydration occurs over a long period of time as ice crystal formation in the medium concentrates the extracellular sucrose, facilitating both cellular dehydration and blastocoel shrinkage. The rapid dehydration that occurs in less than a minute for during vitrification does not however allow time for a complete collapse of the blastocoel, according to them. Therefore, the re-expansion of vitrified/warmed blastocysts appears to be more rapid when compared with slow frozen/thawed blastocysts. As re-expansion had been shown to be the most critical morphological correlate of clinical success of frozen-thawed blastocysts, vitrification might be more advantageous in terms of morphological selection of the blastocysts for transfer, especially if this appears in a more timely manner. Another indirect benefit of faster re-expansion after warming could be the ease of selecting blastocysts according to ICM and Td quality, since these morphological characteristics can be clearly seen in a well-expanded blastocyst.

Ebner et al. suggested a four-part score for vitrified/warmed blastocysts to evaluate prediction of certain morphological parameters that might be more closely correlated with implantation, pregnancy, and live birth [43]. This grading system was based on re-expansion, hatching, extensive cytoplasmic granulation, and the presence of necrotic foci. The study was performed on 129 vitrification/warming cycles, where the overall survival rate of the blastocysts was 74 %. The report showed that early blastocysts showed better survival when compared with expanded/hatching blastocysts ($P<0.01$). Of the morphological parameters analyzed, those that were significantly predictive of implantation, pregnancy, and live birth outcomes were immediate re-expansion ($P<0.05$) and hatching ($P<0.001$).

Conclusions

The predictive value of morphological grading systems has undoubtedly assisted in the selection of the most viable human blastocysts for transfer. However, as such assessments are not directly linked to complex physiological parameters, they provide limited information. It is proposed that combining morphological criteria with noninvasive techniques using metabolic, genetic, and epigenetic markers will undoubtedly increase the success of assisted reproduction, resulting in single blastocyst transfer becoming an excellent strategy for achieving conception in infertile couples [44]. Furthermore, time-lapse analysis of human embryos under in vitro culture conditions may further enable us to quantitate some of the more complex events of embryo development [45]. It is envisaged that using this kind of combined approach for blastocyst analysis will further increase the chances of implantation and live birth outcomes for all couples seeking infertility treatment, beyond current methods of analysis.

References

1. Adashi EY, Barri PN, Berkowitz R, et al. Infertility therapy-associated multiple pregnancies (births): an ongoing epidemic. Reprod Biomed Online. 2003;7:515–42.
2. Menezo YJ, Guerin JF, Czyba JC. Improvement of human early embryo development in vitro by coculture on monolayers of Vero cells. Biol Reprod. 1990;42:301–6.
3. Bongso A, Ng SC, Fong CY, Ratnam S. Cocultures: a new lead in embryo quality improvement for assisted reproduction. Fertil Steril. 1991;56:179–91.
4. Lopata A. The neglected human blastocyst. J Assist Reprod Genet. 1992;9:508–12.
5. Gardner DK, Surrey E, Minjarez D, et al. Single blastocyst transfer: a prospective randomized trial. Fertil Steril. 2004;81:551–5.
6. Papanikolaou EG, D'Haeseleer E, Verheyen G, et al. Live birth rate is significantly higher after blastocyst transfer than after cleavage-stage embryo transfer when at least four embryos are available on day 3 of embryo culture. A randomized prospective study. Hum Reprod. 2005;20:3198–203.
7. Papanikolaou EG, Camus M, Kolibianakis EM, et al. In vitro fertilization with single blastocyst-stage versus single cleavage-stage embryos. N Engl J Med. 2006;354:1139–46.

8. Papanikolaou EG, Camus M, Fatemi HM, et al. Early pregnancy loss is significantly higher after day 3 single embryo transfer than after day 5 single blastocyst transfer in GnRH antagonist stimulated IVF cycles. Reprod Biomed Online. 2006;12:60–5.
9. Bavister BD. Culture of preimplantation embryos: facts and artifacts. Hum Reprod Update. 1995;1:91–148.
10. Leese HJ. Metabolic control during preimplantation mammalian development. Hum Reprod Update. 1995;1:63–72.
11. Pool TB. Recent advances in the production of viable human embryos in vitro. Reprod Biomed Online. 2002;4:294–302.
12. Gardner DK, Lane M. Embryo culture systems. In: Gardner DK, editor. In vitro fertilization a practical approach. New York: Informa Healthcare; 2007. p. 221–82.
13. Gardner DK, Lane M, Calderon I, Leeton J. Environment of the preimplantation human embryo in vivo: metabolite analysis of oviduct and uterine fluids and metabolism of cumulus cells. Fertil Steril. 1996;65:349–53.
14. Brison DR, Houghton FD, Falconer D, et al. Identification of viable embryos in IVF by non-invasive measurement of amino acid turnover. Hum Reprod. 2004;19:2319–24.
15. Katz-Jaffe M, Schoolcraft WB, Gardner DK. Analysis of protein expression (secretome) by human and mouse preimplantation embryos. Fertil Steril. 2006; 86:678–85.
16. Larman M, Katz-Jaffe MG, Sheehan CB, Gardner DK. 1,2-propanediol and the type of cryopreservation procedure adversely affect mouse oocyte physiology. Hum Reprod. 2007;22:250–9.
17. Blake DA, Farquhar CM, Johnson N, Proctor M. Cleavage stage versus blastocyst stage embryo transfer in assisted conception (review). Cochrane Database Syst Rev. 2007;4:CD002118.
18. Dokras A, Sargent I, Barlow D. Human blastocyst grading: an indicator of developmental potential? Hum Reprod. 1993;8:2119–27.
19. Balaban B, Urman B, Sertac A, Alatas C, Aksoy S, Mercan R. Blastocyst quality affects the success of blastocyst stage embryo transfer. Fertil Steril. 2000; 74:282–7.
20. Balaban B, Yakin K, Urman B. Randomized comparison of two different blastocyst grading systems. Fertil Steril. 2006;85:559–63.
21. Gardner DK, Schoolcraft WB. In vitro culture of human blastocysts. In: Jansen R, Mortimer D, editors. Towards reproductive certainty: fertility and genetics beyond 1999. Camforth, UK: Parthenon Publishing; 1999. p. 378–88.
22. Gardner DK, Lane M, Stevens J, Schlenker T, Schoolcraft WB. Blastocyst score affects implantation and pregnancy outcome: towards a single blastocyst transfer. Fertil Steril. 2000;73:1155–8.
23. Gardner DK, Stevens J, Sheehan CB, Schoolcraft WB. Morphological assessment of the human blastocyst. In: Elder K, Cohen J, editors. Analysis of the human embryo. New York.: Taylor & Francis; 2007. p. 79–87.
24. Gardner DK, Surrey E, Minjarez D, Leitz A, Stevens J, Schoolcraft WB. Single blastocyst transfer: a prospective randomized trial. Fertil Steril. 2004;81551–5.
25. Shapiro BS, Harris DC, Richter KS. Predictive value of 72-hour blastomere cell number on blastocyst development and success of subsequent transfer based on the degree of blastocyst development. Fertil Steril. 2000;73:582–6.
26. Zaninovic N, Berrios R, Clarke N, Bodine Z, Ye L, Veeck L. Blastocyst expansion, inner cell mass (ICM) formation, and trophoectoderm (TM) quality: is one more important for implantation? Fertil Steril. 2001;76:S8.
27. Richter KS, Harris DC, Daneshmand ST, Sapiro BS. Quantitative grading of a human blastocyst: optimal inner cell mass size and shape. Fertil Steril. 2001;76: 1157–67.
28. Marek DE, Langley MT, Weiand AC, Nackley KM, Doody KJ. Blastocyst inner cell mass grade predicts outcome for single embryo transfer in fresh cycles. Fertil Steril. 2004;82:S0015–282.
29. Shapiro BS, Daneshmand ST, Garner FC, Aguirre M, Thomas S. Large blastocyst diameter, early blastulation, and low preovulatory serum progesterone are dominant predictors of clinical pregnancy in fresh autologous cycles. Fertil Steril. 2008;90:302–9.
30. Rehman KS, Bukulmez O, Langley M, Carr BR, Nackley AC, Doody KM, et al. Late stages of embryo progression are a much better predictor of clinical pregnancy than early cleavage in intracytoplasmic sperm injection and in vitro fertilization cycles with blastocyst-stage transfer. Fertil Steril. 2007;87:1041–52.
31. Matsuura K, Hayashi N, Takiue C, et al. Blastocyst quality scoring based on morphologic grading correlates with cell number. Fertil Steril. 2010;94:1135–7.
32. Ahlstrom A, Westin C, Reismer E, Wikland M, Hardarson T. Trophoectoderm morphology: an important parameter for predicting live birth after single blastocyst transfer. Hum Reprod. 2011;26: 3289–96.
33. Alpha Scientists in Reproductive Medicine; ESHRE Special Interest Group Embryology. Istanbul consensus workshop on embryo assessment: proceedings of an expert meeting. Reprod Biomed Online. 2011;22: 632–646.
34. Alpha Scientists in Reproductive Medicine; ESHRE Special Interest Group Embryology. Istanbul consensus workshop on embryo assessment: proceedings of an expert meeting. Hum Reprod. 2011;26:1270–1283.

35. Cohen J, Simons RF, Edwards RG, Fehilly CB, Fishel SB. Pregnancies following the frozen storage of expanding human blastocysts. J In Vitro Fert Embryo Transf. 1985;2:59–64.
36. Fehilly CB, Cohen J, Simons RF, Fishel SB, Edwards RG. Cryopreservation of cleaving embryos and expanded blastocysts in the human: a comparative study. Fertil Steril. 1985;44:638–44.
37. Vanderzwalmen P, Bertin G, Debauche C, et al. Vitrification of human blastocysts with the Hemi-straws carrier: application of assisted hatching and thawing. Hum Reprod. 2003;18:1504–11.
38. Van den Abbeel E, Camus M, Verheyen G, et al. Slow controlled-rate freezing of sequentially cultured human blastocysts: an evaluation of two freezing strategies. Hum Reprod. 2005;20:2939–45.
39. Desai N, Goldfarb J. Examination of frozen cycles with replacement of a single thawed blastocyst. Reprod Biomed Online. 2005;11:349–54.
40. Shu Y, Watt J, Gerbardt J, Dasig J, Appling J, Behr B. The value of fast blastocoel re-expansion in the selection of a viable thawed blastocyst for transfer. Fertil Steril. 2009;91:401–6.
41. Balaban B, Urman B, Ata B, et al. A randomized controlled study of human day 3 embryo cryopreservation by slow freezing or vitrification: vitrification is associated with higher survival, metabolism, and blastocyst formation. Hum Reprod. 2008;23:1976–82.
42. Stehlik E, Stehlik J, Katayama KP, Kuwayama M, Jambor V, Brohammer R, et al. Vitrification demonstrates significant improvement versus slow freezing of human blastocysts. Reprod Biomed Online. 2005;11:53–7.
43. Ebner T, Vanderzwalmen P, Shebi O, Urdl W, Moser M, Zech NH, et al. Morphology of vitrified/warmed day-5 embryos predicts rates of implantation, pregnancy and live birth. Reprod Biomed Online. 2009;19:72–8.
44. Urman B, Yakin K, Ata B, Balaban B. How can we improve current blastocyst grading systems? Curr Opin Obstet Gynecol. 2007;19:273–8.
45. Meseguer M, Herrero J, Tejera A, Hilligsoe KM, Ramsing NB, Remhi J. The use of morphokinetics as a predictor of embryo implantation. Hum Reprod. 2011;26:2658–71.

Real-Time Imaging Strategies to Improve Morphological Assessment

5

María Cruz, Manuel Muñoz, and Marcos Meseguer

With more than four million babies and counting, in vitro fertilization (IVF) is a well-established choice for couples who otherwise could not have children; for some, it is their only option. It has been more than three decades since a physician produced the first successful pregnancy through IVF [1]. But the success rate for a live birth still remains disappointingly low, on average round 30 %, mainly due to the low probability of an individual embryo successfully implanting in the uterus and producing a child. For this reason, IVF clinics generally transfer more than one embryo per cycle, in the hope of increasing the probability of success. While this approach has helped to maintain IVF pregnancy rates at an acceptable level, it has also led to a dramatic rise in the number of multiple pregnancies and the subsequent risk of complications for both the mother and developing fetuses. Multiple pregnancies are prevented by transferring fewer embryos to the mother's uterus each cycle; however, restricting the number of embryos transferred has a negative impact on the likelihood of a patient becoming pregnant each cycle. The reason for this is that the embryos produced in a typical IVF cycle are extremely variable in terms of their ability to form a viable pregnancy. In cases of single embryo transfer (SET) it is therefore essential that the embryo chosen for transfer is the one having the greatest potential to form a pregnancy and produce a healthy child.

IVF technology allows for observation of early actions of human fertilization and embryogenesis. Nevertheless, concerns about excessive embryo handling have limited the frequency of microscopic observations outside the controlled incubation environment, thus the knowledge of growth rates and morphological changes have been deduced largely from morphological appearance of embryos at a few discrete static points. Such "freeze frame" images of the active processes of growth and development necessarily limit the information available to the observer and short-lived events may be missed entirely [2]. Additionally, most of the grading systems currently used for assessing embryo quality are made on the basis of morphological evaluation conducted in the IVF laboratory and although there are a large number of published studies, there is no consensus about the most accurate method for embryo quality estimation. Grading based only on these qualitative criteria is very subjective and may be one of the main causes of the interobserver variance introduced in these methods. In view of these considerations, researchers have been looking for an innovative way to improve the chances of a pregnancy by selecting only the strongest and healthiest embryos.

M. Cruz
IVI Alicante, Alicante, Spain

M. Muñoz
Instituto Valenciano de Infertilidad, Alicante, Spain

M. Meseguer (✉)
IVF Unit, Clinical Embryology Laboratory, Instituto Valenciano de Infertilidad, Valencia 46015, Spain
e-mail: marcos.meseguer@ivi.es

D.K. Gardner et al. (eds.), *Human Gametes and Preimplantation Embryos: Assessment and Diagnosis*,
DOI 10.1007/978-1-4614-6651-2_5,

Time Lapse Imaging

Image analysis may be a way to overcome the subjectivity of the existing rating systems if it could provide quantitative evaluation of key aspects of embryo development. The technology for recording embryo development has become progressively user-friendly and as its value became clear, the technology improved. Imaging development is now carried out digitally, with images captured at specific time intervals through specialized image-capture software installed on a computer. In combination with image processing software, digital time-lapse imaging makes processing, editing, annotating, and viewing the developmental sequence forwards and backwards veritably easier [3]. Time-lapse analysis records a series of still images of a developing embryo over time and when aligned and assembled into an animated sequence, time-lapse images reveal surprisingly dynamic events, which could be captured with no other methods.

Mammalian embryos were studied using time-lapse cinematography for the first time in 1929 [4]. Rabbit blastocysts were examined and it was found that mature blastocysts can periodically contract and expand; similar characteristic contractions were found later in blastocysts of other mammalian species including humans. Other important discoveries made with the use of time-lapse cinematography are data on the time course of embryo cleavage, durations of individual cell cycles, critical stages of preimplantation development, and many other processes. Optimal conditions for culturing early embryos accompanied by long-term time-lapse are certainly of prime importance in terms of obtaining complete information on the development of individual embryos along with directly estimating their quality [5].

Time-lapse image acquisition can minimize disturbance to the culture environment by integrating the incubation and embryo evaluation into one system. This has advanced the fertilization processes and development of early human embryos. The opportunity to follow the dynamic developmental patterns of individual embryos will give embryologists useful information for embryo selection and allows a phenomenon observed at a specific time point to be linked directly to an embryo's developmental capacity and implantation potential [6].

In essence, micro-cinematography offers unique possibilities for noninvasive studies of early embryogenesis in humans. One of the new generations of combined incubator-microscope structures is the Embryoscope (Unisense FertiliTech, Aarhus, Denmark), which provides an integrated monitoring system consisting of a safe, controlled culture environment including automated time-lapse high resolution image acquisition. A number of other systems have also been adapted to video monitoring including Auxogyn EEVA™ system and PRIMO Vision System. The imaging systems therefore allow retrospective detection and testing for critical events during early embryo development, thus one of the first objectives related with this new technology was to validate its clinical use.

Built-in Time-Lapse Incubation

It has been previously discussed that embryo selection at static routine timepoints is not always associated with a higher implantation or pregnancy rate, therefore other criteria should be considered in the recognition of embryos with a good prognosis. Time-lapse image analysis has rendered more information of human embryonic development and growth behavior in comparison with conventional practice or intermittent observation. It offers the potential for morphological evaluation to be carried out without the need to remove embryos from the optimized gas and temperature conditions inside the incubator; this should reduce environmental stress experienced by the embryo and may lead to some improvements in embryo viability and pregnancy rates as a result. In a recent study, it has been shown that embryos in the combined culture and monitoring system are not affected by the continuous observation associated with the Embryoscope (Fig. 1) [7]. It can therefore be concluded that this technology provides new openings to get detailed and precise information about morphological characteristics and cleavage status.

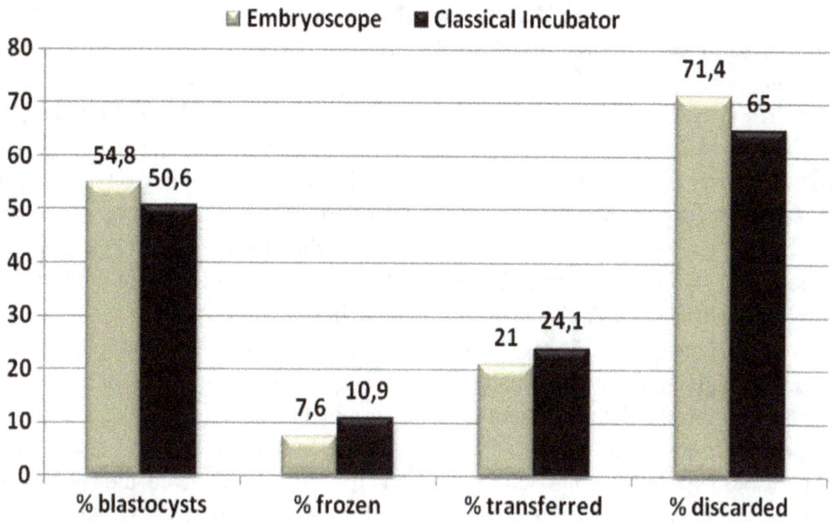

Fig. 5.1 Comparison of blastocyst development and the proportion of transferred, frozen, and discarded embryos when cultured in the embryoscope vs. classical incubator

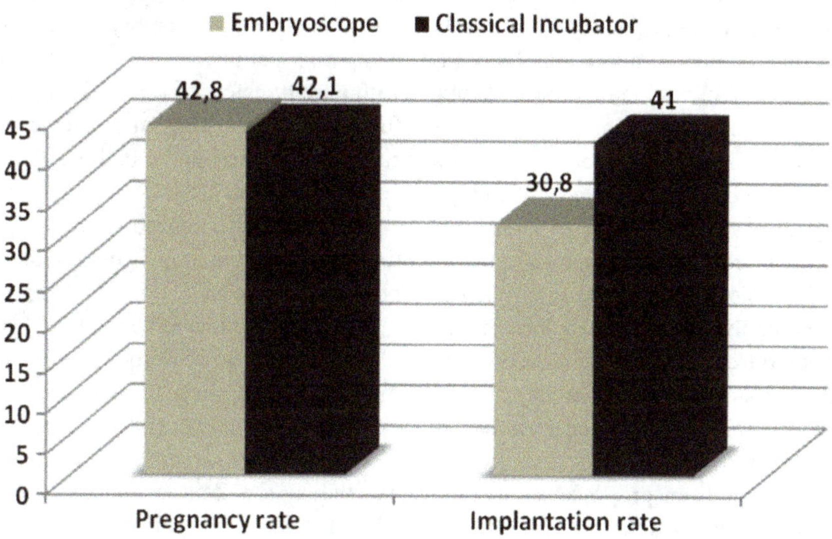

Fig. 5.2 Reproductive outcomes as assessed by Clinical Pregnancy Rate and Implantation Rate (Positive Fetal Heart Beat) of embryos cultured in the embryoscope vs. classical incubator and transferred on Day 3. No significant differences were observed between both groups

At this point it is important to bring to light that embryos cultured in an incubator with an integrated time-lapse system are periodically exposed to light when digital images are acquired and it is clear that light exposure is an unnatural stress to embryos and might affect embryo development [8]. Despite the risk of impaired development in these culture surroundings, authors did not find significant differences between embryos cultured with the time-lapse video system and embryos submitted to discontinuous observations in a conventional incubator. Blastocyst rate and percentage of viable embryos were similar between the two culture systems (Embryoscope or standard incubator). The reproductive outcomes were also the same between the two groups, confirming the usefulness of this new technology (Fig. 2). Studies assessing embryo culture in a time-lapse monitoring system will allow us to detect new valuable selection parameters in order to improve embryo selection.

Morphokinetics for Embryo Selection: A Time-Lapse Study

Accurate selection of viable embryos for transfer is a key factor in the success of IVF. However, the definition of "optimal" embryos and how to select such embryos with high developmental potential remains an open question. The estimation of embryo competence prior to transfer is notoriously subjective so one possible approach to further increase the pregnancy rate following IVF relies on the association between embryo development and rate of cleavage [9]. Cleavage-stage development is a dynamic process in which embryo morphology may change significantly over a time span of even a few hours, thus conventional grading practices may not detect subtle differences between individual embryos such as the time to progress from one cleavage division to the next. Compared with assessment of embryo morphology, embryo progression is a less-well studied concept reflecting dynamic changes (growth and development) of the embryo over time. Progression thus encompasses information from serial embryo evaluations over time whereas morphology is a snapshot of the embryo at one point in time, probably most crucially on the day of embryo transfer [10]. One aspect of embryo progression that has been proposed as an early marker of embryo quality is the presence of early cleavage, referring to the timing of the first and second blastomere divisions to reach the two- and four-cell stages.

The timing of the first zygotic cleavage has been successfully used in human IVF programs to identify embryos of superior quality and represents a noninvasive marker of embryo developmental potential [11]. Studies in animal models point to a connection between timing of completion of the first cell cycle and developmental potential and it has been observed that morulae and blastocysts developed from slowly dividing embryos gave rise to a lower fetal development after transfer than those embryos which developed from more rapidly dividing cleavage stages [12]. The idea that such an association also exists in human comes from the finding that patients who produced early cleavage had higher pregnancy and implantation rates than those who did not [13–15]. These studies were corroborated by others who also found that blastocysts from early cleaving embryos were of higher quality than their later counterparts and this was attributable specifically to difference in the timing of the first cleavage rather than variations in the rate of progression of subsequent cell cycles [16, 17].

One limitation of these studies implied that many transfers involved more than one embryo and included both early and late cleaving embryos thus it is difficult to obtain conclusive evidences that the implantation could be attributed to early cleavage. However, in one interesting study, Van Montfoort compared embryo transfers that were composed entirely of early cleaving embryos with pure transfers of late cleaving embryos and found significantly higher pregnancy rates in the early cleavage group in both single and double embryo transfers [18].

A key reflection in most studies related to the timing of cell divisions is the limited number of observations, which restricts temporal assessment of a given phenomenon to a determination if an event occurred before or after a particular time point. In a study of morphological grading carried out for day-3 embryos, the existence of moderate intraobserver variability was confirmed and the authors demonstrated substantial differences between embryologists in the morphological scores given to a group of embryos [19]. In addition, the dynamic and gradual nature of change in cellular morphology can obscure events that only become visible when images are condensed into a continuous and coherent movie. It is inevitable that in some circumstances this variability will affect the decision of which embryos are selected for transfer and will have, as a result, direct impact on the probability of IVF success. Current classification scores only analyze morphology at a few predefined points during embryo development leading to a subsequent lack of information about what happened between the examined time points. Thus, nonstop monitoring might provide one strategy to collect a complete representation of embryo developmental kinetics.

The search for prognostic factors predicting embryo development and the outcome of IVF treatment attracts considerable research attention and one such predictive factor is the proper timing of early embryo development which can be measured using noninvasive, automated approaches. When coupled to software analysis this can yield objective and consistent data and thus avoid subjective classification of embryo characteristics. Time-lapse video cinematography overcomes the limitations of intermittent observations by providing a higher resolution and continuous image in which the various components of the cells can be recognized and followed during the entire course of the record period; for instance, a correlation exists between a higher pregnancy rate and the synchronous reappearance of nuclei in the two blastomeres formed after the first division and human embryo development to blastocyst stage was strictly correlated with some specific interval timings in the first stages of development [20, 21].

In a recent study, our own group examined the existence of a correlation between morphokinetic parameters and implantation and ongoing pregnancy rates in order to generate and evaluate a tool for the selection of viable embryos based on the exact timing of embryo development events together with morphological parameters by using a time-lapse monitoring system [22]. This compelling study investigated the integer chronologic pattern of development with morphologic features with the purpose of describing correlations between time taken to reach each developmental milestone and the implantation potential of that specific embryo. It identified an optimal range for each variable which was correlated with a significantly higher probability of implantation; these correlations formed the basis for a proposed hierarchical classification procedure to select viable embryos for transfer with a high implantation potential.

A retrospective analysis was conducted, with an external monitor (EmbryoViewer, Unisense Fertilitech, Aarhus, Denmark), using image analysis software in which exact timings of embryo divisions were annotated and six discriminative morphokinetic parameters were identified: the consecutive embryo divisions from zygote to 5-cell stage (t2, t3, t4, and t5); the duration of the second cell cycle (cc2=t3-t2) representing the time of division from a two-cell embryo until division to a three-cell embryo; and the second synchrony (s2) defined as the transition from a two-cell embryo to a four-cell embryo (s2=t4-t3). For each of these variables two timing intervals were selected with the highest frequency of implanting embryos and this was combined with morphologic exclusion criteria such as first cleavage asymmetry, abrupt first division to more than two cells and multinucleation on day 2 of development. Thus the conclusion was the possibility of identifying an optimal timing range within embryos that have a greater probability to implant (Fig. 3). Observed variations in the timing of embryonic development may be related to culture conditions that can affect embryo metabolism and/or sperm paternal effect which may influence the length of the S-phase in the cell cycle [23, 24].

Up to date, human embryo research on morphokinetic development has been limited by the small number of samples produced under diverse experimental conditions; in fact, the majority of studies using time-lapse image analysis only included measurements from early stages of development, and although an interesting link has been described to human embryo development between digital images and molecular data from the zygote to blastocyst stage, the results were provided from frozen-thawed zygotes and may not be comparable with studies with fresh embryos [17, 21, 25–29].

The description of important differences in the chronology of development between implanting and nonimplanting embryos can significantly improve the chance of implantation when comparing embryos with slower/faster development. These data support the hypothesis in which embryo viability depends on a tightly regulated sequence of cellular events that begin at the time of the fertilization and also confirms the presence of an optimal time interval for all the embryo cell

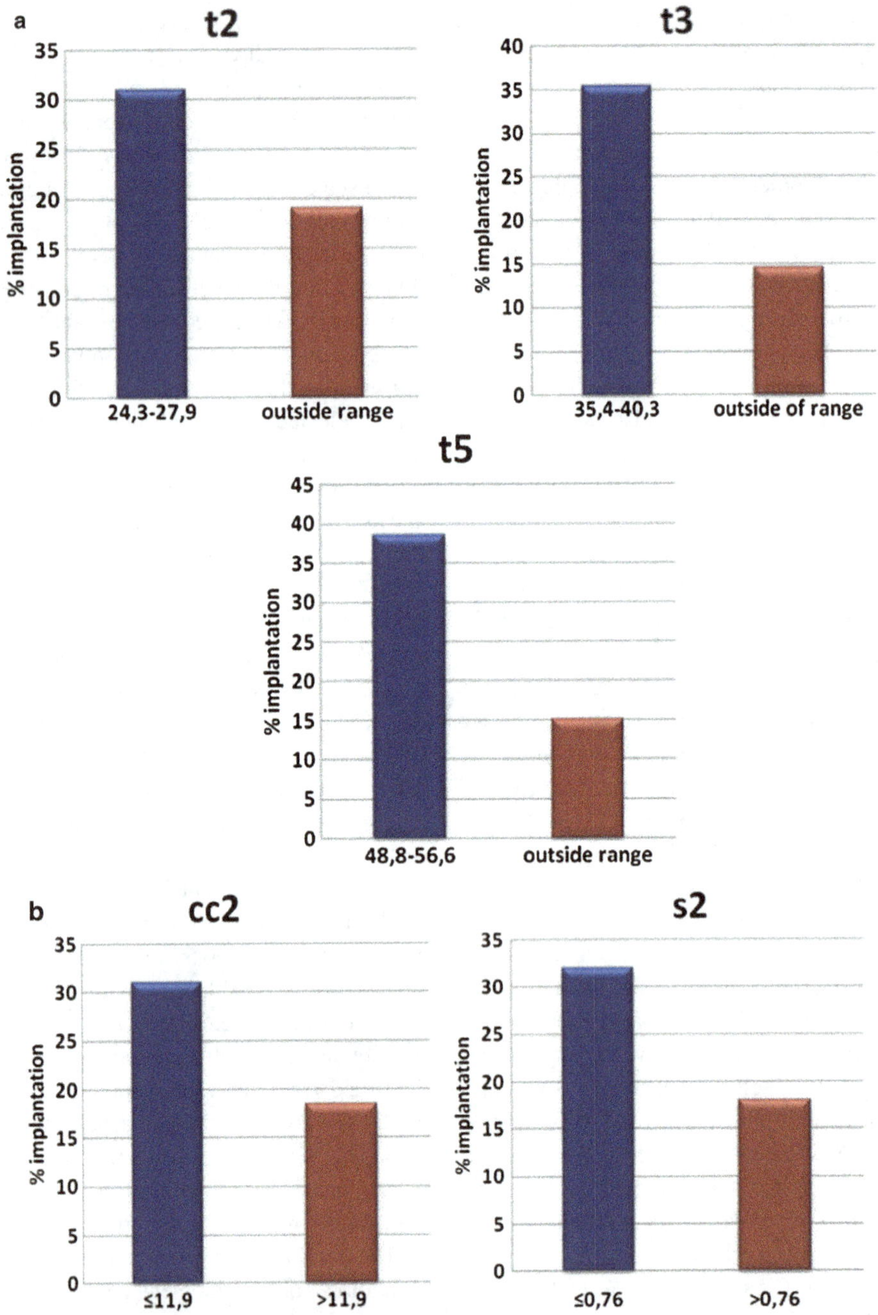

Fig. 5.3 (**a**) Percentage of implanting embryos with cell division times inside or outside ranges. We determined the timing of cleavage timings to a 2-, 3-, and 5-cell embryo (t2, t3, and t5). (**b**) Percentage of implanting embryos with cell division times inside or outside ranges. We also determined a variable related to duration of cell cycles named cc2, second cell cycle, duration of the time as a 2-blastomere (t3-t2) and s2 synchrony in division from 2-blastomere embryo to 4-blastomere embryo

divisions; although it is generally accepted that early cleavages are better than later cleavages, it has been demonstrated that cell division could occur "too early" and impair embryo competence.

According to the kinetic parameters evaluated, t5, cc2, and s2 seem to be important indicators which are significantly correlated with embryo implantation. Perhaps, later divisions could be even more indicative of embryo viability but as long as the embryo development progresses, it is more difficult to precise exact timings both manually and through digital image analysis. When an embryo has to be evaluated, it is easier to count two cells rather than counting eight cells, the more cells in the embryo, the more they tend to cover each other and distinguishing embryo fragmentation becomes harder in the first stages of development. The data from our study monitors embryo development until day 3 of culture and in doing so provides additional information that will improve the ability to select the more competent embryos for transferring; moreover, by using implantation rate as the main end-point it is possible to examine not only embryo competence for blastocyst formation but also following processes like hatching and successful implantation.

The correlation established between morphokinetics data and embryo implantation could be considered the starting point to build a decision tree in order to improve the selection of embryos with the highest implantation potential. This hierarchical classification includes six categories from A to F. The categorization starts with a morphological screening of all embryos in a cohort to discard nonviable embryos which are not being considered for transfer (class F); subsequently, the model excludes embryos that fulfill any of the exclusion criteria (class E). The successive levels follow a strict hierarchy based on the binary timing variables t5, cc2, and s2. If the value of T5 falls inside the optimal range (48.8–56.6 h), the embryo is categorized as A or B; if the value of T5 falls outside the optimal range, the embryo is classified as C or D. If s2 is within the optimal range (≤0.76 h), embryo is A or C depending on T5; in a similar way, if s2 >0.76 h, embryo is B or D depending also on T5. Finally, the embryo is cataloged with the extra plus (+) if CC2 ≤11.9 h (A+/B+/C+/D+) or with a minus (−) if CC2 >11.9 h (A−/B−/C−/D−) (Fig. 4). Depending on its cataloging, embryo implantation potential dramatically decreases from class A+ (66 %) to class E (8 %).

Conclusions

In summary, these data demonstrate that a time-lapse embryo monitoring system in a clinical setting provides novel information about developmental parameters that differ between implanting and nonimplanting embryos. An embryo can belong to both the best morphology and the best time-lapse category and still fail so it is not rare that unsuccessful embryos have the same morphokinetic profile as implanting embryos; by contrast, the morphokinetics data facilitate rejecting embryos with lower implantation potential because their variances are larger than implanting embryos. In conclusion, this categorized scheme could be helpful in improving embryo selection.

As previously mentioned, image analysis may add objectivity to the process of embryo selection and consequently lead to an improvement of the IVF process. An automatic system might stimulate different grading systems and the combined scores could lead to a final single status; also, image analysis techniques would allow storage of accurate measurements of several embryo characteristics that could be used for improving the knowledge about early embryo development and lead to further refinements of morphological grading systems. For example, Richter showed that blastocysts with relative large and/or slight oval inner mass cell are more likely to implant than other blastocysts [30]. With a full automatic segmentation and quantification of embryos morphological features, more findings of this kind will hopefully be found.

However, embryo image analysis poses some challenges to the image analysis community. Many of the morphological features analyzed are not always well perceived immediately thus an accurate evaluation of a three dimensional embryo would require an automatic system to analyze several images of the same embryo taken through different planes of focus in order to quantify the features needed [31].

Time-lapse image analysis is an exciting, powerful, and noninvasive technique for observing

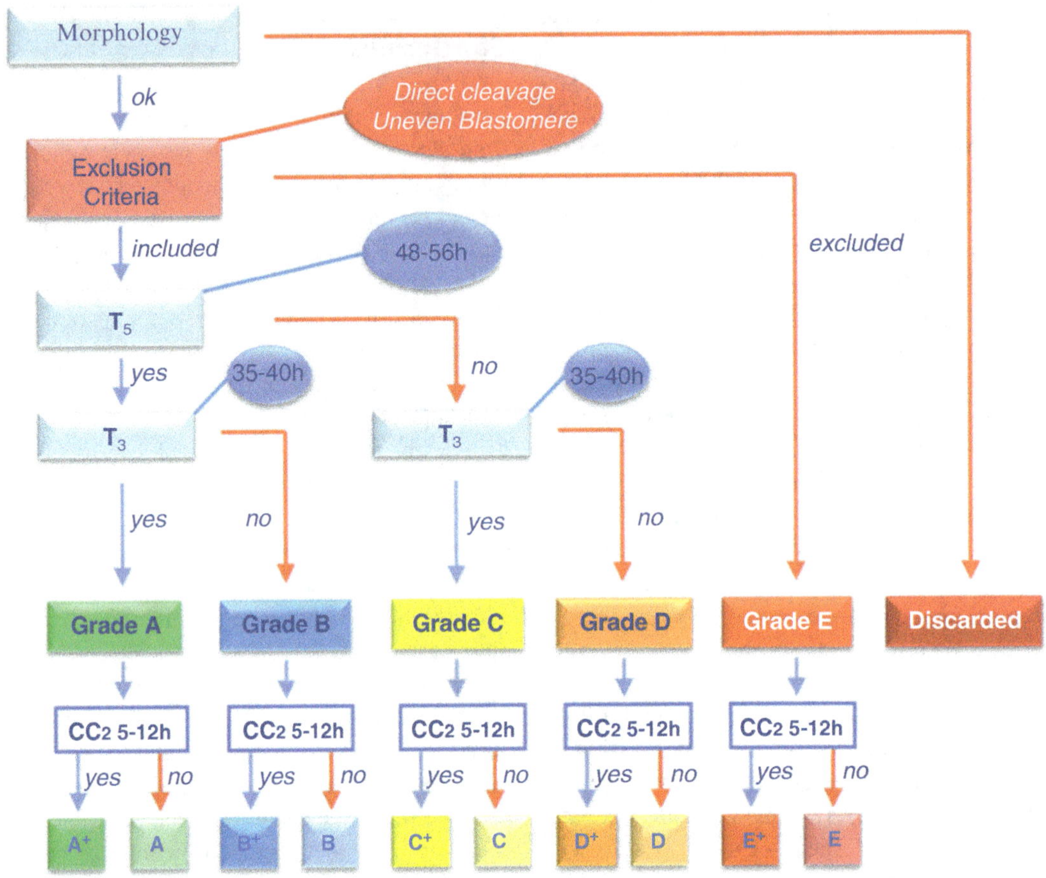

Fig. 5.4 Hierarchical classification of embryos

cellular activity during fertilization and embryogenesis in a coherent, uninterrupted manner. The technology to perform analysis in real time has improved dramatically and the morphological and chronological analysis of reproduction can potentially make important contributions to assisted reproductive technology. It is likely that the use of automated systems will save the embryologist staff a significant amount of time and the availability of 24 h observation may allow IVF procedures to be conducted in a more flexible manner throughout the day. Computer-assisted embryo evaluation will improve and streamline the IVF procedure, reducing costs and increasing the ability of embryologists to identify the embryo most likely to produce a child. Advances of this type will be vital for clinics to transition to efficient SET and eliminate high order multiple pregnancies.

References

1. Steptoe PC, Edwards RG. Birth after the reimplantation of a human embryo. Lancet. 1978;2(8085):366.
2. Payne D, Flaherty SP, Barry MF, Matthews CD. Preliminary observations on polar body extrusion and pronuclear formation in human oocytes using time-lapse video cinematography. Hum Reprod. 1997;12(3):532–41.
3. Ezin M, Fraser S. Time-lapse imaging of the early avian embryo. Methods Cell Biol. 2008;87:211–36.
4. Lewis WH, Gregory PW. Cinematographs of living developing rabbit-eggs. Science. 1929;69(1782):226–9.
5. Karnaukhov AV, Sviridova-Chailakhyan TA, Karnaukhova EV, Panchenko MM, Bogdanenko EV, Chailakhyan LM. Time-lapse cinematography study of preimplantation mouse embryo development. Dokl Biol Sci. 2009;426:306–10.
6. Yamagata K, Suetsugu R, Wakayama T. Long-term, six-dimensional live-cell imaging for the mouse preimplantation embryo that does not affect full-term development. J Reprod Dev. 2009;55(3):343–50.

7. Cruz M, Gadea B, Garrido N, et al. Embryo quality, blastocyst and ongoing pregnancy rates in oocyte donation patients whose embryos were monitored by time-lapse imaging. J Assist Reprod Genet. 2011;28(7):569–73.
8. Nakahara T, Iwase A, Goto M, et al. Evaluation of the safety of time-lapse observations for human embryos. J Assist Reprod Genet. 2010;27(2–3):93–6.
9. McKiernan SH, Bavister BD. Timing of development is a critical parameter for predicting successful embryogenesis. Hum Reprod. 1994;9(11):2123–9.
10. Rehman KS, Bukulmez O, Langley M, et al. Late stages of embryo progression are a much better predictor of clinical pregnancy than early cleavage in intracytoplasmic sperm injection and in vitro fertilization cycles with blastocyst-stage transfer. Fertil Steril. 2007;87(5):1041–52.
11. Lechniak D, Pers-Kamczyc E, Pawlak P. Timing of the first zygotic cleavage as a marker of developmental potential of mammalian embryos. Reprod Biol. 2008;8(1):23–42.
12. Lonergan P, Khatir H, Piumi F, Rieger D, Humblot P, Boland MP. Effect of time interval from insemination to first cleavage on the developmental characteristics, sex ratio and pregnancy rate after transfer of bovine embryos. J Reprod Fertil. 1999;117(1):159–67.
13. Sakkas D, Shoukir Y, Chardonnens D, Bianchi PG, Campana A. Early cleavage of human embryos to the two-cell stage after intracytoplasmic sperm injection as an indicator of embryo viability. Hum Reprod. 1998;13(1):182–7.
14. Sakkas D, Percival G, D'Arcy Y, Sharif K, Afnan M. Assessment of early cleaving in vitro fertilized human embryos at the 2-cell stage before transfer improves embryo selection. Fertil Steril. 2001;76(6):1150–6.
15. Shoukir Y, Campana A, Farley T, Sakkas D. Early cleavage of in-vitro fertilized human embryos to the 2-cell stage: a novel indicator of embryo quality and viability. Hum Reprod. 1997;12(7):1531–6.
16. Salumets A, Hyden-Granskog C, Makinen S, Suikkari AM, Tiitinen A, Tuuri T. Early cleavage predicts the viability of human embryos in elective single embryo transfer procedures. Hum Reprod. 2003;18(4):821–5.
17. Fenwick J, Platteau P, Murdoch AP, Herbert M. Time from insemination to first cleavage predicts developmental competence of human preimplantation embryos in vitro. Hum Reprod. 2002;17(2):407–12.
18. Van Montfoort AP, Dumoulin JC, Kester AD, Evers JL. Early cleavage is a valuable addition to existing embryo selection parameters: a study using single embryo transfers. Hum Reprod. 2004;19(9):2103–8.
19. Baxter Bendus AE, Mayer JF, Shipley SK, Catherino WH. Interobserver and intraobserver variation in day 3 embryo grading. Fertil Steril. 2006;86(6):1608–15.
20. Lemmen JG, Agerholm I, Ziebe S. Kinetic markers of human embryo quality using time-lapse recordings of IVF/ICSI-fertilized oocytes. Reprod Biomed Online. 2008;17(3):385–91.
21. Wong CC, Loewke KE, Bossert NL, et al. Non-invasive imaging of human embryos before embryonic genome activation predicts development to the blastocyst stage. Nat Biotechnol. 2010;28(10):1115–21.
22. Meseguer M, Herrero J, Tejera A, Hilligsoe KM, Ramsing N, Remohi J. The use of morphokinetics as a predictor of embryo implantation. Hum Reprod. 2011;26(10):2658–71.
23. Escrich L, Grau N, Meseguer M, Pellicer A, Escriba MJ. Morphologic indicators predict the stage of chromatin condensation of human germinal vesicle oocytes recovered from stimulated cycles. Fertil Steril. 2010;93(8):2557–64.
24. Eid LN, Lorton SP, Parrish JJ. Paternal influence on S-phase in the first cell cycle of the bovine embryo. Biol Reprod. 1994;51(6):1232–7.
25. Mio Y. Morphological analysis of human embryonic development using time-lapse cinematography. J Mamm Ova Res. 2006;23:27–35.
26. Mio Y, Maeda K. Time-lapse cinematography of dynamic changes occurring during in vitro development of human embryos. Am J Obstet Gynecol. 2008;199(6):660.e1–e5.
27. Maeda K. The beginning of human life under time-lapse cinematography. Period Biol. 2009;111(3):323–7.
28. Nagy ZP, Liu J, Joris H, Devroey P, Van Steirteghem A. Time-course of oocyte activation, pronucleus formation and cleavage in human oocytes fertilized by intracytoplasmic sperm injection. Hum Reprod. 1994;9(9):1743–8.
29. Lundin K, Bergh C, Hardarson T. Early embryo cleavage is a strong indicator of embryo quality in human IVF. Hum Reprod. 2001;16(12):2652–7.
30. Richter KS, Harris DC, Daneshmand ST, Shapiro BS. Quantitative grading of a human blastocyst: optimal inner cell mass size and shape. Fertil Steril. 2001; 76(6):1157–67.
31. Filho ES, Noble JA, Wells D. A review on automatic analysis of human embryo microscope images. Open Biomed Eng J. 2010;4:170–7.

Limitations and Benefits of Morphologic Embryo Assessment Strategies: How Far Can Morphological Assessment Go in the Identification of Viable Embryos?

6

Denny Sakkas and David K. Gardner

Morphological assessment has been the primary tool of the embryologist for selecting which embryo(s) to replace. Since the early years of in vitro fertilization (IVF), it was noted that embryos cleaving faster and those of better morphological appearance were more likely to lead to a pregnancy. Indeed, Edwards et al. noted only a few years after the birth of Louise Brown "that cleavage rates on a certain day and overall embryo morphology were valuable in choosing which embryo to transfer" [1]. In 1986 one of the initial large studies ($N = 1{,}539$ embryos) examining the utility of embryo morphology was published by Cummins et al. [2]. It was reported that embryo quality scores were valuable in predicting success. Indeed Cummins et al. [2] calculated an embryo development rating based on the ratio between the time at which embryos were observed at a particular stage after insemination and the time at which they would be expected to reach that stage of a hypothetical "ideal" growth rate with a cell cycle length of 11.9 h. Using this scoring system, "normally" growing embryos scored 100; however, the scoring system appears to have never been assessed prospectively. The following year a study by Puissant et al. [3] reported the grading of embryos based on the amount of anucleate fragments expelled during early cleavage and on developmental speed. They found that embryos endowed with a high score were more often associated with pregnancy and in particular with the occurrence of multiple pregnancy. Interestingly, they already proposed that in the event of a high score: "It might be warranted to replace only two embryos when these conditions are fulfilled."

In addition to the classical parameters of cell number and fragmentation, numerous other characteristics have now been examined including pronuclear (PN) morphology, early cleavage to the 2-cell stage, top quality embryos on successive days, and various forms of sequential assessment of embryos (see reviews by refs. [4–6]). One could therefore make a case that morphological assessment systems have evolved over the past decade. Furthermore, the ability to culture and assess blastocyst stage embryos has also significantly improved the ability to select embryos on the basis of morphology [7]. The main question is however "How far can morphological assessment of the cleavage stage embryo go in the identification of viable embryos?"

Pronucleate Oocyte

The many transformations that take place during the fertilization process make this a dynamic stage to assess. The oocyte contains the majority of the developmental materials, maternal mRNA

D. Sakkas (✉)
Boston IVF, 130 Second Avenue,
Waltham, MA 02451, USA
e-mail: dsakkas@bostonivf.com

D.K. Gardner
Department of Zoology, University of Melbourne,
Melbourne, VIC, Australia

D.K. Gardner et al. (eds.), *Human Gametes and Preimplantation Embryos: Assessment and Diagnosis*,
DOI 10.1007/978-1-4614-6651-2_6,

and proteins, for ensuring that the embryo reaches the 4–8-cell stage. In human embryos, embryonic genome activation has been shown to occur between the 4- and 8-cell stage [8]. The quality of the oocyte therefore, plays the lead role for determining embryo development and subsequent viability.

A number of studies have postulated that embryo quality can be predicted at the pronucleate oocyte stage. Separate studies by Tesarik and Scott [9, 10] had concentrated on the predictive value of the nucleoli. Tesarik and Greco [9] postulated that the normal and abnormal morphology of the pronuclei were related to the developmental fate of human embryos. They retrospectively assessed the number and distribution of nucleolar precursor bodies (NPB) in each pronucleus of fertilized oocytes that led to embryos that implanted. The characteristics of viable embryos were then compared to those that led to failures in implantation. The features that were shared by zygotes that had the 100 % implantation success were: (1) the number of NPB in both pronuclei never differed by more than 3, and (2) the NPB were always polarized or not-polarized in both pronuclei but never polarized in one pronucleus and not in the other. Pronucleate oocytes not showing the above criteria were more likely to develop into preimplantation embryos that had poor morphology and/or experienced cleavage arrest. The presence of at least one embryo, which had shown the above criteria at the pronuclear stage in those transferred, led to a pregnancy rate of 50 % (22/44) compared to only 9 % (2/23) when none were present. A further study by Scott and Smith [11] devised an embryo score on day 1 based on the alignment of pronuclei and nucleoli, the appearance of the cytoplasm, nuclear membrane breakdown, and cleavage to the 2-cell stage. Patients who had an overall high embryo score (≥15) had a pregnancy and implantation rate of 71 % (34/48) and 28 % (49/175), respectively, compared to only 8 % (4/49) and 2 % (4/178) in the low embryo score group. It is interesting to note that in the embryo scoring system initially described by Scott and Smith [11], embryos that had already cleaved to the 2-cell stage by 25–26 h post-insemination were assigned an additional score of 10. This represents a sizeable part of the overall score considering that high-quality embryos were judged to be those scoring ≥15, i.e., in order to be high quality the embryo had to exhibit early cleavage.

Table 6.1 The use of pronuclear scoring and early 2-cell cleavage in predicting pregnancy outcome

Stage of assessment	Predictive (reference numbers)	Not Predictive (reference numbers)
Pronuclear scoring	[10, 76–78]	[14, 79–81]
Early 2-cell cleavage	[25, 26, 28, 29, 82–85]	[73]

A selection of studies indicating predictability or no predictability in using these techniques

Subsequent studies examining similar pronuclear attributes, defined as the “Z-score” [10, 12]. This have been reviewed by Scott [12]. However, although the use of the Z-score has some supporters, there are just as many detractors (Table 1). Initial studies on pronucleate assessment suffered because of small sample sizes and because the technique was never rigorously evaluated using single embryo transfer (SET). In a study using SET [13] a total of 1,520 zygotes were analyzed according to a classification system based on the number and distribution of NPB. In the comparative analysis, none of the six different PN scoring classes produced superior quality embryos or higher pregnancy rates in 144 single embryo transfers. In a recent larger study [14] the authors did not find any statistically significant correlation between the Z-score of 1,032 embryos transferred in 393 embryo transfers and the implantation rate or the pregnancy outcome. In particular, the best Z-score identified (Z1, 7.2 %) did not seem to correlate with embryo implantation rate or pregnancy outcomes any better than those with worse scores (Z2, 6.9 % and Z3, 85.9 %). Nicoli et al. [14] concluded that Z-score alone cannot be considered a better tool than standard morphologic criteria for identifying, controlling, or selecting embryos with a better chance of successful ongoing pregnancy.

Cleavage Stage Embryos

Sequential Analysis of Cleavage and Morphology

The most widely used criteria for selecting the best embryos for transfer have been based on cell number and morphology [2]. A vast number of variations on this theme have been published and the main change that has happened in the past decade is a greater focus on sequential assessment of the embryo. This has come about because of the understanding that a static assessment of a particular embryo is less informative (Fig. 1). As discussed by Bavister [15] one of the most critical factors in determining selection criteria is to ascertain strict time points to compare the embryos.

In a series of key studies Gerris et al. [16] and Van Royen et al. [17] employed sequential criteria to select single embryos for transfer. The necessary characteristics of their "top" quality embryos were established by examining retrospectively embryos that had a very high implantation potential [17]. Such "top" quality embryos had the following characteristics: 4 or 5 blastomeres on day 2 and at least 7 blastomeres on day 3 after fertilization, an absence of multinucleated blastomeres, and <20 % of fragments on days 2 and 3 after fertilization. When these criteria were utilized in a prospective randomized clinical trial comparing single and double embryo transfers (DET), it was found that in 26 single embryo transfers where a top quality embryo was available an implantation rate of 42.3 % and ongoing pregnancy rate of 38.5 % was obtained. In a preliminary study of 27 DET an implantation rate of 48.1 % and ongoing pregnancy rate of 74 % was obtained. A larger study analyzing the outcome of 370 consecutive single top quality embryo transfers in patients younger than 38 years for pregnancy showed that the ongoing pregnancy rate after single top quality embryo transfer was 36.5 % (135/370) [18].

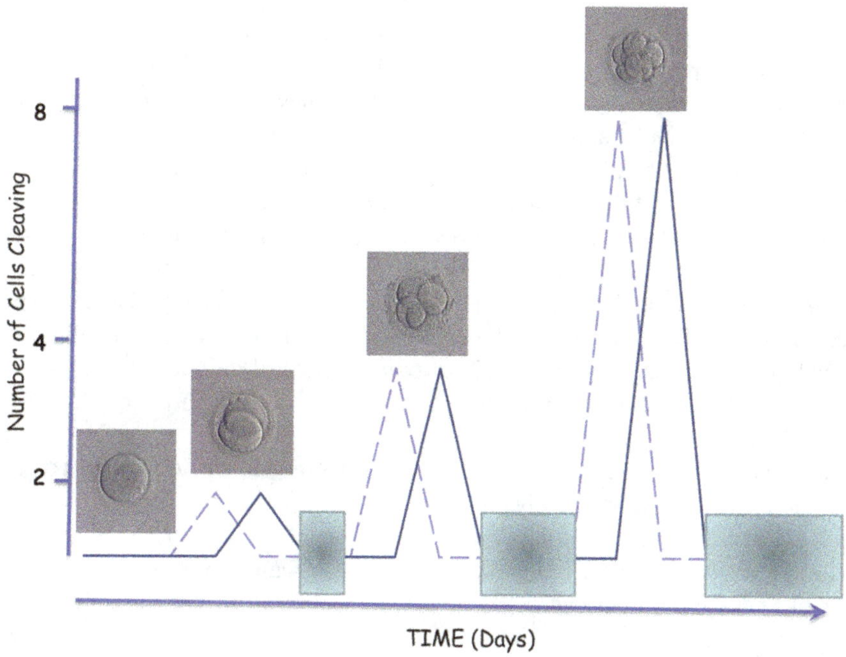

Fig. 6.1 The impact of scoring times on cleavage stage embryo development. A slower (*solid line*) and faster (*dashed line*) cleaving embryo can not be distinguished when scored at specific time points in their development (*rectangular boxes*) therefore not allowing the embryologist to distinguish cleavage rates. Selecting specific times of expected cleavage as times of assessment can help distinguish the faster and slower cleaving embryos more efficiently

Many groups have now reported the use of sequential scoring systems (see review by Skiadas and Racowsky [19]). One type of scoring system is the Graduated Embryo Score (GES): a value of up to 100 which includes investigation of nucleolar alignment along the pronuclear axis, regular cleavage, and degree of fragmentation at the first cell division, and cell number and morphology on day 3. It was determined that the transfer of one or more embryos with a GES ≥70 predicted pregnancy and implantation rates better than a single morphologic evaluation on day 3 [20, 21]. It was also found that a high GES score up to day 3 was more predictive of blastocyst development. In a further study, using a sequential embryo assessment score, it was found that even though an embryo had the best developmental markers on days 1, 2, and 3 it was still only likely to reach the blastocyst stage only 50 % of the time [22].

Recently a larger data set has been reported examining the sequential growth of 4,042 embryos individually cultured from day 1 to 5/6 [23]. Pronuclear morphology on day 1, and early cleavage, cell number, and fragmentation rate on day 2 were evaluated for each zygote. Interestingly, early cleavage and cell number on day 2 were the most powerful parameters to predict the development of a good morphology blastocyst at day 5. Overall the study found that parameters of early development were not helpful in predicting their implantation ability and that transfer of a good morphology blastocyst was still associated with high implantation and live birth rates. The more complex sequential embryo assessment schemes, including the GES, have yet to be tested in a single embryo transfer setting as has the Top Quality Embryo Scoring system described above, therefore it is hard to gauge their true benefit. Recently, however Racowsky et al. [24] have investigated the benefits of scoring embryos on more than 1 day and concluded that day 2 or 3 evaluations alone are sufficient for morphological selection of cleavage stage embryos.

Early Cleavage to the Two-Cell Stage

The issue of using a static assessment of embryo development has always been one that has plagued embryologists. To address this issue, Sakkas and colleagues determined that at particular times assessment of cleavage could be more discerning in identifying which embryos were cleaving faster than others. For example, a 4-cell embryo scored in the morning of day 2 is clearly not the same as one that only developed into a 4-cell in the afternoon of day 2. Therefore, cleavage to the 2-cell stage at 25 h post-insemination or microinjection was chosen as the critical time point for selecting embryos [25–27]. The most impressive data investigating the usefulness of early cleaving (EC) 2-cell embryos is that supported by single embryo transfer [28, 29]. In one of these studies Salumets et al. [28], showed that when transferring single embryos a significantly higher clinical pregnancy rate was observed after the transfer of early cleaving (50 %) rather than non-early cleaving (26.4 %) embryos. Van Montfoort et al. [29] also found in a retrospective analysis of 165 SETs that a significantly higher pregnancy rate was observed after transfer of single EC embryos compared to single non-EC embryos (46 % vs. 18 %). This result was verified in DET when two early cleavers were present when compared to DET with two non-EC embryos (45 % vs. 25 %). Logistic regression analysis showed that EC was an independent predictor for pregnancy. A number of studies have also found that the embryos that cleave early to the 2-cell stage have also been reported to have a significantly higher blastocyst formation rate [22, 23, 28, 29]. In conclusion, a number of studies on early embryo cleavage on day 2 have proven useful, although there is one that did not find it of benefit (Table 1).

Fragmentation and Multinucleation

More detail has recently been placed on assessment of fragmentation within the embryos and multinucleation in individual blastomeres. It is generally held that increasing percentages of fragmentation within an embryo leads to lower pregnancy rates [3, 30, 31]. The assessment of fragmentation is however hindered by the observations that fragments are extruded and absorbed by blastomeres [32]. As with other aspects of morphology this infers that examining embryos at particular times may alter the outcomes of assessment. The fluidity and transient nature of some of these fragments brings into question how we can truly examine them morphologically. Of interest it appears that the removal of fragments may be beneficial [33, 34]. Furthermore, fragmentation is influenced by the culture system, the presence of serum and/or ambient oxygen, leading to greater embryo trauma. Subsequently, a certain percentage of fragmentation observed is an artifact of the culture system employed.

Another morphological detail that is drawing more attention is the presence of multinuclei in individual blastomeres. Multinucleated embryos can be observed most efficiently on days 2 or 3 as afterwards their observation is difficult. The frequency of multinucleation has been assessed in a number studies with varying reports about the incidence; however, their impact in general is considered to be detrimental [35–39]. Significantly, both fragmentation and multinucleation have both been correlated to the presence of chromosomal abnormalities in embryos [33, 40, 41].

Development to the Blastocyst Stage

A perplexing fact is that with the commercial availability of sequential culture media systems, and the ability to routinely perform blastocyst culture in many IVF clinics, the majority of transfers are still performed at the cleavage stages. There is still an argument as to whether day 5 or 2/3 transfers differ [42–50] even though the most recent Cochrane report ruled in favor of day 5 transfers [51]. This recent Cochrane report concluded that their examination of the available trials provided evidence to suggest that there is now a significant difference in pregnancy and live birth rates in favor of blastocyst transfer with good prognosis patients, with high numbers of 8-cell embryos on day 3 being the most favored subgroup for whom there is no difference in cycle cancellation.

Morphologically the assessment of a good blastocyst has consistently shown the greatest impact on influencing implantation rates [7, 43, 47, 52–66]. As with the scoring of embryos during the cleavage stages, time and morphology play an important part in selecting the best blastocyst. Although many scoring assessment schemes exist for blastocysts, they are largely based on assessing the expansion state of the blastocyst and on the consistency of the inner cell mass (ICM) and trophectoderm cells [67]. Using one such grading system Gardner and Schoolcraft determined that when two high scoring blastocysts (>3AA), i.e., expanded blastocoel with compacted ICM and cohesive trophectoderm epithelium, are transferred a clinical pregnancy and implantation rate of >80 % and 69 % can be attained [68]. When two blastocysts not achieving these scores (<3AA) are transferred, the clinical pregnancy and implantation rate are significantly lower, 50 % and 33 % [69]. Although reduced from the values obtained with top scoring blastocysts, it is evident that early blastocysts on day 5 still have high developmental potential. It is important to note that to date the strongest criteria of morphological assessment appears to be the selection of a high-quality blastocyst on day 5 of development [23, 68]. In addition to this data looking at individual components of the blastocysts has also proved effective. Ahlstrom et al. [70] examined morphological parameters of 1,117 fresh day 5 single blastocyst transfers and their live birth outcome in a retrospective analysis and found that degree of blastocoel expansion, appearance of the trophectoderm (TE), and the ICM all had a significant effect on live birth. However, once adjusted for known significant confounders, it was shown that TE was the only statistically significant-independent predictor of live birth outcome. Their study indicated for the first time the predictive strength of TE grade over ICM for selecting the best blastocyst for embryo replacement.

Interestingly, another indication of the importance of blastocyst development as a morphological marker is the fact that many studies examining earlier morphological markers adopt blastocyst development as an endpoint [20, 22, 23]. Recently, a day 4 scoring system was also successfully developed and implemented. Day 4 SETs were found to be a viable option or alternative to day 5 SETs with no difference in pregnancy rates [71].

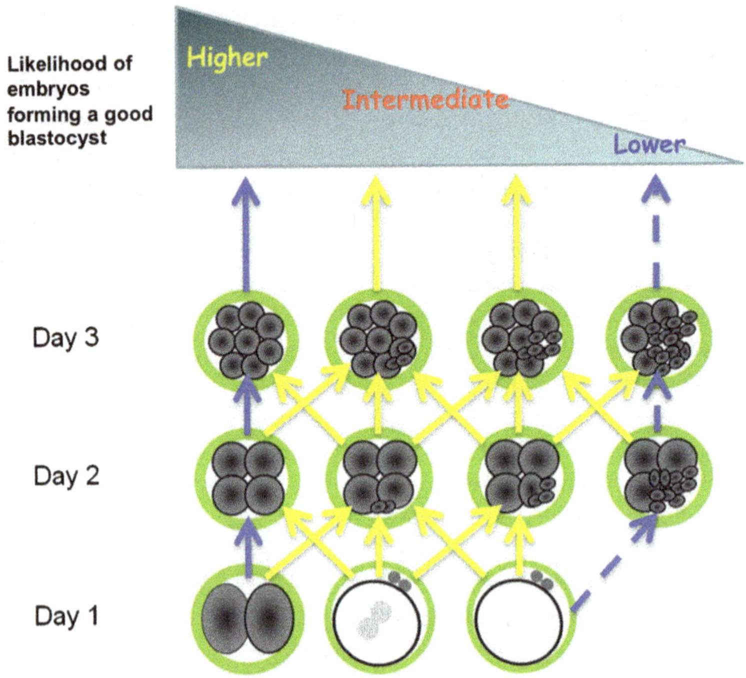

Fig. 6.2 An embryo can take various paths to becoming a blastocyst on day 5. Although the likelihood of forming a blastocyst is higher when an embryo is top quality on days 1, 2, and 3 (*solid blue arrows*), it can still take numerous other morphological paths to form a similar looking blastocyst (*yellow arrows*) or even have poor morphology (*dashed blue arrows*) and form a blastocyst

It is also of note that an embryo may not pass any of the earlier hurdles of development on days 1, 2, or 3 but still form a high-grade blastocyst on day 5. A number of studies have shown that preselection of the best embryos on day 3 does not always predict embryos that would have been transferred on day 5 as blastocysts [6, 22, 47, 72]. An embryo can therefore take numerous paths to become a blastocyst and this may not always be reflected in its morphology on days 1, 2, or 3 (Fig. 2).

Problems with Morphology

Although morphology has been used almost exclusively for embryo selection over the past 30 years, it is still a very subjective technique. As a technique it has never truly been validated and many clinics come across cases in which poor quality embryos are replaced and lead to live births. One of the only attempts at an international standardization has been the creation of web sites with photographic documentation of embryos and quality control assessment (for example: www.fertaid.com). Therefore, in relation to cleavage stage embryos little progress appears to have been made in their assessment, and in comparison to some of the early assessment papers published in the early 1980s, we are generating few new conclusions.

A significant advance in the IVF laboratory over the past decade has been the ability to grow blastocysts, whose morphological assessment appears to give great benefit in embryo selection [51]. Unfortunately, although day 5 blastocyst culture remains as one of the strongest indicators of all morphological parameters [73], the reality is that most practicing IVF centers still choose to perform the majority of transfers on an earlier day, although this appears to be changing slowly.

In conclusion, although assessment of specific morphological parameters at specific times has been shown to greatly increase the success of embryo selection, such knowledge does not provide information regarding the actual physiology of the embryo. The advent of real-time morphology [74, 75] may or may not change this, and its role may still be limited in providing a selection tool. Indeed some of the initial strategies are examining de-selection rather than prospective selection (see Chap. 5 by Meseguer and colleagues). The data from Wong et al. does indicate that time-lapse image analysis and gene expression profiling do correlate [75]. Therefore, it is envisaged that we may move away from the traditional morphological parameters we have relied on for many years and other methods of assessment, such as real-time imaging, genetic, proteomic, and/or metabolic analysis will provide more relevant information to assist in the selection of the one embryo for transfer.

References

1. Edwards R, Fishel S, Cohen J. Factors influencing the success of in vitro fertilization for alleviating human infertility. J In Vitro Fert Embryo Transf. 1984;1:3–23.
2. Cummins J, Breen T, Harrison K, Shaw J, Wilson L, Hennessey J. A formula for scoring human embryo growth rates in in vitro fertilization: its value in predicting pregnancy and in comparison with visual estimates of embryo quality. J In Vitro Fert Embryo Transf. 1986;3:284–95.
3. Puissant F, Van RM, Barlow P, Deweze J, Leroy F. Embryo scoring as a prognostic tool in IVF treatment. Hum Reprod. 1987;2(8):705–8.
4. De Neubourg D, Gerris J. Single embryo transfer—state of the art. Reprod Biomed Online. 2003;7(6): 615–22.
5. Sakkas, D. Evaluation of embryo quality: A strategy for sequential analysis of embryo development with the aim of single embryo transfer. In: Laboratory and Clinical Perspectives, Gardner D, Weissman A, Howles C, Shoham Z (Eds), Martin Dunitz Press, London; 2001. p. 223.
6. Sakkas D, Gardner DK. Noninvasive methods to assess embryo quality. Curr Opin Obstet Gynecol. 2005;17(3):283–8.
7. Gardner DK, Surrey E, Minjarez D, Leitz A, Stevens J, Schoolcraft WB. Single blastocyst transfer: a prospective randomized trial. Fertil Steril. 2004;81(3): 551–5.
8. Braude P, Bolton V, Moore S. Human gene expression first occurs between the four- and eight-cell stages of preimplantation development. Nature. 1988;332: 459–61.
9. Tesarik J, Greco E. The probability of abnormal preimplantation development can be predicted by a single static observation on pronuclear stage morphology. Hum Reprod. 1999;14:318–23.
10. Scott L, Alvero R, Leondires M, Miller B. The morphology of human pronuclear embryos is positively related to blastocyst development and implantation. Hum Reprod. 2000;15(11):2394–403.
11. Scott LA, Smith S. The successful use of pronuclear embryo transfers the day following oocyte retrieval. Hum Reprod. 1998;13(4):1003–13.
12. Scott L. Pronuclear scoring as a predictor of embryo development. Reprod Biomed Online. 2003;6(2): 201–14.
13. Salumets A, Hyden-Granskog C, Suikkari AM, Tiitinen A, Tuuri T. The predictive value of pronuclear morphology of zygotes in the assessment of human embryo quality. Hum Reprod. 2001;16(10):2177–81.
14. Nicoli A, Valli B, Di GR, Di TB, Gallinelli A, La Sala GB. Limited importance of pre-embryo pronuclear morphology (zygote score) in assisted reproduction outcome in the absence of embryo cryopreservation. Fertil Steril. 2007;88(4 Suppl):1167–73.
15. Bavister B. Culture of preimplantation embryos: facts and artefacts. Hum Reprod Update. 1995;1:91–148.
16. Gerris J, De Neubourg D, Mangelschots K, Van Royen E, Van de Meerssche M, Valkenburg M. Prevention of twin pregnancy after in-vitro fertilization or intracytoplasmic sperm injection based on strict embryo criteria: a prospective randomized clinical trial. Hum Reprod. 1999;14(10):2581–7.
17. Van Royen E, Mangelschots K, De Neubourg D, Valkenburg M, Van de Meerssche M, Ryckaert G, et al. Characterization of a top quality embryo, a step towards single-embryo transfer. Hum Reprod. 1999;14(9):2345–9.
18. De Neubourg D, Gerris J, Mangelschots K, Van Royen E, Vercruyssen M, Elseviers M. Single top quality embryo transfer as a model for prediction of early pregnancy outcome. Hum Reprod. 2004;19(6): 1476–9.
19. Skiadas CC, Racowsky C. Development rate, cumulative scoring and embryonic viability. In: Cohen J, Elder KT, editors. Human embryo evaluation & selection. London: Informa Healthcare; 2007. p. 101–21.
20. Fisch JD, Rodriguez H, Ross R, Overby G, Sher G. The Graduated Embryo Score (GES) predicts blastocyst formation and pregnancy rate from cleavage-stage embryos. Hum Reprod. 2001;16(9):1970–5.
21. Fisch JD, Sher G, Adamowicz M, Keskintepe L. The graduated embryo score predicts the outcome of assisted reproductive technologies better than a single day 3 evaluation and achieves results associated with blastocyst transfer from day 3 embryo transfer. Fertil Steril. 2003;80(6):1352–8.
22. Neuber E, Rinaudo P, Trimarchi JR, Sakkas D. Sequential assessment of individually cultured human embryos as an indicator of subsequent good quality blastocyst development. Hum Reprod. 2003;18(6): 1307–12.

23. Guerif F, Le Gouge A, Giraudeau B, Poindron J, Bidault R, Gasnier O, et al. Limited value of morphological assessment at days 1 and 2 to predict blastocyst development potential: a prospective study based on 4042 embryos. Hum Reprod. 2007;22(7): 1973–81.
24. Racowsky C, Ohno-Machado L, Kim J, Biggers JD. Is there an advantage in scoring early embryos on more than one day? Hum Reprod. 2009;24(9):2104–13.
25. Shoukir Y, Campana A, Farley T, Sakkas D. Early cleavage of in-vitro fertilized human embryos to the 2-cell stage: a novel indicator of embryo quality and viability. Hum Reprod. 1997;12(7):1531–6.
26. Sakkas D, Shoukir Y, Chardonnens D, Bianchi PG, Campana A. Early cleavage of human embryos to the two-cell stage after intracytoplasmic sperm injection as an indicator of embryo viability. Hum Reprod. 1998;13(1):182–7.
27. Sakkas D, Percival G, D'Arcy Y, Sharif K, Afnan M. Assessment of early cleaving in vitro fertilized human embryos at the 2-cell stage before transfer improves embryo selection. Fertil Steril. 2001;76(6):1150–6.
28. Salumets A, Hyden-Granskog C, Makinen S, Suikkari AM, Tiitinen A, Tuuri T. Early cleavage predicts the viability of human embryos in elective single embryo transfer procedures. Hum Reprod. 2003;18(4):821–5.
29. Van Montfoort AP, Dumoulin JC, Kester AD, Evers JL. Early cleavage is a valuable addition to existing embryo selection parameters: a study using single embryo transfers. Hum Reprod. 2004;19(9):2103–8.
30. Alikani M, Calderon G, Tomkin G, Garrisi J, Kokot M, Cohen J. Cleavage anomalies in early human embryos and survival after prolonged culture in-vitro. Hum Reprod. 2000;15(12):2634–43.
31. Antczak M, Van Blerkom J. Temporal and spatial aspects of fragmentation in early human embryos: possible effects on developmental competence and association with the differential elimination of regulatory proteins from polarized domains. Hum Reprod. 1999;14(2):429–47.
32. Hardarson T, Lofman C, Coull G, Sjogren A, Hamberger L, Edwards RG. Internalization of cellular fragments in a human embryo: time-lapse recordings. Reprod Biomed Online. 2002;5(1):36–8.
33. Alikani M, Cohen J, Tomkin G, Garrisi GJ, Mack C, Scott RT. Human embryo fragmentation in vitro and its implications for pregnancy and implantation. Fertil Steril. 1999;71(5):836–42.
34. Keltz MD, Skorupski JC, Bradley K, Stein D. Predictors of embryo fragmentation and outcome after fragment removal in in vitro fertilization. Fertil Steril. 2006;86(2):321–4.
35. Hardarson T, Hanson C, Sjogren A, Lundin K. Human embryos with unevenly sized blastomeres have lower pregnancy and implantation rates: indications for aneuploidy and multinucleation. Hum Reprod. 2001; 16(2):313–8.
36. Pickering SJ, Taylor A, Johnson MH, Braude PR. An analysis of multinucleated blastomere formation in human embryos. Hum Reprod. 1995;10(7):1912–22.
37. Royen EV, Mangelschots K, Vercruyssen M, Neubourg DD, Valkenburg M, Ryckaert G, et al. Multinucleation in cleavage stage embryos. Hum Reprod. 2003;18(5): 1062–9.
38. Van Royen E, Mangelschots K, Vercruyssen M, De Neubourg D, Valkenburg M, Ryckaert G, et al. Multinucleation in cleavage stage embryos. Hum Reprod. 2003;18(5):1062–9.
39. Yakin K, Balaban B, Urman B. Impact of the presence of one or more multinucleated blastomeres on the developmental potential of the embryo to the blastocyst stage. Fertil Steril. 2005;83(1):243–5.
40. Kligman I, Benadiva C, Alikani M, Munne S. The presence of multinucleated blastomeres in human embryos is correlated with chromosomal abnormalities. Hum Reprod. 1996;11(7):1492–8.
41. Staessen C, Van SA. The genetic constitution of multinuclear blastomeres and their derivative daughter blastomeres. Hum Reprod. 1998;13(6):1625–31.
42. Bungum M, Bungum L, Humaidan P, Yding AC. Day 3 versus day 5 embryo transfer: a prospective randomized study. Reprod Biomed Online. 2003;7(1):98–104.
43. Estes SJ, Hoover LM, Smith SE, Somkuti SG, Schinfeld JS, Barmat LI. Comparison of pregnancy, implantation, and multiple gestation rates for day 3 versus day 5 embryo transfers. J Assist Reprod Genet. 2003;20(10):409–12.
44. Kolibianakis EM, Zikopoulos K, Verpoest W, Camus M, Joris H, Van Steirteghem AC, et al. Should we advise patients undergoing IVF to start a cycle leading to a day 3 or a day 5 transfer? Hum Reprod. 2004;19(11):2550–4.
45. Racowsky C, Jackson KV, Cekleniak NA, Fox JH, Hornstein MD, Ginsburg ES. The number of eight-cell embryos is a key determinant for selecting day 3 or day 5 transfer. Fertil Steril. 2000;73(3):558–64.
46. Rienzi L, Ubaldi F, Iacobelli M, Ferrero S, Minasi MG, Martinez F, et al. Day 3 embryo transfer with combined evaluation at the pronuclear and cleavage stages compares favourably with day 5 blastocyst transfer. Hum Reprod. 2002;17(7):1852–5.
47. Rijnders PM, Jansen CA. The predictive value of day 3 embryo morphology regarding blastocyst formation, pregnancy and implantation rate after day 5 transfer following in-vitro fertilization or intracytoplasmic sperm injection. Hum Reprod. 1998;13(10): 2869–73.
48. Blake D, Proctor M, Johnson N, Olive D. Cleavage stage versus blastocyst stage embryo transfer in assisted conception. Cochrane Database Syst Rev. 2002;2:CD002118.
49. Blake D, Proctor M, Johnson N, Olive D. Cleavage stage versus blastocyst stage embryo transfer in assisted conception. Cochrane Database Syst Rev. 2005;4:CD002118.
50. Blake DA, Proctor M, Johnson NP. The merits of blastocyst versus cleavage stage embryo transfer: a Cochrane review. Hum Reprod. 2004;19(9):2174.
51. Blake DA, Farquhar CM, Johnson N, Proctor M. Cleavage stage versus blastocyst stage embryo trans-

fer in assisted conception. Cochrane Database Syst Rev. 2007;4:CD002118.

52. Balaban B, Urman B, Alatas C, Mercan R, Aksoy S, Isiklar A. Blastocyst-stage transfer of poor-quality cleavage-stage embryos results in higher implantation rates. Fertil Steril. 2001;75(3):514–8.
53. Balaban B, Urman B, Sertac A, Alatas C, Aksoy S, Mercan R. Blastocyst quality affects the success of blastocyst-stage embryo transfer. Fertil Steril. 2000;74(2):282–7.
54. Bolton VN, Wren ME, Parsons JH. Pregnancies after in vitro fertilization and transfer of human blastocysts. Fertil Steril. 1991;55(4):830–2.
55. Gardner DK, Schoolcraft WB. Culture and transfer of human blastocysts. Curr Opin Obstet Gynecol. 1999;11(3):307–11.
56. Gardner DK, Schoolcraft WB, Wagley L, Schlenker T, Stevens J, Hesla J. A prospective randomized trial of blastocyst culture and transfer in in-vitro fertilization. Hum Reprod. 1998;13(12):3434–40.
57. Gardner DK, Lane M. Culture of viable human blastocysts in defined sequential serum-free media. Hum Reprod. 1998;13 Suppl 3:148–59.
58. Jones GM, Trounson AO, Lolatgis N, Wood C. Factors affecting the success of human blastocyst development and pregnancy following in vitro fertilization and embryo transfer. Fertil Steril. 1998;70(6):1022–9.
59. Menezo YJ, Sakkas D, Janny L. Co-culture of the early human embryo: factors affecting human blastocyst formation in vitro. Microsc Res Tech. 1995; 32(1):50–6.
60. Milki AA, Fisch JD, Behr B. Two-blastocyst transfer has similar pregnancy rates and a decreased multiple gestation rate compared with three-blastocyst transfer [see comments]. Fertil Steril. 1999;72(2):225–8.
61. Olivennes F, Hazout A, Lelaidier C, Freitas S, Fanchin R, de Ziegler D, et al. Four indications for embryo transfer at the blastocyst stage. Hum Reprod. 1994;9(12):2367–73.
62. Sakkas D, Percival G, D'Arcy Y, Lenton W, Sharif K, Afnan M. Blastocyst transfer for patients with multiple assisted reproduction treatment failures: preliminary experience. Hum Fertil (Camb). 2001;4(2): 104–8.
63. Schoolcraft WB, Gardner DK, Lane M, Schlenker T, Hamilton F, Meldrum DR. Blastocyst culture and transfer: analysis of results and parameters affecting outcome in two in vitro fertilization programs. Fertil Steril. 1999;72(4):604–9.
64. Toledo AA, Wright G, Jones AE, Smith SS, Johnson-Ward J, Brockman WW, et al. Blastocyst transfer: a useful tool for reduction of high-order multiple gestations in a human assisted reproduction program. Am J Obstet Gynecol. 2000;183(2):377–82.
65. Van der Auwera I, Debrock S, Spiessens C, Afschrift H, Bakelants E, Meuleman C, et al. A prospective randomized study: day 2 versus day 5 embryo transfer. Hum Reprod. 2002;17(6):1507–12.
66. Marek D, Langley M, Gardner DK, Confer N, Doody KM, Doody KJ. Introduction of blastocyst culture and transfer for all patients in an in vitro fertilization program. Fertil Steril. 1999;72(6):1035–40.
67. Gardner DK, Schoolcraft WB. In vitro culture of human blastocysts. In: Jansen R, Mortimer D, editors. Towards reproductive certainty: infertility and genetics beyond. Carnforth: Parthenon Press; 1999. p. 378.
68. Gardner DK, Lane M, Stevens J, Schlenker T, Schoolcraft WB. Blastocyst score affects implantation and pregnancy outcome: towards a single blastocyst transfer. Fertil Steril. 2000;73(6):1155–8.
69. Gardner DK, Stevens J, Sheehan CB, Schoolcraft WB. Morphological assessment of the human blastocyst. In: Elder KT, Cohen J, editors. Analysis of the human embryo. London: Taylor & Francis; 2007. p. 79–87.
70. Ahlstrom A, Westin C, Reismer E, Wikland M, Hardarson T. Trophectoderm morphology: an important parameter for predicting live birth after single blastocyst transfer. Hum Reprod. 2011;26(12): 3289–96.
71. Feil D, Henshaw RC, Lane M. Day 4 embryo selection is equal to Day 5 using a new embryo scoring system validated in single embryo transfers. Hum Reprod. 2008;23(7):1505–10.
72. Milki AA, Hinckley MD, Gebhardt J, Dasig D, Westphal LM, Behr B. Accuracy of day 3 criteria for selecting the best embryos. Fertil Steril. 2002;77(6): 1191–5.
73. Rehman KS, Bukulmez O, Langley M, Carr BR, Nackley AC, Doody KM, et al. Late stages of embryo progression are a much better predictor of clinical pregnancy than early cleavage in intracytoplasmic sperm injection and in vitro fertilization cycles with blastocyst-stage transfer. Fertil Steril. 2007;87(5):1041–52.
74. Meseguer M, Herrero J, Tejera A, Hilligsoe KM, Ramsing NB, Remohi J. The use of morphokinetics as a predictor of embryo implantation. Hum Reprod. 2011;26(10):2658–71.
75. Wong CC, Loewke KE, Bossert NL, Behr B, De Jonge CJ, Baer TM, et al. Non-invasive imaging of human embryos before embryonic genome activation predicts development to the blastocyst stage. Nat Biotechnol. 2010;28(10):1115–21.
76. Balaban B, Urman B, Isiklar A, Alatas C, Aksoy S, Mercan R, et al. The effect of pronuclear morphology on embryo quality parameters and blastocyst transfer outcome. Hum Reprod. 2001;16(11):2357–61.
77. Senn A, Urner F, Chanson A, Primi MP, Wirthner D, Germond M. Morphological scoring of human pronuclear zygotes for prediction of pregnancy outcome. Hum Reprod. 2006;21(1):234–9.
78. Scott L, Finn A, O'Leary T, McLellan S, Hill J. Morphologic parameters of early cleavage-stage embryos that correlate with fetal development and delivery: prospective and applied data for increased pregnancy rates. Hum Reprod. 2007;22(1):230–40.
79. James AN, Hennessy S, Reggio B, Wiemer K, Larsen F, Cohen J. The limited importance of pronuclear scoring of human zygotes. Hum Reprod. 2006;21(6): 1599–604.

80. Chen C, Kattera S. Comparison of pronuclear zygote morphology and early cleavage status of zygotes as additional criteria in the selection of day 3 embryos: a randomized study. Fertil Steril. 2006;85(2):347–52.
81. Payne JF, Raburn DJ, Couchman GM, Price TM, Jamison MG, Walmer DK. Relationship between pre-embryo pronuclear morphology (zygote score) and standard day 2 or 3 embryo morphology with regard to assisted reproductive technique outcomes. Fertil Steril. 2005;84(4):900–9.
82. Terriou P, Giorgetti C, Hans E, Salzmann J, Charles O, Cignetti L, et al. Relationship between even early cleavage and day 2 embryo score and assessment of their predictive value for pregnancy. Reprod Biomed Online. 2007;14(3):294–9.
83. Hesters L, Prisant N, Fanchin R, Mendez Lozano DH, Feyereisen E, Frydman R, et al. Impact of early cleaved zygote morphology on embryo development and in vitro fertilization-embryo transfer outcome: a prospective study. Fertil Steril. 2008;89(6):1677–84.
84. Lundqvist M, Johansson U, Lundkvist O, Milton K, Westin C, Simberg N. Does pronuclear morphology and/or early cleavage rate predict embryo implantation potential? Reprod Biomed Online. 2001;2(1):12–6.
85. Platteau P, Fenwick J, Murdoch AP, Herbert C. Time from insemination to first cleavage predicts developmental competence of human preimplantation embryos in vitro. Hum Reprod. 2002;17(2):407–12.

Sperm Morphologic Characteristics and Their Impact on Embryo Quality and Pregnancy Outcome

7

Bhushan K. Gangrade and Ashok Agarwal

The successful outcome following in vitro fertilization and embryo transfer (IVF-ET) depends on a large number of variables ranging from maternal age, cause of infertility, number and maturity of oocytes, sperm characteristics, embryo quality, and ultimately the quality of embryo transfer. In the order of significance the two parameters that influence the outcome of IVF most are the age of the female patient (or the egg donor) followed by the quality of the embryo(s) transferred. It is well established that the morphological characteristics and the quality of the embryos are largely dependent on the oocyte [1–4]. A combination of sperm characteristics such as concentration, morphology, and motility offers some predictive value as it relates to the fertilization of oocytes in vitro; however, their importance in predicting embryo morphology is controversial. In fact the contribution of sperm to the process of reproduction can be divided into three steps: (1) transfer of paternal genome to the oocyte; (2) activation of the oocyte; and (3) transfer of centriole/centrosome to the oocyte to assist in the organization of mitotic spindle. It is only logical to assume that any abnormality or defect in the spermatozoon fertilizing the oocyte will be reflected in the embryonic development and pregnancy outcome following transfer of the embryo. The term "embryo quality" generally refers to the morphological assessment of the embryo; however, in terms of implantation potential the embryo quality suitably includes criteria such as the rate of embryonic cleavage and its genetic (chromosomal) status. Several publications have analyzed the relationship between sperm morphology and implantation and/or pregnancy outcome with little or no mention of embryo quality. Since successful implantation and clinical pregnancies are indirect indication of potentially good quality embryos, these studies have been included in this review.

B.K. Gangrade (✉)
IVF Laboratory, Center for Reproductive Medicine, Orlando, FL, USA
e-mail: bhushan.gangrade@integramed.com

A. Agarwal
Clinical Andrology Laboratory and Reproductive Tissue Bank, Glickman Urological and Kidney Institute, Cleveland, OH, USA

Center for Reproductive Medicine, Cleveland Clinic, Cleveland, OH, USA

Sperm Morphology

The normal human spermatozoon is identified with its oval shaped head that is covered with an acrosome extending to over one third of the head, a midpiece shorter than one third of the width of the head, and a long tail flagellum extending beyond the base of the midpiece. In terms of measurement the length and the width of the head should be 4.0–5.0 and 2.5–3.5 μm, respectively. The midpiece should measure 2.0–2.5 μm in length and less than 1 μm in width. The tail should be slender, straight, and approximately 45 μm in length.

D.K. Gardner et al. (eds.), *Human Gametes and Preimplantation Embryos: Assessment and Diagnosis*, DOI 10.1007/978-1-4614-6651-2_7,

Determination of normal sperm morphology is an integral part of semen analysis. Over the years the reference ranges for normal sperm in ejaculate as outlined in WHO Manual has been revised multiple times and the criteria for classifying sperm as morphological normal has changed over time. Thus the classification of semen sample under the category of teratozoospermia has inherent limitations. Various reproductive laboratories follow different WHO standards for the analysis of sperm samples and this further compounds the morphological classification of sperm. The Kruger's strict morphology criteria is one of the most rigorous sperm classification systems and according to this even slight deviation from normal shape and measurement categorizes the sperm cell as abnormal [5]. Based on the strict morphology criteria ejaculates with less than 4 % morphologically normal sperm have poor prognosis for pregnancy and the use of such sperm sample in IVF may result in severely reduced fertilization and increased incidence of failed fertilization [6–8]. Despite its strict categorization, Kruger's system has limitations and its significance in evaluating the fertility potential of the male has been supported as well as questioned [9–11].

Sperm Morphology and Chromosomal/Chromatin Abnormalities

Human sperm exhibit wide variations in the morphology ranging from defects in acrosome, head, midpiece, and tail. Human ejaculate is a complex mixture, among several other components, of morphologically normal and abnormal spermatozoa. Based on high fertility potential of men who have high proportion of normal shaped sperm, it is instinctively logical to assume that morphologically normal sperm are also normal in terms of chromosome number. By the same token, it is also reasonable to think that morphological defects in the sperm are a reflection of genetic make-up and morphologically abnormal spermatozoa are chromosomally abnormal. This perception of positive correlation between normal sperm morphology and normal haploid chromosomal status has been largely found to be untrue. Human sperm karyotype analysis of pronucleus following hamster egg penetration found no significant association between the proportions of morphologically and chromosomally abnormal sperm suggesting sperm morphology is not a good indicator of chromosomal normality [12]. There is also a lack of association between sperm morphology and karyotype in infertile men [13–15]. Despite the absence of direct correlation between sperm morphology and chromosomal content, a two- to threefold increase in numerical chromosomal abnormalities in infertile men with teratozoospermia as compared with normal fertile donors has been reported [16–19]. Sperm with certain specific morphological defects exhibit a significant correlation with chromosomal complement. Macrocephallic (large head) sperm display a high rate of aneuploidy or polyploidy [20, 21]. Other sperm defects such as multiple tails, multinucleated head, and microcephaly (pin head) are also associated with significantly elevated numerical chromosomal aberrations [22, 23].

The normal haploid chromosomal constitution of sperm does not necessarily imply that such sperm are essentially capable of fertilizing karyotypically normal oocytes to produce genetically normal embryos. Spermatozoa have been shown to have fragmentation and damage in the DNA strands and there is a negative correlation between the degree of DNA damage in sperm nucleus and fertility in men [24]. Spermatozoa with DNA fragmentation are capable of fertilizing oocytes at the rate similar to sperm with intact DNA and there is no correlation between sperm morphology and the integrity of DNA. There are conflicting reports on the effect of damaged sperm DNA on embryonic cleavage [25–27]. Sperm with fragmented DNA form embryos that exhibit slow cleavage and reduced blastocyst formation [25, 26]. Moreover, a high incidence of spontaneous pregnancy loss appears to be a direct consequence of damaged DNA in sperm population. Couples with high proportion (over 30 %) of spermatozoa with denatured DNA in the ejaculate have high incidence of multinucleated embryos following ICSI as compared those who show lower incidence of sperm DNA damage [27]. Multinucleated human embryos are known to be associated with a reduced implantation and pregnancy rate. Injection of sperm with vacuoles which are not visible at the magnifications commonly used for ICSI may have a negative effect on fertilization, implantation, and pregnancy [28]. Identification and selection of normal sperm without vacuoles and other defects for ICSI has been suggested to enhance successful outcome [28, 29].

In general the individual sperm defects such as head, midpiece, and tail defects are not associated with chromosomal abnormalities. The incidence of numerical or structural chromosomal aberrations in morphologically abnormal sperm is comparable to those observed in normal spermatozoa [30].

Globozoospermia in Assisted Conception

Globozoospermia is a rare cause of male infertility characterized by the presence in the ejaculate of round headed sperm lacking acrosomal cap. The incidence of globozoospermia has been reported to be less than 0.1 % in infertile men [31, 32]. In patients with absolute globozoospermia there is complete failure of fertilization in IVF primarily due to the failure of sperm to attach and penetrate zona pellucida. Using sperm injection (ICSI) suboptimum fertilization (0–37 %) and pregnancies have been achieved in patients with globozoospermia [33–37]. There is however little direct information available regarding the quality of embryos produced from round headed sperm injection. The activation of oocytes using calcium ionophore augments the fertilization rate of injected oocytes; however, several investigators have reported fertilization and successful pregnancies following ICSI with round headed sperm without assisted oocyte activation [33, 38–40]. The reason for failed or reduced fertilization by round sperm is the asynchronous chromosome condensation of the sperm nucleus. The round sperm injected in the oocyte undergo premature chromosome condensation (PCC) in response to chromosome condensing factors present in the ooplasm without activating the oocyte which remains arrested at Metaphase II [41]. The premature chromatin condensation has been attributed to the protamine deficiency in globozoospermic sperm [42]. Globozoospermia is associated with a modest (two- to threefold) increase in the frequency of sex chromosome aneuploidy and also autosomal aneuploidy but if pregnancy is initiated there is no evidence of higher incidence of miscarriage or congenital defects [31, 43–46]. Sperm chromatin integrity and DNA fragmentation in globozoospermia are comparable to sperm populations in normal fertile males [47]. The occurrence of globozoospermia in siblings indicates a genetic origin [43, 48, 49]. The pathogenesis of this syndrome implies defective elongation of sperm head and acrosome formation during spermiogenesis [31]. There is some evidence that globozoospermia may be associated with microdeletions in AZFa and AZFb regions of the Y chromosome [50].

Effect of Teratozoospermia on Embryo Development and Pregnancy

The diminishing pregnancy rates with advancing maternal age are attributed to high frequency of chromosomal aberrations, namely meiotic nondisjunction in Metaphase II oocytes. The introduction of the paternal genome by spermatozoon into the oocyte initiates the complex cycle of events leading to fertilization and embryonic cleavage. There exists a significant correlation between normal sperm parameters, namely concentration, normal morphology, and progressive motility, and the rate of fertilization in IVF. A marked reduction in the fertilization rate is observed in couples when the male partner is diagnosed with teratozoospermia [51]. Interestingly the morphological qualities of embryos in terms of fragmentation, number and appearance of blastomeres, irregular cells, and embryo score are quite similar between normozoospermic and teratozoospermic couples. Embryo implantation, clinical pregnancy and live birth rates between normospermic and teratozospermic groups are also comparable between the two groups [51]. The decrease in the fertilization rate in teratozoospermia is attributed to reduced sperm binding to the zona. The equivalent post-fertilization embryonic development and implantation in teratozoospermia as compared with normospermic group can be explained in two ways:

1. Abnormal sperm especially those with sperm head and acrosome defects fail to penetrate the cumulus and zona pellucida. It is possible that in teratozoospermic samples there are enough normal spermatozoa that are able to penetrate the cumulus and the oocyte is fertilized by a normal sperm. This leads to normal fertilization, development, implantation, and pregnancy.
2. It is possible that morphologically borderline abnormal sperm are also capable of fertilizing the oocyte resulting in normal embryonic development and pregnancy [51].

Contrary to the reports of the lack of association between teratozoospermia, embryo quality, and pregnancy, some investigators have observed a direct link between abnormal sperm parameters with poor embryo morphology [52, 53]. Interestingly there also appears a correlation between the severity of male factor and the timeline of fertilization. In majority of normospermic patients, normal fertilization as evident by the appearance of two pronuclei is noted at approximately 16–18 h post-insemination. In contrast, in patients with moderate male factor, fertilization may be delayed until 42–90 h post-insemination. Moreover male factor-associated delayed fertilization is also accompanied with a significant reduction in embryo quality and the rate of cleavage [53].

The differential influence of oocyte and sperm on early embryonic development has been elegantly analyzed in oocyte donation setting [11]. In this study oocytes from each young donor were divided equally between two recipients and fertilized by standard insemination (no ICSI) using partner's sperm. The embryo quality between two couples who shared oocytes from the same donor was then compared to assess the effect of sperm on morphology and rate of early cleavage. There was a strong correlation in embryo morphology between recipients who shared the oocytes from a single donor. The rate of embryonic cleavage, on the other hand, was strongly correlated with the sperm morphology. Other sperm characteristics such as concentration and progressive motility had no influence on blastomere cleavage or embryo morphology [11]. Even though embryo morphology is a good predictor of pregnancy, the rate of early embryonic cleavage offers a better prognosis of implantation potential of embryos [54].

Insemination by IVF or ICSI and Embryo Quality

The two basic methods of insemination of oocytes are standard insemination (also referred to as the microdrop insemination, standard insemination, or IVF) and intracytoplasmic sperm injection (ICSI). Several investigators have attempted to compare the fertilization rate, embryo development, and pregnancy outcome following insemination by IVF and ICSI [55–58]. During the standard IVF, the oocytes are incubated for 16–20 h with several thousand sperm, evaluated for fertilization and then transferred to the fresh medium for further culture. It is argued that the prolonged incubation with spermatozoa exposes the oocytes to free oxygen radicals released by sperm [59]. The exposure to reactive oxygen species results in the peroxidation of unsaturated fatty acids in the sperm plasma membrane and may negatively affect sperm–oocyte fusion. In addition oxidative stress has been shown to affect the integrity of sperm chromatin and cause extensive damage in DNA strands [60, 61]. Short-term (2 h) coincubation of oocytes with sperm has been shown to yield fertilization rates that are similar to prolonged 20 h sperm exposure [62]. The embryos generated by short-term exposure to spermatozoa exhibit better morphology and less fragmentation than those derived by prolonged overnight incubation with sperm [62]. Embryo implantation and clinical pregnancy rate likewise are significantly higher in the group with short-term exposure to spermatozoa. Brief exposure to sperm while adequate for allowing fertilization limits the exposure of oocytes to metabolic byproducts and free oxygen radicals generated by spermatozoa during prolonged incubation. Insemination with high concentration of sperm also adversely affects early cleavage in the embryo [63]. The ICSI offers comparable or even higher fertilization rates than standard insemination of oocyte, avoids the exposure of oocytes to high concentration of sperm, and produces embryos that are superior in morphology as compared with those generated in IVF [64–66].

Assessment of sperm morphology while useful in predicting fertilization in IVF has little if any predictive value in ICSI. Sperm classified as morphologically abnormal by Kruger's strict or WHO criteria are capable of fertilizing when introduced in the oocyte by ICSI. Comparison of embryos generated following IVF and ICSI shows that sperm morphology does not influence the embryo quality on day 2 or 3 of development [58]. This is logical in view of the fact that early human embryonic cleavage (up to 6–8 cells) is largely under the influence of maternal genome. The development of embryos from eight cells to blastocyst stage should therefore provide better information on the role of sperm in early embryonic development. In fact poor sperm morphology has been attributed to result in lower rate and poor quality blastocyst formation [56].

It is not possible to determine the morphology of the individual sperm that fertilized the oocyte in IVF and therefore studies involving embryo quality or pregnancy outcome in relation to sperm morphology try to correlate the embryo quality with the proportion of normal and abnormal sperm in the washed preparation. Such correlations while certainly provide some insight into the process of embryonic development lack the rigor of studies involving ICSI where it is possible to select the sperm and follow the development of the embryo.

It is interesting that the site of sperm deposition in the oocyte by ICSI does not affect the fertilization rate but influences the rate of embryo development. When sperm are deposited farthest from the anticipated site of spindle (near the polar body), the embryos exhibit less fragmentation and better morphology than those embryos that are generated by depositing sperm close to the mitotic spindle [67]. Interestingly the mode of oolema penetration during ICSI and the amount of suction applied to aspirate the ooplasm also affects the rate of embryo development. Pricking the oolema once and depositing the sperm without sucking ooplasm in the ICSI needle resulted in higher rate of degeneration of oocytes. Slight suction of ooplasm followed by deposition of the sperm in the oocyte produced relatively better quality embryos than no suction, higher suction, or when more than one prick was needed to penetrate the oolema [67].

Injection of isolated sperm head or tail flagellum is capable of causing oocyte activation and formation of two pronuclei. The resulting embryos however exhibit high incidence of mosaicism and abnormal development [68, 69]. Structurally damaged spermatozoa when injected in the oocyte are capable of pronuclear formation but these zygotes fail to undergo embryonic cleavage. This suggests the importance of structural integrity of spermatozoa in normal embryo development.

Developments in the Techniques for the Selection of Normal Sperm for Injection and Their Outcome

As discussed earlier in this chapter, there is little evidence showing a correlation between the poor sperm quality and fertilization rate or embryo quality post-ICSI. One of the explanations for the lack of association between poor semen analysis and pregnancy outcome is that the embryologists selectively choose morphologically normal (or near normal) shaped sperm for ICSI. Excellent fertilization rates following injection of morphologically selected sperm followed by selection and transfer of developmentally and morphologically chosen embryos from a cohort results in superior pregnancy rates in couples with a primary diagnosis of male factor infertility. Certain defects in the sperm head especially the nucleus that are not visible at magnifications commonly employed for ICSI (up to ×400) may be responsible for poor outcome following sperm injection. It has been hypothesized that subtle organelle malformations may be associated with abnormal sperm those are incapable of producing successful pregnancies [29]. It may be possible to recognize normal sperm nucleus with smooth outlines, without nuclear vacuoles and other slight midpiece and tail defects under high magnification. The approach that uses real-time motile sperm organelle morphology examination (MSOME) is based on the premise that assessment of sperm nuclear morphology at higher magnification (>6,000×) offers a means to select sperm with normal nuclear DNA content and organization and also significantly reduced probability of DNA fragmentation [29, 70]. Sperm injection (ICSI) using MSOME has been referred to as intracytoplasmic morphologically selected sperm injection or IMSI. In couples with the male factor diagnosis of severe oligoasthenoteratozoospermia, IMSI resulted in a significantly higher clinical pregnancy rate as compared with conventional ICSI). Furthermore couples with two or more previous failed attempts using ICSI as the method of insemination benefitted most with IMSI. Selection at high optical and digital magnifications of sperm without nuclear imperfections also results in a substantial reduction in miscarriage rate [71]. Based on the studies suggesting the superiority of IMSI over ICSI, this technique may be especially advantageous in couples with severe oligoasthenoteratozoospermia or when only a few oocytes are available for sperm injection and embryo selection based on the number of available embryos is limited.

Another method to select mature genetically normal sperm devoid of DNA fragmentation that has been suggested involves the use of hyaluronic acid (HA). The remodeling of sperm plasma membrane during spermiogenesis results in the appearance of HA receptors on the sperm head. Only mature sperm are capable of binding to HA or zona pellucida. The sperm that bind to a solid phase HA have been shown to exhibit three- to ninefold decreased frequency of chromosomal disomy, diploidy, and sex chromosome disomy [72, 73]. The mature sperm that bind to HA are also devoid of cytoplasmic remnants and exhibit significantly lower incidence of DNA fragmentation [74]. A significant enhancement in the fertilization rate following sperm selection by HA binding has been noted; however, further studies are needed to confirm the effect of such selection on embryo quality, implantation, and pregnancy outcome [75].

Conclusions

The prognostic value of sperm morphology in implantation potential of resulting embryos remains controversial. There is no correlation between the sperm morphology and the chromosomal make up. Likewise the sperm chromatin or DNA integrity is also not reflected in morphology of the spermatozoa. Patients with teratozoospermia have reduced fertilization by IVF and have better prognosis of pregnancy if ICSI is used to fertilize the oocytes. The morphological appearance of embryos and the rate of early cleavage in couples with the diagnosis of teratozoospermia is comparable to those with normal semen analysis. ICSI offers high rate of fertilization in severe oligoasthenoteratozoospermia, the only requirement for fertilization being the availability of one viable sperm per oocyte. There is little diagnostic and predictive value of Kruger's strict sperm morphology involving ICSI cycles. Severe oligoasthenoteratozoospermia may be responsible for poor embryo quality including high degree of fragmentation and slow cleavage. Infertility due to morphologic abnormalities in the sperm such as globozoospermia can be treated with ICSI though fertilization and pregnancy rates are lower than those observed in other male factor categories. The advances in the technique of sperm injection involving selection of motile sperm with normal organelle morphology (IMSI) or HA binding may offer higher pregnancy and lower miscarriage rates but further studies are needed to confirm the superior outcome of these sperm selection procedures.

References

1. Xia P. Intraytoplasmic sperm injection: correlation of oocyte grade based on polar body, perivitelline space and cytoplasmic inclusions with fertilization rate and embryo quality. Hum Reprod. 1997;12:1750–5.
2. Serhal PF, Ranieri DM, Kinis A, Marchant S, Davies M, Khadun IM. Oocyte morphology predicts outcome

of intracytoplasmic sperm injection. Hum Reprod. 1997;12:1267–70.
3. Loutradis D, Drakakis P, Kallianidis K, Milingos S, Dendrinos S, Michalas S. Oocyte morphology correlates with embryo quality and pregnancy rate after intracytoplasmic sperm injection. Fertil Steril. 1999;72:240–4.
4. Weigert M, Hofstetter G, Kaipl D, Gottlich H, Krischker U, Bichler K, et al. The effect of smoking on oocyte quality and hormonal parameters of patients undergoing in vitro fertilization-embryo transfer. J Assist Reprod Genet. 1999;16:287–93.
5. Kruger TF, Menkveld R, Stander FS, Lombard CJ, Van der Merwe JP, van Zyl JA, et al. Sperm morphologic features as a prognostic factor in in vitro fertilization. Fertil Steril. 1986;46:1118–23.
6. Kruger TF, Acosta AA, Simmons KF, Swanson RJ, Matta JF, Veeck LL, et al. New method of evaluating sperm morphology with predictive value for human in vitro fertilization. Urology. 1987;30:248–51.
7. Kruger TF, Acosta AA, Simmons KF, Swanson RG, Matta JF, Oehninger S. Predective of abnormal sperm morphology in in vitro fertilization. Fertil Steril. 1988;49:112–7.
8. Grow DR, Oehninger S, Seltman HJ, Toner JP, Swanson RJ, Kruger TF, et al. Sperm morphology as diagnosed by strict criteria: probing the impact of teratozoospermia on fertilization rate and pregnancy outcome in a large in vitro fertilization population. Fertil Steril. 1994;62:559–67.
9. Kobayashi T, Jinno M, Sugimura K, Nozawa S, Sugiyama T, Lida E. Sperm morphological assessment based on strict criteria and in-vitro fertilization outcome. Hum Reprod. 1991;7:983–6.
10. Check JH, Adelson HG, Schubert BR, Bollendorf A. Evaluation of sperm morphology using Kruger's strict criteria. Arch Androl. 1992;28:15–7.
11. Salumets A, Suikkari AM, Molos T, Soderstrom-Anttila V, Tuuri T. Influence of oocytes and spermatozoa on early embryonic development. Fertil Steril. 2002;78:1082–7.
12. Martin RH, Rademaker A. The relationship between sperm chromosomal abnormalities and sperm morphology in human. Mutat Res. 1988;207:159–64.
13. Rives N, Saint Clair A, Mazurier S, Sibert L, Simeon N, Joly G, et al. Relationship between clinical phenotype, semen parameters and aneuploidy frequency in sperm nuclei of 50 infertile males. Hum Genet. 1999;155:266–72.
14. Vegetti W, Van Assche E, Frias A, Verheyne G, Bianchi MM, Bonduelle M, et al. Correlation between semen parameters and sperm aneuploidy rates investigated by fluorescence in situ hybridization in infertile men. Hum Reprod. 2000;15:351–65.
15. Vivelle S, Mollard R, Bach ML, Falquet C, Gerlinger P, Warter S. Do morphological reflect chromosomal aneuploidies? Hum Reprod. 2000;15:2563–6.
16. Templado C, Hoang T, Greene C, Rademaker A, Chernos J, Martin RH. Aneuploid spermatozoa in infertile men: teratozoospemia. Mol Reprod Dev. 2002;61:200–4.
17. Harkonen K, Suominen J, Lahdetie J. Aneuploidy in spermatozoa of infertile men with teratozoospermia. Int J Androl. 2001;24:197–205.
18. Calogero AE, De Palma A, Grazioso C, Barone N, Romeo R, Rappazzo G, et al. Aneuploidy rate in spermatozoa of selected men with abnormal semen parameters. Hum Reprod. 2001;16:1172–9.
19. Hristova R, Ko E, Greene C, Rademaker A, Chernos J, Martin RH. Chromosome abnormalities in sperm from infertile men with asthenoteratozoospermia. Biol Reprod. 2002;66:1781–3.
20. Benzacken B, Gavelle FM, Martin-Pont B, Dupuy O, Lievre N, Hugues JN, et al. Familial sperm polyploidy induced by genetic spermatogenesis failure: case report. Hum Reprod. 2001;16:2646–51.
21. In't Veld PA, Broekmans FJ, deFrance HF, Pearson PL, Pieters MH, van Kooij RJ. Intracytoplasmic sperm injection (ICSI) and chromosomally abnormal spermatozoa. Hum Reprod. 1997;12:752–4.
22. Devillard F, Metzler-Guillemain C, Pelletier R, DeRobertis C, Bergues U, Hennebicq S, et al. Polyploidy in large-headed sperm: FISH study of three cases. Hum Reprod. 2002;17:1292–8.
23. Bernardini L, Borini A, Preti S, Conte N, Flamigni C, Capitanio GL, et al. Study of aneuploidy in normal and abnormal germ cells from semen of fertile and infertile men. Hum Reprod. 1988;13:3406–13.
24. Larson KL, DeJonge CJ, Barnes AM, Jost LK, Evenson DP. Sperm chromatin structure assay parameters as predictor of failed pregnancy following assisted reproductive techniques. Hum Reprod. 2000; 15:1717–22.
25. Seli E, Gardner DK, Schoolcraft WB, Moffatt O, Sakkas D. Extent of nuclear DNA damage in ejaculated spermatozoa impacts on blastocyst development after in vitro fertilization. Fertil Steril. 2004;82:378–83.
26. Virro MR, Larson-Cook KL, Evenson DP. Sperm chromatin structure assay (SCSA) parameters are related to fertilization, blastocyst development and ongoing pregnancy in in vitro fertilization and intracytoplasmic sperm injection cycle. Fertil Steril. 2004;81:1289–95.
27. Zini A, Merian J, Kader K, Jarvi K, Laskin CA, Cadesky K. Potential adverse effect of sperm DNA damage on embryo quality after ICSI. Hum Reprod. 2005;12:3476–80.
28. Braga DP, Setti AS, Figueira RCS, Nichi M, Martinhago CD, Iaconelli A, et al. Sperm organelle morphologic abnormalities: contributing factors and effects on intracytoplasmic sperm injection cycles outcomes. Urology. 2011;78:786–91.
29. Bartoov B, Berkovitz A, Eltes F, Kogosowski A, Menezo Y, Barak Y. Real-time fine morphology of motile human sperm cells is associated with IVF-ICSI outcome. J Androl. 2002;23:1–8.
30. Sun F, Ko E, Martin RH. Is there a relationship between sperm chromosome abnormalities and sperm morphology? Reprod Biol Endocrinol. 2006;4:1.
31. Dam AH, Feenstra I, Westphal JR, Ramos L, van Golde RJ, Kremer JA. Globozoospermia revisited. Hum Reprod Update. 2007;13:63–75.

32. Koscinski I, Ellnati E, Fossard C, Redin C, Muller J, Velez de la Calle J, et al. DPY19L2 deletion as a major cause of globozoospermia. Am J Hum Genet. 2011;88:344–50.
33. Trokoudes KM, Danos N, Kalogirou L, Vlachou R, Lysiotis T, Georghiades N, et al. Pregnancy with spermatozoa from a globozoospermic man after intracytoplasmic sperm injection treatment. Hum Reprod. 1995;10:880–2.
34. Liu J, Nagy Z, Joris H, Tournaye H, Devroey P, Van Steirteghem A. Successful fertilization and establishment of pregnancies after intracytoplasmic sperm injection in patients with globozoospermia. Hum Reprod. 1995;10:626–9.
35. Battaglia DE, Koehler JK, Klein NA, Tucker MJ. Failure of oocyte activation after intracytoplasmic sperm injection using round-headed sperm. Fertil Steril. 1997;68:118–22.
36. Rybouchkin AV, Van der Straeten F, Quatacker J, De Sutter P, Dhont M. Fertilization and pregnancy after assisted oocyte activation and intracytoplasmic sperm injection in a case of round-headed sperm associated with deficient oocyte activation capacity. Fertil Steril. 1997;68:1144–7.
37. Tejera A, Molla M, Muriel L, Remohi J, Pellicer A, De Pablo J. Successful pregnancy and childbirth after intracytoplasmic sperm injection with calcium ionophone oocyte activation in a globozoospermic patient. Fertil Steril. 2008;90:1202e1–4.
38. Dirican EK, Sik AI, Vicdan K, Sozen EN, Suludere ZE. Clinical pregnancies and livebirths achieved by intracytoplasmic injection of round headed acrosomeless spermatozoa with and without oocyte activation in familial globozoospermia: a case report. Asian J Androl. 2008;10:332–6.
39. Lundin K, Sjogren A, Nilsson L, Hamberger L. Fertilization and pregnancy after intracytoplasmic microinjection of acrosomeless of spermatozoa. Fertil Steril. 1994;62:1266–7.
40. Stone S, O'Mahony F, Khalaf Y, Taylor A, Braude P. A normal livebirth after intracytoplasmic sperm injection for globozoospermia without assisted oocyte activation. Hum Reprod. 2000;15:139–41.
41. Schmiady H, Schulze W, Scheiber I, Pfuller B. High rate of premature chromosome condensation in human oocytes following microinjection with round-headed sperm: case report. Hum Reprod. 2005;20:1319–23.
42. Deemeh MR, Tavalee M, Razavi S, Esfahani MH. Evaluation of protamine deficiency and DNA fragmentation in two globozoospermia patients undergoing ICSI. Iran J Fertil Steril. 2007;1:85–8.
43. Carrell DT, Emery BR, Liu L. Characterization of aneuploidy rates, protamine levels, ultrastructure, and functional ability of round-headed sperm from two siblings and implications for intracytoplasmic sperm injection. Fertil Steril. 1999;71:511–6.
44. Carrell DT, Wilcox AL, Udoff LC, Thorp C, Campbell B. Chromosome 15 aneuploidy in the sperm and conceptus of a sibling with variable familial expression of round-headed sperm syndrome. Fertil Steril. 2001;76:1258–60.
45. Martin RH, Greene C, Rademaker A. Sperm chromosome aneuploidy analysis in a man with globozoospermia. Fertil Steril. 2003;79:1662–4.
46. Ditzel N, El-Danasouri I, Just w, Sterzik K. Higher aneuploidy rates of chromosomes 13, 16, and 21 in a patient with globozoospermia. Fertil Steril. 2005;84: 217–8.
47. Larson KL, Brannian JD, Singh NP, Burbach JA, Jost LK, Hansen KP, et al. Chromatin structure in globozoospermia: a case report. J Androl. 2001;22: 424–31.
48. Florke-Gerloff S, Topfer-Peterson E, Muller-Estrel W, Mansouri A, Schatz R, Schirre C. Biochemical and genetic investigation of round-headed spermatozoa in infertile men including two brothers and their father. Andrologia. 1984;16:187–202.
49. Kilani Z, Ismail R, Ghunaim S, Mohamed H, Hughes D, Brewis I, et al. Evaluation and treatment of familial globozoospermia in five brothers. Fertil Steril. 2004;82:1436–9.
50. Zeyneloglu HB, Baltaci V, Duran HE, Erdemli E, Batioglu S. Achievement of pregnancy in globozoospermia with Y chromosome microdeletion after ICSI. Hum Reprod. 2002;17:1833–6.
51. Terriou P, Giorgetti C, Auquier P, Hans E, Spach JL, Salzmann J, et al. Teratozoospermia influences fertilization rate in vitro but not embryo quality. Hum Reprod. 1997;12:1069–72.
52. Parinaud J, Mieusset R, Vieitez G, Labal B, Richoilley G. Influence of sperm parameters on embryo quality. Fertil Steril. 1993;60:888–92.
53. Ron-El R, Nachum H, Herman A, Golan A, Caspi E, Soffer E. Delayed fertilization and poor embryonic development associated with impaired semen quality. Fertil Steril. 1991;55:338–44.
54. Shoukir Y, Campana A, Farley T, Sakkas D. Early cleavage of in vitro fertilized human embryos to the 2-cellstage: a novel indicator of embryo quality and viability. Hum Reprod. 1997;12:1531–6.
55. Lundin K, Soderlund B, Hamberger L. The relationship between sperm morphology and rates of fertilization, pregnancy and spontaneous abortion in an in-vitro fertilization/intracytoplasmic sperm injection programme. Hum Reprod. 1997;12:2676–81.
56. Dumoulin J, Coonen E, Bras M, Van Wissen L, Ignoul-Vanvulchelen R, Bergers-Jansen J. Comparison of in vitro development of embryos originating from either conventional in-vitro fertilization or intracytoplasmic sperm injection. Hum Reprod. 2000;15: 402–9.
57. Yoeli R, Ashkenazi J, Orvieb R, Levy T, Ben-Rafel Z, Bar-Hava I. Pregnancy potential of embryos from in vitro fertilization compared to intracytoplasmic sperm injection. Gynecol Endocrinol. 2000;14: 253–7.
58. Kellerman LM, Windt ML, Lombard CJ. The effect of sperm morphology and testicular spermatozoa on

embryo quality. S Afr J Obstet Gynecol. 2007;13: 46–50.
59. Aitken RJ, Clarkson JS. Cellular basis of defective sperm function and its association with the genesis of reactive oxygen species by human spermatozoa. J Reprod Fertil. 1987;81:459–69.
60. Moustafa MH, Sharma RK, Thornton J, Masche E, Abden-Hafez M, Thomas A, et al. Relationship between ROS production and DNA denaturation in spermatozoa from patients examined for infertility. Hum Reprod. 2004;19:129–38.
61. Mahfouz R, Sharma R, Thiyagarajan A, Kale V, Gupta S, Sabanegh E, et al. Semen characteristics and sperm DNA fragmentation in infertile men with low and high levels of seminal reactive oxygen species. Fertil Steril. 2010;94:214–6.
62. Kattera S, Chen C. Short coincubation of gametes in in vitro fertilization improves implantation and pregnancy rates; a prospective, randomized, controlled study. Fertil Steril. 2003;80:1017–21.
63. Dumoulin JC, Bras M, Land JA, Pieters MH, Enginsu ME, Geraedts JP, et al. Effect of the number of inseminated spermatozoa on subsequent human and mouse embryonic development in vitro. Hum Reprod. 1992; 7:1010–3.
64. Oehninger S, Kruger TF, Simon T, Jones D, Mayer J, Lanzendorf S, et al. A comparative analysis of embryo implantation potential in patients with severe teratozoospermia undergoing in-vitro fertilization with a high insemination concentration or intracytoplasmic sperm injection. Hum Reprod. 1996;11:1086–9.
65. Yang D, Shahata MA, Al-Bader M, Al-Natasha SD, Al-Flamerzia M, Al-Shawaf T. Intracytoplasmic sperm injection improving embryo quality: comparison of the sibling oocyte of non-male-factor couples. J Assist Reprod Genet. 1996;13:351–5.
66. Khamsi F, Yavaas Y, Roberge S, Wong JC, Lacanna IC, Endman M. Intracytoplasmic sperm injection increases fertilization and good quality embryo formation in patients with non-male factor indications for in vitro fertilization: a prospective randomized study. Fertil Steril. 2001;75:342–7.
67. Nagy ZP, Liu G, Joris G, Bocken G, Desmet B, van Ranst A, et al. The influence of the site of sperm deposition and mode of oolema breakage at intracytoplasmic sperm injection on fertilization and embryo development rates. Hum Reprod. 1995;10: 3171–7.
68. Colombero T, Moomjy M, Silis S, Rosenwaks Z, Palermo D. The role of structural integrity of the fertilizing spermatozoon in early human embryogenesis. Zygote. 1999;7:157–63.
69. Moomjy M, Colombero LT, Veeck L, Rosenwaks Z, Palermo D. Sperm integrity is critical for normal mitotic division and early embryonic development. Mol Hum Reprod. 1999;5:836–44.
70. Berkovitz A, Eltes F, Yaari S, Katz N, Barr I, Fisman A, et al. The morphological normalcy of the sperm nucleus and pregnancy rate of intracytoplasmic injection with morphologically selected sperm. Hum Reprod. 2005;20:185–90.
71. Antinori M, Licata E, Dani G, Cerusico F, Versaci C, d'Angelo D, et al. Intracytoplasmic morphologically selected sperm injection: a prospective randomized trial. Reprod Biomed Online. 2008;16:835–41.
72. Jakab A, Sakkas D, Delpoano E, Cayli S, Kovanci E, Ward D, et al. Intracytoplasmic sperm injection: a novel selection method for sperm with normal frequency of chromosomal aneuploidies. Fertil Steril. 2005;84:1665–73.
73. Huszar G, Jakab A, Sakkas D, Ozenci CC, Cayli S, Delpiano E, et al. Fertility testing and ICSI sperm selection by hyaluronic acid binding: clinical and genetic aspects. Reprod Biomed Online. 2007;14: 650–63.
74. Cayli S, Sakkas D, Vigue L, Demir R, Huszar G. Cellular maturity and apoptosis in human sperm: creatine kinase, caspase-3 and Bclx expression in mature and diminished maturity spermatozoa. Mol Hum Reprod. 2004;10:365–72.
75. Nasr-Esfahani MH, Razavi S, Vahdati AA, Fathi F, Tavalaee M. Evaluation of sperm selection procedure based on hyaluronic acid binding ability on ICSI outcome. J Assist Reprod Genet. 2008;25:197–203.

8 Objective Biomarkers of Sperm Development and Fertility: Assessment of Sperm-Zona Pellucida Binding Ability and Hyaluronic Acid-Mediated Selection of Sperm for ICSI Fertilization

Gabor Huszar

Intracytoplasmic sperm injection, or ICSI, had been introduced in the mid-90s, for treatment of male infertility patients with low sperm concentration and motility [1]. ICSI may also be used in non-oligozoospermic men, either in those with unexplained male infertility, characterized by normal seminal sperm concentration and motility yet diminished fertilizing potential. Another group of patients are treated with ICSI in order to increase pregnancy success, particularly in couples who failed to achieve pregnancy in previous IVF cycles. A key issue of ICSI is sperm quality which depends on the method of sperm selection, and it may be assessed by the objective sperm biomarkers that have been the primary focus of the Huszar laboratory in the past two decades [2].

Regarding ICSI sperm selection, it should be recognized that due to the historically known incidence of various adverse genetic outcome following physiological fertilization, one would prefer to select and use for ICSI a sperm that would exhibit properties of sperm normally binding to the zona pellucida of oocytes, and, thus, participate in physiological conception by intercourse or conventional IVF. Also, with the advent of scientific ICSI sperm selection, the ongoing research on sperm biochemical markers of and function has became more prominent [2].

G. Huszar (✉)
Sperm Physiology Laboratory, Department of Obstetrics, Gynecology, and Reproductive Sciences, Yale School of Medicine, 333 Cedar Street, Suite 302 FMB, PO Box 208063, New Haven, CT, USA
e-mail: Gabor.Huszar@Yale.edu

Beyond Routine Sperm Analysis: Sperm Biochemical Markers

A major approach in the discovery of sperm biochemical markers is based on the recognition that there are objective biomarkers of sperm integrity and function that focus on elements of spermatogenesis and spermiogenesis that cause arrested sperm development. One of the first recognized markers was cytoplasmic retention which was assessed by the excess cytoplasm in sperm; biochemically this was measured by increased sperm creatine phosphokinase (CK) activity [3]. The variation in CK activity in semen samples is well documented, as well as the fact that sperm recovered from pellets following density gradient centrifugation, had substantially lower CK content [4]. A logistic regression analysis of 180 couples with oligozoospermic husbands treated with intrauterine insemination (IUI) indicated that the increased levels of CK activity (excess cytoplasmic retention) in oligospermic men predicted a lower likelihood for causing pregnancy [5].

The association between arrested cytoplasmic extrusion and diminished sperm fertilizing function was also established by experiments using CK-immunocytochemistry of individual sperm–hemizona complexes; only the sperm with clear heads without cytoplasmic retention were able to bind to the hemizona [6]. This important finding led to the recognition of spermiogenetic remodeling of the sperm plasma membrane, that is related

D.K. Gardner et al. (eds.), *Human Gametes and Preimplantation Embryos: Assessment and Diagnosis*, DOI 10.1007/978-1-4614-6651-2_8, © Springer Science+Business Media New York 2013

to the discovery of the formation of the sperm receptors for the zona pellucida and also for hyaluronic acid that is a key element of the contemporary ICSI sperm selection [2, 7].

Other aspects of the sperm biochemical markers, including (a) developmentally regulated protein expression of the HspA2 protein in human sperm (b) persistent histones which indicate abnormal histone-transition protein-protamine replacement process; (c) apoptotic processes; (d) reactive oxygen species (ROS), and (e) Sperm DNA chain integrity will all be discussed with the benefits of the novel ICSI sperm selection method facilitated by sperm-hyaluronic acid binding [2, 8–10].

Sperm Testing: DNA Chain Integrity

Over the past two decades, a number of tests have been introduced for the analysis of sperm nuclear DNA fragmentation [11, 12]. In general, single-stranded DNA damage provides a better prognosis and is easier to repair than double-stranded DNA damage [11–20]. Double-stranded DNA damage is more likely to lead to failure of paternal contribution of sperm to the embryo [21].

Some controversy still exists regarding which DNA test is best [22]. A recent study reported by Borini et al. showed that sperm DNA fragmentation values in aliquots of the same sperm fraction used for IVF, measured by TUNEL, were significantly correlated with pregnancy outcome [23]. This is in contrast to the results reported by Bungum et al. who found no correlation between sperm DNA fragmentation values in IVF samples, as measured by the SCSA test, and pregnancy outcome [12].

SCSA Issues

Regarding SCSA, Evenson et al. published data in which they used flow cytometry measurements of heated sperm nuclei to reveal a significant decrease in resistance to in situ denaturation of spermatozoal DNA in samples from bulls, men with diminished fertility [24]. The SCSA test has been more extensively studied to date from the clinical point of view [24–29]. The degree of DNA damage is measured by flow cytometry and is expressed as a DNA Fragmentation Index or DFI. Previous studies indicate that a DFI value >27 % is associated with pregnancy failure in ART [30, 31]. However, recent reports challenge the predictive value of the SCSA test [32, 33]. Independently from the SCSA values, various studies have emphasized the importance of DNA integrity in human fertility success [22, 34, 35]. The single final determinant of pregnancy success is the quality of the sperm DNA in the actual fertilizing spermatozoa.

We suggest that a possible reason for the discrepancy between the SCSA studies is the variability of sperm concentrations within the samples studied. In other words, for fertilization to occur there is a minimal threshold number of normal fertile sperm that is necessary. If this amount of fertile sperm is present (the threshold level depends on the conception model), the additional presence of non-fertile sperm, whether 20, 40, or 70 % of the total sperm content is not a relevant factor.

Sperm Preparation by Gradient Centrifugation

The two phase gradient centrifugation and fractionations of sperm is based on the specific gravity differences between normally developed spermatozoa (as the biomarkers indicate, completed cytoplasmic retention, in the head there are only DNA and the plasma membrane), as opposed to sperm affected by arrested development (excess cytoplasm in the sperm head). Normal sperm will sediment in the pellet whereas the lighter, arrested development, sperm with cytoplasmic retention will remain at the interface or on the top phase of the gradient media.

In 1988, a paper by Aitken and Clarkson demonstrated that centrifugal pelleting of unselected sperm fractions from human ejaculates caused the production of ROS (superoxide and hydroxyl radicals) within the pellet [36]. ROS production has induced irreversible damage to the spermatozoa and impairment of their fertilizing ability.

Superoxide radicals cause peroxidation of sperm plasma membrane phospholipids and elevated superoxide production, through a membrane-bound NADPH oxidase system, which has been implicated in defective sperm function at the cellular level [37, 38].

Various other studies have emphasized the importance of DNA integrity in human fertility success [22, 34, 35]. Independently from the SCSA values, the single final determinant of pregnancy success is the quality of the sperm DNA within the actual fertilizing spermatozoa.

Regarding the question whether all sperm (developed or with arrested development) are equally affected by ROS propagation three related biomarker issues were addressed in the Huszar laboratory [6]. First, a relationship was found between cytoplasmic retention as measured by creatine phosphokinase activity and ROS production: thus, retention of the excess cytoplasm was proportional with the ROS production. The second point was the fact that sperm fractions sedimented through Percoll gradient centrifugation showed lower ROS production and residual cytoplasmic content. Third, in order to study whether the iatrogenic cause of increased ROS production indeed propagate from spermatozoa-to-spermatozoa, the following experiments were performed. Semen pairs (with low and high ROS) were studied by first assessing sperm destruction by ROS following measurement of malonyldialdehide (MDA), an end product of sperm lipid peroxidation. First, the two semen samples were assayed independently, and the mixture of the two samples were also subjected to MDA assessment. All three semen fractions (A, B, and A+B) were than centrifuged for 10 min, and the sperm pellets were incubated at 37°C for 30 min, in order to provide close sperm-to-sperm contact in the experiments. Further, the MDA has been remeasured in all three samples. The data indicated that the aggregate (A+B) MDA levels were in the range of the original starting two semen samples (A and B) before the mixing, centrifugation, and incubation of the two semen samples, whether the initial MDA measurements were low or high [6].

Thus, it appeared that in the case of iatrogenic ROS damage, the propagation of the ROS production, does not apparently apply to the normally developed sperm without cytoplasmic retention. Further, based on the data, Huszar and colleagues concluded that the increased sperm MDA levels and ROS production is apparently not an "acquired," but an "inborn" error of spermatogenesis and spermiogenesis [6]. The data, with respect to "inborn errors," and the role of objective biochemical markers in the detection of sperm function and fertility, have been confirmed with numerous further studies [2, 8, 39–42].

Scientific Basis of Hyaluronic Acid-Mediated Sperm Selection

The hyaluronic acid-based sperm selection is based on the recognition of molecular and cellular aspects of sperm development, particularly the attributes that are generally present in normally developed spermatozoa selected by nature for spontaneous fertilization. Conversely, it is now well established that the presence of some sperm attributes indicate failed development and diminished fertilizing potential and/or deficient sperm paternal contribution [2].

The recognitions of such positive or negative sperm characteristics have evolved in the past 15–20 years in the Huszar laboratory. Biomarkers have been identified, and their role in sperm fertilizing potential, implantation, and success in causing pregnancy has been examined. In the first approach, sperm creatine kinase content and activity were assessed, which reflects the presence of surplus cytoplasm, due to incomplete sperm cytoplasmic extrusion which is a key event of spermiogenesis [5, 43, 44]. Indeed, it has been observed that normal spermatozoa which completed cytoplasmic extrusion are the only ones that are able to bind to the zona pellucida or to hemizonae (these are unfertilized human oocytes which were bisected in order to avoid inadvertent fertilization) [45].

This experiment provided three novel conclusions of paramount importance: (1) Sperm that failed to undergo cytoplasmic extrusion are unable to bind to the zona pellucida, and (2) Sperm–oocyte interaction during fertilization is directed and regulated by the attributes of the spermatozoa. (3) Another key element in the contemporary sperm research has been the recognition of the sperm plasma membrane remodeling, simultaneously with cytoplasmic extrusion in terminal spermiogenesis. This remodeling facilitates the formation of the zona pellucida and hyaluronic acid-binding site(s) in spermatozoa. Thus, sperm that fail to undergo the plasma membrane remodeling process are unable to recognize the zona pellucida or the layer of hyaluronic acid, and thus the fertilizing potential of such sperm are diminished [2].

ICSI Sperm Selection in Men with Excessive Semen ROS Production

Sperm preparation for assisted reproduction in men with high seminal ROS may improve sperm quality with media containing antioxidants such as reduced glutathione, catalase/EDTA [46–48]. Such approach may protect gametes from high oxidative stress.

In case of oxidative stress-related infertility, the appropriate treatment strategy is the elimination of the underlying cause, whether lifestyle and environmental factors that enhance oxidative stress, or use of sperm for IVF-ICSI arising from the testicular sperm extraction (TESE sperm). It is also advisable to avoid using cryopreserved spermatozoa which are very sensitive to DNA damage [49].

Regarding the utilization of TESE sperm, is it established that sperm originating in the adluminal area are protected from oxidative attack, whereas most ROS initiated DNA fragmentation occurs during epididymal storage [50]. There were significant improvements in sperm DNA quality in TESE samples compared to the cauda epididymis or ejaculated sperm [51, 52].

Another approach is offered by the hyaluronic acid-mediated sperm selection for single sperm for IVF/ICSI. The rationale is as follows: (a) A close correlation has been shown between ROS production and cytoplasmic retention which represent arrested gamete development. (b) Sperm selection by HA binding is also helpful as hyaluronic acid-bound sperm is also devoid of cytoplasmic retention, of excess persistent histones, DNA fragmentation and the apoptotic process [6]. Thus, sperm selection by prioritizing of normally developed spermatozoa with low or no ROS production is an appropriate and practical solution [2].

In line with the above discussion regarding ROS damaged sperm, most negative effects may be avoided by using testicular sperm. A number of reports indicate that sperm DNA damage is significantly lower in the seminiferous tubules. The use of testicular sperm in couples with repeated pregnancy failure in ART, and high sperm DNA fragmentation, resulted in a significant increase in pregnancy rates [51]. However, due to the lack of motility, testicular sperm are not appropriate for hyaluronic acid-binding-mediated selection.

Sperm Chromatin Maturation and Its Importance

The formation of normally developed mature spermatozoa is a unique process involving a series of developmental steps in both the nuclear and cytoplasmic compartments including histone-transition protein-protamine replacement. In this process, first somatic histones are replaced by testis-specific histone variants which are then replaced by transition proteins (TP1 and TP2) in a process that involves extensive DNA rearrangement and remodeling [53]. A greater than tenfold compaction of sperm chromatin is achieved during the final phases of spermatogenesis when the normally occurring histone that is bound to DNA is almost completely replaced by protamine 1 and protamine 2 [54].

Earlier studies showed an association between diminished histone-transition protein-protamine exchanges that may be detected by aniline blue staining due to the excess persistent lysine-rich histones [55–60]. Accordingly, based on the variations in sperm maturity, staining intensity was light, intermediate, and dark tone, and represents sperm with mature, moderately immature, and severely immature developmental status,

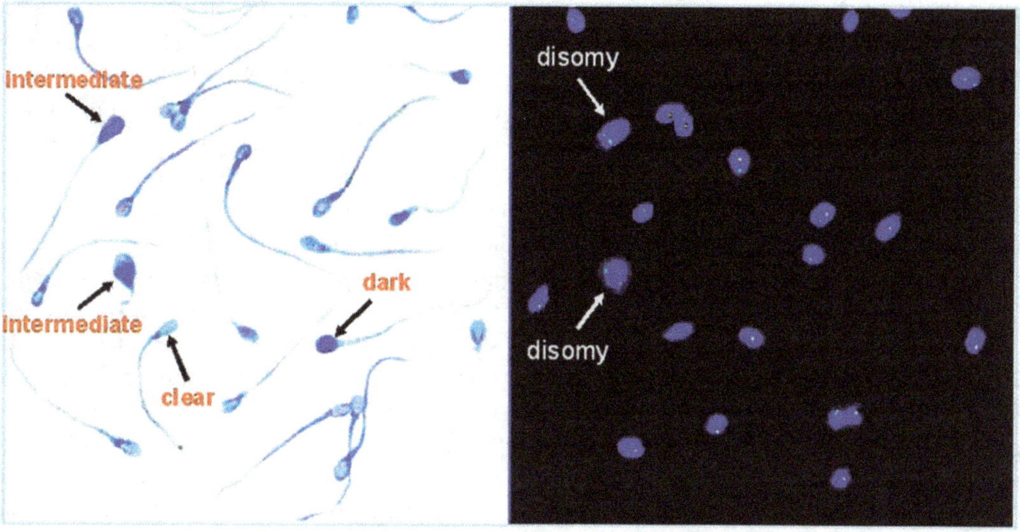

Fig. 8.1 Double staining of human spermatozoa with aniline blue (*left panel*) and fluorescence in situ hybridization (FISH, *right panel*), using FISH probes for chromosome Y (*red*), chromosome X (*green*), and chromosome 17 (*yellow*). Please observe on the *left panel* the spermatozoa with various amounts of persistent histones stained with aniline blue (quantified as light, intermediate, and dark), and the respective FISH results on the *right panel*. Light sperm (low levels of persistent histones) show normal chromosomal pattern, sperm with intermediate staining (more of persistent histones) show a higher frequency of sperm with disomies, finally dark sperm (high levels of persistent histones) don't exhibit FISH signal. We suggest that the lack of FISH signal in dark sperm is a consequence of the extensive DNA chain fragmentation in sperm cells which affected by retardation of the histone-transition protein-protamine developmental sequence. Thus, the FISH probes do not find long DNA chains to attach (from Ovari et al. [63], with permission)

respectively. This requirement for histone-to-protamine exchange in order to maintain chromatin integrity facilitates the correct folding of DNA and preserves DNA chain integrity [42].

It is clear that sperm chromatin is essential for sperm function and subsequent embryonic development because defects in sperm chromatin are linked to natural reproductive malfunctions like spontaneous abortion as well as assisted reproductive failure [12, 56, 59, 61]. Protamine replacement of histones and transition proteins may also facilitate the modulation of the expression pattern of the genome, as well as the imprinting pattern of the gamete. This methylation pattern lends variability to the paternal genome during zygotic gene expression events with individual consequences in developmental factors and epigenetic variations. There are several studies on the impact of sperm chromatin methylation levels in IVF success regarding both fertilization and pregnancy rates. Some support the idea that children conceived by ART do not show a higher degree of imprinting variability and that DNA methylation and the state of chromatin development are important [61, 62].

The relationship between persistent histones and DNA degradation was highlighted in a recent report from the Huszar laboratory. In individual spermatozoa with dark aniline blue staining, representing extensive levels of persistent histones, there was a lack of fluorescence in situ hybridization (FISH) chromosome signal [63]. Thus, deficiency in sperm chromatin development, improper DNA folding, and consequentially diminished DNA chain integrity caused diminished FISH probe binding, as there were limited number of long DNA sequences for FISH probe binding (Fig. 1). In addition, environmental stress also can disturb chromatin maturation, and ultimately lead to an abnormal chromatin structure that is incompatible with fertility [10, 64].

HSPA2 Chaperon Protein Sperm Biomarker and Clinical Applications

Another key biomarker identified in human sperm is the chaperone protein HspA2 [8, 65, 66]. This protein is homologous to the HSP70 which has been found in the mouse system [67–69]. Measurements of HspA2 levels in human sperm fractions have indicated that HspA2, which is part of the synaptonemal complex and also a key element of intracellular transport of DNA repair enzymes and other housekeeping elements in the developing spermatozoa, is very important indicator of sperm fertilizing potential [65]. HspA2 is also involved in the control of sperm DNA chain integrity and aneuploidy frequency. In the clinical arena, the markers of sperm creatine kinase and HspA2 levels were tested with respect to pregnancy success in blinded studies of IUI or IVF couples. The data indicated that the sperm CK content (a measure of excess cytoplasm in sperm) and HspA2 levels provide an objective measure of sperm fertilizing potential. The first study was conducted on couples with oligozoospermic husbands who were treated with IUI. When sperm CK content of couples with pregnancy success and lack of pregnancy were compared, the data indicated that there was no relationship between pregnancy success and sperm concentration, motility, or the amount of sperm inseminated. The important factor was sperm creatine kinase activity, reflecting sperm cytoplasmic content. The lower CK activity patients who had undergone cytoplasmic extrusion showed significantly higher pregnancy rates compared to those who had high creatine kinase activity and cytoplasmic retention. This indicated that the sperm biomarker CK reflecting extra cytoplasm, which is a negative factor with respect to fertility and pregnancy occurrence, whereas sperm concentration, motility, and total motile sperm are not contributing to the relationship between sperm developmental integrity and fertility, whether due to the fertilization process or to sperm paternal contribution [4].

The predictive value of sperm creatine kinase and HspA2 levels were also tested in the IVF setting. Similar to the IUI study, when the sperm creatine kinase activity was high in the samples, the pregnancy success has declined in spite of comparable sperm concentration and motility in the semen samples with high CK and low HspA2 levels. In a blind collaborative study between Yale and Norfolk, we have analyzed IVF cycles in 82 couples and found that if the sperm creatine kinase activity in the husband's sample was high, the couples did not achieve pregnancy [70]. In a subsequent study where sperm HspA2 was measured, we had a similar experience. With low HspA2 levels, there was lack of pregnancies. In both of these studies, there were about 15 % of men who were normozoospermic with normal sperm concentration and motility, yet they did not achieve pregnancy either in the creatine kinase-focused or in the HspA2 chaperone protein-focused IVF groups [65]. This is the basis for the idea of "unexplained male infertility" concept (diminished fertility in spite of normal sperm concentration and motility) that was developed in the Huszar laboratory during the 1990s.

The discovery of the HspA2 chaperone in sperm has led our group to the biomarkers of sperm development and sperm genetic integrity. First, HspA2 is part of the synaptonemal complex of the developing sperm cell and, thus, the low levels of chaperone protein are leading to problems with respect to chromosomal aneuploidies, including disomies and diploidies. This phenomenon of the relationship between cytoplasmic retention and low HspA2 levels, as they are related to increase in chromosomal aneuploidies, was well demonstrated by the report of [71]. When the spermatozoa were sorted by gradient centrifugation, sperm with cytoplasmic retention, which have decreased specific gravity due to the presence of cytoplasm, were compared to the developed spermatozoa which completed cytoplasmic extrusion. The spermatozoa with extra surplus cytoplasm exhibited a two and a half times higher incidence of chromosomal aneuploidies. Indeed, in the lighter sperm fraction, there was a close correlation ($r=0.05$, $p<0.002$) between residual cytoplasm and disomies of the 17 and Y chromosomes, as well as the XY sex-chromosome disomies.

The other key enlightenment regarding sperm biomarkers, the remodeling of sperm plasma membrane during spermiogenesis, was another substantial contribution by the Huszar laboratory: we have assessed in the same sperm fractions the amount of residual cytoplasm and also the presence of the enzyme galactosyltransferase, a unique sperm marker signifying the development of the sperm plasma membrane. There was a very close and significant inverse correlation (r=>–0.9) indicating that the spermatozoa which have surplus cytoplasm, and low HspA2 levels, also exhibit arrested sperm plasma membrane remodeling, Thus, sperm with the increased creatine kinase activity, indicating the failure of cytoplasmic extrusion, are unable to recognize and bind to the zona pellucida. These data are very important because they indicated that the sperm plasma membrane remodeling is a key in the formation of the zona pellucida binding sites and development of sperm fertilizing potential [72].

Sperm Plasma Membrane Remodeling and Formation of the Zona Pellucida and the Newly Recognized Hyaluronic Acid (HA) Receptor

Hyaluronic acid or hyaluronan, is a complex bioactive agent, which is well represented in the female reproductive tract. It is part of the cervical mucus spinkbarkheit during ovulation, and it is also a component of the cumulus oophorus which surrounds the oocytes. We recognized the sperm-hyaluronic acid interaction via observing that in the presence of hyaluronic acid, human sperm exhibited a substantially increased tail cross-beat frequency. Further, when we applied solid-state hyaluronic acid to a glass slide or a plastic surface, some of the sperm attached to it headfirst: the sperm progress was diminished secondary to the head attachment, yet the tail beating frequency increased and was maintained, sometimes even for days [4, 7]. We have made the hypothesis, and proved it, that during sperm plasma membrane remodeling in spermiogenesis, along with the formation of the zona pellucida receptors, receptors for hyaluronic acid are also formed. The common origin of the zona pellucida and hyaluronic acid receptor on sperm indicates that sperm binding to hyaluronic acid would also bind to the zona pellucida. Thus, the idea was conceived that we may select spermatozoa that would be participating in zona pellucida binding via a hyaluronan-mediated sperm selection [58].

The observations regarding the common origin of the zona pellucida and hyaluronic acid receptor lead to two inventions important for sperm assessment and ICSI sperm selection. Regarding Andrology, there is now a semen test (in addition to assessment of sperm concentration, motility, and morphology), which predicts what percent of sperm in an ejaculate would have zona binding properties (thus normally developed) leading to fertilizing potential. This is a very important advance and opportunity for physicians and patients [2]. The individual hyaluronic acid-bound spermatozoa are removable and may be used for intracytoplasmic sperm injection. This provides the opportunity to the embryologist to have ICSI fertilization with sperm which normally would have been fertilized in the zona pellucida-mediated physiological circumstances during intercourse or conventional IVF. As discussed below, the shape and biochemical properties, as well as genetic attributes of HA-selected sperm are comparable to that of the zona pellucida-bound sperm that may perform the fertilization following physiological sperm-zona pellucida interaction.

In the past few years, both HA-mediated devices, the sperm-hyaluronic acid-binding assessment in the Andrology laboratory, and the ICSI sperm selection device, the so-called PICSI dish (an IVF Petri dish that carries an HA-spot), has been increasingly accepted and used worldwide [73]. Indeed, the hyaluronic acid-binding score in the semen sperm provides a direction for the best approach in the fertility treatment of the couple, whether natural intercourse, or assisted reproduction with IUI, IVF, or ICSI with hyaluronic acid-mediated sperm selection. The sperm selected with the HA-mediated approach were shown to improve the fertilization rates, embryo quality, implantation rates, and most important, caused a major reduction in spontaneous miscarriage rates, most likely due to the superior DNA integrity in the HA-selected sperm (Fig. 2) [2, 74]. The published data indicate that men with low HA-binding score, after the HA-mediated sperm selection, achieve approximately 30 % higher pregnancy rates compared to the men with similar HA-binding score treated with ICSI using eye-selected spermatozoa.

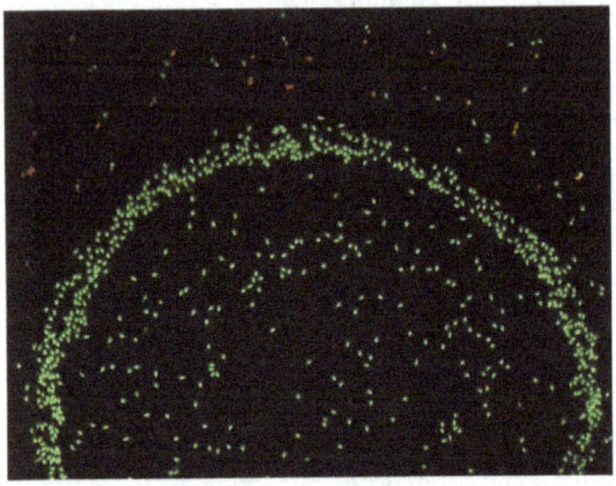

Fig. 8.2 Acridine orange-stained spermatozoa in the perimeter and center regions of the hyaluronic acid (HA) sperm selection area of HA-coated sperm selection Petri dish (PICSI dish). The perimeter area with mixed orange (fragmented DNA) and green sperm (sperm with intact high integrity DNA) shows the DNA integrity in the initial semen sperm fraction. However, the hundreds of green sperm with high integrity DNA in the center region of the dish, demonstrate the selection power of the hyaluronic acid with respect to sperm DNA integrity (from Yagci et al. [74], with permission)

Attributes of Hyaluronan-Bound Sperm

As discussed above, sperm with normal development and hyaluronan binding properties (reflecting the completion of plasma membrane remodeling) show an inverse correlation with DNA degradation, diminished histone-protamine transition, or excess persistent histones and dark aniline blue staining [2]. Further biomarkers are the presence or absence of caspase 3 and apoptotic changes, and the positive correlation between aneuploidy and abnormal sperm forms [75]. The viability studies indicate that all HA-bound spermatozoa are viable, which is a great advantage for ICSI selection (Fig. 3). However, it is also true that normal sperm morphology does not assure of low frequency of chromosomal aneuploidy. This was established by studies in the Huszar laboratory demonstrating that the shape properties of sperm in the native or decondensed and denatured states (necessary for the method of FISH) have remained identical. This finding was confirmed in several

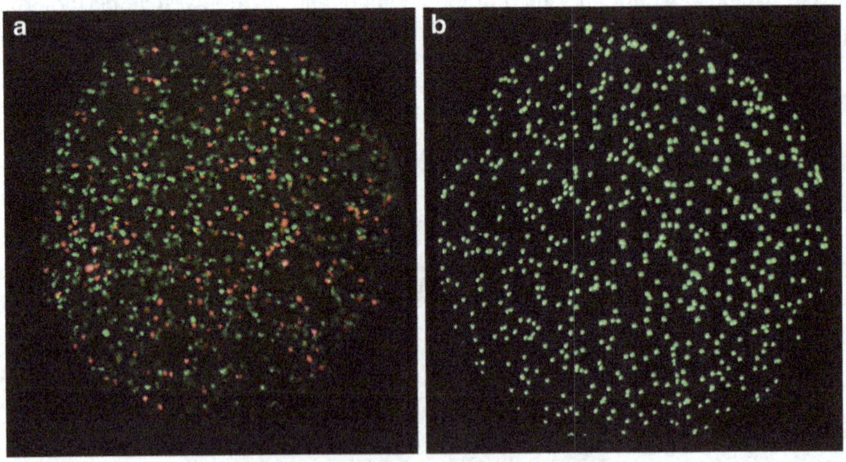

Fig. 8.3 Viable sperm are exclusively selected by HA binding. Sperm treated with the FertiLight kit (sperm membrane permeable Cyber green DNA viability stain and the red propidium iodide, which stains nonviable sperm) were applied to HA-coated slides. After 15 min the slides were gently rinsed, in order to remove unbound sperm. (**a**) Semen sperm fraction (*red* and *green*). (**b**) Hyaluronic acid-bound sperm fraction after the rinsing step (exclusively viable green sperm) (from Huszar et al. [58], with permission)

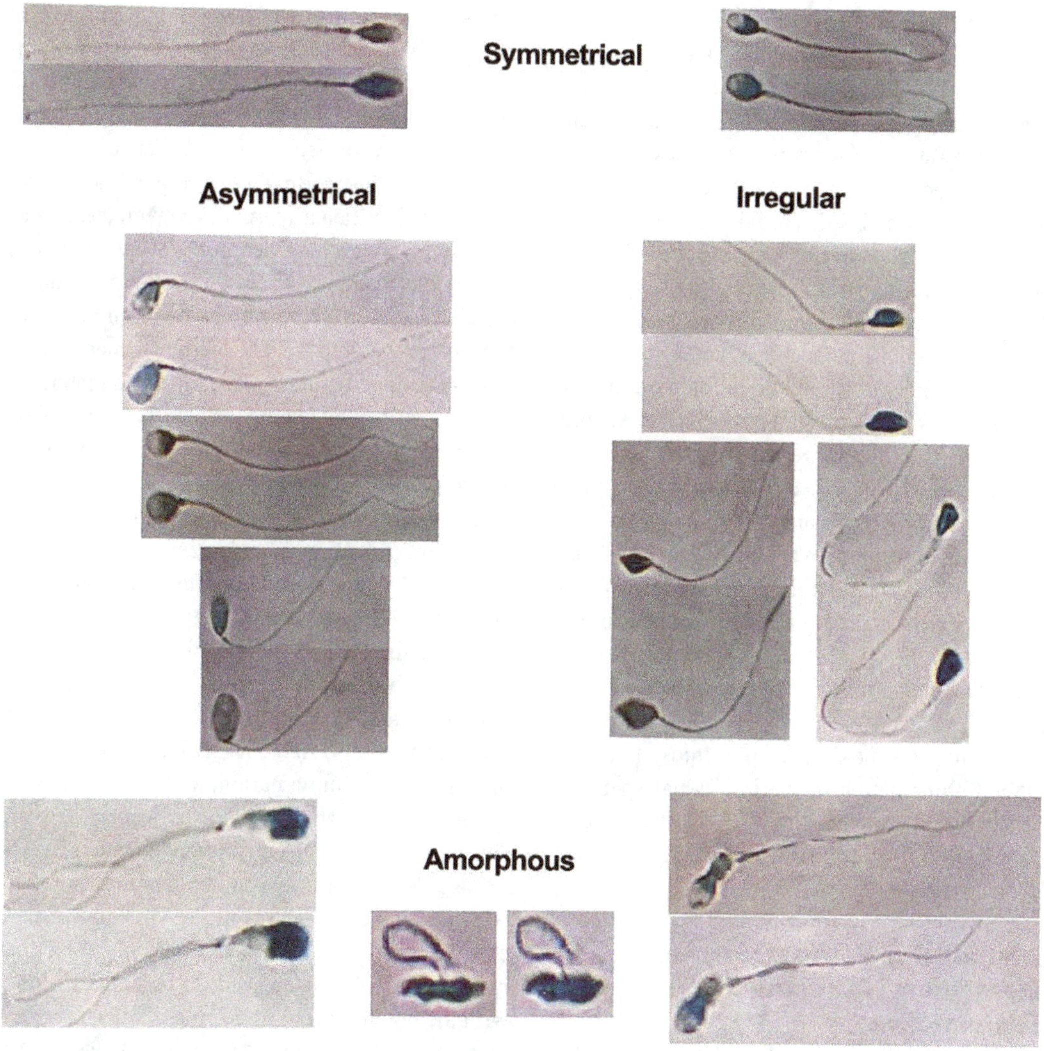

Fig. 8.4 Pre- and post-decondensation sperm images of various shape types. Sperm were classified according to their head shape properties as symmetrical, asymmetrical, irregular, and amorphous. Please observe the maintenance of sperm shape in the native vs. decondensed state in all sperm types. Magnification ×1,500 (from Celik-Ozenci et al. [77], with permission)

sperm types, including normal, abnormal, and irregular shapes in which the minor details and aspects of sperm shape were examined thoroughly in sperm of native and decondensed shapes (Fig. 4). With this methodological advancement we could study shape and aneuploidy within the same spermatozoa with high fidelity [76].

The relationship between sperm aneuploidy, sperm development, and morphology is controversial. Referring again to the relationship between cytoplasmic retention and sperm aneuploidy frequency, which was well established by Kovanci et al. [71], the relationship between low HspA2 content in sperm (a chaperone protein which is present in the synaptonemal complex) and residual cytoplasm representing arrested spermiogenesis well explains the potential relationship. However, it is unclear how general this relationship is, because not all sperm with abnormal sperm morphology has shown to carry aneuploidies [76]. Thus, sperm shape and aneuploidy status may be examined in the same spermatozoa [77].

Indeed individual spermatozoa, which show perfect Tygerberg morphology, and were evaluated with computerized morphometry for ideal shape, still have aneuploidies. The data indicated with several representative pictures that the decondensed sperm maintains their morphology exactly as it was in the initial non-decondensed state. Although there was some relationship between abnormal morphology and aneuploidies, the approach also demonstrated that aneuploidy may be found in perfectly normal spermatozo [76, 77]. Finally, it should be pointed out that the double-stained sperm study by Sati et al. indicated that cytoplasmic retention, DNA fragmentation, thus, the sperm chromatin packaging or sperm morphology, or any other sperm attributes of arrested development similarly and to a high extent (70–80 %) affect the same spermatozoa, as well as embryo propagation, if such sperm is used for ICSI [42]. Due to the common origin of DNA fragmentation and arrested sperm maturation, no matter what sperm attributes the investigators may be looking at, it is most likely the DNA fragmentation in the individual spermatozoa is the key element that affects the paternal contribution to embryo development.

Relationship Between Sperm Biomarkers Within the Same Spermatozoa

Regarding the features of arrested sperm development and other biomarkers reflecting sperm development, genetic aspects, aneuploidies, sperm shape, chromatin evolvement, and DNA chain integrity, the work of Sati et al. provided a major insight into very complex and far reaching features [42]. An inventive sequential methodological approach (aniline blue staining of individual sperm fields, recording of the sperm fields, and destaining, followed by application of a second sperm biomarker) facilitated the study of double-stained spermatozoa, including (1) aniline blue staining coupled with CK immunostaining (increased histone retention and cytoplasmic retention), (2) aniline blue staining and DNA fragmentation (histone retention and DNA fragmentation studied by in situ DNA nick translation), (3) along with aniline blue staining and immunostaining with caspase-3 (increased histone retention and apoptotic process), (4) and the particularly relevant finding of the inverse correlation between persistent histones and normal Tygerberg Kruger sperm morphology. When a spermatozoa with these morphological or biochemical probes were studied in the double staining process, there was about an approximately 80 % agreement between the staining patterns, scored as light (normal), intermediate (underdeveloped), and dark (diminished maturity), with the various biochemical nuclear and cytoplasmic probes arising from early or late spermiogenesis or spermatogenesis (Fig. 5).

Thus, abnormal sperm morphology and the underlying retention of cytoplasm and persistent histones, DNA chain fragmentation, aneuploidies, and the limited ability of the embryo for repair of the inborn deficiencies caused by the adverse sperm attributes mutually signal abnormal spermatozoa which is expected to provide lower fertilization rates, lesser embryonic development, lesser implantation, and higher rates of spontaneous abortion due to the arrested sperm development and DNA chain fragmentation [9, 21, 23, 42, 78–83]. This is a potential point where the ICSI sperm selection via the HA-mediated process and by IMSI sperm morphology selection may overlap. The issue needs to be studied, along with the potential inhibitory role of nuclear vacuoles, as well as the relationship between the known biochemical biomarkers and vacuoles. The relationship between sperm shape and sperm development, due to the cytoplasmic retention, has been already demonstrated. Thus, once we understand the relationship between the already identified sperm biomarkers and perhaps the nuclear vacuoles in sperm, we may have a more extended and comprehensive global picture how sperm shape or nuclear structure might support (if indeed it does?) IMSI sperm selection, and to what extent maybe or may not be compared to hyaluronan-mediated sperm selection. It is also of interest that the sperm morphology features, according to the Tygerberg criteria, have little prognostic value with respect to the IMSI morphology and were not predictive with respect to

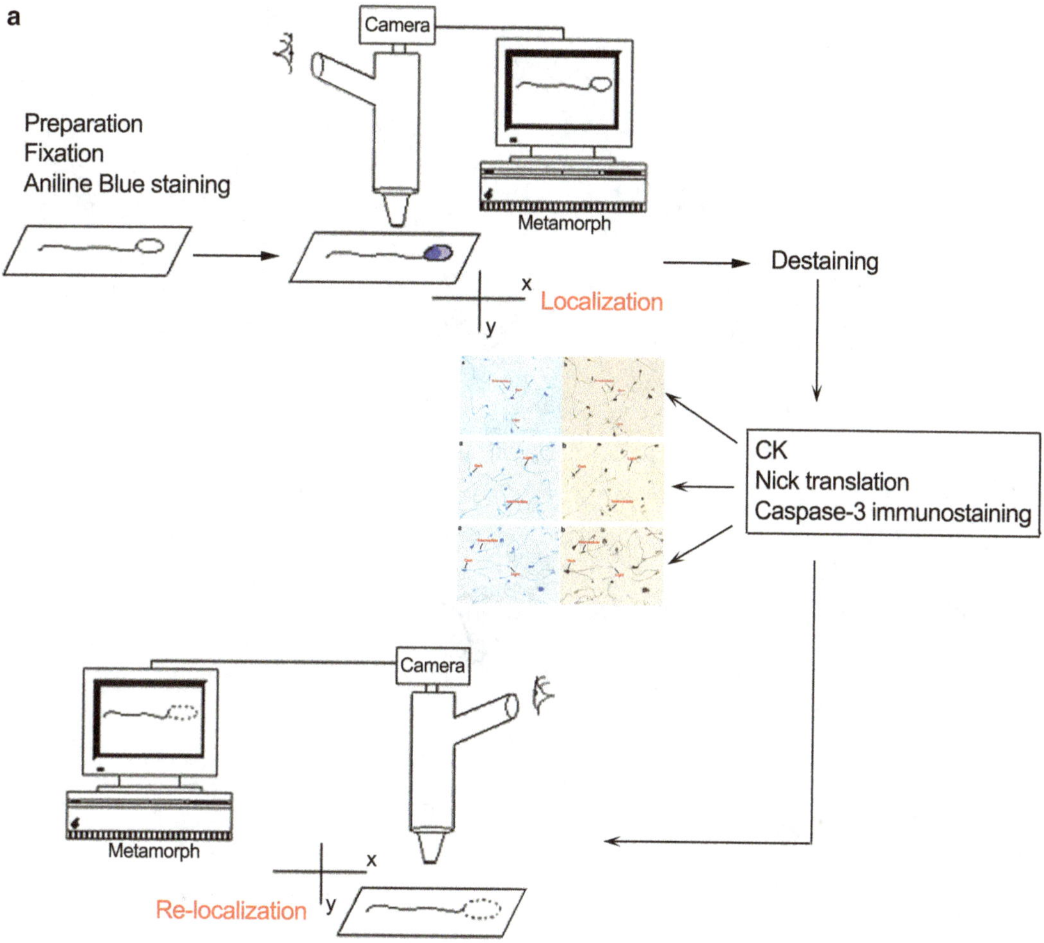

Fig. 8.5 Studies focusing upon the relationships between the sperm biochemical markers within double probed individual spermatozoa. (**a**) A flow chart of experimental design. Aniline blue staining pattern of individual sperm is recorded by the Metamorph program. Subsequently the sperm are distained from aniline blue, and the same sperm are restrained with a second probe (examples: CK-creatine phophokinase for surplus cytoplasm, DNA nick translation for fragmentation, Caspase-3 for apoptosis). The images of sperm in the fields treated with the two probes are than compared, and the staining pattern of the individual sperm are quantified as light, intermediate, and dark (Sati et al. [42], with permission). (**b**) Aniline blue staining (*panel A*) and creatine kinase (*panel B*) immunostaining of the same spermatozoa. Note the substantial similarity in the patterns of light-, intermediate-, and dark aniline blue staining and CK in the individual double-stained spermatozoa. (**c**) Aniline blue staining (**a**) and caspase-3 immunostaining (**b**) of the same individual spermatozoa. Note the similarity in the light-, intermediate-, and dark-staining patterns of the respective sperm in the aniline blue and the apoptotic marker, caspase-3 panels. Also, caspase-3 immunostaining is present in the mid-piece of intermediate-type spermatozoa, whereas in dark spermatozoa with more extensive developmental arrest both the head and the mid-piece are stained (**a, b**). (**d**) Aniline blue staining of persistent histones (**a**) and in situ DNA nick translation for DNA chain fragmentation (**b**) of the same double-stained spermatozoa. Note the high degree of similarity in the staining patterns of the light-, intermediate, and dark staining with the two probes in the respective spermatozoa. This indicates the relationship between excess persistent histones (arrested histone-intermediate) protein-protamine developmental sequence and extent of sperm DNA fragmentation. (**e**) Aniline blue staining (**a**) and (**b**) creatine kinase immunostaining (or other markers of cytoplasmic retention) reveal an inverse correlation between persistent histones and normal Tygerberg (Kruger) sperm morphology

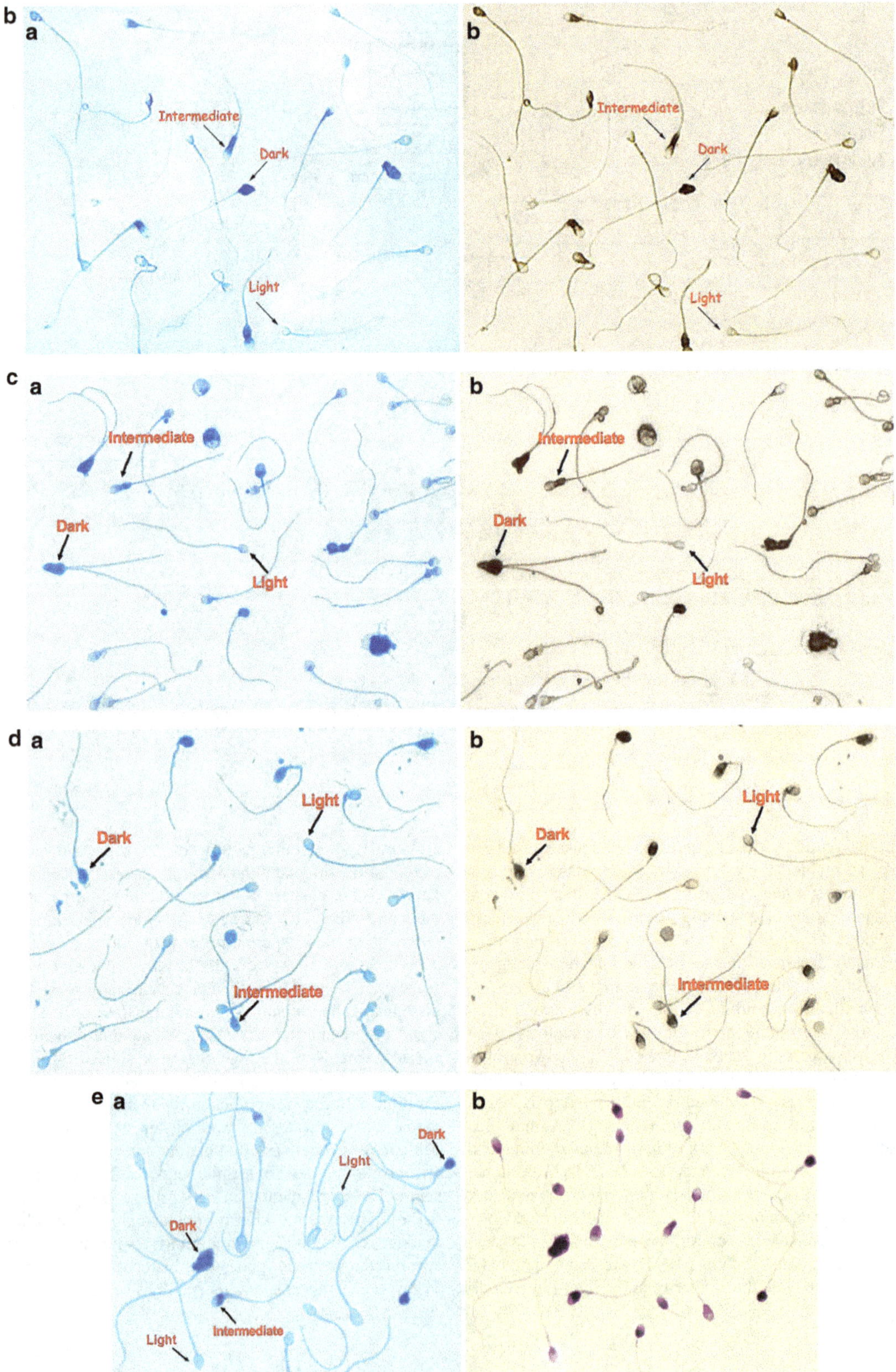

Fig. 8.5 (continued)

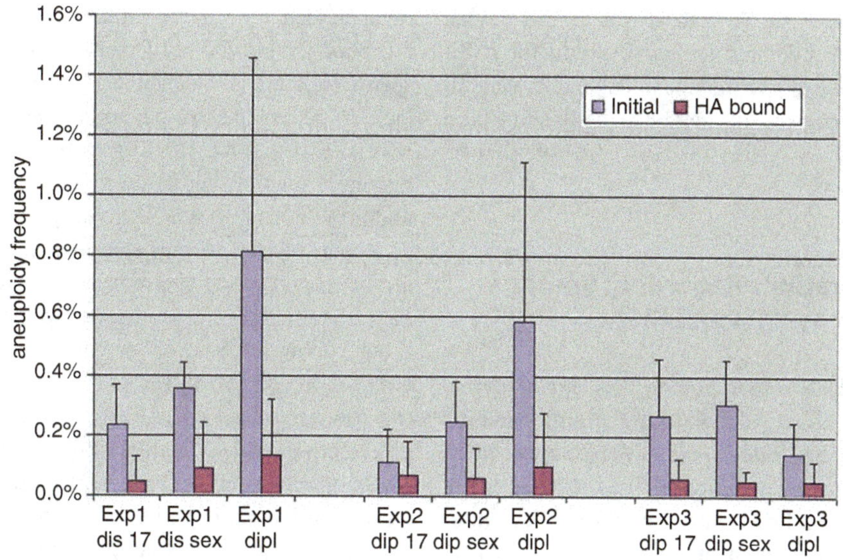

Fig. 8.6 Sperm aneuploidy frequencies before and after hyaluronic acid-mediated sperm selection. Sperm aneuploidy frequencies in the initial semen (*blue bars*) and in the respective HA-bound/selected sperm fractions (*red bars*). The three bar-groups represent experiments with 12 oligozoospermic men, 12 men with very high sperm concentrations (>100 million sperm/mL, further enriched with gradient centrifugation), and 10 husbands of couples treated with ICSI. In each man we have evaluated the FISH pattern (FISH probes for X, Y, and 17 chromosomes) in close to 5,000 sperm, 162,210 sperm in all. *Exp* experiment; *dis 17* chromosome 17 disomy; *dis sex* sex-chromosome disomy; *dipl* diploidy

ICSI outcome of embryo development, embryo morphology, or implantation rates.

Obviously, the discovery of the sperm plasma membrane remodeling and the formation of the zona pellucida and hyaluronic acid receptors, and the association between the lack of spermiogenetic development and sperm plasma membrane remodeling along with the increased DNA fragmentation, chromosomal aneuploidies, and other sperm attributes that may affect development, the duration of life time, or cancer rates of the offspring, generated major concerns regarding the long-term public health effect of ICSI fertilization with spermatozoa that was never selected by Nature for sperm–oocyte interaction or fertilization, as a fertilizing sperm. It should also be pointed out that the sperm preparation techniques which thought to be minimizing the ICSI injection of developmentally dysfunctional spermatozoa are a false hope. One point which brings this concept home is the fact that the diminished HA binding, which of course is related to increased levels of spermatozoa with arrested development, shows an inconsistency with sperm concentration and motility vs. HA binding. More impressive evidence comes from the work of Jakab et al. [84]. In this report, the efficiency of HA binding in purifying sperm specimens with respect to sperm with chromosomal aneuploidies were demonstrated. Indeed, in 10 men who had a sperm concentration of over 100 million sperm/ml, and the sperm had been further purified with a density gradient, the sperm pellet has shown diploidy and sex and 17 disomy frequencies of *0.9*, *0.2*, and *0.1*, whereas the chromosomal aneuploidy frequencies in the respective HA-bound spermatozoa were all in the 0.1–0.2 % normal aneuploidy frequency range (Fig. 6).

Another supportive idea with respect to DNA fragmentation of spermatozoa is demonstrated most recently by the paper of Yagci et al., in which a sperm fraction studied with Acridine Orange stain, and showing close to 50–50 % sperm with green and red fluorescence (high DNA chain integrity or fragmented DNA attributes, respectively), whereas the HA-selected sperm in the PICSI dish which is the device for the HA-mediated sperm selection for ICSI, the hundreds of spermatozoa observable were all of Acridine green fluorescence, indicating high integrity DNA chains in those HA-bound spermatozoa [74].

Considerations Regarding Sperm Selected by IMSI and PICSI

With respect to a morphologically defined normal nucleus without vacuoles, higher implantation and pregnancy rates were achieved with IMSI in couples with previous ICSI failures [85–87]. The improved IMSI outcome by the injection of spermatozoa without nuclear defects is related, perhaps, to improved chromatin status and reduced aneuploidy rates [88, 89].

A negative feature of the IMSI sperm selection method is the fact that it is a time-consuming procedure which may require 90–120 min [85]. It is also suspected that during this long period on the heated microscopic stage, the sperm cell and nucleus deterioration are enhanced along with an ROS generation process, and will cause sperm DNA chain degradation, particularly in those sperm which are underdeveloped or damaged. In comparison, the HA selection of spermatozoa with the PICSI dish may take only a few minutes.

Further, the PICSI dish provides a spacious area for sperm selection. It is equipped with lines of orientation, and all spermatozoa are within the same depth of microscopic focus range. Thus, the embryologist has a good opportunity to compare the available spermatozoa with respect to shape (morphology) and also HA binding, as well as the important specific response of the fully developed sperm to hyaluronic acid contact; 2–4 times increased cross-beat frequency. The motility arrest and the tail-beat response highlights the methodological advantage of HA-mediated sperm selection which is an efficient noninvasive process, and the fully completed sperm plasma membrane remodeling which also characterizes the biochemical attributes of "best" spermatozoa with respect to lack of cytoplasmic retention, lack of apoptotic process, high DNA chain integrity, high incidence of sperm with normal Tygerberg morphology, similar to the zona pellucida-bound sperm. Further, the biochemical probes include the lack of excess histone retention which indicates normal chromatin maturation with respect to the histone-transition protein-protamine sequence and promotes normal DNA folding [62, 64].

Regarding the various sperm attributes which are beneficial in the sperm selection process, we have identified several biomarkers which may promote sperm fertilization potential and paternal contribution of sperm. These biomarkers, including low creatine kinase content as a reflection of the completion of cytoplasmic extrusion, low levels of persistent histones, which reflect normal chromatin maturation with respect to progression from histones to intermediate proteins to protamine. The normal chromatin progression affects sperm function as well as normal DNA folding, and reduces the vulnerability to DNA fragmentation [62, 64]. We test for DNA integrity with the very highly accurate method of in situ DNA nick translation, and also with the sperm acridine orange fluorescence in situ. Further, we are testing for the presence of apoptotic agent caspase-3 which reflects potential DNA degradation due to apoptosis [90].

The major biomarker which distinguishes the spermatozoa selected by Hyaluronic acid-mediated binding compared to those used for eye-selected sperm used by in vitro ICSI fertilization is the binding, or lack of binding, to hyaluronic acid. This property represents the extent of sperm development or arrest of sperm development (with respect to the spermiogenetic plasma membrane remodeling) and the presence or absence of the zona pellucida and hyaluronic acid receptors, formation of which are simultaneously facilitated by the sperm membrane remodeling during terminal spermiogenesis.

On the other hand, the IMSI method does not consider sperm function or sperm biomarkers. It is strictly a pragmatic approach looking at sperm morphology or nuclear sperm morphology. Sperm morphology or sperm nuclear morphology of high magnification provides a moderately higher level of fertilization or implantation, but it does lack two features: (1) There is no objective measure of comparison between ICSI candidates (such as the sperm-HA-binding score), and the parameters used in sperm selection (morphology and nuclear morphology), and mid-piece attributes are not standardized. Further, there is controversy between various IVF centers as to what morphological features are relevant and how they may affect fertility and pregnancy outcome [91]. All is known that the observation of morphological attributes at sperm selection improve fertilization, implantation rates, and somewhat diminish the spontaneous abortion rates. (2) At the present time, as opposed to the HA-sperm ICSI selection, there are no organized studies performed focusing upon DNA integrity, aneuploidy, or other sperm genetic studies in connection with the IMSI methods. Thus, it is unclear how IMSI provides improvement with respect to the IMSI-selected spermatozoa or how IMSI-selected sperm provides any assurance for the future public health ICSI concerns regarding the individual development and aneuploidy frequency of the offspring, as well as life span, and future cancer incidence in the post-IMSI offspring population [92, 93].

The sperm selection by hyaluronic acid binding is based on the events related to sperm plasma membrane remodeling. The advantage of the HA-mediated selection of the best sperm, or the de-selection of sperm with various negative attributes, such as abnormal morphology, apoptotic process, DNA fragmentation, increased aneuploidy frequency, cytoplasmic retention, and low concentration of the chaperone protein HspA2, all of which were shown adversely affect fertilization potential and paternal contribution of spermatozoa to the embryo and thus cause a decline in fertilization rates, embryo development, implantation rates, and pregnancy success in line with the increased frequency of these adverse sperm attributes [2, 74, 84].

Other shortcomings of the IMSI studies: that there are no objective parameters for comparisons other than the sperm shape, which may be interpreted very differently from IVF Center to IVF Center [91]. As opposed to IMSI, the HA-mediated sperm selection, the semen may be evaluated with the sperm-HA-binding score, and the data indicate that the benefits of the HA-mediate sperm selection can be measured directly based on the sperm-HA-binding score [73, 94]. At a score of 80 % binding (8 of 10 sperm) sperm are well developed and completed plasma membrane remodeling; there is little or no benefit of HA-mediated sperm selection. However, in the population in which the HA-binding score is 60 % or lower (less than 6 of 10 binds to HA, and could be as low as 2), higher pregnancy rates were reported [95]. This is well coordinated with the fact that those spermatozoa which are able to bind to HA, thus, during spermatogenesis and spermiogenesis showed normal development all the way downstream to the key event of sperm plasma membrane remodeling and formation of the zona pellucida and HA-binding sites. In the poorly binding sperm samples, due to the lower frequency of the good spermatozoa which are greatly enhanced by HA-mediated sperm selection, there is the expected improvement in higher pregnancy and lower miscarriage rates. Indeed, this is well demonstrated by the multicenter study of Worrilow et al. which indicates a 10–30 % improvement in pregnancy rates and consequential decline in the spontaneous miscarriages that are both inversely correlated with the sperm-HA-binding score of the male partners.

ICSI Clinical Results: Comparison of HA-Mediated and Conventional, Eye-Selected Methods for ICSI Sperm Selection

There are now numerous laboratories that have initiated hyaluronic acid-mediated sperm selection in the past few years. It is important that none of the groups practicing the HA-sperm selection reported any adverse effects regarding fertilization or embryo development. In one 2005 ESHRE presentation, preliminary data on 18 pregnancies were reported. Comparing ICSI results with visually selected ICSI sperm ($N=84$) vs. HA-selected ICSI sperm ($N=18$): there were no differences in fertilization rates, proportion of good grade embryos, pregnancy and miscarriage rates, or take home baby rates. Again, there were no adverse findings during the cycles [96].

A similar study was performed on 20 unselected couples treated with ICSI in which at least eight MII oocytes were recovered. The sibling oocytes were injected either with HA-selected or visually selected spermatozoa ($N = 146$ and 145). The fertilization rates (72.9 and 66.9 %), oocyte degeneration rates (9.6 and 13.8 %), rates of embryo cleavage, embryo quality, embryo transfer, and embryo cryopreservation rates were all similar [97]. In a related publication, Park, Uhm et al. reported improvements with HA-selected sperm in porcine IVF [98]. Porcine embryos were produced by IVF, ICSI, and ICSI performed with HA-selected sperm. The HA-mediated sperm selection was superior to visual sperm selection in producing chromosomally normal embryos, and increasing ICSI efficiency by reducing the early embryonic mortality and thus enhancing ICSI success rates.

A related clinical aspect of the sperm biomarkers of sperm development and fertility is the enhancement of sperm with normal morphology in the HA-bound sperm fraction. Studies in the Huszar laboratory indicated that there was a two to threefold enrichment of Tygerberg normal sperm in the HA-bound fraction compared to the respective semen sperm fraction [99]. This enhancement, interestingly, agreed with the finding of the Tygerberg group with respect to the enrichment of normal morphology sperm in the zona pellucida bound vs. semen sperm fraction [100]. This is a further indication that sperm binding to the zona pellucida and to hyaluronic acid is not distinguishable from the point of view of the spermatozoa.

A number of recent studies have indicated that HA-bound sperm used in the ICSI procedure (the so called physiological ICSI) may lead to increased fertilization and implantation rates [94, 101]. In the Parmegiani study 293 couples were treated with HA-ICSI vs. 86 couples treated with conventional ICSI (historical control group). All outcome measures of fertilization, embryo quality, implantation, and pregnancy were the same or improved in the HA-mediated sperm selection group. The implantation rate was increased from 10.3 % in conventional ICSI to 17.1 % in the HA group. A smaller clinical trial assessing the same technology by Worillow et al. has also shown that clinical pregnancy rates are improved when using HA-selected sperm compared to conventional ICSI. Furthermore, the sperm-HA-binding score (the proportion of sperm that underwent plasma membrane remodeling in spermatogenesis and binds to hyaluronic acid) is an important diagnostic indicator. Men with <55 % binding score would particularly benefit from the HA-mediated sperm selection, as their ICSI pregnancy success rates were improved by 15–30 % [95]. Thus, it is important that in IVF programs, the Andrology Laboratory performs the sperm-HA-binding test for the husbands of IVF-ICSI couples, as the HA-binding score provides the information on the proportion of sperm with attributes of incomplete development, such as DNA fragmentation, chromosomal aneuploidies, persistent histones, cytoplasmic retention, and lack of HA-binding ability. The IVF team should triage the couples according to their HA-binding score in order to perform IUI, IVF or conventional ICSI, or ICSI with HA-mediated sperm selection.

All these supporting data from various laboratories led to a recent multicenter trial. Among the couples enrolled, 802 men had hyaluronic acid-binding score of <65 % (approximately 200 eligible couples). These men were treated in two arms, one received conventional ICSI, and the other group had hyaluronic acid-mediated ICSI sperm selection. However, it is an essential point that the pairs matched with conventional or hyaluronan-mediated ICSI sperm selection had comparable hyaluronic acid-binding scores. The couples treated with the hyaluronic acid-mediated vs. conventional ICSI sperm selection approach showed improved results. Implantation rates: 37.4 % vs. 30.7 %, clinical pregnancy rates: 50.8 % vs. 37.9 %, pregnancy loss: 2 % vs. 16.8 %, $P = 0.02$. This is an important study because of the strong points: (1) This is so far the largest patient population dealing with the benefits of the hyaluronic acid-mediated sperm selection; (2) the multicenter participation and the double blinded design; (3) the use of the sperm-hyaluronan binding score based matching of the randomized eye-selected and hyaluronic acid selected sperm used for ICSI; (4) confirmation of the increased pregnancy rates and statistically significant reduction in the spontaneous pregnancy loss in the group with hyaluronic acid-mediated sperm selection [73]. More confirmatory data are expected from the recently (2012) organized UK-multicenter HA-sperm selection trial (11 venues) with the direction of Dr. David Miller in Leeds.

Conclusions

We can conclude that at the present stage of the ICSI sperm selection science, the data support a preference for the hyaluronic acid-mediated sperm selection. However, regarding IMSI, studies focusing upon a more rigorous and valid comparison will have to be conducted regarding the presence and size of nuclear vacuoles in sperm populations which are simultaneously studied for hyaluronic acid-binding score, as well as the nuclear and cytoplasmic sperm biomarkers developed in the Huszar laboratory, including hyaluronic acid binding, DNA integrity, chromosomal aneuploidies, cytoplasmic retention, and chromatin structure. Evaluation of these parameters will provide a basis for a valid comparison of the sperm selection approaches primarily utilized in the present time.

Acknowledgments The multiple contributions of Leyla Sati, Ph.D. to the editorial aspects of this article are greatly appreciated.

References

1. Palermo G, Joris H, et al. Pregnancies after intracytoplasmic injection of single spermatozoon into an oocyte. Lancet. 1992;340(8810):17–8.
2. Huszar G, Jakab A, et al. Fertility testing and ICSI sperm selection by hyaluronic acid binding: clinical and genetic aspects. Reprod Biomed Online. 2007;14(5):650–63.
3. Huszar G, Corrales M, Vigue L. Correlation between sperm creatine phosphokinase activity and sperm concentrations in normospermic and oligospermic men. Gamete Res. 1988;19:67–754.
4. Huszar G, Vigue L. Spermatogenesis-related change in the synthesis of the creatine kinase B-type and M-type isoforms in human spermatozoa. Mol Reprod Dev. 1990;25(3):258–62.
5. Huszar G, Vigue L, et al. Sperm creatine phosphokinase activity as a measure of sperm quality in normospermic, variablespermic, and oligospermic men. Biol Reprod. 1988;38(5):1061–6.
6. Huszar G, Vigue L. Correlation between the rate of lipid peroxidation and cellular maturity as measured by creatine kinase activity in human spermatozoa. J Androl. 1994;15(1):71–7.
7. Sbracia M, Grasso J, et al. Hyaluronic acid substantially increases the retention of motility in cryopreserved/thawed human spermatozoa. Hum Reprod. 1997;12(9):1949–54.
8. Huszar G, Stone K, et al. Putative creatine kinase M-isoform in human sperm is identified as the 70-kilodalton heat shock protein HspA2. Biol Reprod. 2000;63(3):925–32.
9. Seli E, Sakkas D. Spermatozoal nuclear determinants of reproductive outcome: implications for ART. Hum Reprod Update. 2005;11(4):337–49.
10. Aoki VW, Emery BR, et al. Protamine levels vary between individual sperm cells of infertile human males and correlate with viability and DNA integrity. J Androl. 2006;27(6):890–8.
11. Perreault SD, Aitken RJ, et al. Integrating new tests of sperm genetic integrity into semen analysis: breakout group discussion. Adv Exp Med Biol. 2003;518:253–68.
12. Bungum M, Humaidan P, et al. Sperm DNA integrity assessment in prediction of assisted reproduction technology outcome. Hum Reprod. 2007;22(1):174–9.
13. Bianchi PG, Manicardi GC, et al. Effect of deoxyribonucleic acid protamination on fluorochrome staining and in situ nick-translation of murine and human mature spermatozoa. Biol Reprod. 1993;49(5):1083–8.
14. Gorczyca W, Traganos F, et al. Presence of DNA strand breaks and increased sensitivity of DNA in situ to denaturation in abnormal human sperm cells: analogy to apoptosis of somatic cells. Exp Cell Res. 1993;207(1):202–5.
15. Manicardi GC, Bianchi PG, et al. Presence of endogenous nicks in DNA of ejaculated human spermatozoa and its relationship to chromomycin A3 accessibility. Biol Reprod. 1995;52(4):864–7.
16. Hughes CM, Lewis SE, et al. A comparison of baseline and induced DNA damage in human spermatozoa from fertile and infertile men, using a modified comet assay. Mol Hum Reprod. 1996;2(8):613–9.
17. Fernandez JL, Vazquez-Gundin F, et al. DNA breakage detection-FISH (DBD-FISH) in human spermatozoa: technical variants evidence different structural features. Mutat Res. 2000;453(1):77–82.
18. Tomlinson MJ, Moffatt O, et al. Interrelationships between seminal parameters and sperm nuclear DNA damage before and after density gradient centrifugation: implications for assisted conception. Hum Reprod. 2001;16(10):2160–5.

19. Fernandez JL, Muriel L, et al. The sperm chromatin dispersion test: a simple method for the determination of sperm DNA fragmentation. J Androl. 2003;24(1):59–66.
20. Virro MR, Larson-Cook KL, et al. Sperm chromatin structure assay (SCSA) parameters are related to fertilization, blastocyst development, and ongoing pregnancy in in vitro fertilization and intracytoplasmic sperm injection cycles. Fertil Steril. 2004;81(5):1289–95.
21. Sakkas D, Alvarez JG. Sperm DNA fragmentation: mechanisms of origin, impact on reproductive outcome, and analysis. Fertil Steril. 2010;93(4):1027–36.
22. Barratt CL, Aitken RJ, et al. Sperm DNA: organization, protection and vulnerability: from basic science to clinical applications–a position report. Hum Reprod. 2010;25(4):824–38.
23. Borini A, Tarozzi N, et al. Sperm DNA fragmentation: paternal effect on early post-implantation embryo development in ART. Hum Reprod. 2006;21(11):2876–81.
24. Evenson DP, Darzynkiewicz Z, et al. Relation of mammalian sperm chromatin heterogeneity to fertility. Science. 1980;210(4474):1131–3.
25. Evenson DP. Flow cytometry of acridine orange stained sperm is a rapid and practical method for monitoring occupational exposure to genotoxicants. Prog Clin Biol Res. 1986;207:121–32.
26. Evenson DP. Flow cytometric analysis of male germ cell quality. Methods Cell Biol. 1990;33:401–10.
27. Evenson D, Jost L. Sperm chromatin structure assay: DNA denaturability. Methods Cell Biol. 1994;42(Pt B):159–76.
28. Evenson D, Jost L, et al. Comparative sperm chromatin structure assay measurements on epiillumination and orthogonal axes flow cytometers. Cytometry. 1995;19(4):295–303.
29. Evenson DP, Larson KL, et al. Sperm chromatin structure assay: its clinical use for detecting sperm DNA fragmentation in male infertility and comparisons with other techniques. J Androl. 2002;23(1):25–43.
30. Larson KL, DeJonge CJ, et al. Sperm chromatin structure assay parameters as predictors of failed pregnancy following assisted reproductive techniques. Hum Reprod. 2000;15(8):1717–22.
31. Larson-Cook KL, Brannian JD, et al. Relationship between the outcomes of assisted reproductive techniques and sperm DNA fragmentation as measured by the sperm chromatin structure assay. Fertil Steril. 2003;80(4):895–902.
32. Gandini L, Lombardo F, et al. Full-term pregnancies achieved with ICSI despite high levels of sperm chromatin damage. Hum Reprod. 2004;19(6):1409–17.
33. Bungum M, Humaidan P, et al. The predictive value of sperm chromatin structure assay (SCSA) parameters for the outcome of intrauterine insemination, IVF and ICSI. Hum Reprod. 2004;19(6):1401–8.
34. Spano M, Seli E, et al. The significance of sperm nuclear DNA strand breaks on reproductive outcome. Curr Opin Obstet Gynecol. 2005;17(3):255–60.
35. Zini A, Libman J. Sperm DNA damage: clinical significance in the era of assisted reproduction. CMAJ. 2006;175(5):495–500.
36. Aitken RJ, Clarkson JS. Significance of reactive oxygen species and antioxidants in defining the efficacy of sperm preparation techniques. J Androl. 1988;9(6):367–76.
37. Alvarez JG, Touchstone JC, et al. Spontaneous lipid peroxidation and production of hydrogen peroxide and superoxide in human spermatozoa. Superoxide dismutase as major enzyme protectant against oxygen toxicity. J Androl. 1987;8(5):338–48.
38. Aitken RJ, Clarkson JS. Cellular basis of defective sperm function and its association with the genesis of reactive oxygen species by human spermatozoa. J Reprod Fertil. 1987;81(2):459–69.
39. Spano M, Cordelli E, et al. Nuclear chromatin variations in human spermatozoa undergoing swim-up and cryopreservation evaluated by the flow cytometric sperm chromatin structure assay. Mol Hum Reprod. 1999;5(1):29–37.
40. Sakkas D, Manicardi GC, et al. The use of two density gradient centrifugation techniques and the swim-up method to separate spermatozoa with chromatin and nuclear DNA anomalies. Hum Reprod. 2000;15(5):1112–6.
41. Morrell JM, Moffatt O, et al. Reduced senescence and retained nuclear DNA integrity in human spermatozoa prepared by density gradient centrifugation. J Assist Reprod Genet. 2004;21(6):217–22.
42. Sati L, Ovari L, et al. Double probing of human spermatozoa for persistent histones, surplus cytoplasm, apoptosis and DNA fragmentation. Reprod Biomed Online. 2008;16(4):570–9.
43. Huszar G, Vigue L, et al. Sperm creatine kinase activity in fertile and infertile oligospermic men. J Androl. 1990;11(1):40–6.
44. Huszar G, Vigue L. Incomplete development of human spermatozoa is associated with increased creatine phosphokinase concentration and abnormal head morphology. Mol Reprod Dev. 1993;34(3):292–8.
45. Huszar G, Vigue L, et al. Creatine kinase immunocytochemistry of human sperm-hemizona complexes: selective binding of sperm with mature creatine kinase-staining pattern. Fertil Steril. 1994;61(1):136–42.
46. Griveau JF, Le Lannou D. Effects of antioxidants on human sperm preparation techniques. Int J Androl. 1994;17(5):225–31.
47. Donnelly ET, McClure N, et al. Glutathione and hypotaurine in vitro: effects on human sperm motility, DNA integrity and production of reactive oxygen species. Mutagenesis. 2000;15(1):61–8.
48. Chi HJ, Kim JH, et al. Protective effect of antioxidant supplementation in sperm-preparation medium against oxidative stress in human spermatozoa. Hum Reprod. 2008;23(5):1023–8.

49. Donnelly ET, Steele EK, et al. Assessment of DNA integrity and morphology of ejaculated spermatozoa from fertile and infertile men before and after cryo-preservation. Hum Reprod. 2001;16(6):1191–9.
50. Steele EK, McClure N, et al. A comparison of DNA damage in testicular and proximal epididymal spermatozoa in obstructive azoospermia. Mol Hum Reprod. 1999;5(9):831–5.
51. Greco E, Scarselli F, et al. Efficient treatment of infertility due to sperm DNA damage by ICSI with testicular spermatozoa. Hum Reprod. 2005;20(1):226–30.
52. Suganuma R, Yanagimachi R, et al. Decline in fertility of mouse sperm with abnormal chromatin during epididymal passage as revealed by ICSI. Hum Reprod. 2005;20(11):3101–8.
53. Ward WS, Coffey DS. DNA packaging and organization in mammalian spermatozoa: comparison with somatic cells. Biol Reprod. 1991;44(4):569–74.
54. Braun RE. Packaging paternal chromosomes with protamine. Nat Genet. 2001;28(1):10–2.
55. Dadoune JP. The nuclear status of human sperm cells. Micron. 1995;26(4):323–45.
56. Filatov MV, Semenova EV, et al. Relationship between abnormal sperm chromatin packing and IVF results. Mol Hum Reprod. 1999;5(9):825–30.
57. Steger K. Transcriptional and translational regulation of gene expression in haploid spermatids. Anat Embryol (Berl). 1999;199(6):471–87.
58. Huszar G, Ozenci CC, et al. Hyaluronic acid binding by human sperm indicates cellular maturity, viability, and unreacted acrosomal status. Fertil Steril. 2003;79 Suppl 3:1616–24.
59. Aoki VW, Moskovtsev SI, et al. DNA integrity is compromised in protamine-deficient human sperm. J Androl. 2005;26(6):741–8.
60. Ramos L, van der Heijden GW, et al. Incomplete nuclear transformation of human spermatozoa in oligo-astheno-teratospermia: characterization by indirect immunofluorescence of chromatin and thiol status. Hum Reprod. 2008;23(2):259–70.
61. Miller D, Brinkworth M, et al. Paternal DNA packaging in spermatozoa: more than the sum of its parts? DNA, histones, protamines and epigenetics. Reproduction. 2010;139(2):287–301.
62. Aoki VW, Carrell DT. Human protamines and the developing spermatid: their structure, function, expression and relationship with male infertility. Asian J Androl. 2003;5(4):315–24.
63. Ovari L, Sati L, et al. Double probing individual human spermatozoa: aniline blue staining for persistent histones and fluorescence in situ hybridization for aneuploidies. Fertil Steril. 2010;93(7):2255–61.
64. Carrell DT, Emery BR, et al. Altered protamine expression and diminished spermatogenesis: what is the link? Hum Reprod Update. 2007;13(3):313–27.
65. Ergur AR, Dokras A, et al. Sperm maturity and treatment choice of in vitro fertilization (IVF) or intracytoplasmic sperm injection: diminished sperm HspA2 chaperone levels predict IVF failure. Fertil Steril. 2002;77(5):910–8.
66. Cayli S, Jakab A, et al. Biochemical markers of sperm function: male fertility and sperm selection for ICSI. Reprod Biomed Online. 2003;7(4):462–8.
67. Allen JW, Dix DJ, et al. HSP70-2 is part of the synaptonemal complex in mouse and hamster spermatocytes. Chromosoma. 1996;104(6):414–21.
68. Dix DJ, Allen JW, et al. Targeted gene disruption of Hsp70-2 results in failed meiosis, germ cell apoptosis, and male infertility. Proc Natl Acad Sci USA. 1996;93(8):3264–8.
69. Eddy EM. Role of heat shock protein HSP70-2 in spermatogenesis. Rev Reprod. 1999;4(1):23–30.
70. Huszar G, Vigue L, et al. Sperm creatine phosphokinase M-isoform ratios and fertilizing potential of men: a blinded study of 84 couples treated with in vitro fertilization. Fertil Steril. 1992;57(4):882–8.
71. Kovanci E, Kovacs T, et al. FISH assessment of aneuploidy frequencies in mature and immature human spermatozoa classified by the absence or presence of cytoplasmic retention. Hum Reprod. 2001;16(6):1209–17.
72. Huszar G, Sbracia M, et al. Sperm plasma membrane remodeling during spermiogenetic maturation in men: relationship among plasma membrane beta 1,4-galactosyltransferase, cytoplasmic creatine phosphokinase, and creatine phosphokinase isoform ratios. Biol Reprod. 1997;56(4):1020–4.
73. Worrilow K, Eld S, et al. Prospective, multi-center, double-blind, randomized clinical trial evaluating the use of hyaluronan-bound sperm in ICSI: statistically significant improvement in clinical outcomes. In: ASRM annual meeting, Orlando, FL; 2011.
74. Worrilow KC, Eid S, et al. Use of hyaluronan in the selection of sperm for intracytoplasmic sperm injection (ICSI): significant improvement in clinical outcomes–multicenter, double-blinded and randomized controlled trial. Hum Reprod. 2013; 28(2):306–14.
75. Gergely A, Kovanci E, et al. Morphometric assessment of mature and diminished-maturity human spermatozoa: sperm regions that reflect differences in maturity. Hum Reprod. 1999;14(8):2007–14.
76. Celik-Ozenci C, Jakab A, et al. Sperm selection for ICSI: shape properties do not predict the absence or presence of numerical chromosomal aberrations. Hum Reprod. 2004;19(9):2052–9.
77. Celik-Ozenci C, Catalanotti J, et al. Human sperm maintain their shape following decondensation and denaturation for fluorescent in situ hybridization: shape analysis and objective morphometry. Biol Reprod. 2003;69(4):1347–55.
78. Simon L, Lutton D, et al. Sperm DNA damage measured by the alkaline Comet assay as an independent predictor of male infertility and in vitro fertilization success. Fertil Steril. 2011;95(2):652–7.
79. Ebner T, Moser M, et al. Presence, but not type or degree of extension, of a cytoplasmic halo has a significant influence on preimplantation development and implantation behaviour. Hum Reprod. 2003;18(11):2406–12.

80. Zini A, Boman JM, et al. Sperm DNA damage is associated with an increased risk of pregnancy loss after IVF and ICSI: systematic review and meta-analysis. Hum Reprod. 2008;23(12):2663–8.
81. Avendano C, Franchi A, et al. DNA fragmentation of normal spermatozoa negatively impacts embryo quality and intracytoplasmic sperm injection outcome. Fertil Steril. 2010;94(2):549–57.
82. Menezo Y, Dale B, et al. DNA damage and repair in human oocytes and embryos: a review. Zygote. 2010;18(4):357–65.
83. Simon L, Brunborg G, et al. Clinical significance of sperm DNA damage in assisted reproduction outcome. Hum Reprod. 2010;25(7):1594–608.
84. Jakab A, Sakkas D, et al. Intracytoplasmic sperm injection: a novel selection method for sperm with normal frequency of chromosomal aneuploidies. Fertil Steril. 2005;84(6):1665–73.
85. Antinori M, Licata E, et al. Intracytoplasmic morphologically selected sperm injection: a prospective randomized trial. Reprod Biomed Online. 2008; 16(6):835–41.
86. Franco Jr JG, Baruffi RL, et al. Significance of large nuclear vacuoles in human spermatozoa: implications for ICSI. Reprod Biomed Online. 2008;17(1):42–5.
87. Souza Setti A, Ferreira RC, et al. Intracytoplasmic sperm injection outcome versus intracytoplasmic morphologically selected sperm injection outcome: a meta-analysis. Reprod Biomed Online. 2010; 21(4):450–5.
88. Garolla A, Fortini D, et al. High-power microscopy for selecting spermatozoa for ICSI by physiological status. Reprod Biomed Online. 2008;17(5):610–6.
89. Boitrelle F, Ferfouri F, et al. Large human sperm vacuoles observed in motile spermatozoa under high magnification: nuclear thumbprints linked to failure of chromatin condensation. Hum Reprod. 2011; 26(7):1650–8.
90. Cayli S, Sakkas D, et al. Cellular maturity and apoptosis in human sperm: creatine kinase, caspase-3 and Bcl-XL levels in mature and diminished maturity sperm. Mol Hum Reprod. 2004;10(5):365–72.
91. Perdrix A, Travers A, et al. Assessment of acrosome and nuclear abnormalities in human spermatozoa with large vacuoles. Hum Reprod. 2011;26(1):47–58.
92. Simpson JL, Lamb DJ. Genetic effects of intracytoplasmic sperm injection. Semin Reprod Med. 2001; 19(3):239–49.
93. Bonduelle M, Liebaers I, et al. Neonatal data on a cohort of 2889 infants born after ICSI (1991–1999) and of 2995 infants born after IVF (1983–1999). Hum Reprod. 2002;17(3):671–94.
94. Parmegiani L, Cognigni GE, et al. Efficiency of hyaluronic acid (HA) sperm selection. J Assist Reprod Genet. 2010;27(1):13–6.
95. Worrilow K, Huynh H. The clinical impact associated with the use of PICSI derived embryos. In: Annual meeting of ASRM, Atlanta; 2009.
96. Sanchez M, Aran B, et al. Preliminary clinical and FISH results on hyaluronic acid sperm selection to improve ICSI. 21st Annual meeting of European Society for Human Reproduction & Embryology (ESHRE), 19–22 June, Copenhagen, Denmark. Hum Reprod. 2005;20 Suppl 1:556.
97. Janssens R, Verheyen G, et al. Use of PICSI dishes for sperm selection in clinical ICSI practice: results of a pilot study. In: Annual meeting of the Belgian Society Reproductive Medicine, Brussels; 2006.
98. Park CY, Uhm SJ, et al. Increase of ICSI efficiency with hyaluronic acid binding sperm for low aneuploidy frequency in pig. Theriogenology. 2005;64(5): 1158–69.
99. Prinosilova P, Kruger T, et al. Selectivity of hyaluronic acid binding for spermatozoa with normal Tygerberg strict morphology. Reprod Biomed Online. 2009;18(2):177–83.
100. Menkveld R, Franken DR, et al. Sperm selection capacity of the human zona pellucida. Mol Reprod Dev. 1991;30(4):346–52.
101. Nasr-Esfahani MH, Razavi S, et al. Evaluation of sperm selection procedure based on hyaluronic acid binding ability on ICSI outcome. J Assist Reprod Genet. 2008;25(5):197–203.

Additional Reading

Huszar G, Patrizio P, et al. Cytoplasmic extrusion and the switch from creatine kinase B to M isoform are completed by the commencement of epididymal transport in human and stallion spermatozoa. J Androl. 1998; 19(1):11–20.

9 Selecting the Best Sperm and Its Implications in Clinical Practice

Juan G. Alvarez

If we ask the question of what is the main function of the spermatozoon, the consensus would be that it is to introduce an intact normal DNA into the oocyte. The sperm DNA is the manual of instructions of the paternal genome that once fused with that of the oocyte gives place to the embryo's genome, responsible for normal embryo and fetal development. The presence of breaks in the DNA strands of the embryonic genome or of modifications in its nucleotides, coming from the paternal genome that had not been repaired by the oocyte or the embryo, is not compatible with normal embryo or fetal development. This would be equivalent to the missing pages in the manual of instructions or if these pages were blurred and thus could not be read correctly. Once the DNA has been introduced into the oocyte by the fertilizing spermatozoon, the highly packed sperm chromatin must be decondensed and the protamines substituted by histones. This requires the reduction by GSH of the disulfide bonds that crosslink the sperm nuclear protamines. Thereafter, pronuclear formation will proceed. To that end, the sperm must release its proximal centriole into the oocyte in order for pronuclear alignment and mitotic spindle formation to take place after fertilization.

In order for the embryo's genome to be read and expressed, it is necessary that the oocyte-activating factor (OAF) that the fertilizing spermatozoon carries in its nuclear membrane and that has been characterized as a phospholipase C_{zeta}, induce calcium release from intracellular stores leading to the activation of inositol phosphate- and diacyl glycerol (DAG)-mediated signal transduction mechanisms, protein phosphorylation, the expression of specific gene expression factors, and the activation of the so-called master genes in the embryo's genome that will set in motion the development of an embryo.

The spermatozoon is a highly specialized cell designed for the transport of its DNA into the oocyte. The teleological function of the complex self-propelling mechanisms that the axoneme microtubules of the sperm flagellum represent, and the biochemical drill that the sperm's acrosome constitutes, have been developed and perfected through millions of years of evolution to facilitate the transport of the sperm DNA into the oocyte. Therefore, the axoneme, as well as the acrosome can be considered as mere accessories developed for sperm's primary function of introducing the DNA into the oocyte. However, the transport of spermatozoa from the seminiferous tubules to the ampullary region of the oviduct entails a significant risk of sperm DNA damage. That is precisely why the sperm chromatin is packed in the head of the spermatozoon in a very singular way that includes the presence of specific nuclear proteins, the so-called protamines, that substitute the histones present in somatic cells, and the fact that the protamines are extensively

J.G. Alvarez (✉)
Department of Maile Infertility, Centro ANDROGEN, La Coruña, Spain
e-mail: jalvarez@androgen.es

D.K. Gardner et al. (eds.), *Human Gametes and Preimplantation Embryos: Assessment and Diagnosis*, DOI 10.1007/978-1-4614-6651-2_9, © Springer Science+Business Media New York 2013

cross-linked with disulfide bonds thus providing a kind of a seal that protects the sperm DNA against potential damage during sperm transport to the oviduct. Nevertheless, despite this evolutionary feature of sperm chromatin packing, the risk still remains and, in fact, clinical studies show that significant DNA damage may occur in the epididymis leading to sperm DNA fragmentation and nucleotide modification. As a last resort, the oocyte and the embryo are equipped with DNA repair mechanisms designed to repair sperm DNA damage. From the biological standpoint, a term pregnancy is a significant investment and, therefore, through evolution a number of mechanisms have been developed in order to warrant the birth of a healthy offspring. However, the oocyte's capacity to repair damage in the sperm DNA has some limitations since it can mainly repair single-stranded DNA damage with some limited ability to repair double-stranded DNA damage.

In addition to the integrity of the sperm DNA, a normal sperm chromosomal composition and structure is of paramount importance for normal embryo and fetal development. It is well known that synaptic anomalies during meiosis may lead to telomere defects, sperm aneuploidy, and embryo aneuploidy.

The main objectives of this chapter are (1) to identify the most relevant biochemical and biological markers to be used for sperm selection in assisted reproductive technologies and (2) to establish the criteria and recommendations of methodologies to be used for the selection of the best spermatozoa. Most of the applications described in this chapter are mainly directed to ICSI.

Biochemical Markers for Sperm Selection

The biochemical markers considered key for the development of the sperm selection methodologies and diagnostic tests to be used in assisted reproductive technologies are chromatin structure, chromosomal composition and structure, activity of the oocyte-activating factor, and functionality of the sperm proximal centriole.

Chromatin Structure

Normal chromatin structure is a *sine qua non* condition for normal fertilization and for normal embryo and fetal development. As mentioned before, normal embryo and fetal development is going to depend, at least in part, on the integrity of the DNA introduced by the fertilizing spermatozoon. With regard to fertilization, once the spermatozoon is microinjected into the oocyte, sperm chromatin decondensation must take place for normal male pronuclear formation to occur. Failure of chromatin to decondense may either be related to defects in chromatin packing or to failure of the oocyte to reduce the disulphide bonds of sperm protamines through the oocyte' endogenous supply of reduced glutathione (GSH) [1, 2]. Normal activity of glutathione reductase and subsequent generation of GSH is going to depend on a normal supply of NADPH through the pentose-phosphate pathway. Glutathione reductase uses NADPH as a substrate to produce GSH. Since sperm chromatin decondensation capability cannot be evaluated prior to ICSI and, on the other hand, it depends on the endogenous supply of GSH, sperm chromatin decondensation can only be predicted *a posteriori* after fertilization failure occurs. As it will be described later on in this chapter, the other two factors that may be involved in fertilization failure are (1) lack of activity of the oocyte-activating factor or (2) a defective sperm proximal centriole.

A well-preserved sperm DNA, on the other hand, is going to determine, to a great extent, normal embryo and fetal development, especially if the fertilizing spermatozoon carries DNA damage that affects essential sequences, such as exons, and if this damage cannot be repaired by the oocyte and/or the embryo [3–5]. Should these two conditions be met, embryo development, particularly after embryo implantation, would be compromised. Since most of the sperm DNA damage takes place in the epididymis, two different approaches could be used to select sperm with intact DNA: (1) use of testicular sperm; and (2) select from the ejaculate spermatozoa with low levels of DNA damage [6–10].

The recommended methodologies derived from these two approaches will be described in the last section of this chapter.

Chromosomal Composition and Structure

In addition to the presence of structural damage in sperm's DNA stands, another important biochemical marker to consider is the amount and quality of the genetic information present in the male's genome. This amount of genetic information should be very precise: *not more, not less*. Since sperm's chromosomal composition is haploid, either diploidies or nullosomies should be absent. An excess of genetic information, such as disomy or polyploidy, or a shortage of genetic information such as nullisomy, may lead to embryo aneuploidy and failed pregnancy or miscarriage. The presence of sperm aneuploidies in the paternal genome is also going to interfere with embryo and fetal development. In this case, either excess pages have been added to the manual or some pages have been omitted while in press. Errors in the meiotic process can result in an increased rate of aneuploid or diploid sperm, affecting the fertilizing ability of these spermatozoa [11–13]. Numerous studies using Fluorescene In Situ Hybridization (FISH) analysis have demonstrated an increase in the rate of aneuploid and diploid sperm in infertile men [14–16]. Although the percentage of spermatozoa carrying aneuploidies in ejaculated sperm from normozoospermic males, as assessed by FISH is below 0.5 %, and it is considered abnormal when this percentage exceeds 0.5 %, the predictive value of an abnormal FISH test result, in terms of pregnancy outcome, is relatively high. This predictive value cannot be explained only based on the fact that the oocyte has been fertilized by an aneuploid spermatozoon.

The only logical explanation for this apparent paradox would be that sperm aneuploidy correlates with another defect that is present in a high percentage of ejaculated mature spermatozoa, e.g., a telomeric defect, that is not measured and that is transmitted to the embryo [17]. Sperm aneuploidy, to a great extent, reflects defects in the process of meiosis. That is: defects of synapsis of the bivalents during prophase and metaphase of meiosis I would lead to sperm aneuploidy. However, the seminiferous tubules epithelium is equipped with checkpoints to identify primary spermatocytes with synaptic anomalies. Once defective primary spermatocytes are identified at these checkpoints, the cells are earmarked for the induction of apoptosis and their elimination by the Sertoli cell [18]. If these checkpoints work properly, these spermatozoa should not reach the ejaculate. However, sometimes primary spermatocytes with synaptic anomalies are not recognized at these checkpoints and, as a result of that, aneuploid spermatozoa appear in the ejaculate.

In the first scenario, there is a defect of meiosis related to synaptic anomalies, and yet aneuploid sperm do not appear in the ejaculate. Therefore, if we were to perform a study of FISH in semen, the test result would be normal (<0.5 %) and yet there is defect of meiosis. In sharp contrast, in the second scenario, because the checkpoints fail to recognize defective primary spermatocytes with synaptic anomalies, aneuploid spermatozoa will be released into the lumen of the seminiferous tubules and thus the presence of aneuploid sperm in the ejaculate would be alerting us of a defect of meiosis. Therefore, in this second scenario, the study of FISH in semen would yield an abnormal test result and it won't be necessary to perform a testicular biopsy for a study of meiosis. However, in the first case, since the FISH test result is normal, we would have to perform a study of meiosis in testicular biopsy to see whether meiosis is normal or not.

What is then the connection between defects of synapsis in the bivalents during meiosis, telomeric defects and sperm and embryo aneuploidy? It turns out that since the synapsis of bivalents takes place by direct contact of both telomeric ends, should a telomeric defect be present it might affect the synapsis of the bivalents. Can this defect be present and yet sperm aneuploidy rate in ejaculated spermatozoa be <0.5 %? The answer to this question, although it has not been confirmed experimentally in human IVF, may be affirmative: it is possible that telomeric defects present in sperm chromosomes in a relatively high proportion of ejaculated spermatozoa, even from the gradient pellet which are those used for ICSI, are transmitted to the embryo after fertilization and be responsible for the relatively high rate of embryo aneuploidy observed in males with meiotic anomalies, and yet the rate of sperm aneuploidy be relatively low [19–23]. Since technologies directed to select telomeric defect-free spermatozoa have not yet been developed, rather than resorting to the selection of these spermatozoa, we would have to resort to the selection of euploid embryos by Preimplantational Genetic Screening (PGS), preferably using probes for all chromosomes either by array-CGH technology or by FISH on day-3 embryos.

Activity of the Oocyte-Activating Factor

The OAF is a phospholipase C_{zeta} that cleaves the phosphate bond of phosphatidylinositol with the release of inositol 1,4,5 triphosphate (IP3) and DAG [24]. The OAF is responsible for the initiation of the early events of fertilization involving the release of calcium from intracellular stores leading to the activation of IP3 and DAG-mediated signal transduction mechanisms including protein phosphorylation and binding of gene expression factors to the master genes responsible for setting in motion embryo development. Since the OAF is located in the nuclear membrane of the spermatozoon, membrane damage in sperm may lead to damage of the OAF and failed fertilization. Since currently, the activity of OAF in the spermatozoon to be injected by ICSI cannot be measured, as in the case of sperm chromatin decondensation, the activity of the OAF can only be assessed in a functional manner using the mouse oocyte-activating test, as it will be described in the last section of this chapter.

Functionality of the Sperm Proximal Centriole

The sperm proximal centriole is responsible for the alignment of both male and female pronuclei and the formation of the mitotic spindle [25]. The proximal centriole is located within the connecting piece next to the basal plate of the sperm head. This centriole displays a pin-wheel-like structure of nine triplet microtubules surrounded by pericentriolar components. Shortly after sperm penetration of the oocyte, a sperm aster is formed from the proximal centriole that allows pronuclear apposition. In addition to this pronuclear apposition guiding function, it also serves as a railroad system for the transport of signal transduction molecules. A defective sperm centriole may also be responsible for failed fertilization. As in the case of the OAF, since the functionality of the sperm centriole cannot be assessed in the spermatozoon to be microinjected by ICSI, it can only be assessed using the mouse oocyte-activating test, as it will be described in the last section of this chapter.

Selection Criteria

Based on the biochemical and biological markers selected, the established criteria for sperm selection would be (1) genomic criteria; (2) morphological criteria; and (3) functional criteria.

Genomic Criteria for Selection of the Best Spermatozoa

DNA Integrity

As previously indicated, the selection of spermatozoa with low levels of DNA damage can be accomplished following two different strategies: (1) use of testicular sperm before damage in the epididymis takes place; and (2) selection of ejaculated spermatozoa with low levels of DNA damage. Concerning the second strategy, three different main methodologies can be applied: (1) Annexin-V columns; (2) IMSI; and (3) Confocal light-scattering absorption spectroscopy (CLASS) technology.

Use of Testicular Sperm. Sperm DNA damage observed in ejaculated spermatozoa is produced, for the most part, in the epididymis [3, 7]. That is supported by the fact that in 90 % of the cases, the levels of DNA damage observed in ejaculated spermatozoa are significantly higher than those observed in testicular sperm [3, 6–9]. This DNA damage may either be induced directly by the impact of free radicals on the DNA strands or indirectly through the activation of sperm endonucleases [3]. Since oxygen radicals exported into the extracellular medium have a very short lifespan of the order of nano- to microseconds, in order for extracellular damage to take place, immature sperm must be in close contact with mature sperm. And this is precisely what occurs in the epididymis where sperm are highly packed. In a recent study carried out in infertility patients, it was found that co-incubation of sperm suspensions with PMA-activated polymorphonuclear leukocytes in vitro produces a significant increase in the production of oxygen radicals by immature sperm [26]. The authors of this study conclude that proinflammatory factors produced by activated leukocytes amplify oxygen radical production by immature sperm by two to three orders of magnitude. Therefore, in patients in whom there may be an increase in the levels of proinflammatory factors in the epididymis, e.g., inflammatory or infectious processes, an increase in DNA damage may take place [27]. This explains, at least in part, the beneficial effects of antibiotics in patients with high levels of sperm DNA damage in ejaculated sperm [27].

Since more than 90 % of the DNA is comprised of introns and DNA damage in the fertilizing spermatozoa may be repaired by the oocyte and/or the embryo, the use of testicular sperm should mostly be applied to those couples in which non-repairable DNA damage affects essential sequences, e.g., exons. Since currently, there are no tests available to assess non-repairable sperm DNA damage, and this type of damage should be mostly found in couples with repeated IVF failure without an apparent cause, the use of testicular sperm should be recommended only to these couples and to couples with recurrent miscarriage [3].

Annexin-V Columns. A method recently introduced for the separation and isolation of non-apoptotic and apoptotic sperm is the Annexin-V-conjugated microbeads (ANMB Microbead Kit, Miltenyl Biotec, Germany) coupled to Magnetically Activated Cell Sorting (MACS) columns [28–30]. The principle in which these columns are based is that apoptotic spermatozoa express phosphatidylserine in the outer leaflet of the sperm membrane and bind to Annexin-V. When a magnetic field is applied to the columns, those sperm bound to Annexin-V conjugated to the magnetic microbeads are retained in the column while non-apoptotic sperm go through the column [28]. A recent report by Rawe et al., in which several modifications in the methodology reported by Grunenwald et al., have been introduced, resulting in a significant reduction in the levels of DNA damage with excellent sperm recovery in the negative fraction [31]. Application of this methodology to couples with repeated pregnancy failure without an apparent cause has resulted in the birth of healthy offspring [31]. Tagging cell surface apoptotic markers is part of the screening of genomically defective primary spermatocytes, that are more likely to be aneuploid or have some other structural defects affecting the sperm chromosomes, hence as some of these cells may escape these checkpoints it is conceivable that the Annexin-V columns, in addition to reducing the percentage of spermatozoa with DNA damage, may also help reduce the percentage of aneuploid sperm. This application needs to be tested and validated experimentally.

Confocal Light Absorption Scattering Spectroscopy Microscopy. Confocal Light Absorption Scattering Spectroscopy (CLASS) is a novel technology that allows for the noninvasive visualization of live cells of subcellular structures with diameters between 0.1 and 10 μm using light in the visible spectrum [32]. Therefore, the CLASS technology could be applied to the visualization of sperm chromatin and also for noninvasive embryo selection. These subcellular structures can be identified by two main modes: (1) direct visualization by confocal microscopy or (2) through their specific spectrum. With regard to the applications of the spectral mode in assisted reproductive technologies, a spectroscope would be attached to the inverted microscope and the spectrum of subcellular structures, such as the sperm chromatin, be collected in less than a second. In order to develop the application of the CLASS technology for the selection of spermatozoa with intact DNA, spectral data should be collected concerning chromatin damage in individual spermatozoa exposed to different types of free radicals (ROS and NOS), nucleases, radiation, etc. These spectral data would be incorporated into a library and used for comparison for sperm chromatin evaluation during ICSI. However, caution must be exercised concerning the potential deleterious effects of using these noninvasive technologies, since iatrogenic damage may be induced under some unanticipated conditions. Since time of sperm selection and visible light exposure in the case of the CLASS technology would be limited to about one second, this drawback is more likely to apply to the IMSI technology where sperm selection time is significantly higher.

Chromatin Decondensation

As previously mentioned, the assessment of chromatin decondensation can only be assessed *a posteriori* after failed fertilization is observed. To this end, oocytes are evaluated using the DAPI fluorochrome to stain the condensed pronuclei.

Sperm Aneuploidy Rate and Meiotic Alterations

As indicated previously, defects in synapsis or recombination are normally caught by meiotic checkpoints. Genetically defective germ cells are earmarked for apoptosis followed by cell cycle arrest and elimination by the Sertoli cell. However, some germ cells may be able to escape this screening process and progress through meiosis, resulting in an increased proportion of sperm in the ejaculate with chromosomal abnormalities. Therefore, errors in the meiotic process can result in an increased rate of aneuploid or diploid sperm, affecting the fertilizing ability of these spermatozoa [11–13]. Numerous studies using FISH analysis have demonstrated an increase in the rate of aneuploid and diploid sperm in infertile men [14–16]. Also, a correlation has been suggested between an increase in disomic/diploid sperm and recurrent miscarriage [33, 34]. However, synaptic defects in germ cells are not always correlated with sperm aneuploidy. This may be due to: (1) the normal functioning of the meiotic checkpoints by which these cells are eliminated; (2) to a process of selective elimination of aneuploid sperm in the epididymis, as previously suggested by Blanco et al.; or (3) to the fact that only a limited number of chromosomes are usually evaluated when FISH analysis is performed in ejaculated sperm [35].

The recommended methodology to be used for the assessment of genomic anomalies related to sperm aneuploidy or telomeric defects are the study of FISH in semen and the study of meiosis in testicular biopsy. Should the FISH test result be abnormal, PGS for all chromosomes, either by array-CGH or FISH on day-3 embryos is recommended. If the FISH test result is normal, a study of meiosis in testicular biopsy should be performed. If abnormal, PGS should be recommended. In a recent observational study reported by García et al., in couples with repeated pregnancy failure after IVF with an apparent cause, the presence of synaptic anomalies in testicular biopsy in these couples was associated with implantation rates of 4 % and pregnancy rates of 8.9 %. When PGS for 12 chromosomes was performed in these couples, implantation and pregnancy rates increased to 40 % and 55 %, respectively [17].

Morphological Criteria

Phase-Contrast Microscopy

Following the introduction of the Tygerberg criteria in the early 1990s, a significant improvement in fertilization and pregnancy rates in IVF was observed. According to these criteria, when sperm selection during ICSI at 400× was based on the presence of an oval-shaped sperm head, a longitudinal diameter between 3.5 and 4.5 μm, a sperm width of 2.5–3.5 μm and an axial insertion of the flagellum in the head. Solely based on the implementation of these criteria, a significant improvement in IVF outcome could be observed.

Although the presence of normal forms as general rule is associated with low rates of sperm aneuploidy, this cannot be generalized. In a report by Burrello et al., it was shown that if normal forms were associated with low rates of aneuploidy in ejaculated spermatozoa from normozoospermic males, in oligozoospermic males, normal forms were associated with relatively high rates of sperm aneuploidy [36]. Therefore, normal sperm forms can only be used as selection criteria for euploid sperm when using normozoospermic semen samples. Since non-axial insertion of the flagellum has been reported to be associated with ultrastructural defects of the sperm proximal centriole, sperm selection during ICSI can be used as morphological criteria for the selection of sperm with a functional proximal centriole, at least as a general approach. Another example is the presence of sperm with globozoospermia. It has been shown that microinjection of sperm with type I globozoospermia also resulted in either partial or total failure of oocyte fertilization, but in this case due to lack of activity of the OAF [37].

Hyaluronic Acid Binding Assay

Since binding of sperm to hyaluronic acid has been related to higher sperm quality, in terms of sperm morphology and sperm maturity, the hyaluronic binding assay can be used for the selection of morphological normal spermatozoa for ICSI [38]. In addition, since the hyaluronic acid binding assay (HBA) has also been reported to be associated with an improvement in the enrichment of sperm with intact DNA and lower rates of aneuploidy, it could also used as a method for the selection of genomically normal sperm. In fact, some reports have suggested the potential utility of hyaluronic acid binding in the selection of sperm with normal morphology and lower rates of aneuploidy [39, 40]. Furthermore, since finding of sperm with none or a low number of small vacuoles during IMSI may be a time-consuming task, preselection of morphologically normal spermatozoa using the HBA may be of significant benefit during sperm election by IMSI. Should HBA result in an enrichment of sperm with a reduced nuclear malformation according to IMSI, this will significantly increase the efficiency of IMSI by reducing the time employed in sperm selection during IMSI. The recommended format for the HBA application for selection in ICSI is the Sperm Slow® test. However, in these studies only a limited number of chromosomes were evaluated. Therefore, further studies are required in order to validate these observations in terms of both improved morphology, as assessed by IMSI, and lower aneuploidy rate through the analysis of all 23 chromosomes, respectively. The Hyaluronic Acid Binding tests are covered in more detail in Chap. 8.

Intracytoplasmic Morphologically Selected Sperm Injection (IMSI)

The technique of Intracytoplasmic Morphologically Selected Sperm Injection (IMSI) has been recently introduced for the selection of sperm for ICSI. Several publications report that the selection of spermatozoa with normal head morphology at high magnification is positively associated with pregnancy rates after day-3 embryo transfer in couples with repeated implantation failures and in patients with high levels of sperm DNA fragmentation [41–44]. Berkovitz et al. analyzed more specifically the impact of nuclear vacuoles in the head of spermatozoa on pregnancy outcome [45]. They concluded that spermatozoa with normal nuclear shape and with large vacuoles negatively influence pregnancy and implantation rates as compared with a control group containing spermatozoa with normal head morphology. Furthermore, they demonstrated an association between defective spermatozoa and higher early abortion rates, despite no apparent decrease in embryo quality on day-3. However, the relationship between the number of vacuoles in the head region of sperm and DNA fragmentation has yet to be established although a recent report by Gosalvez et al. indicates that lower rates of sperm DNA damage are associated with sperm with less than two small vacuoles. Preliminary results reported in this study indicate that sperm with $\leq$1 small vacuole have the chromatin intact while sperm with $\geq$2 vacuoles have DNA damage (J. Gosalvez, personal communication) (Fig. 1).

However, these preliminary results should be confirmed in larger series of cases in order to validate the application of IMSI for the selection

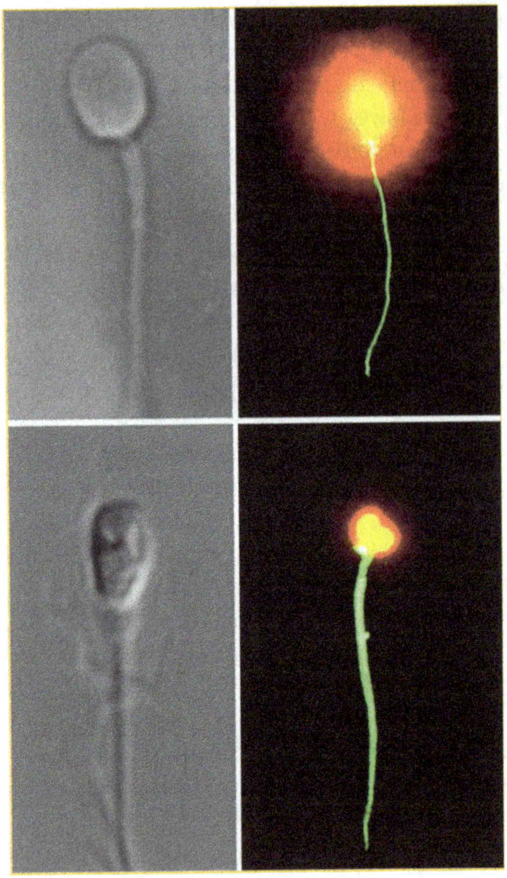

Fig. 9.1 The upper panels correspond to a sperm cell with no vacuoles as visualized by IMSI (*upper left*) with intact chromatin (*upper right*), as measured by the Halosperm test. The *lower panels* correspond to a defective sperm cell with large vacuoles as visualized by IMSI (*lower left*) with fragmented DNA (*lower right*)

of spermatozoa with low levels of DNA damage. Since one of the main indications proposed for the use of IMSI in assisted reproductive technologies is in patients with teratozoospermia and the percentage of spermatozoa with less than two small vacuoles is exceedingly low in these patients, future studies should focus on the correlation between sperm DNA damage and the presence of less than four to five small vacuoles in order for this methodology to be of any significant clinical use in IVF.

Functional Criteria

Mouse Oocyte Activation Test

A heterologous ICSI of human sperm into mouse oocytes (mouse oocyte activation test, MOAT) for diagnosing sperm- or oocyte-related activation deficiencies has been reported [37]. According to this test, motile human sperm are immobilized by touching their tails with a blunt injection needle against the bottom of the dish. After deep invagination of the oocyte membrane with the injection needle (inner diameter 5–6 mm) through the slit made by PZD, the oolemma is broken by gentle suction. Cytoplasm is aspirated and then returned into the oocyte together with the spermatozoon. In the negative control, sham injection of injection medium (KSOM-HEPES þ PVP) is performed. Oocyte activation is assessed around 44 h post-hCG by examining the percentage of two-cell formation (number of two cells versus the number of surviving injected oocytes). As a standard, the positive control must show >90 % two-cell formation while both the negative control and medium control groups must show <10 % two-cell formation before MOAT results can be considered as reliable [37]. In those cases in which a potential oocyte activation defect is found with the MOAT, assisted oocyte activation using the Ca2þ ionophore could be an efficacious way of managing rare cases of fertilization failure after ICSI. In fact, the MOAT can differentiate between sperm- and oocyte-related factors in fertilization failure thus having some prognostic value. The best results can be expected when the MOAT test indicates a deficiency of the sperm oocyte-activating factor as in cases of globozoospermia [37]. When the MOAT is normal it is assumed that the fertilization failure is due to an undisclosed oocyte factor. Poor or absent fertilization in these cases could also be the result of some transient biological reasons or technical imperfections. Although optimal results can be obtained with freshly obtained oocytes, frozen mouse or hamster oocytes can also be used.

Conclusion

Based on the selection criteria established herein, a number of techniques can be used for the selection and isolation of the best spermatozoa. Using the genomic criteria of DNA integrity, five main techniques are proposed which include TESA, the Annexin-V columns, HBA assay, IMSI, and the CLASS technology. Since the performance characteristics of sperm DNA fragmentation testing are relatively poor using the tests currently available (low sensitivity, low specificity, and low positive and negative predictive values), the use of these techniques in assisted reproductive technologies, rather than based on the test result of these tests, should be solely based on clinical indications. The main indication for the use of these selection techniques should be idiopathic pregnancy failure in IVF and recurrent miscarriage. Although preliminary results suggest that IMSI may have some applications in the selection of sperm with intact DNA, additional studies are required to confirm these preliminary findings. The same applies to the HBA assay. Although the applications of the CLASS technology in the selection of sperm with intact chromatin are very promising, this technique is still under development and, therefore, we should wait until its safety and efficacy are fully confirmed. Although the applications of the HBA assay and IMSI in the selection of spermatozoa with intact chromatin are yet to be validated, these techniques have been shown to have positive outcomes on the selection of morphologically normal spermatozoa. Based on either morphological (e.g., teratozoospermia) or clinical criteria (idiopathic pregnancy failure in IVF), these techniques certainly have great utility in the selection of the best spermatozoa for assisted reproductive technologies.

Using the genomic criteria of sperm aneuploidy and meiotic alterations, two main techniques are proposed for sperm selection: the study of FISH in semen and the study of meiosis in testicular biopsy. Should the test result of any of these studies be abnormal, PGS for all chromosomes, either by array-CGH or FISH on day-3 embryos should be recommended. Finally, although it cannot be considered a sperm selection technique per se, the MOAT could be used as a diagnostic test to evaluate the functionality of the proximal centriole and of the oocyte-activating factor in cases of failed fertilization in conventional IVF and ICSI.

References

1. Huret JL. Nuclear chromatin decondensation of human sperm: a review. Arch Androl. 1986;16:97–109.
2. Reyes R, Rosado A, Hernandez O, Delgado NM. Heparin and glutathione: physiological decondensing agents of human sperm nuclei. Gamete Res. 1989;23:39–47.
3. Sakkas D, Alvarez JG. Sperm DNA fragmentation: mechanisms of origin, impact on reproductive outcome, and analysis. Fertil Steril. 2010;93:1027–36.
4. Matsuda Y, Tobari I. Chromosomal analysis in mouse eggs fertilized in vitro with sperm exposed to ultraviolet light and methyl and ethyl methansulfonate. Mutat Res. 1988;198:131–44.
5. Brandriff B, Pedersen RA. Repair of the ultraviolet-irradiated male genome in fertilized mouse eggs. Science. 1981;211:1431–3.
6. Steele EK, McClure N, Maxwell RJ, Lewis SE. A comparison of DNA damage in testicular and proximal epididymal spermatozoa in obstructive azoospermia. Mol Hum Reprod. 1999;5:831–5.
7. Ollero M, Gil-Guzman E, Lopez MC, Sharma RK, Agarwal A, Larson K, et al. Characterization of subsets of human spermatozoa at different stages of maturation: implications in the diagnosis and treatment of male infertility. Hum Reprod. 2011;16:1912–21.
8. Greco E, Scarselli F, Iacobelli M, Rienzi L, Ubaldi F, Ferrero S, et al. Efficient treatment of infertility due to sperm DNA damage by ICSI with testicular spermatozoa. Hum Reprod. 2005;20:226–30.
9. Alvarez JG. Efficient treatment of infertility due to sperm DNA damage by ICSI with testicular sperm. Hum Reprod. 2005;20:2031–2.
10. Moskovtsev SI, Jarvi K, Mullen JB, Cadesky KI, Hannam T, Lo KC. Testicular spermatozoa have statistically significant lower DNA damage compared with ejaculated spermatozoa in patients with unsuccessful oral antioxidant treatment. Fertil Steril. 2010;93:1142–6.
11. Egozcue J, Sarrate Z, Codina-Pascual M, Egozcue S, Oliver-Bonet M, Blanco J, et al. Meiotic abnormalities in infertile males. Cytogenet Genome Res. 2005;111(3–4):337–42.
12. Martin RH. Meiotic chromosome abnormalities in human spermatogenesis. Reprod Toxicol. 2006;22:142–7.

13. Ferguson KA, Wong EC, Chow V, Nigro M, Ma S. Abnormal meiotic recombination in infertile men and its association with sperm aneuploidy. Hum Mol Genet. 2007;16:2870–9.
14. Aran B, Blanco J, Vidal F, Vendrell J, Egozcue S, Barri P, et al. Screening for abnormalities of chromosomes X, Y, and 18 and for diploidy in spermatozoa from infertile men participating in an in vitro fertilization-intracytoplasmic sperm injection program. Fertil Steril. 1999;72:696–701.
15. Vendrell JM, Garcia F, Veiga A, Calderon G, Egozcue S, Egozcue J, et al. Meiotic abnormalities and spermatogenic parameters in severe oligoasthenozoospermia. Hum Reprod. 1999;14:375–8.
16. Pang M, Hoegerman S, Cuticchia A, Moon S, Doncel G, Acosta Giorlandino C, et al. Spermatozoa with chromosomal abnormalities may result in a higher rate of recurrent abortion. Fertil Steril. 1998;70: 576–7.
17. Garcia F, Alvarez JG, Velilla E, Fernandez S, Lopez-Teijon M. Clinical value of the study of meiosis in testicular biopsy. Rev J Androl. (in press).
18. Billig H, Chun SY, Eisenhauer K, Hsueh AJ. Gonadal cell apoptosis: hormone-regulated cell demise. Hum Reprod Update. 1996;2:103–17.
19. Hande MP, Samper E, Lansdorp P, Blasco MA. Telomere length dynamics and chromosomal instability in cells derived from telomerase null mice. J Cell Biol. 1999;144:589–601.
20. Shakirov EV, Surovtseva YV, Osbun N, Shippen DE. The Arabidopsis Pot1 and Pot2 proteins function in telomere length homeostasis and chromosome end protection. Mol Cell Biol. 2005;25:7725–33.
21. Shore D. Telomeric chromatin: replicating and wrapping up chromosome ends. Curr Opin Genet Dev. 2001;11:189–98.
22. Greider CW. Telomere length regulation. Annu Rev Biochem. 1996;65:337–65.
23. Artandi SE, Chang S, Lee SL, Alson S, Gottlieb GJ, Chin L, et al. Telomere dysfunction promotes non-reciprocal translocations and epithelial cancers in mice. Nature. 2000;406:641–5.
24. Swann K, Saunders CM, Rogers NT, Lai FA. PLCζ(zeta): a sperm protein that triggers Ca^{2+} oscillations and egg activation in mammals. Semin Cell Dev Biol. 2006;17:264–73.
25. Schatten H, Sun QY. The role of centrosomes in fertilization, cell division and establishment of asymmetry during embryo development. Semin Cell Dev Biol. 2010;21:174–84.
26. Saleh RA, Agarwal A, Kandirali E, Sharma RK, Thomas AJ, Nada EA, et al. Leukocytospermia is associated with increased reactive oxygen species production by human spermatozoa. Fertil Steril. 2002;78:1215–24.
27. Gallegos G, Ramos B, Santiso R, Goyanes V, Gosálvez J, Fernández JL. Sperm DNA fragmentation in infertile men with genitourinary infection by Chlamydia trachomatis and Mycoplasma. Fertil Steril. 2008;90: 328–34.
28. Grunewald S, Paasch U, Glander HJ. Enrichment of non-apoptotic human spermatozoa after cryopreservation by immunomagnetic cell sorting. Cell Tissue Bank. 2001;2:127–33.
29. Said TM, Grunewald S, Paasch U, Glander HJ, Baumann T, Kriegel C, et al. Advantage of combining magnetic cell separation with sperm preparation techniques. Reprod Biomed Online. 2005;10:740–6.
30. Said T, Agarwal A, Grunewald S, Rasch M, Baumann T, Kriegel C, et al. Selection of nonapoptotic spermatozoa as a new tool for enhancing assisted reproduction outcomes: an in vitro model. Biol Reprod. 2006; 74:530–7.
31. Rawe VY, Boudri HU, Alvarez Sedó C, Carro M, Papier S, Nodar F. Healthy baby born after reduction of sperm DNA fragmentation using cell sorting before ICSI. Reprod Biomed Online. 2010;20:320–3.
32. Itzkan I, Qiu L, Fang H, Zaman MM, Vitkin E, Ghiran IC, et al. Confocal light absorption and scattering spectroscopic microscopy monitors organelles in live cells with no exogenous labels. Proc Natl Acad Sci USA. 2007;104:17255–60.
33. Giorlandino C, Calugi G, Iaconianni L, Santoro ML, Lippa A. Spermatozoa with chromosomal abnormalities may result in a higher rate of recurrent abortion. Fertil Steril. 1998;70:576–7.
34. Rubio C, Simón C, Blanco J, Vidal F, Mínguez Y, Egozcue J, et al. Implications of sperm chromosome abnormalities in recurrent miscarriage. J Assist Reprod Genet. 1999;16:253–8.
35. Blanco J, Farreras A, Egozcue J, Vidal F. Meiotic behavior of the sex chromosomes in a 45, X/46, X, r(Y)/46, X, dic r(Y) patient whose semen was assessed by fluorescence in situ hybridization. Fertil Steril. 2003;79:913–8.
36. Burrello N, Arcidiacono G, Vicari E, Asero P, Di Benedetto D, De Palma A, et al. Morphologically normal spermatozoa of patients with secretory oligo-astheno-teratozoospermia have an increased aneuploidy rate. Hum Reprod. 2004;19:2298–302.
37. Heindryckx B, De Gheselle S, Gerris J, Dhont M, De Sutter P. Efficiency of assisted oocyte activation as a solution for failed intracytoplasmic sperm injection. Reprod Biomed Online. 2008;17:662–8.
38. Huszar G, Ozkavukcu S, Jakab A, Celik-Ozenci C, Sati GL, Cayli S. Hyaluronic acid binding ability of human sperm reflects cellular maturity and fertilizing potential: selection of sperm for intracytoplasmic sperm injection. Curr Opin Obstet Gynecol. 2006;18: 260–7.
39. Jakab A, Sakkas D, Delpiano E, Cayli S, Kovanci E, Ward D, et al. Intracytoplasmic sperm injection: a novel selection method for sperm with normal frequency of chromosomal aneuploidies. Fertil Steril. 2005;84:1665–73.
40. Huszar G, Jakab A, Sakkas D, Ozenci CC, Cayli S, Delpiano E, et al. Fertility testing and ICSI sperm selection by hyaluronic acid binding: clinical and genetic aspects. Reprod Biomed Online. 2007;14: 650–63.

41. Bartoov B, Berkovitz A, Eltes F, et al. 2003 Pregnancy rates are higher with intracytoplasmic morphologically selected sperm injection than with conventional intracytoplasmic injection. Fertil Steril. 2003;80:1413–9.
42. Berkovitz A, Eltes F, Lederman H, et al. How to improve IVF–ICSI outcome by sperm injection? Reprod Biomed Online. 2006;12:634–8.
43. Junca AM, Cohen-Bacrie P, Hazout A. Improvement of fertilisation and pregnancy rate after intracytoplasmic fine morphology selected sperm injection. Fertil Steril. 2004;82 Suppl 2:S173.
44. Berkovitz A, Eltes F, Ellenbogen A, et al. Does the presence of nuclear vacuoles in human sperm selected for ICSI affect pregnancy outcome? Hum Reprod. 2006;21:1787–90.
45. Hazout A, Dumomt-Hassant M, Junca AM, et al. High-magnification ICSI overcomes paternal effect resistant to conventional ICSI. Reprod Biomed Online. 2006;12:19–25.

The Origins of Aneuploidy in Human Embryos

10

Elpida Fragouli and Joy Delhanty

Humans as a species are not as efficient in reproducing compared to other mammals. Specifically, a couple of proven fertility will achieve a viable pregnancy in only 20–25 % of all natural cycles [1, 2]. This rate decreases during in vitro fertilisation (IVF) cycles as only approximately 13 % of all morphologically normal embryos transferred will go on to produce a live birth [3]. One of the main causes of these relatively low reproductive success rates seen in humans is numerical chromosome abnormalities (aneuploidy). The advent of IVF and associated diagnostic methods such as preimplantation genetic diagnosis (PGD) and screening (PGS) enabled a detailed investigation of the chromosome content of human gametes and embryos. Such investigations clearly showed that the incidence of numerical chromosome abnormalities was high and as would be expected had an adverse impact on the progress of embryo development and viability [4, 5].

Embryonic aneuploidy can have a meiotic origin with chromosome malsegregation taking place during gametogenesis, and a post-zygotic origin with abnormalities occurring after fertilisation. Direct analysis of the human female gamete using a variety of cytogenetic methods has shown that the majority of meiotically derived aneuploidies arise during oogenesis. The close relationship between advancing female age and increasing aneuploidy rates was also confirmed, as more than 50 % of oocytes generated by women over the age of 40 years were demonstrated to be chromosomally abnormal [6–12]. Graphs illustrating the changing oocyte aneuploidy rate with advancing maternal age are a mirror image of those showing the declining implantation rate of IVF embryos with age, suggesting that the increase in meiotic errors might explain the reduced success rate of IVF treatments for women in their late 30s and 40s.

The contribution of aneuploidy of male meiotic origin to the embryo is not as clear. Several studies have been carried out and examined the chromosome complement of sperm generated by fertile as well as infertile men. What was concluded was that the incidence of chromosome anomalies ranged between 3 and 5 % in the sperm of fertile men, but significantly (approximately threefold) increased in the sperm obtained by infertile men [13].

Two different preimplantation development stages have been examined in order to establish the frequency of aneuploidy arising after fertilisation. These are the cleavage stage, which is reached 3 days after fertilisation when the embryo consists of 6–8 totipotent cells called blastomeres, and the blastocyst stage. Embryos become

E. Fragouli (✉)
Nuffield Department of Obstetrics and Gynaecology, University of Oxford, Oxford, UK

Reprogenetics UK, Oxford, UK
e-mail: elpida.fragouli@obs-gyn.ox.ac.uk

J. Delhanty
Fetal and Maternal Medicine, Institute for Women's Health, University College, 86-96 Chenies Mews, London, UK

D.K. Gardner et al. (eds.), *Human Gametes and Preimplantation Embryos: Assessment and Diagnosis*, DOI 10.1007/978-1-4614-6651-2_10, © Springer Science+Business Media New York 2013

blastocysts 5–6 days after fertilisation and consist of two different cell types, the outer trophectoderm (TE) and the inner cell mass (ICM). Studies investigating these two different preimplantation development stages have suggested that post-zygotic chromosome anomalies take place even more frequently compared to the meiotic ones, especially at the cleavage stage [14–17]. A result of post-zygotic anomalies is chromosome mosaicism, the presence of two or more karyotypically distinct cell lines within the same embryo.

During this chapter, the data obtained from cytogenetic investigations of human oocytes, sperm and also embryos at the cleavage and blastocyst stage of preimplantation development will be summarised. In addition, the different mechanisms leading to aneuploidy of meiotic and post-zygotic origin will be described and their frequencies and impact on embryonic survival will be discussed.

Aneuploidy of Female Meiotic Origin

It has been demonstrated that the vast majority of meiotic chromosome abnormalities in the embryo originate from the oocyte. As they mature, both the male and female gametes begin a specialised cellular division called meiosis. As a result, the diploid chromosome number is reduced by half, leading to the formation of haploid gametes.

Meiosis is separated into two different divisions, meiosis I (MI) and II (MII). The whole process starts with the replication of DNA during S phase, leading to the generation of two sister chromatids. During MI the homologous chromosomes align, and exchange of material between the chromatids of different homologues may occur. At the end of MI, bivalents separate, with homologues travelling to opposite poles of the meiotic spindle, one entering the first polar body (PB) while the other stays in the oocyte. During MI, sister chromatids are held together, and it is not until MII that they are finally separated, one of the chromatids passing into the second PB, the other remaining in the oocyte. The end result is the generation of haploid gametes, sperm cells in the male and an oocyte and two PBs in the female. Figure 1 describes the normal segregation of chromosomes during meiosis.

There are three different stages during which a chromosome could malsegregate and cause aneuploidy in the embryo. These are the initial set of premeiotic mitotic divisions, MI and MII. Two different mechanisms of oocyte chromosome malsegregation have been described, whole chromosome nondisjunction and unbalanced chromatid predivision.

Whole chromosome nondisjunction occurs in MI as well as MII and is the result of homologous chromosomes not segregating to opposite poles of the meiotic spindle, but instead moving together towards the same pole. As a result, an oocyte with an extra chromosome is generated whereas the corresponding PB (either the first or second) is missing this chromosome, or vice versa. Risk factors associated with this aneuploidy-causing mechanism depend on the chromosome and the meiotic division, but generally include the number and positioning of the chiasmata in relation to the centromere (too proximal or too distal). It is also believed that female age has differing effects on the various recombination patterns predisposing to nondisjunction [11, 18].

Unbalanced chromatid predivision was described when a group of researchers in their analysis of metaphase II oocytes noticed that some cells consisted of an extra one or two single chromatids [19, 20]. This observation led them to suggest that imbalance can result from premature division (predivision) of the chromosome centromere after which chromatids segregate at random, potentially moving to the same pole at anaphase of MII [19, 20]. Both whole chromosome nondisjunction and unbalanced chromatid predivision are illustrated in Figs. 2 and 3 respectively.

Both whole chromosome and single chromatid malsegregation have been shown to be active and responsible for anomalies of female meiotic origin. The difference between them is that whole chromosome nondisjunction will produce an aneuploid oocyte and subsequent embryo in all cases, whereas a single chromatid abnormality will result to embryonic aneuploidy in 50 % of cases, depending initially on whether the unattached

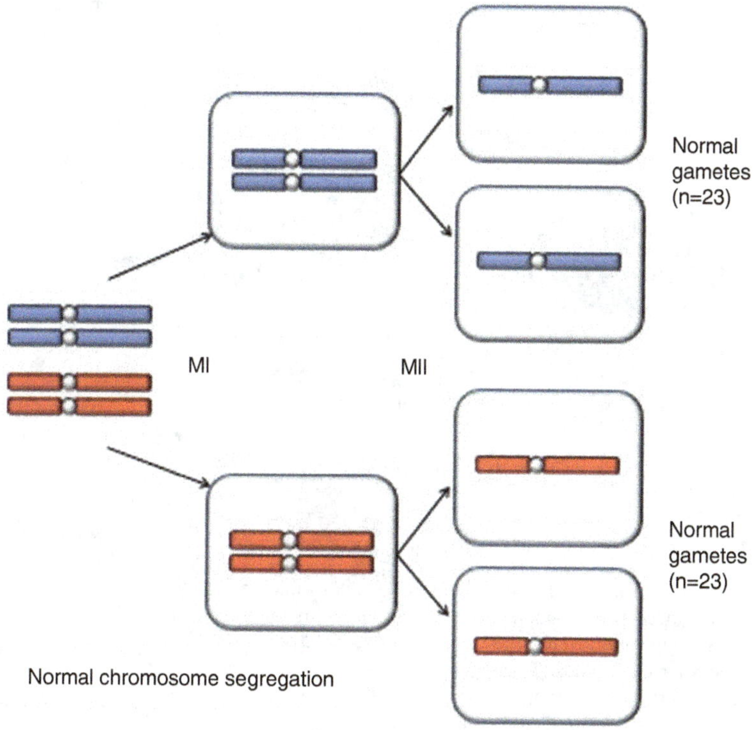

Fig. 10.1 Normal chromosome segregation during meiosis. Meiosis is made up of two divisions, MI and MII. During prophase I, the 46 chromosomes condense and form 23 homologous pairs of bivalents. Formation of chiasmata and exchange of genetic material between homologues follows. During metaphase I, these bivalents align on the metaphase plate orientated by attachment to the spindle. They then disjoin and segregate to the resulting daughter cells at anaphase I and telophase I. MI is a reduction division, whereas MII is a mitotic type of division during which chromosomes align once again on the metaphase II spindle. Separation and segregation of sister chromatids to opposite poles follows at anaphase II and telophase II. Cytokinesis produces four haploid products. (From Fragouli E, Wells D, Delhanty JD. Chromosome abnormalities in the human oocyte. Cytogenet Genome Res. 2011;133 (2–4):107–18, with permission.)

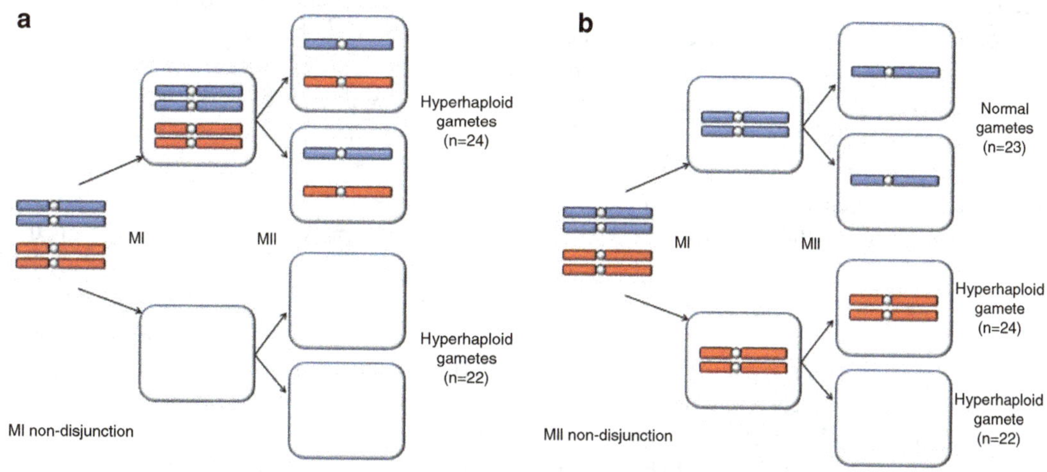

Fig. 10.2 Whole chromosome non-disjunction. The first aneuploidy-causing mechanism could take place during MI (**a**) and also MII (**b**). It involves the segregation of entire chromosomes towards the same pole of the meiotic spindle which leads to the formation of disomic and nullisomic gametes. (From Fragouli E, Wells D, Delhanty JD. Chromosome abnormalities in the human oocyte. Cytogenet Genome Res. 2011;133 (2–4):107–18, with permission.)

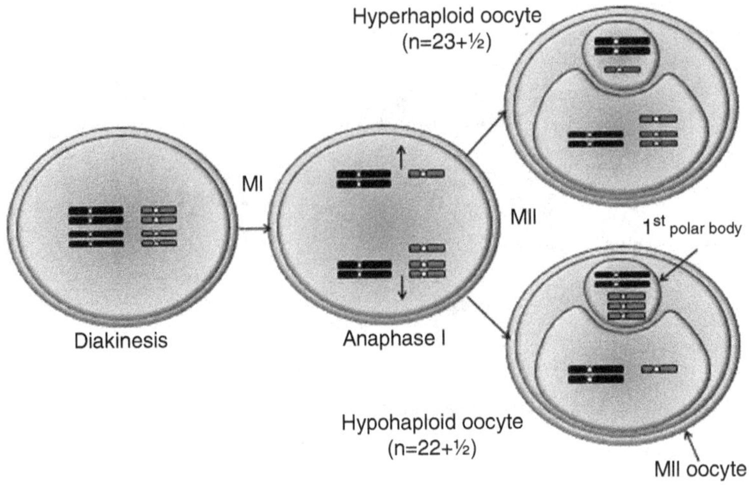

Fig. 10.3 Unbalanced chromatid predivision. This second aneuploidy-causing mechanism could take place only during MI and involves the premature separation of a chromosome into its sister chromatids. These are subsequently distributed at random during anaphase I. Unbalanced chromatid predivision could have as an effect the formation of gametes which have either an extra or a missing chromatid. (From Fragouli E, Wells D, Delhanty JD. Chromosome abnormalities in the human oocyte. Cytogenet Genome Res. 2011;133 (2–4):107–18, with permission.)

chromatids segregate to opposite spindle poles or move together towards the same pole, and finally on events at anaphase II after fertilisation. As with whole chromosome nondisjunction, absent or altered recombination, combined with advancing maternal age, predispose oocytes to become aneuploid via random segregation of single chromatids.

To elucidate the causal mechanisms of maternally derived aneuploidy, researchers employed several different cytogenetic methods to examine human oocytes and/or their corresponding PBs. The following sections will summarise findings for MI and MII obtained with the use of classical and molecular cytogenetic methods.

Meiosis I

Classical cytogenetic techniques such as G and R-banding, along with various molecular methods such as fluorescence in situ hybridisation (FISH), spectral karyotyping (SKY) and comparative genomic hybridisation [metaphase, (CGH) or array (aCGH)] have been employed for the study of MI. For this purpose, oocytes arrested at the metaphase II stage of development and, whenever available, their corresponding first PBs have been examined.

The largest data set of karyotyped metaphase II oocytes was reported by Pellestor et al. [8]. Specifically, a total of 1,397 oocytes were analysed with the use of R-banding. These were donated by 792 women undergoing IVF with an average age of ~34 years (age range 19–46 years). Of all the examined oocytes, chromosome errors were scored in 10.8 %. This investigation confirmed the expected relationship between advancing female age and global aneuploidy rate. It was also concluded that advancing age had a more pronounced effect on the predivision and unbalanced segregation of single chromatids [8]. This study along with data obtained from similar investigations clearly showed that smaller chromosomes, belonging to groups D–G, were more frequently participating in aneuploidy events [8, 21–24]. The poor morphology of oocyte metaphase preparations, however, made the exact identification of individual chromosomes difficult. The use of a different molecular cytogenetic method, FISH, solved this problem.

FISH is advantageous over classical karyotyping methods because it can yield results regardless of the quality of the cell under analysis. Using FISH, it was not only possible to examine the chromosomes of the metaphase II oocyte, but also those of the even more challenging first PB. The chromosomes targeted were selected on the basis of data obtained from the analysis of miscarriages and abnormal live births, and generally included smaller size ones (starting from 13 onwards).

A combination of the larger chromosomes 1, 9, 12 and X and the smaller 13, 16, 18 and 21 were investigated during the course of two different studies carried out by our group [25, 26]. A three-round FISH protocol was employed and a total of 236 spare, mostly unfertilised oocytes and their corresponding first PBs were analysed. These were donated by 124 patients, whose average maternal age was 32.5 years (age range 22–44 years). Only gains of chromosomes were scored, as it was considered that chromosome loss could be due to the spreading of the oocyte and/or PB on the microscope slide. The hyperploidy rate was calculated to be approximately 4 %, the smaller chromosomes 13, 16, 18 and 21 were mostly affected, and both whole chromosome nondisjunction and unbalanced chromatid predivision were identified to be active. Moreover, a third aneuploidy-causing mechanism was observed, involving the presence of a trisomic cell line in the gonads of some patients (germinal/gonadal mosaicism) [25, 26].

The use of alternative cytogenetic methods such as SKY enabled the analysis of all 23 chromosomes of human oocytes. Sandalinas and colleagues employed SKY to examine 47 fresh non-inseminated metaphase II oocytes, donated by 16 patients with a female age range of 24–48 years [6]. A total of 9 whole chromosome nondisjunction events were observed, along with 11 errors involving single chromatids. Chromosomes 9, 11, 12, 14, 18, 20, 21 and 22 were affected. More importantly, 12 different oocytes with balanced chromatid predivision were observed. It was therefore confirmed that this type of abnormality is real and not an artefact of oocyte ageing in culture, and it is closely associated with advancing female age and decreasing chromosome size [6].

Even though classical karyotyping, FISH and SKY are all capable of accurately examining the chromosomes of human oocytes, their main disadvantage is that they all require the spreading of a single cell arrested in metaphase on a microscope slide, risking in this way the artefactual loss of chromosomes. Clearly an alternative cytogenetic method, which could not only avoid spreading but could examine all 23 chromosomes as well, was needed. Ultimately, this was achieved by a combination of whole genome amplification (WGA) and CGH [27, 28]. CGH is related to FISH and employs simultaneous hybridisation of differentially labelled DNA samples (sample DNA: green; chromosomally normal reference DNA: red) to normal metaphase chromosomes. The ratio of green:red fluorescence along the length of each chromosome indicates whether there has been any gain or loss of chromosomal material in the test sample.

The first application of this approach took place in a clinical context, and involved the chromosome complement analysis of ten first PBs biopsied from oocytes generated by a 40-year old IVF patient with a history of repeated implantation failure (RIF) [29]. CGH was further validated and used to examine larger sets of metaphase II oocytes and their corresponding first PBs, by our group and others [9, 10]. During our investigation, 107 oocyte-PB complexes were analysed via CGH. These were donated by 46 women who were undergoing routine IVF procedures, and whose average age was 32.5 years (range 18–42 years). It was evident from the obtained results that aneuploidy frequently affected even the larger chromosomes (1–12), as well as the smaller ones. Both aneuploidy-causing mechanisms, i.e. whole chromosome nondisjunction and unbalanced predivision of single chromatids were observed, and the resulting aneuploidy rate was 22 %. Interestingly, the larger chromosomes (1–12) participated solely in whole chromosome nondisjunction events, whereas a combination of whole chromosome and single chromatid anomalies were seen for smaller chromosomes (13 onwards) and

Table 10.1 Studies examining the incidence of oocyte aneuploidy after completion of the first meiotic division (MI)

Study	Average female age (age range)	Method used	No. of oocytes examined	No. of first PBs examined	MI aneuploidy rate
Pellestor et al. [8]	33.7 years (19–46 years)	R-banding	1,397	Not examined	10.8 %
Cupisti et al. [26]	32.5 years (22–44 years)	FISH	236	88	7.6 % (3.8 % hyperploidy)
Sandalinas et al. [6]	35 years (24–48 years)	SKY	47	Not examined	38 %
Gutierrez-Mateo et al. [9]	33.2 years (21–41 years)	CGH	30	30	48 %
Fragouli et al. [10]	32.5 years (18–42 years)	CGH	93	107	22 %

chromosome X. CGH was also capable of accurately detecting structural abnormalities resulting from chromosome breakage. Additionally, evidence of age-independent factors influencing aneuploidy of MI origin was provided, with certain patients exhibiting unexpectedly high frequencies of abnormal oocytes [10].

In summary, studies using a variety of cytogenetic methods to examine human oocytes have uniformly shown that even though all chromosomes can be affected by MI malsegregation errors, there seems to be a preferential involvement of the smaller ones. Combining data obtained in a research and clinical setting suggests that for an average female age of 32 years, the expected MI aneuploidy rate is in the range of 22 % and can increase to over 45 % for women of an average age of 40 years or more [9, 10, 30, 31]. Table 1 shows a summary of results obtained during the analysis of metaphase II oocytes using methods such as karyotyping, FISH and CGH.

Meiosis II

Mature oocytes are arrested at the metaphase stage of the second meiotic division (MII). At this stage oocytes consist of 23 chromosomes with sister chromatids held together at the centromeres. Fertilisation leads to resumption of MII, followed by centromere separation. As a result, 23 chromatids remain in the fertilised oocyte, while the other 23 move to the second PB, which is extruded soon after oocyte activation. As it would be difficult to directly examine the fertilised oocyte, data on the incidence of MII aneuploidy has been obtained almost exclusively from the investigation of the second PB. FISH, CGH and recently aCGH, have all been used to examine MII [7, 12, 32, 33].

Verlinsky and colleagues have reported FISH results from large numbers of first as well as second PBs [7, 32]. Five different chromosomes were targeted, namely 13, 16, 18, 21 and 22 in a single hybridisation round. It was shown for the first time that women of advanced reproductive age generate oocytes carrying an almost equal amount of MI and MII chromosomes errors (41.8 % and 37.3 % respectively). They also reported findings on the meiotic origin of abnormalities affecting chromosomes 16 and 18 that contradict data obtained from analysis of spontaneous abortion material. Specifically, such studies demonstrated that most abnormalities affecting chromosome 16 have an MI origin, and those affecting 18 originate during MII [34–36], whereas the complete opposite was observed from the FISH analysis of first and second PBs. Another important finding was that almost one third (32.5 %) of oocytes classified as abnormal due to an MI chromatid error led to the formation of apparently normal zygotes, following segregation of the chromatid to the second PB in MII [7, 32].

FISH analysis of second PBs provided a valuable insight into the frequency and type of MII chromosome malsegregation errors. However, as with MI, PBs were spread on microscope slides,

Table 10.2 Studies examining the incidence of oocyte aneuploidy after completion of the second meiotic division (MII)

Study	Average female age (age range)	Method used	No. of first PBs examined	MII aneuploidy rate (%)
Kuliev and Verlinsky [32]	38.5 years (19–46 years)	FISH	7,103	37.3
Fragouli et al. [12]	39.8 years (35–44 years)	CGH	117	45.8

risking the artefactual loss of chromosome material, and only 5 of the 23 chromosomes were examined. In a more recent investigation, CGH was applied to analyse first and second PBs biopsied from a total of 117 zygotes generated by couples with a poor reproductive history [12]. The total meiotic aneuploidy rate was 65.5 % and this was seen for an average maternal age of 39.8 years. It was evident from the obtained results that anomalies of MII origin occurred slightly more frequently, compared to those taking place during MI (45.8 % and 36.5 % respectively), and as with the FISH data, the mechanism of MII 'correction' of MI chromatid errors was also observed. Combining the MI and MII cytogenetic data predicted that 60 % of abnormalities would lead to a trisomy in the resulting embryo. The fact that chromosome losses in the PBs were more frequent than gains suggests that anaphase lag or chromosome failure to congress on the spindle is a significant aneuploidy-causing mechanism. Additionally, it was demonstrated that MII malsegregation errors affected chromosomes from all groups, but the smaller 16, 21, 22, 15 and 19 were found to more frequently participate in aneuploidy events [12]. A summary of the data obtained from the cytogenetic analysis of first and second PBs is shown on Table 2.

It can therefore be concluded that both MI and MII are prone to mistakes in chromosome segregation, at least in older women. Additionally, even though aneuploidy events can affect the larger chromosomes, it is the smaller ones that seem to be preferentially involved during both meiotic divisions. It is also very clear that advancing female age has a significant adverse effect on both meiotic divisions, but MII may be more susceptible to age-related errors than MI.

Aneuploidy of Male Meiotic Origin

Estimates of sperm aneuploidy have been arrived at by two methods. First, by fusing sperm with hamster eggs when all the chromosomes may be visualised; secondly by FISH analysis of the nucleus when a few chromosomes at a time may be analysed. The first method is very labour intensive, the second less so, but many thousand sperm need to be analysed to obtain a reliable result. Templado and colleagues reviewed aneuploidy levels in healthy men from 30 FISH studies that used a minimum of five donors and employed strict scoring criteria and obtained a lower estimate of total aneuploidy of 4.5 % (2× disomy of 2.26 %) [35]. This figure was more than double that found by sperm karyotyping. Disomy for the autosomes is about 0.1 % on average but ranges between 0.03 (chromosome 8) and 0.47 (chromosome 22). Most authors investigating a limited range of chromosomes found that chromosome 21 (0.17 %) has an increased disomy frequency and that the sex chromosomes at 0.27 % have the highest, reflecting the significant male component in causing Down and Klinefelter syndromes and the sole male origin of the XYY cases. However, the studies revealed a considerable level of interindividual variability making it clear that certain men are far more prone to the production of sperm with unbalanced chromosomes than others. A doubling of sperm disomy for the chromosome pair involved was seen in fathers of offspring with Down, Turner and Klinefelter syndromes which had been shown to be of paternal origin [35]. Variability has also been observed in male meiotic cells; the frequency of unpaired sex chromosomes at MI in spermatocytes ranged between 3.2 and 43.7 % in fertile men [37]. The rate of sex chromosome abnormalities seen at MI of meiosis (mean 27.4 %) is far higher than the 0.5 % seen in spermatozoa. This difference can be explained by the arrest of chromosomally abnormal (asynapsed) cells by the activation of meiotic checkpoints that operate with much greater efficiency in males than in females [38].

How does the mechanism of origin of sperm aneuploidy compare with that in female gametes? Clearly errors in chromosome segregation, as in females, may result from failure to pair properly initially, altered or reduced recombination, or failure to maintain chromatid cohesion beyond anaphase I of meiosis. As with autosomal trisomies, sex chromosome trisomy is clearly linked with reduced recombination of the XY bivalent [11]. Recently, for the first time, the two types of nondisjunction seen in oocytes, that involving whole chromosomes and premature separation of chromatids, have been seen in metaphase I and II of male meiosis [39]. Premature separation of chromatids was the more frequent type in that study, seen in MII spermatocytes as extra or missing chromatids of chromosomes 21, X or Y. Very recently, evidence for the existence of a postmeiotic checkpoint that monitors numerical abnormalities was found by the application of Multiplex fluorescence in situ hybridisation (M-FISH) to metaphase I and II spermatocytes from three fertile donors [40]. This technique allows identification of each and every chromosome by a combination of different fluorochromes. As expected, the frequency of numerical abnormalities (disomy) at MII (14.5 %) was found to be far higher than that seen at MI (trisomy) (1.3 %). A significant proportion of spermatocytes at MI (27.7 %) were seen to display a low chiasma count, with small chromosomes present as two univalents. The chromosomes most frequently involved were X, Y and 21 and these were also those most frequently exhibiting disomy at MII.

The conclusion was that achiasmate nondisjunction of whole chromosomes and premature separation of chromatids appear as the main mechanisms generating aneuploidy in human male meiosis and that both contribute equally. Since the level of disomy observed in spermatocytes II is about threefold higher than that seen in spermatozoa the existence of a postmeiotic checkpoint is postulated [40]. The detection of spermatocytes II with separated sister chromatids is the first evidence that balanced predivision, seen in fresh oocytes, also occurs in male meiosis and may lead to aneuploid sperm by random segregation [6]. In conclusion, it appears that there are many similarities between the mechanisms leading to aneuploidy in the two sexes; however in contrast to the situation in females, it has not been possible to obtain definitive evidence for a paternal age effect [41].

Sperm Aneuploidy and Male Infertility

About 5 % of infertile men have a chromosomal abnormality; these subjects will clearly be at increased risk of producing aneuploid sperm. However, the efficiency of the meiotic cell cycle checkpoints that detect unpaired segments of DNA ensures that most prospective aneuploid gametes undergo apoptosis; a lowered sperm count is the result. In men with a normal somatic karyotype, an inverse correlation between sperm aneuploidy and sperm concentration has been well documented [42]. Analysis of sperm chromosomal content in 46 male carriers of reciprocal translocations shows that a mean of 40 % of sperm have a normal or balanced complement (by FISH) with a range between 19 and 77 % [43]. The risk is highly dependent upon the type of chromosomes involved (acrocentric vs. metacentric) and the position of the breakpoints. In contrast the sperm of Robertsonian translocation carriers have a majority of normal or balanced types, mean 85 %, range 60–96 % [44]. Couples where the male is the carrier of a chromosomal rearrangement may opt for PGD if they are unsuccessful in achieving a normal pregnancy, but follow-up studies on embryos not transferred clearly show that post-zygotic mitotic anomalies are at least as important as errors in meiotic segregation in causing embryonic aneuploidy [45, 46]. The high proportion of errors developing during cleavage in embryos from such couples is probably related to their reproductive failure.

Germline Mosaicism: Inherited Aneuploidy

Germinal or germline mosaicism may be defined as genetic abnormality of premeiotic origin in an otherwise normal organism. It can be the result of mosaicism that affects a proportion of the premeiotic germ cells and will thus lead to recurrent genetic abnormality of the same type in the offspring. This type could also be described as gonadal mosaicism. Alternatively, if the error occurred during one of the mitotic divisions prior to the onset of meiosis it could be confined to a single gamete. The term germline mosaicism covers both types. It has generally been considered to be a rare phenomenon.

Evidence for the existence of chromosomal germline mosaicism is obtained from both genetic and cytological studies. Recurrent aneuploid conceptions of the same type may be due to chance, especially if the mother is of advanced age [47]. However, careful analysis using both karyotyping and molecular studies in 151 families with Down syndrome offspring identified 8 families with germline mosaicism. In all cases the mother was younger than 35 years. Thus the prevalence of germinal mosaicism in young couples with a Down syndrome child was estimated to be 5.3 % [48].

Mosaicism for Chromosomal Rearrangements

Most cases of this type of mosaicism are revealed because of a history of repeated conceptions with similar cytogenetic abnormalities but in other cases a single conception with an unbalanced karyotype can result in the identification of the presence of a low level of balanced cells in a parent. In one interesting case, a couple were referred for PGD with a history of recurrent miscarriage. Two cycles of IVF for PGD were carried out; in all, 4 of 13 embryos were found to have a partial duplication of chromosome 21q. The same duplication was then detected by FISH analysis in 6 % of sperm nuclei, thereby proving paternal gonadal mosaicism for the duplication [49].

Cytological Proof of Germinal Mosaicism

The application of PGD led to the first cytological proof of gonadal mosaicism for trisomy 21 in the case of a couple with normal lymphocyte chromosomes that had a history of 3 conceptions with Down syndrome and one normal child [50]. The couple was referred for PGD; of 7 preimplantation embryos tested 4 had trisomy 21 and 3 of 4 unfertilised oocytes were abnormal. In 3 of the oocytes there was either an extra chromosome or chromatid 21; a crucial observation was that in one oocyte an extra chromatid was found in both the MII and in the first PB. This provided the first direct evidence of a maternal trisomic germ cell line and showed that the extra chromosome 21 had precociously divided into two chromatids before completion of MI.

Studies on Oocytes

The great majority of studies on metaphase II oocytes have been carried out without the analysis of the corresponding first PB. In this situation it is not possible to determine whether any extra chromosomal material present has arisen due to a meiotic error or is caused by a premeiotic trisomic cell. The other option is to analyse oocytes at the MI stage; no studies of this kind have so far been published. Thus it is very difficult to obtain a reliable estimate of the frequency of germinal mosaicism in the human female. Four studies that do provide some information, since oocyte/first PB doublets were analysed, are listed in Table 3. With the exception of Mahmood et al. all studies used either oocytes collected at GV or MI (and allowed to mature to the MII/first PB stage—IVM) or a mixture of these and oocytes that had failed to show evidence of fertilisation after IVF or ICSI [25]. By far the highest frequency of

Table 10.3 Examples of germinal mosaicism in studies of first polar bodies and metaphase II oocytes

Study	No. of oocyte/PB pairs examined	Method used	No. of oocyte/PBs with nonreciprocal results	No. of patients/age	Chromosomes affected
Mahmood et al. [25]	57 IVF/ICSI or unexposed	FISH up to 7 chromosomes	3	2 Age 26 and 31	21 and 13 21
Pujol et al. [51]	54 IVM	FISH with 9 chromosomes	11	9 Ages 31–38	1,13(5),15,16, 17(3),21,22(2),X
Gutierrez-Mateo et al. [9]	42 Mixed IVM and IVF/ICSI	CGH on PBS FISH on oocytes 7 chromosomes	4	4 Ages 36–42	4,13,16,18
Fragouli et al. [10]	39 Mixed IVM and IVF/ICSI	CGH	1	1 Age 32	13

germinal mosaicism (20 %) was seen by Pujol et al.; virtually all of their samples were IVM [51]. For the other three studies, the average frequency was about 6 %. It is to be expected that a higher frequency of this type of aneuploidy will be found in IVM oocytes, since preexisting chromosomal anomalies will lead to delay in completing the cell cycle.

Studies on Spermatocytes

Metaphase I of meiosis is more easily studied in the male. In their study of material from three fertile donors, Uroz and Templado found 1.3 % of MI spermatocytes to be trisomic [40]. Four of the 317 spermatocytes I contained an extra chromosome (18, 19, 22 or Y); this was considered to be caused by preexisting aneuploidy in the germ cells.

Direct Studies on Cells from Foetal Ovaries and Testes

An alternative cytological approach to search for evidence of germinal mosaicism was used by Hultén et al. [52]. Ovarian cells from eight phenotypically normal female foetuses (14–22 weeks gestation) were analysed by FISH using two chromosome 21 specific probes that mapped to different locations. The number of cells studied per case varied between 967 and 2,200 and consisted of premeiotic and stromal cells as well as those of meiotic origin. Mosaicism for trisomy 21 was detected in all the foetal ovaries with frequencies varying between 0.2 and 0.88 % (average 0.54 %), affecting all cell types. This is not an unexpected finding considering that levels of chromosomal mosaicism in human cleavage stage embryos reach 60–70 % even in those of good quality [53]. Interestingly, when investigated by the same group using the same strategy, testicular cells from four normal male foetuses failed to show a single example of trisomy 21 mosaicism [54]. The difference is again likely to be due to the stringent control of the cell cycle during spermatogenesis; testicular cells with additional (unpaired) chromosomes are likely to be arrested in development and to undergo apoptosis [55].

Mechanisms Leading to Aneuploidy in Cases of Germinal Mosaicism

An extra chromosome in a proportion of premeiotic germ cells can lead to aneuploidy via two mechanisms. During prophase of meiosis I, to accommodate the extra chromosome either a trivalent is formed with all three chromosomes associated, or a bivalent plus a univalent [56]. After trivalent formation, secondary (or inevitable) nondisjunction follows when one daughter cell receives a single chromosome and the other receives the remaining two bodies. There is thus a

50 % aneuploidy risk from a trivalent. In the other situation of a bivalent plus univalent, the evidence is that the aneuploidy risk is 100 %. Observations on mammalian meiosis show that the univalent positions itself at MI in a way that the kinetochore of each sister chromatid is orientated towards opposite spindle poles [57, 58]. The chromosome then splits into two chromatids, and one passes to each daughter cell, either the MII oocyte or the first PB, as observed in cases of germinal mosaicism in humans [50]. The combined effect of these two mechanisms is that even a low percentage of premeiotic trisomic cells significantly elevates the risk of an aneuploid conception and consequent embryonic or foetal death or disability, independently of maternal age.

Aneuploidy of Post-zygotic Origin

One day after fertilisation and under the control of the maternal genome, the zygote starts dividing mitotically into smaller cells called blastomeres. To begin with, these cells are spherical and totipotent, but very soon the mitosis becomes asynchronous and totipotency is lost [59]. Embryonic genome activation takes place approximately 3 days after fertilisation, during the cleavage stage of preimplantation development [60]. Compaction follows soon afterwards, which eventually causes the embryo to undergo its first cellular differentiation into TE which will form the extra-embryonic tissues, and ICM which will form the embryo proper. The embryo is now called a blastocyst and this stage of preimplantation development is reached 5–6 days after fertilisation. Prior to implanting, the blastocyst releases enzymes which open a hole in the membrane surrounding it (zona pellucida), causing it to hatch and begin the process of implantation to the maternal uterus [61, 62].

Chromosome abnormalities occur very frequently after fertilisation and have an important contribution to embryonic aneuploidy. The cleavage and blastocyst stages of preimplantation development have been examined cytogenetically and the following sections will summarise the findings obtained during such investigations.

Cleavage Stage

Following fertilisation on day 0, the embryo enters the cleavage stage that lasts until day 3, when it should contain about 8 cells. Cell division during this time interval is thus under the control of stored maternal mRNA transcripts. The development and application of molecular cytogenetic methods for single cell analysis from 1993 onwards allowed the acquisition of data that revealed the full extent of chromosomal anomalies at the cleavage stage. In stark contrast to the situation in postnatal life, 60 % of an average set of embryos created by IVF will contain at least one aneuploid cell by day 3 but the majority will consist mainly of abnormal cells. Prior to the application of molecular methods, traditional karyotyping had been used to analyse cleavage embryos [22]. Abnormality rates between 25 and 40 % were seen with diploid/aneuploid mosaics the most common type. Jamieson et al., found that full chromosome aneuploidy at that stage mirrored the situation in spontaneous abortions, with selective involvement of the smaller chromosomes [61].

As soon as interphase FISH analysis was developed for use in PGD, the karyotyping data was confirmed; aneuploidy and chromosomal mosaicism were common in the spare embryos from PGD cases [4]. Application of the technique to donated IVF embryos in general showed that abnormally developing or arrested embryos are frequently uniformly aneuploid or polyploid while an equal number are mosaic [63, 64]. More unexpected was the finding that normally developing embryos are also often abnormal; although rarely aneuploid throughout, 30–50 % were mosaics [65, 66]. Further data from PGD cycles showed that even fertile couples produced embryos that had highly abnormal chromosome complements, with anomalies affecting several chromosomes, varying in a random fashion from cell to cell, designated chaotic mosaics. Moreover, it became clear that certain couples were prone to the production of such embryos while others produced none of this type [14]. In general, IVF couples will have 5 % of their embryos in the chaotic category but in those with a history of RIF the proportion is much higher [67, 68].

Essentially, it was found that the greater the number of FISH probes used the higher the rate of mosaicism detected, raising the possibility that by day 3 all embryos created by IVF are mosaic. The answer came with another technical advance, that of single cell analysis by CGH. The whole genome had first to be amplified (WGA) to provide sufficient DNA for analysis. The great advantage of CGH is that the copy number of every chromosome is determined and any imbalance detected. WGA and CGH were then applied to all the single cells from a series of good quality cleavage embryos—12 in each series [28, 69]. There was good agreement between the two sets of data; in both sets 25 % were completely euploid with no anomalies detected. Overall, five embryos were aneuploid throughout, with seven the result of a meiotic error. Two thirds were mosaic in both sets of data; the majority were diploid/aneuploid but half of these had at least 50 % of cells abnormal. The new application of CGH allowed the detection of partial aneuploidy, the product of chromosome breakage, confirmed by the appearance of reciprocal products in sister cells in some cases. This was observed in about 10 % of embryos in these series and also later in a much larger diagnostic cohort [70]. If the chromosomal fragments are acentric they will be lost at the next cell division unless they become translocated to another chromosome; the resulting haploinsuffiency will be highly detrimental to the embryo.

When Does Mosaicism Originate and What Is Its Effect?

The evidence indicates that the first three cleavage divisions are the most prone to mitotic errors that lead to mosaicism. Bielanska et al. analysed 216 embryos available after routine IVF treatment and found that the frequency of mosaics increased from 15 % (2–4 cell stage) to 49 % (5–8 cells) and 58 % by day 4 (morula stage) [71]. They further concluded that mosaicism affecting a high proportion of cells, or of a chaotic type, interferes with development of the embryo to blastocyst. Various other publications support this finding. Katz-Jaffe et al. made use of single cell multiplex fluorescent PCR to distinguish between meiotic and mitotic errors in blastomeres from embryos diagnosed with chromosome 21 aneuploidy [16]. Twenty-five embryos were identified to be carrying an error of meiotic origin, while the remaining 13 were mosaic. The timing of the errors was 38 % first division, 31 % second division, and 19 % third division with the others (12 %) an error at MI. Most of the mosaics in fact were derived from diploid zygotes. Overall, evidence suggests that mosaicism interferes with development to a greater degree than uniform aneuploidy. Developmental arrest may affect embryos with fully chaotic or widespread mosaicism but in those with anomalies confined to one chromosome there is likely to be death or a reduction in proliferation of the aneuploid cells. Depending upon the initial proportion of abnormal cells, the rapid growth of the embryo between days 3 and 5 may allow normal cells to predominate and an embryo diagnosed as aneuploid from a single cell on day 3 may be able to lead to a viable pregnancy [72].

Correlation of Aneuploidy Mechanisms with Types of Infertility

Most of the recently published information on the chromosome status of the cleavage stage embryo has come from the analysis of large series of aneuploidy screening (PGS) cases (e.g. Munne et al.) [73]. However, few of these include full follow up of the abnormal embryos after diagnosis. As a result, embryos are designated 'aneuploid' based upon the result from a single cell that cannot provide information about the origin of the aneuploidy. This seems to lead to an overestimate of the contribution of meiotic errors. An interesting variation in the proportion of embryos with meiotic errors according to referral reason was found in a comprehensive follow-up study after PGS carried out by our group (Mantzouratou et al. and unpublished data) [67]. A total of 700 embryos that had been diagnosed as abnormal by single cell analysis on day 3 was followed up by applying the diagnostic probe set for six chromosomes (13,15,16,18,21 and 22) to individual cells in the remainder of the embryos on day 5. The recurrent miscarriage group had the highest proportion of meiotic errors, 24 % for an average maternal age of 37.6 years, with the lowest proportion in the RIF group, 8.9 %, average maternal age 36 years. An intermediate value of 20.4 % was found for the advanced maternal age group (over 40 years, average 42). The embryos from couples with RIF were more prone to post-zygotic errors, especially complex errors of the chaotic type. This latter finding was confirmed by another study [68].

Cytogenetic Mechanisms Leading to Mosaicism

Since interphase FISH analysis has a known error rate, the most efficient studies to investigate the mechanisms leading to mosaic aneuploidy have used sets of two probes per chromosome that hybridise to different loci. An early, unpublished study (Conn and Delhanty 1995) used paired probes for chromosomes 13,18 and 21 on cells from 37 very good quality 3-day-old embryos (6–8 cells). Eight embryos were mosaic for these chromosomes; in four cases this was a result of chromosome loss, in one chromosome gain, and in the other three to mitotic nondisjunction (MND). Two probes for each of chromosomes 1,11, and 18 were used in the study by Daphnis et al. mentioned in the section on blastocysts, below [74]. Chromosome loss was again the most common mechanism. Interestingly, the incidence of MND has been found to be maternal age dependent [15].

Blastocyst Stage

Reaching and surviving the blastocyst stage poses a number of potential challenges to the developing embryo. Hence, embryos that successfully achieve this developmental milestone are thought to be of very good quality and have an excellent implantation potential. However, studies using various cytogenetic methods to examine the chromosome complement of blastocysts have shown that both aneuploidy and the phenomenon of mosaicism persist to this final stage of development before implantation.

Clouston and colleagues attempted to analyse all 23 pairs of chromosomes of 438 human blastocysts with the use of classical G-banding [75, 76]. The results obtained showed that in their majority (68 %) these embryos were euploid. The remaining blastocysts were classified as aneuploid, and abnormalities of meiotic and post-zygotic origin were scored. A variety of chromosomes, including 2, 3, 4, 5, 6, 7, one acrocentric chromosome (13, 15), 17 and 22 were seen to participate in aneuploidy events [75, 76].

As with the cleavage stage though, most of the data concerning the chromosome status of blastocysts, have been obtained with the use of FISH. Two different investigations used a combination of immunosurgery to separate TE and ICM from a total of 131 embryos which were classified as aneuploid during day-3 PGS, but went on to form blastocysts [77, 78]. FISH was used to target chromosomes 13, 16, 18, 21, X and Y. The analysis of these embryos showed that both ICM and TE could tolerate a variety of aneuploidies, including tetraploidy, mosaicism and complex abnormalities involving multiple chromosomes, trisomies and monosomies. It was also evident from both studies that there was no preferential allocation of chromosome errors to the TE cells [77, 78].

Many other studies used FISH to examine non-transferred blastocysts, which were either diagnosed as aneuploid via day-3 PGS or had not undergone screening and were donated for research [63, 74, 79–81]. All these studies confirmed that chromosome abnormalities and mosaicism occur at the blastocyst stage, but their incidence is not as frequent as it is during the earlier cleavage stage. The main mosaicism-causing mechanism was identified to be chromosome loss most likely via anaphase lag. This was followed by chromosome gain, whereas MND (leading to monosomic and trisomic cell lines within the same embryo) was not as frequently observed [63, 74].

The use of FISH enabled the accurate identification of ploidy changes, such as triploidy and haploidy, as well. Interestingly, the most prevalent form of ploidy error seen were mosaic diploid-tetraploid blastocysts [63, 74, 82]. The presence of tetraploid cells is considered to represent the start of trophoblast differentiation, and for this reason mosaic diploid-tetraploid blastocysts are not generally considered abnormal [80].

The recent development of more comprehensive molecular cytogenetic methodology such as CGH (metaphase and array) or SNP microarrays enabled an accurate and reliable analysis of the blastocyst chromosomes and provided definitive evidence on the different types and frequency of anomalies that survive to this stage of preimplantation development. During one such study, a combination of metaphase and array CGH and also FISH took place to analyse three different parts obtained from the same blastocyst [17]. Forty-two percent of the 52 blastocysts which were investigated were euploid in every cell. Of the ones characterised as abnormal, 25 % carried the same chromosome error in all of the cells, suggesting a meiotic origin, whereas the remaining embryos had varying degrees of mosacism. Most of these mosaics contained different abnormalities in every cell, but we did observe a few (10 %) diploid-aneuploid mosaic embryos, which contained a majority of normal cells. The fate of such embryos, as far as their ability to implant is concerned is not currently known [17].

Another investigation which used SNP microarrays to analyse 50 blastocysts reported very similar findings to our study [72]. Specifically, mosaicism was also observed in various degrees in 24 % of the embryos, with the remaining 76 % being either completely normal or uniformly abnormal [72]. Combination of the data from both the abovementioned studies, indicate that approximately 30 % of blastocyst embryos are mosaic, but only a small proportion of these contain a diploid cell line as a majority.

The use of more comprehensive methods for the analysis of blastocysts demonstrated that aneuploidy affects chromosomes of all sizes and groups, with 22, 16, 15, 21 and X being the ones to malsegregate most frequently. Additionally, monosomies seemed to be in excess of trisomies (514 vs. 494 respectively), confirming FISH observations about chromosome loss being the main aneuploidy-causing mechanism during this stage of development [83]. It was also clear that even though most (60 %) aneuploid blastocysts tend to carry a single chromosome error in them, there are others (15 %) with multiple errors, which are capable of reaching the final stage of preimplantation development. Similarly to findings obtained for oocytes and cleavage stage embryos, CGH of blastocysts detected several partial abnormalities, mostly affecting pieces of the larger autosomes (i.e. 1–11 and X), but also the smaller 16 and 20 [83].

Analysis of TE and ICM's coming from the same embryos showed an identical chromosome complement for both parts [84, 85]. These findings agreed with previous FISH investigations, and suggest that TE biopsy, undertaken in a clinical PGS setting, can generally be relied upon to provide a good indication of the chromosomal status of the ICM and therefore of the foetus [77, 78]. As a result, screening of embryos on day-5 to identify ones that are chromosomally normal has been increasingly used by many IVF clinics, and has shown some very encouraging clinical outcomes [86, 87]. Data obtained from such analysis suggest that the expected blastocyst aneuploidy rate for an average female age of 38 years is 56 % (Fragouli et al. and unpublished) [31]. In agreement with observations during female meiosis and cleavage stage (to an extent), advancing female age seems to be closely related to increasing aneuploidy rates at the blastocyst stage as well. Data obtained for 191 women who underwent CGH screening of blastocysts revealed that the aneuploidy rate in younger patients (age range: 29–34 years, average age: 32.3 years) was 46.5 %, whereas in an older group (age range: 35–50, average age: 40) it was 60.6 %, and this difference was found to be highly statistically significant (Fisher's exact test, $P=0.0007$) [83]. Table 4 illustrates results obtained during the cytogenetic analysis of embryos at the final stage of preimplantation development, using different methods.

Table 10.4 Analysis of the chromosome complement of human blastocysts with the use of FISH or CGH

Study	No. of embryos examined	Average female age (age range)	Method used	Chromosomes examined	No. of euploid embryos	No. of uniformly aneuploid blastocysts	No. of mosaic embryos	
							Mosaic diploid-aneuploid	Mosaic aneuploid/chaotic
Ruangvutilert et al. [79]	19	32.6 years (27–41 years)	FISH	13, 18, 21, X, Y	2	0	8	9
Coonen et al. [63]	299	33 years	FISH	18, X, Y	74	0	Not specified	221
Daphnis et al. [74]	42	33.7 years (19–41 years)	FISH	1, 11, 18, X, Y	66	6	19	0
Fragouli et al. [17]	52	36 years (24–42 years)	CGH, aCGH, FISH	All chromosomes	22	13	7	10

Conclusions

The exceptionally high incidence of chromosomal anomalies in human preimplantation embryos is the outcome of the accumulated risk of errors that may occur at various stages during gametogenesis and embryogenesis. In rare cases an error may exist or arise in the premeiotic germ cells; much more commonly it may arise during the first or second meiotic division in the male or female. More efficient cell cycle checkpoints in the male ensure that the incidence of aneuploidy in the male gamete is low compared to that in the female. Hence most errors of meiotic origin come from the female. Chromosomal mosaicism affects the majority of 3-day-old embryos created by IVF and this persists to a lesser degree to the blastocyst stage on day 5. With the exception of women over the age of 40 and some that are particularly prone to meiotic errors, embryos from all other groups will have predominantly post-zygotic mitotic errors. Couples experiencing repetitive implantation failure are particularly likely to produce highly abnormal (chaotic) embryos by post-zygotic mechanisms.

References

1. Edwards RG, Brody SA. Principles and practice of assisted human reproduction. Philadelphia: Saunders; 1995. p. 65–80.
2. Bonde JP, Ernst E, Jensen TK, et al. Relation between semen quality and fertility: a population based study of 430 first-pregnancy planners. Lancet. 1998;352:1172–7.
3. Centers for Disease Control and Prevention. 2006 Assisted reproductive technology success rates: preliminary data national summary and fertility clinic reports. 2008. Available at http://www.cdc.gov/art/art2006/index.htm.
4. Delhanty JD, Griffin DK, Handyside AH, et al. Detection of aneuploidy and chromosomal mosaicism in human embryos during preimplantation sex determination by fluorescent in situ hybridisation (FISH). Hum Mol Genet. 1993;2:1183–5.
5. Munne S, Lee A, Rosenwaks Z, et al. Diagnosis of major chromosome aneuploidies in human preimplantation embryos. Hum Reprod. 1993;8:2185–91.
6. Sandalinas M, Marquez C, Munne S. Spectral karyotyping of fresh, non-inseminated oocytes. Mol Hum Reprod. 2002;8:580–5.
7. Kuliev A, Cieslak J, Ilkevitch Y, et al. Chromosomal abnormalities in a series of 6,733 human oocytes in preimplantation diagnosis for age-related aneuploidies. Reprod Biomed Online. 2003;6:54–9.
8. Pellestor F, Andreo B, Arnal F, et al. Maternal aging and chromosomal abnormalities: new data drawn from in vitro unfertilized human oocytes. Hum Genet. 2003;112:195–203.
9. Gutierrez-Mateo C, Benet J, Wells D, et al. Aneuploidy study of human oocytes first polar body comparative genomic hybridization and metaphase II fluorescence in situ hybridization analysis. Hum Reprod. 2004;19:2859–68.
10. Fragouli E, Wells D, Thornhill A, et al. Comparative genomic hybridization analysis of human oocytes and polar bodies. Hum Reprod. 2006;21:2319–28.
11. Hassold T, Hall H, Hunt P. The origin of human aneuploidy: where we have been, where we are going. Hum Mol Genet. 2007;16:R203–8.
12. Fragouli E, Alfarawati S, Goodall NN. The cytogenetics of polar bodies: insights into female meiosis and the diagnosis of aneuploidy. Mol Hum Reprod. 2011;17:286–95.
13. Harton GL, Tempest HG. Chromosomal disorders and male infertility. Asian J Androl. 2012;14:32–9.
14. Delhanty JD, Harper JC, Ao A, et al. Multicolour FISH detects frequent chromosomal mosaicism and chaotic division in normal preimplantation embryos from fertile patients. Hum Genet. 1997;99:755–60.
15. Munne S, Sandalinas M, Escudero T, et al. Chromosome mosaicism in cleavage- stage human embryos: evidence of a maternal age effect. Reprod Biomed Online. 2002;4:223–32.
16. Katz-Jaffe MG, Trounson AO, Cram DS. Mitotic errors in chromosome 21 of human preimplantation embryos are associated with non-viability. Mol Hum Reprod. 2004;10:143–7.
17. Fragouli E, Alfarawati S, Daphnis DD, et al. Cytogenetic analysis of human blastocysts with the use of FISH, CGH and aCGH: scientific data and technical evaluation. Hum Reprod. 2011;26:480–90.
18. Delhanty JD. Mechanisms of aneuploidy induction in human oogenesis and early embryogenesis. Cytogenet Genome Res. 2005;111:237–44.
19. Angell RR. Predivision in human oocytes at meiosis I: a mechanism for trisomy formation in man. Hum Genet. 1991;86:383–7.
20. Angell RR, Xian J, Keith J, et al. First meiotic division abnormalities in human oocytes: mechanism of trisomy formation. Cytogenet Cell Genet. 1994;65:194–202.
21. Pellestor F. Frequency and distribution of aneuploidy in human female gametes. Hum Genet. 1991;86:283–8.
22. Zenzes MT, Casper RF. Cytogenetics of human oocytes, zygotes and embryos after in vitro fertilisation. Hum Genet. 1992;88:367–75.
23. Kamiguchi Y, Rosenbusch B, Sterzik K, et al. Chromosomal analysis of unfertilized human oocytes prepared by a gradual fixationair drying method. Hum Genet. 1993;90:533–41.

24. Lim AS, Ho AT, Tsakok MF. Chromosomes of oocytes failing in-vitro fertilization. Hum Reprod. 1995;10: 2570–5.
25. Mahmood R, Brierley CH, Faed MJ, et al. Mechanisms of maternal aneuploidy: FISH analysis of oocytes and polar bodies in patients undergoing assisted conception. Hum Genet. 2000;106:620–6.
26. Cupisti S, Conn CM, Fragouli E, et al. Sequential FISH analysis of oocytes and polar bodies reveals aneuploidy mechanisms. Prenat Diagn. 2003;23: 663–8.
27. Wells D, Sherlock JK, Handyside AH, et al. Detailed chromosomal and molecular genetic analysis of single cells by whole genome amplification and comparative genomic hybridisation. Nucleic Acids Res. 1999;27:1214–8.
28. Wells D, Delhanty JD. Comprehensive chromosomal analysis of human preimplantation embryos using whole genome amplification and single cell comparative genomic hybridisation. Mol Hum Reprod. 2000;11:1055–62.
29. Wells D, Escudero T, Levy B, et al. First clinical application of comparative genomic hybridisation and polar body testing for preimplantation genetic diagnosis of aneuploidy. Fertil Steril. 2002;78:543–9.
30. Pellestor F, Anahory T, Hamamah S. The chromosomal analysis of human oocytes. Hum Reprod Update. 2005;11:15–32.
31. Fragouli E, Katz-Jaffe M, Alfarawati S, et al. Comprehensive chromosome screening of polar bodies and blastocysts from couples experiencing repeated implantation failure. Fertil Steril. 2010;94:875–87.
32. Kuliev A, Verlinsky Y. Meiotic and mitotic nondisjunction: lessons from preimplantation genetic diagnosis. Hum Reprod Update. 2004;10:401–7.
33. Geraedts J, Montag M, Magli MC, et al. Polar body array CGH for prediction of the status of the corresponding oocyte. Part I: clinical results. Hum Reprod. 2011;26:3173–80.
34. Fisher JM, Harvey JF, Morton NE, et al. Trisomy 18: studies of the parent and cell division of origin and the effect of aberrant recombination on nondisjunction. Am J Hum Genet. 1995;56:669–75.
35. Hassold T, Merrill M, Adkins K, et al. Recombination and maternal age-dependent nondisjunction: molecular studies of trisomy 16. Am J Hum Genet. 1995; 57:867–74.
36. Templado C, Vidal F, Estop A. Aneuploidy in human spermatozoa. Cytogenet Genome Res. 2011;133: 91–9.
37. Uroz L, Rajmil O, Templado C. Meiotic chromosome abnormalities in fertile men: are they increasing? Fertil Steril. 2011;95:141–6.
38. Burgoyne PS, Mahadevaiah SK, Turner JM. The consequences of asynapsis for mammalian meiosis. Nat Rev Genet. 2009;10:207–16.
39. Uroz L, Rajmil O, Templado C. Premature separation of sister chromatids in human male meiosis. Hum Reprod. 2008;23:982–7.
40. Uroz L, Templado C. Meiotic non-disjunction mechanisms in human fertile males. Hum Reprod. 2012; 27(5):1518–24.
41. Fonseka KGL, Griffin DK. Is there a paternal age effect for aneuploidy? Cytogenet Genome Res. 2011;133:280–91.
42. Miharu N. Chromosome abnormalities in sperm from infertile men with normal somatic karyotypes: oligospermia. Cytogenet Genome Res. 2005;111: 347–51.
43. Benet J, Oliver-Bonet M, Cifuentes P, et al. Segregation of chromosomes in sperm of reciprocal translocation carriers. Cytogenet Genome Res. 2005;111:281–90.
44. Roux C, Tripogney C, Morel F, et al. Segregation of chromosomes in sperm of Robertsonian translocation carriers. Cytogenet Genome Res. 2005;111:291–6.
45. Iwarsson E, Malmgren H, Inzunza J, et al. Highly abnormal cleavage divisions in preimplantation embryos from translocation carriers. Prenat Diagn. 2000;20:1038–47.
46. Simopoulou M, Harper JC, Fragouli E, et al. Preimplantation genetic diagnosis of chromosome abnormalities: implications from the outcome for couples with chromosomal rearrangements. Prenat Diagn. 2003;23:652–62.
47. Robinson WP, McFadden DE, Stephenson MD. The origin of abnormalities in recurrent aneuploidy/polyploidy. Am J Hum Genet. 2001;69:1245–54.
48. Kovaleva NV, Tahmasebi-Hesari M. Gonadal mosaicism. Down Syndr News. 2007;14:23.
49. Somprasit C, Aguinaga M, Cisneros PL, et al. Paternal gonadal mosaicism detected in a couple with recurrent abortions undergoing PGD: FISH analysis of sperm nuclei proves valuable. Reprod Biomed Online. 2004;9:225–30.
50. Cozzi J, Conn CM, Harper J, et al. A trisomic germ cell line and precocious chromatid separation leads to recurrent trisomy 21 conception. Hum Genet. 1999;104:23–8.
51. Pujol A, Boiso I, Benet J, et al. Analysis of nine chromosome pairs in first polar bodies and metapahse II oocytes for the detection of aneuploidies. Eur J Hum Genet. 2003;11:325–36.
52. Hultén MA, Patel SD, Tankimanova M, et al. On the origin of trisomy 21 Down syndrome. Mol Cytogenet. 2008;1:21.
53. Mantzouratou A, Delhanty JD. Aneuploidy in the human cleavage stage embryo. Cytogenet Genome Res. 2011;133:141–8.
54. Hultén MA, Patel SD, Westgren M, et al. On the paternal origin of trisomy 21 Down Syndrome. Mol Cytogenet. 2010;3:4.
55. Morelli M, Cohen P. Not all germ cells are created equal: aspects of sexual dimorphism in mammalian meiosis. Reproduction. 2005;130:761–81.
56. Speed RM. Meiotic configurations in female trisomy 21 foetuses. Hum Genet. 1984;66:176–80.
57. LeMaire-Adkins R, Radke K, et al. Lack of checkpoint control at the metaphase/anaphase transition: a mechanism of meiotic nondisjunction in mammalian females. J Cell Biol. 1997;139:1611–9.
58. Kourznetsova A, Lister L, Nordenskjöld M, et al. Bi-orientation of achiasmatic chromosomes in meiosis I oocytes contributes to aneuploidy in mice. Nat Genet. 2007;39:966–8.

59. Heikinheimo O, Gibbons WE. The molecular mechanisms of oocyte maturation and early embryonic development are unveiling new insights into reproductive medicine. Mol Hum Reprod. 1998;4:745–56.
60. Braude P, Bolton V, Moore S. Human gene expression occurs between the four- and eight-cell stages of preimplantation development. Nature. 1988;332:459–61.
61. Edwards RG, Beard HK. Oocyte polarity and cell determination in early mammalian embryos. Mol Hum Reprod. 1997;3:863–905.
62. Jamieson ME, Coutts JRT, Conner JM. The chromosome constitution of human preimplantation embryos fertilised in vitro. Hum Reprod. 1994;9:709–15.
63. Coonen E, Derhaag JG, Dumoulin JC, et al. Anaphase lagging mainly explains chromosomal mosaicism in human preimplantation embryos. Hum Reprod. 2004;19:316–24.
64. Munné S, Grifo J, Cohen J. Chromosome abnormalities in human arrested preimplantation embryos fertilized *in vitro*: a multiprobe FISH study. Am J Hum Genet. 1994;55:150–9.
65. Harper JC, Coonen E, Handyside AH, et al. Mosaicism of autosomes and sex chromosomes in morphologically normal, monospermic preimplantation human embryos. Prenat Diagn. 1995;15:41–9.
66. Munné S, Sultan KM, Weier HU, Grifo JA, Cohen J, Rosenwaks Z. Assessment of numeric abnormalities of X, Y, 18, and 16 chromosomes in preimplantation human embryos before transfer. Am J Obstet Gynecol. 1995;172:1191–9.
67. Mantzouratou A, Mania A, Fragouli E, et al. Variable aneuploidy mechanisms in embryos from couples with poor reproductive histories undergoing preimplantation genetic screening. Hum Reprod. 2007;22:1844–53.
68. Voullaire L, Collins V, Callaghan T, et al. High incidence of complex chromosome abnormality in cleavage embryos from patients with repeated implantation failure. Fertil Steril. 2007;87:1053–8.
69. Voullaire L, Slater H, Williamson R, et al. Chromosome analysis of blastomeres from human embryos by using comparative genomic hybridisation. Hum Genet. 2000;106:210–7.
70. Voullaire L, Wilton L, McBain J, et al. Chromosome abnormalities identified by comparative genomic hybridization in embryos from women with repeated implantation failure. Mol Hum Reprod. 2002;8:1035–41.
71. Bielanska M, Tan SL, Ao A. Chromosomal mosaicism throughout human preimplantation development *in vitro*: incidence, type, and relevance to embryo outcome. Hum Reprod. 2002;17:413–9.
72. Northrop LE, Treff NR, Levy B, et al. SNP microarray based 24 chromosome aneuploidy screening demonstrates that cleavage stage FISH poorly predicts aneuploidy in embryos that develop to morphologically normal blastocysts. Mol Hum Reprod. 2010;16:590–600.
73. Munné S, Bahçe M, Sandalinas M, et al. Differences in chromosome susceptibility to aneuploidy and survival to first trimester. Reprod Biomed Online. 2004;8:81–90.
74. Daphnis DD, Delhanty JD, Jerkovic S, et al. Detailed FISH analysis of day 5 human embryos reveals the mechanisms leading to mosaic aneuploidy. Hum Reprod. 2005;20:129–37.
75. Clouston HJ, Fenwick J, Webb AL, et al. Detection of mosaic and non-mosaic chromosome abnormalities in 6- to 8-day old human blastocysts. Hum Genet. 1997;101:30–6.
76. Clouston HJ, Herbert M, Fenwick J, et al. Cytogenetic analysis of human blastocysts. Prenat Diagn. 2002;22:1143–52.
77. Evsikov S, Verlinsky Y. Mosaicism in the inner cell mass of human blastocysts. Hum Reprod. 1998;13:3151–5.
78. Magli MC, Jones GM, Gras L, et al. Chromosome mosaicism in day 3 aneuploid embryos that develop to morphologically normal blastocysts in vitro. Hum Reprod. 2000;15:1781–6.
79. Ruangvutilert P, Delhanty JD, Serhal P, et al. FISH analysis on day 5 post-insemination of human arrested and blastocyst stage embryos. Prenat Diagn. 2000;20:552–60.
80. Sandalinas M, Sadowy S, Alikani M, et al. Developmental ability of chromosomally abnormal human embryos to develop to the blastocyst stage. Hum Reprod. 2001;16:1954–8.
81. Santos MA, Teklenburg G, Macklon NS, et al. The fate of the mosaic embryo: chromosomal constitution and development of Day 4, 5 and 8 human embryos. Hum Reprod. 2010;25:1916–26.
82. Bielanska M, Jin S, Bernier M, et al. Diploid- aneuploid mosaicism in human embryos cultured to the blastocyst stage. Fertil Steril. 2005;84:336–42.
83. Fragouli E, Wells D. Aneuploidy in the human blastocyst. Cytogenet Genome Res. 2011;133:149–59.
84. Fragouli E, Lenzi M, Ross R, et al. Comprehensive molecular cytogenetic analysis of the human blastocyst stage. Hum Reprod. 2008;23:2596–608.
85. Johnson DS, Cinnioglu C, Ross R, et al. Comprehensive analysis of karyotypic mosaicism between trophectoderm and inner cell mass. Mol Hum Reprod. 2010;16:944–9.
86. Schoolcraft WB, Fragouli E, Stevens J, et al. Clinical application of comprehensive chromosomal screening at the blastocyst stage. Fertil Steril. 2010;94:1700–6.
87. Schoolcraft WB, Treff NR, Stevens JM, et al. Live birth outcome with trophectoderm biopsy, blastocyst vitrification, and single-nucleotide polymorphism microarray-based comprehensive chromosome screening in infertile patients. Fertil Steril. 2011;96:638–40.
88. Ruangvutilert P, Delhanty JD, Serhal P, Simopoulou M, Rodeck CH, Harper JC. FISH analysis on day 5 post-insemination of human arrested and blastocyst stage embryos. Prenat Diagn. 2000;20:552–560.

Additional Reading

Jones KT. Meiosis in oocytes: predisposition to aneuploidy and its increased incidence with age. Hum Reprod Update. 2008;14:143–58.

Preimplantation Genetic Screening and Diagnosis Using Fluorescent In Situ Hybridization (FISH)

11

Tsilya Gerasimova and Maria D. Lalioti

Preimplantation Genetic Diagnosis (PGD) is the screening of embryos at the cleavage or blastocyst stage in order to select and transfer only the *desired* embryo. The main indications of PGD are monogenic disorders and aneuploidy. Additionally, PGD can be employed to distinguish a male from a female embryo or to choose a HLA-matched embryo to a child requiring bone marrow or cord blood transplant. The European Society of Human Reproduction and Embryology (ESHRE) classifies PGD into two categories [1]: high-risk PGD for patients at high risk of transmitting a genetic or chromosomal abnormality to their children, which includes single gene defects, namely autosomal recessive, autosomal dominant and X-linked disorders, as well as chromosomal abnormalities (translocations, small deletions, etc.); and low-risk PGD (or PGS for Preimplantation Genetic Screening) for sex selection, and for infertile patients undergoing in vitro fertilization (IVF) IVF with the aim of increasing the IVF pregnancy rates. Patients that fall into this category are those of advanced maternal age (AMA) and repeated IVF failure and couples with normal karyotypes who have experienced repeated miscarriages.

PGD is performed in very early stage embryos before implantation, and therefore, it requires the use of In Vitro Fertilization (IVF) despite the fact that a great proportion of patients are not infertile. For example, the majority of patients seeking PGD for single gene disorders are fertile and thus the pregnancy success rates after PGD are higher than other groups of patients [2].

This chapter presents the use of Fluorescent In Situ Hybridization (FISH) in embryo aneuploidy screening, the efficiency, and the technical challenges of the method. New methodology for aneuploidy screening is briefly discussed and is covered in other chapters.

Embryo Biopsy and Fixation

PGD can be performed either on one blastomere biopsied from the embryo 3 days after fertilization, or a group of cells removed from the blastocyst on day 5 after fertilization, or, even in the polar bodies extruded from oocytes during meiosis (Fig. 1). Polar body biopsy can only test for conditions inherited from the mother and can only speculate on the chromosomal complement of the oocyte, depending on what is found in the polar body. For example, if the polar body contains an extra copy of X chromosome, it is assumed that the oocyte lacks one X. However, a reciprocal error on meiosis II may correct the meiosis I error and result in a normal embryo [3]. Therefore, this method is not as accurate as blastomere biopsy.

Following IVF, the embryos to be tested are cultured for 3 days and are expected to have undergone 2–4 cell divisions and consist of 4–10 cells. At this stage all blastomeres are known to be

T. Gerasimova • M.D. Lalioti (✉)
Department of Obstetrics, Gynecology and Reproductive Sciences, Yale School of Medicine, New Haven, CT, USA
e-mail: maria.lalioti@yale.edu

D.K. Gardner et al. (eds.), *Human Gametes and Preimplantation Embryos: Assessment and Diagnosis*, DOI 10.1007/978-1-4614-6651-2_11, © Springer Science+Business Media New York 2013

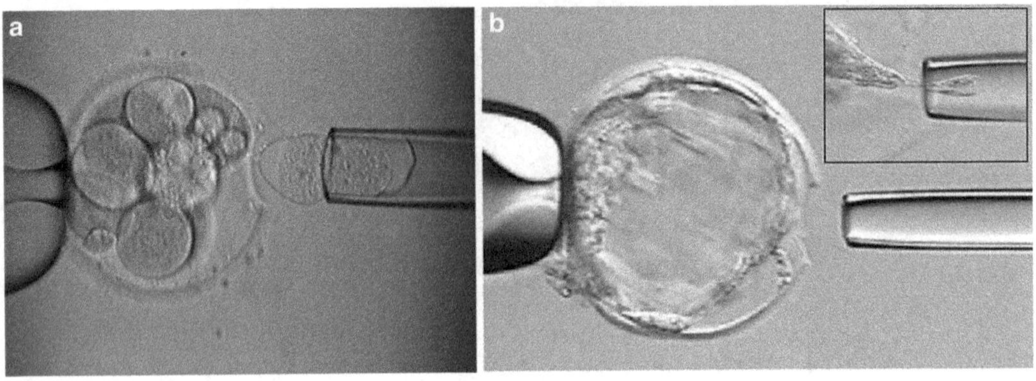

Fig. 11.1 Embryo biopsy for PGD. (**a**) Blastomere biopsy. (**b**) Blastocyst biopsy (Courtesy of Dr. Denny Sakkas, Boston IVF)

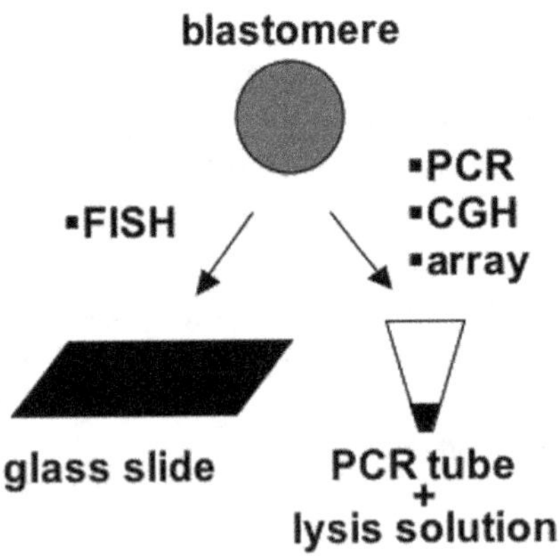

Fig. 11.2 Processing of biopsied cell. Depending on the indication for PGD, the biopsied blastomere is fixed on a glass slide or placed in a PCR tube containing lysis solution

identical and totipotent. The biopsy is performed by a trained embryologist in two steps: first, an opening is made in the zona pellucida surrounding the oocyte with a laser; a biopsy pipette is entered through the opening and one blastomere is removed for analysis (Fig. 1). The rest of the embryo is then returned in the incubator to continue its development while the genetic analysis is performed. Alternatively, a blastocyst biopsy removes cells from the trophectoderm that gives rise to extraembryonic tissues and the placenta.

The biopsy procedure is the same regardless of the indication. However, further processing of the cell is dependent on the molecular technique used to diagnose the condition needed and will be discussed below (Fig. 2).

In most cases, fertilization of embryos to be tested by PGD is done using Intracytoplasmic Sperm Injection (ICSI) and not regular oocyte insemination with sperm, in order to prevent the presence of spermatozoa in proximity to the oocyte. If present during biopsy, these spermatozoa could be transferred in the analysis tube together with the blastomere and introduce significant error especially in those methods involving PCR (polymerase chain reaction). For the same reason, the oocyte has to be completely stripped of its cumulus cells prior to ICSI.

When biopsied at the cleavage stage, any embryo testing should be completed within 48 h from the biopsy, to allow direct transfer of the embryo to the mother, without the need for embryo cryopreservation. More recently, improvement of embryo freezing methods has contributed to higher viability of cryopreserved biopsied embryos and has allowed PGD to be performed in later stages of embryo development, such as the blastocyst stage [4]. Embryo biopsy is an invasive method and should be only performed by well-trained embryologists. Examination and medical follow-up of children up to 2 years of age have not shown any increase in congenital abnormalities due to PGD/PGS.

PGD for Chromosomal Rearrangements

Chromosomal rearrangements include balanced translocations, inversions, or deletions. In balanced translocations, two chromosomes have exchanged fragments in a precise manner and

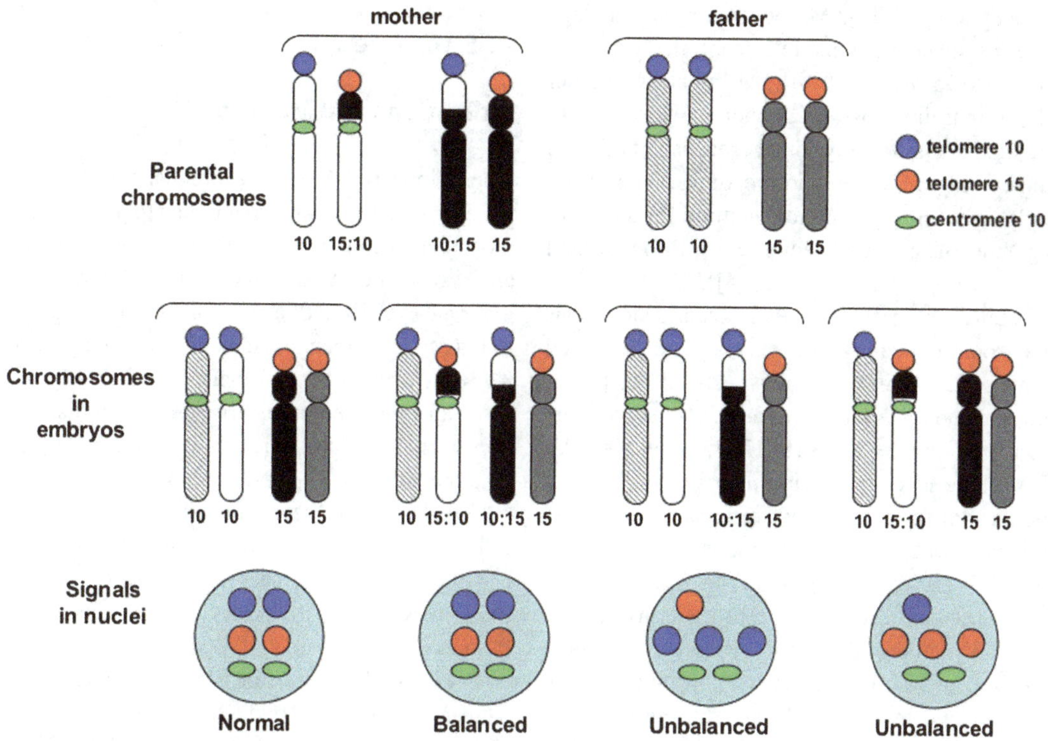

Fig. 11.3 Schematic representation of a balanced translocation between chromosomes 10 and 15. The maternal chromosomes are shown on the *top*. The chromosome 10 is *white* and the chromosome 15 is *black*. The paternal chromosome 10 is shown cross-hatched and the paternal chromosome 15 is *grey* (to distinguish from the maternal chromosomes). The possible segregation of these two chromosomes in the embryos is shown on the *middle*. The specific probes for telomere 10, telomere 15, and centromere 10 are depicted with *blue*, *red*, and *green circles* and *ovals*, respectively. Corresponding signals in blastomeres are shown on the *bottom*. Two dots from each probe indicate normal and balanced embryos. Any other combination of signals indicates excess or lack of chromosomal material

therefore the carrier parent contains the correct amount of genetic material. Patients carrying a chromosomal rearrangement have an increased risk for chromosomally unbalanced conceptions. During meiosis, upon separation of chromosomal pairs, a gamete, and subsequently the resulting embryo, can contain a mix of normal and translocated chromosomes that can result in a surplus or lack of genetic material (Fig. 3). Depending on the genes carried by the affected genomic portion, these abnormalities are often incompatible with life and result in miscarriage or elective pregnancy termination due to extensive fetal abnormalities. Approximately 1–2 % of pregnancy losses are due to previously undiagnosed balanced translocations carried by one of the parents.

PGD can be performed to select the normal or balanced embryos and avoid the transfer of embryos carrying unbalanced rearrangements, therefore increasing the chance of a normal pregnancy. Traditionally, these cases are performed with FISH with probes specific for the two affected chromosomes (Fig. 3). The embryos are biopsied on day 3 after fertilization and the blastomere is fixed on a glass slide with methanol-acetic acid that dissolves the cytoplasm and exposes the DNA of the nucleus. The fixed blastomeres are hybridized with the probes chosen within the rearranged chromosomes (Fig. 3).

Several studies have shown that PGD for translocation carriers resulted in higher live birth rates per embryo transfer compared to natural conceptions [5–13]. Moreover, the miscarriage rate of these patients fell from the expected 62–75 to 15 % [10, 12, 13]. It is not clear whether the remaining lost pregnancies were due to misdiagnosis or any other reason, including aneuploidy of other chromosomes. Therefore, PGD is definitely a reliable method for the management of cases with reciprocal or Robertsonian translocations (reviewed in [14]).

However, in cases of PGD for translocations the total percentage of normal and balanced embryos is lower than the expected 50 % (25 % normal and 25 % balanced) and the observed rate can be as low as 15 % [8, 12, 15]. This is most likely due to errors during meiosis, and in particular during the step of pairing and crossover (chiasmata) between homologous chromosomes, which is critical for meiosis [16]. Chromosomal pairing is hampered because of the translocation and the extend of the defect depends on the type (reciprocal vs. Robertsonian) and size of the translocated fragments. As a result translocation carriers produce fewer transferable embryos [2]. More recently, the application of microarrays to whole genome screening, discussed below, provides the possibility for testing of chromosomal imbalances in combination with a comprehensive chromosomal analysis [13, 17–21].

PGD for Aneuploidy

Indications and Method

Approximately 20 % of all pregnancies result in miscarriage. A proportion of them are due to chromosomal aneuploidy and depends on maternal age. Losses due to aneuploidy increase with the maternal age: 57 % of abnormal karyotypes found in fetuses of women less than 35 years of age, and 82 % in women 35 and older [22, 23] (Fig. 4). Most aneuploid embryos arise from non-disjunction errors in maternal meiosis I, which depend on maternal age [24, 25], reviewed in [26].

Besides natural conceptions, the success of IVF is also heavily dependent on maternal age. For these reasons, it seemed reasonable to use PGS in women with AMA and repeated IVF failure.

PGS is performed using FISH on a blastomere from a day 3 embryo which is fixed on a glass slide, as is also done for translocations. Most PGS protocols target specifically the nine most common aneuploidies seen in spontaneous abortions or birth (X, Y, 13, 15, 16, 17, 18, 21, 22). Other centers test up to 12 chromosomes in 3 consecutive hybridizations [27]. DNA probes for

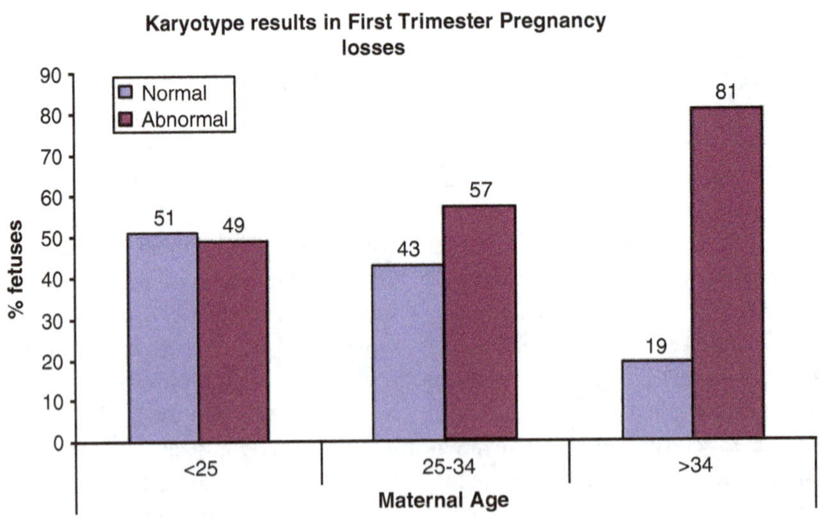

Fig. 11.4 Effect of gestational age and maternal age on karyotypes of spontaneous pregnancy losses (Data from Hogge et al. 2003 and Ljunger et al. 2005)

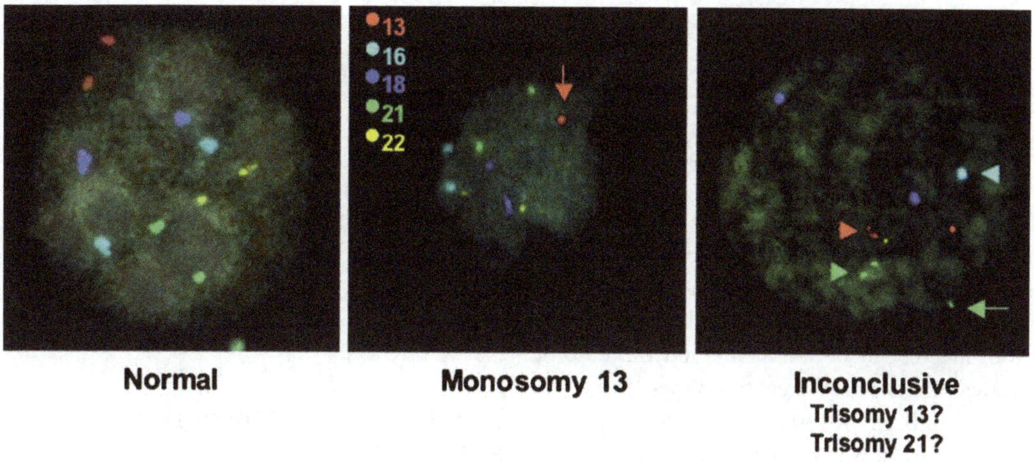

Fig. 11.5 FISH on blastomeres from day 3 embryos. Blastomeres from day 3 (8-cell) embryos were biopsied, fixed, and hybridized with commercial PB (Vysis) probe combination. The probes corresponding to chromosomes 13, 16, 18, 21, and 22 are labeled with *red*, *aqua*, *blue*, *green*, and *yellow* fluorophores, respectively. The *left panel* shows a normal blastomere with two signals for each chromosome. The *middle panel* shows a blastomere carrying only one signal for chromosome 13 (*red arrow*). The *right panel* depicts an embryo with monosomy 16 (*aqua arrow-head*) and inconclusive signals for chromosomes 13 and 21. One of the red signals is split (*arrow-head*). There are two green signals near each other (*green arrow-head*) and one green signal on the border of the cell (*green arrow*)

the 9–12 chromosomes to be tested are labeled with different fluorochromes, hybridized to the slide in 2–3 successive hybridizations and the signals are visualized using a microscope (Fig. 5).

Efficacy of PGD Using FISH

Significant improvement of IVF success and pregnancy rates was reported in AMA and poor prognosis patients, although these were not randomized controlled studies [15, 27–31]. The benefits for younger patients (<35) were not as clear [28].

However, none of the above mentioned studies was a randomized control trial (RCT) and the first such study was published in 2007 showing not only no benefit, but a possible detrimental effect of using PGS [32]. A previous study had shown similar results [33], but its failure had been attributed to the biopsy of 2 rather than 1 blastomere, a method that was shown to be detrimental to the embryo [34]. The 2007 RCT was criticized for numerous technical flaws and suboptimal application of PGS [35]. However, subsequent RCTs agreed with the first and failed to support the use of PGS for 7–9 chromosomes to improve pregnancy rates [36–41]. A further meta-analysis confirmed that the PGS does not result in increased pregnancy rate [42]. One of the studies of PGS for 9 chromosomes showed a trend towards lower miscarriage rate in AMA patients that translates in higher "take-home" baby rates [4].

Following the above studies, ESHRE and ASRM societies have issued guidelines discouraging the use of FISH for aneuploidy screening. Despite the new guidelines, the number of PGD cycles using FISH as the method of diagnosis reported by the ESHRE PGD consortium have only slightly reduced from 67 to 61 % of the overall PGD cycles from before 2007 to 2009 [1, 2].

In contrast with the above studies showing that PGD using FISH is unsuccessful in increasing pregnancy rates, two more recent RCTs show a clear benefit for patients of AMA and patients with previous implantation failures [43, 44]. In patients of AMA, Rubio et al. report 32.3 % vs. 15.5 % ($p=0.0099$) live birth rates per oocyte retrieval for PGD-tested embryos vs. non-tested, respectively. In couples with previous implantation failures, the ongoing pregnancy rates per oocyte retrieval was 48.0 % when tested with FISH vs. 29.5 % without PGD ($p = 0.0363$).

Pitfalls of FISH

In general, there are three major sources of errors that contribute to the overall error rate of a method. The first is due to normal biological variation, the second is due to method limitations, and the third is due to execution flaws.

It has been reported that cleavage-stage embryos present with high mosaicism, but further development to blastocyst may allow for self-correction of earlier aneuploidies [45–47]. The original results showing high mosaicism were obtained using FISH, but a more recent study employing microarray technology has shown that embryo mosaicism is significantly lower than estimated by FISH [48]. Therefore, the argument of error due to mosaicism is no longer valid.

Positioning of chromosomal pairs during the cell cycle may result in a physical distance below the detection capability of the probes used for FISH (Fig. 5). Indeed, monosomies are over-diagnosed in embryos by FISH, but are not confirmed using rehybridization with different probes [38, 49, 50]. Moreover, chromosomal duplication during mitosis is asynchronous [51]. Blastomeres are actively dividing and therefore it is possible that when biopsied one chromosome may have duplicated earlier than others. Such biological variation would explain double signals often detected by FISH (Fig. 5).

FISH for 9–12 chromosomes is not comprehensive enough to cover all possible aneuploidies. Karyotyping of first trimester pregnancy losses and whole genome screening of embryos show that aneuploidy can affect all chromosomes and not only the ones tested by FISH [22, 23, 52–56]. Whole genome screening is currently the method of choice, and the different methods and limitations are briefly discussed below.

FISH is a technically difficult method and is prone to many errors. Errors may arise during the FISH fixation, staining, and evaluation steps. Interestingly, the percentage of non-informative blastomeres vary vastly between studies ranging from 3 to 20 % [32, 41, 49] despite using similar commercial probes. Moreover, additional hybridization rounds with different probes improve the accuracy of the diagnosis [49]. FISH is a method sensitive to operator-bias, or, in other words, a method that requires a high level of technical expertise.

Advances in PGD and Future Perspectives

Whole Genome Screening for Aneuploidy

Due to the above mentioned FISH limitations, several methods of comprehensive whole genome aneuploidy screening are emerging. To distinguish between the different screening methods for aneuploidy, a number of investigators favor the term Comprehensive Chromosome Screening (CCS) when referring to whole genome screening methods [4, 55, 57]. A brief description of these methods is presented here and are covered in other chapters.

The first successful attempt to characterize all 23 chromosomes of a cleavage-stage embryo was done using Comparative Genome Amplification (CGH) [58]. In this method, the DNA of a biopsied blastomere is labeled with a fluorochrome. Another DNA sample from a normal individual is labeled with a different color and the two are mixed and applied on a glass slide carrying chromosomes in metaphase. Any color intensity difference indicates the loss or gain of genetic material. CGH has been successfully performed in polar bodies and cleavage-stage embryos [24, 25, 59, 60]. However, this method is very labor-intensive and unsuitable to routine testing.

Instead, array CGH (aCGH) follows the same principle but is performed in a microarray format. Instead of chromosomes in metaphase, nucleic acid fragments covering the whole genome are dotted (arrayed) on a glass slide. Information is gathered and analyzed with a computer software. Several commercial or custom-made microarray platforms have been tested for Prenatal and PGD [17, 20, 52, 53]. These arrays can detect copy number differences and imbalances of the tested cell. Therefore, they can also be applied in the detection of chromosomal rearrangements such as translocations or microdeletions, but they cannot distinguish a balanced from a normal karyotype.

Another type of microarray for whole genome screening is Single Nucleotide Polymorphism (SNP) arrays, which were originally developed for genetic linkage analysis. They contain several thousands of SNPs found in the Human Genome and therefore they provide extensive coverage of the chromosomes [52, 61]. The analysis of the results requires powerful software and computers, but it generates considerably more information than any other type of array. In addition to aneuploidy they can also detect Uniparental Disomy and the parental origin of each abnormality [61].

All microarray platforms require sophisticated statistics to analyze the results of the hybridization and can provide a vast amount of genomic information about the preimplantation embryos. It remains to be determined how much of this information is helpful for the clinician and the patient, and whether in some cases it may complicate treatment. Whole genome aneuploidy screening shows a significantly lower error rate than FISH [55] and greatly improved results in terms of comprehensive genome screening and pregnancy rates [55].

Blastocyst Biopsy and Embryo Vitrification

Recent advances in embryo freezing and biopsy methods hold great potential for facilitating comprehensive aneuploidy screening. Blastocyst testing showed a 50 % improvement in implantation rates [4]. Another advantage of blastocyst biopsy is increased amount of starting DNA and consequently improved accuracy.

The survival of biopsied embryos after freezing with conventional slow freezing methods is low. Vitrification has been shown to result in very high embryo survival, without adverse effects on the embryo [62]. Vitrification will also be useful for patients seeking PGD for monogenic disorders who often have several normal embryos from one IVF cycle.

Conclusions and Future Perspectives

PGD is a safe and efficient procedure for the screening of embryos in an early stage in order to select and transfer only the unaffected embryos. Aneuploidy screening using FISH is limited to 9–12 chromosomes and is a technically difficult procedure prone to many errors. Thus, aneuploidy screening has passed through a period of reconsideration and is now re-emerging with complete genome screening. However, there is increasing evidence that besides ploidy, gene expression and metabolism contribute to embryo viability [3, 63]. Therefore, a combination of comprehensive screening technologies is likely to significantly improve selection of the normal embryo.

Acknowledgments We thank Dr. C. Rubio (IVI, Valencia, Spain) for sharing PGD results, and Dr. D. Sakkas (Boston IVF, USA) for providing embryo biopsy pictures.

References

1. Goossens V, Harton G, Moutou C, Traeger-Synodinos J, Van Rij M, Harper JC. ESHRE PGD Consortium data collection IX: cycles from January to December 2006 with pregnancy follow-up to October 2007. Hum Reprod. 2009;24:1786–810.
2. Goossens V, Traeger-Synodinos J, Coonen E, De Rycke M, Moutou C, Pehlivan T, et al. ESHRE PGD Consortium data collection XI: cycles from January to December 2008 with pregnancy follow-up to October 2009. Hum Reprod. 2012;27(7):1887–911.
3. Katz-Jaffe MG, McCallie BR, Janesch A, Filipovits JA, Schoolcraft WB, Gardner DK. Blastocysts from patients with polycystic ovaries exhibit altered transcriptome and secretome. Reprod Biomed Online. 2010;21:520–6.
4. Schoolcraft WB, Fragouli E, Stevens J, Munne S, Katz-Jaffe MG, Wells D. Clinical application of comprehensive chromosomal screening at the blastocyst stage. Fertil Steril. 2010;94(5):1700–6.
5. Coonen E, Martini E, Dumoulin JC, Hollanders-Crombach HT, de Die-Smulders C, Geraedts JP, et al. Preimplantation genetic diagnosis of a reciprocal translocation t(3;11)(q27.3;q24.3) in siblings. Mol Hum Reprod. 2000;6:199–206.
6. Scriven PN, O'Mahony F, Bickerstaff H, Yeong CT, Braude P, Mackie Ogilvie C. Clinical pregnancy following blastomere biopsy and PGD for a reciprocal translocation carrier: analysis of meiotic outcomes

and embryo quality in two IVF cycles. Prenat Diagn. 2000;20:587–92.
7. Kyu Lim C, Hyun Jun J, Mi Min D, Lee HS, Young Kim J, Koong MK, et al. Efficacy and clinical outcome of preimplantation genetic diagnosis using FISH for couples of reciprocal and Robertsonian translocations: the Korean experience. Prenat Diagn. 2004;24:556–61.
8. Otani T, Roche M, Mizuike M, Colls P, Escudero T, Munne S. Preimplantation genetic diagnosis significantly improves the pregnancy outcome of translocation carriers with a history of recurrent miscarriage and unsuccessful pregnancies. Reprod Biomed Online. 2006;13:869–74.
9. Verlinsky Y, Cieslak J, Evsikov S, Galat V, Kuliev A. Nuclear transfer for full karyotyping and preimplantation diagnosis for translocations. Reprod Biomed Online. 2002;5:300–5.
10. Sugiura-Ogasawara M, Ozaki Y, Sato T, Suzumori N, Suzumori K. Poor prognosis of recurrent aborters with either maternal or paternal reciprocal translocations. Fertil Steril. 2004;81:367–73.
11. Pujol A, Benet J, Staessen C, Van Assche E, Campillo M, Egozcue J, et al. The importance of aneuploidy screening in reciprocal translocation carriers. Reproduction. 2006;131:1025–35.
12. Fischer J, Colls P, Escudero T, Munne S. Preimplantation genetic diagnosis (PGD) improves pregnancy outcome for translocation carriers with a history of recurrent losses. Fertil Steril. 2009;94(1): 283–9.
13. Fischer J, Colls P, Escudero T, Munne S. Preimplantation genetic diagnosis (PGD) improves pregnancy outcome for translocation carriers with a history of recurrent losses. Fertil Steril. 2010;94:283–9.
14. Lalioti MD. Can preimplantation genetic diagnosis overcome recurrent pregnancy failure? Curr Opin Obstet Gynecol. 2008;20:199–204.
15. Verlinsky Y, Tur-Kaspa I, Cieslak J, Bernal A, Morris R, Taranissi M, et al. Preimplantation testing for chromosomal disorders improves reproductive outcome of poor-prognosis patients. Reprod Biomed Online. 2005;11:219–25.
16. Cheng EY, Hunt PA, Naluai-Cecchini TA, Fligner CL, Fujimoto VY, Pasternack TL, et al. Meiotic recombination in human oocytes. PLoS Genet. 2009;5:e1000661.
17. Kasakyan S, Lohmann L, Aboura A, Quimsiyeh M, Menezo Y, Tachdjian G, et al. De novo complex intra chromosomal rearrangement after ICSI: characterisation by BACs micro array-CGH. Mol Cytogenet. 2008;1:27.
18. Johnson DS, Cinnioglu C, Ross R, Filby A, Gemelos G, Hill M, et al. Comprehensive analysis of karyotypic mosaicism between trophectoderm and inner cell mass. Mol Hum Reprod. 2010;16:944–9.
19. Colls P, Escudero T, Fischer J, Cekleniak NA, Ben-Ozer S, Meyer B, et al. Validation of array comparative genome hybridization for diagnosis of translocations in preimplantation human embryos. Reprod Biomed Online. 2012;24(6):621–9.
20. Alfarawati S, Fragouli E, Colls P, Wells D. First births after preimplantation genetic diagnosis of structural chromosome abnormalities using comparative genomic hybridization and microarray analysis. Hum Reprod. 2011;26:1560–74.
21. Treff NR, Northrop LE, Kasabwala K, Su J, Levy B, Scott Jr RT. Single nucleotide polymorphism microarray-based concurrent screening of 24-chromosome aneuploidy and unbalanced translocations in preimplantation human embryos. Fertil Steril. 2011;95:1606–12 e1-2.
22. Hogge WA, Byrnes AL, Lanasa MC, Surti U. The clinical use of karyotyping spontaneous abortions. Am J Obstet Gynecol. 2003;189:397–400; discussion 400–2.
23. Ljunger E, Cnattingius S, Lundin C, Anneren G. Chromosomal anomalies in first-trimester miscarriages. Acta Obstet Gynecol Scand. 2005;84:1103–7.
24. Fragouli E, Wells D, Thornhill A, Serhal P, Faed MJ, Harper JC, et al. Comparative genomic hybridization analysis of human oocytes and polar bodies. Hum Reprod. 2006;21(9):2319–28.
25. Sher G, Keskintepe L, Keskintepe M, Ginsburg M, Maassarani G, Yakut T, et al. Oocyte karyotyping by comparative genomic hybrydization provides a highly reliable method for selecting "competent" embryos, markedly improving in vitro fertilization outcome: a multiphase study. Fertil Steril. 2007;87(5):1033–40.
26. Hassold T, Hall H, Hunt P. The origin of human aneuploidy: where we have been, where we are going. Hum Mol Genet. 2007;16(Spec No 2):R203–8.
27. Colls P, Goodall N, Zheng X, Munne S. Increased efficiency of preimplantation genetic diagnosis for aneuploidy by testing 12 chromosomes. Reprod Biomed Online. 2009;19:532–8.
28. Munne S, Chen S, Fischer J, Colls P, Zheng X, Stevens J, et al. Preimplantation genetic diagnosis reduces pregnancy loss in women aged 35 years and older with a history of recurrent miscarriages. Fertil Steril. 2005;84:331–5.
29. Platteau P, Staessen C, Michiels A, Van Steirteghem A, Liebaers I, Devroey P. Preimplantation genetic diagnosis for aneuploidy screening in patients with unexplained recurrent miscarriages. Fertil Steril. 2005;83:393–7; quiz 525–6.
30. Rubio C, Rodrigo L, Perez-Cano I, Mercader A, Mateu E, Buendia P, et al. FISH screening of aneuploidies in preimplantation embryos to improve IVF outcome. Reprod Biomed Online. 2005;11:497–506.
31. Rubio C, Simon C, Vidal F, Rodrigo L, Pehlivan T, Remohi J, et al. Chromosomal abnormalities and embryo development in recurrent miscarriage couples. Hum Reprod. 2003;18:182–8.
32. Mastenbroek S, Twisk M, van Echten-Arends J, Sikkema-Raddatz B, Korevaar JC, Verhoeve HR, et al. In vitro fertilization with preimplantation genetic screening. N Engl J Med. 2007;357:9–17.
33. Staessen C, Platteau P, Van Assche E, Michiels A, Tournaye H, Camus M, et al. Comparison of blastocyst transfer with or without preimplantation genetic

diagnosis for aneuploidy screening in couples with advanced maternal age: a prospective randomized controlled trial. Hum Reprod. 2004;19:2849–58.

34. Goossens V, Harton G, Moutou C, Scriven PN, Traeger-Synodinos J, Sermon K, et al. ESHRE PGD Consortium data collection VIII: cycles from January to December 2005 with pregnancy follow-up to October 2006. Hum Reprod. 2008;23:2629–45.
35. Munne S, Gianaroli L, Tur-Kaspa I, Magli C, Sandalinas M, Grifo J, et al. Substandard application of preimplantation genetic screening may interfere with its clinical success. Fertil Steril. 2007;88:781–4.
36. Meyer LR, Klipstein S, Hazlett WD, Nasta T, Mangan P, Karande VC. A prospective randomized controlled trial of preimplantation genetic screening in the "good prognosis" patient. Fertil Steril. 2009;91:1731–8.
37. Blockeel C, Schutyser V, De Vos A, Verpoest W, De Vos M, Staessen C, et al. Prospectively randomized controlled trial of PGS in IVF/ICSI patients with poor implantation. Reprod Biomed Online. 2008;17: 848–54.
38. Hardarson T, Hanson C, Lundin K, Hillensjo T, Nilsson L, Stevic J, et al. Preimplantation genetic screening in women of advanced maternal age caused a decrease in clinical pregnancy rate: a randomized controlled trial. Hum Reprod. 2008;23:2806–12.
39. Twisk M, Mastenbroek S, Hoek A, Heineman MJ, van der Veen F, Bossuyt PM, et al. No beneficial effect of preimplantation genetic screening in women of advanced maternal age with a high risk for embryonic aneuploidy. Hum Reprod. 2008;23:2813–7.
40. Jansen RP, Bowman MC, de Boer KA, Leigh DA, Lieberman DB, McArthur SJ. What next for preimplantation genetic screening (PGS)? Experience with blastocyst biopsy and testing for aneuploidy. Hum Reprod. 2008;23:1476–8.
41. Debrock S, Melotte C, Spiessens C, Peeraer K, Vanneste E, Meeuwis L, et al. Preimplantation genetic screening for aneuploidy of embryos after in vitro fertilization in women aged at least 35 years: a prospective randomized trial. Fertil Steril. 2009;93:364–73.
42. Checa MA, Alonso-Coello P, Sola I, Robles A, Carreras R, Balasch J. IVF/ICSI with or without preimplantation genetic screening for aneuploidy in couples without genetic disorders: a systematic review and meta-analysis. J Assist Reprod Genet. 2009;26:273–83.
43. Rubio C, Mateu E, Bosch E, Mercader A, Milán M, Labarta E, et al. Benefits of PGS in advanced maternal age patient: a prospective randomized trial in the age range between 41–44 years. In: ESHRE annual meeting. Istanbul, Turkey; 2012.
44. Rodrigo L, Rubio C, Buendía P, Bellver J, Vidal C, Giles J, et al. Improved take-home baby rate with Preimplantation Genetic Screening in Implantation Failure couples: a prospective controlled trial in a properly characterized population. In: ESHRE Annual meeting. Istanbul, Turkey; 2012.
45. Daphnis DD, Delhanty JD, Jerkovic S, Geyer J, Craft I, Harper JC. Detailed FISH analysis of day 5 human embryos reveals the mechanisms leading to mosaic aneuploidy. Hum Reprod. 2005;20:129–37.
46. Baart EB, Martini E, van den Berg I, Macklon NS, Galjaard RJ, Fauser BC, et al. Preimplantation genetic screening reveals a high incidence of aneuploidy and mosaicism in embryos from young women undergoing IVF. Hum Reprod. 2006;21:223–33.
47. Li M, DeUgarte CM, Surrey M, Danzer H, DeCherney A, Hill DL. Fluorescence in situ hybridization reanalysis of day-6 human blastocysts diagnosed with aneuploidy on day 3. Fertil Steril. 2005;84:1395–400.
48. Treff NR, Levy B, Su J, Northrop LE, Tao X, Scott Jr RT. SNP microarray-based 24 chromosome aneuploidy screening is significantly more consistent than FISH. Mol Hum Reprod. 2010;16:583–9.
49. Mir P, Rodrigo L, Mateu E, Peinado V, Milan M, Mercader A, et al. Improving FISH diagnosis for preimplantation genetic aneuploidy screening. Hum Reprod. 2010;25:1812–7.
50. Cooper ML, Darilek S, Wun WS, Angus SC, Mensing DE, Pursley AN, et al. A retrospective study of preimplantation embryos diagnosed with monosomy by fluorescence in situ hybridization (FISH). Cytogenet Genome Res. 2006;114:359–66.
51. Anglana M, Apiou F, Bensimon A, Debatisse M. Dynamics of DNA replication in mammalian somatic cells: nucleotide pool modulates origin choice and interorigin spacing. Cell. 2003;114:385–94.
52. Handyside AH, Harton GL, Mariani B, Thornhill AR, Affara NA, Shaw MA, et al. Karyomapping: a Universal Method for Genome Wide Analysis of Genetic Disease based on Mapping Crossovers between Parental Haplotypes. J Med Genet. 2009; 47(10):651–8.
53. Le Caignec C, Spits C, Sermon K, De Rycke M, Thienpont B, Debrock S, et al. Single-cell chromosomal imbalances detection by array CGH. Nucleic Acids Res. 2006;34:e68.
54. Ling J, Zhuang G, Tazon-Vega B, Zhang C, Cao B, Rosenwaks Z, et al. Evaluation of genome coverage and fidelity of multiple displacement amplification from single cells by SNP array. Mol Hum Reprod. 2009;15:739–47.
55. Scott Jr RT, Ferry K, Su J, Tao X, Scott K, Treff NR. Comprehensive chromosome screening is highly predictive of the reproductive potential of human embryos: a prospective, blinded, nonselection study. Fertil Steril. 2012;97:870–5.
56. Van den Veyver IB, Patel A, Shaw CA, Pursley AN, Kang SH, Simovich MJ, et al. Clinical use of array comparative genomic hybridization (aCGH) for prenatal diagnosis in 300 cases. Prenat Diagn. 2009;29:29–39.
57. Fragouli E, Katz-Jaffe M, Alfarawati S, Stevens J, Colls P, Goodall NN, et al. Comprehensive chromosome screening of polar bodies and blastocysts from couples experiencing repeated implantation failure. Fertil Steril. 2010;94(3):875–87.
58. Wells D, Escudero T, Levy B, Hirschhorn K, Delhanty JD, Munne S. First clinical application of comparative genomic hybridization and polar body testing for

preimplantation genetic diagnosis of aneuploidy. Fertil Steril. 2002;78:543–9.
59. Daphnis DD, Fragouli E, Economou K, Jerkovic S, Craft IL, Delhanty JD, et al. Analysis of the evolution of chromosome abnormalities in human embryos from Day 3 to 5 using CGH and FISH. Mol Hum Reprod. 2008;14:117–25.
60. Gutierrez-Mateo C, Benet J, Wells D, Colls P, Bermudez MG, Sanchez-Garcia JF, et al. Aneuploidy study of human oocytes first polar body comparative genomic hybridization and metaphase II fluorescence in situ hybridization analysis. Hum Reprod. 2004;19:2859–68.
61. Johnson N, Speirs V, Curtin NJ, Hall AG. A comparative study of genome-wide SNP, CGH microarray and protein expression analysis to explore genotypic and phenotypic mechanisms of acquired antiestrogen resistance in breast cancer. Breast Cancer Res Treat. 2008;111:55–63.
62. Forman EJ, Li X, Ferry KM, Scott K, Treff NR, Scott Jr RT. Oocyte vitrification does not increase the risk of embryonic aneuploidy or diminish the implantation potential of blastocysts created after intracytoplasmic sperm injection: a novel, paired randomized controlled trial using DNA fingerprinting. Fertil Steril. 2012;98(3):644–9.
63. Seli E, Vergouw CG, Morita H, Botros L, Roos P, Lambalk CB, et al. Noninvasive metabolomic profiling as an adjunct to morphology for noninvasive embryo assessment in women undergoing single embryo transfer. Fertil Steril. 2010;94:535–42.

Single Nucleotide Polymorphisms and Next Generation Sequencing

12

Alan H. Handyside and Dagan Wells

Preimplantation Genetic Diagnosis of Single Gene Disorders Based on DNA Amplification

Single cell analysis for preimplantation genetic diagnosis (PGD) of single gene defects (SGDs) was first used to identify the sex of embryos in a series of couples at risk of various X-linked conditions, which typically only affect males [1]. The use of PCR at the single cell level was still in its infancy and even doubling the typical number of amplification cycles failed to amplify unique target sequences reliably. For this reason, PCR amplification of a Y-linked repeat sequence, present in thousands of copies per cell, was used for identification of male embryos. However, the extreme sensitivity of this protocol and the rapid build-up of amplified DNA products in the laboratory environment, soon led to the appearance of contamination and false positive results in blank (negative) controls. Furthermore, in a minority of single male cells amplification still failed, resulting in a male embryo being identified as female, which lead to the first clinical misdiagnosis following PGD.

A.H. Handyside
The Bridge Centre, London Bridge, London, UK

D. Wells (✉)
Nuffield Department of Obstetrics and Gynaecology, University of Oxford, Oxford, UK

Institute of Reproductive Sciences, Oxford, UK
e-mail: dagan.wells@obs-gyn.ox.ac.uk

The breakthrough, enabling amplification of short unique sequences encompassing the site of the gene mutation, was to use two rounds of PCR amplification, preferably with nested oligonucleotide primers [2, 3]. During the first round of PCR a DNA fragment encompassing the mutation site undergoes a limited amplification. The fragments produced are not amplified to the vast extent necessary for direct visualisation and consequently they pose only a minor contamination risk. The second PCR involves the use of primers that anneal within the initial amplified fragment, producing a smaller 'nested' fragment that has undergone sufficient amplification for subsequent detection. Despite the large amount of amplification, the secondary fragment poses little contamination risk since it lacks the priming sites required for amplification in the initial reaction. Using this strategy, PGD of SGDs using single biopsied cells became possible resulting in the birth of a child free of the common DF508, three base pair deletion of the CFTR gene causing cystic fibrosis [4].

Nested PCR of a short fragment of exon 10 of the CFTR gene, including the sequence around the position of DF508, remains one of the most sensitive and efficient methods of single cell DNA amplification. Nevertheless, in a small percentage of single cells, amplification either fails completely or there is an apparently random failure to amplify one of the two parental alleles. This phenomenon, known as allele dropout (ADO), can cause misdiagnosis of a carrier of an autosomal recessive condition as affected or homozygous normal, or more seriously, in the

D.K. Gardner et al. (eds.), *Human Gametes and Preimplantation Embryos: Assessment and Diagnosis*, DOI 10.1007/978-1-4614-6651-2_12,

case of an autosomal dominant condition, an affected mutation carrier may appear to be unaffected. The incidence of ADO can be minimised by optimising the protocols for cell lysis and amplification, and specifically by raising the denaturation temperature in the first few cycles of the first PCR [5]. However, to date ADO has never been completely eliminated in any targeted or whole genome amplification (WGA) protocol at the single cell level [6].

Multiplex PCR for the Preimplantation Diagnosis of Single Gene Disorders

The combined problems of ADO and contamination prompted the search for DNA markers, which could be used to identify independently the presence of the chromosome carrying the mutant gene, essentially producing a diagnosis with built-in redundancy [7, 8]. In the early 1990s, the intense effort to sequence the human genome led to the discovery and mapping of a highly polymorphic class of markers, known as short tandem repeats (STRs), which are widely distributed throughout the genome and consist of a short sequence of two or more bases repeated a variable number of times. Because the number of repeats is highly polymorphic but relatively stable from one generation to the next, the repeat length can be used as a marker. By selecting a combination of STRs in close proximity to the mutation site, having different repeat lengths (i.e. different alleles) on all four parental chromosomes, it is possible to track the inheritance of each chromosome from parent to embryo. Ideally two or more STRs flanking the proximal and distal boundaries of the gene and, where possible, an intragenic STR are chosen for this purpose. The distance between the flanking STRs and the gene should be minimised (ideally 1 Mb or less), reducing the chance of recombination between the marker and the mutation site during meiosis. Although ADO can potentially affect STR loci as well as the mutation sites, the probability of multiple loci on the same chromosome all being affected in the same cell is very low.

The strategy of using one or more polymorphic markers, combined with mutation detection, has now become the 'gold standard' for single cell analysis [9]. The relatively short length of the STRs (no more than a few hundred base pairs), combined with the sensitivity of fluorescent PCR analysed by capillary electrophoresis using automated sequencers, has facilitated simultaneous amplification of multiple target sequences (multiplex PCR) directly from single cells. Also, mutations are now generally detected by single fluorescent base extension reactions, or minisequencing, using specially designed primers, following the first multiplex PCR [10]. As well as allowing an accurate diagnosis on occasions when ADO affects amplification of the mutation site, STRs also have the capacity to reveal the presence of DNA contaminants. Their highly polymorphic nature means that foreign contaminants will often have combinations of STR alleles that differ from the embryos being tested, resulting in the detection of additional STR alleles not present in the parents.

Multiplex amplification by fluorescent PCR is now so successful that the same principle can be extended to identify the parental origin of more than one region of the genome. For example, the origin of the HLA region of chromosome 6 can be combined with SGD diagnosis to allow the selection of unaffected embryos, which are HLA matched to an existing affected child, for cord blood stem cell transplantation [11, 12]. It is also possible to use STR markers to detect abnormal numbers of chromosomes (aneuploidy), not only for the chromosome affected by the SGD but also for a small number of other chromosomes. Finally, STRs in both the centromeric and subtelomeric regions of chromosomes affected by reciprocal or Robertsonian translocations can be used to test embryos for imbalance of the sections of chromosome involved in the rearrangement [13].

Limitations of Multiplex-PCR Strategies and New Developments

The problem with multiplex fluorescent PCR is that, although the reagents are relatively low in cost, the initial work to identify informative markers for a specific family or inherited condition and optimise their amplification at the single cell level, is time consuming and labour intensive. Furthermore, it may be difficult to identify fully informative closely linked markers in some families, resulting in the testing of numerous potential candidates and a final combination which may only be semi-informative or less closely linked to the mutant gene than desired. For this reason, multiplex panels of markers have been developed for preimplantation genetic haplotyping (PGH) of specific inherited conditions. In the PGH approach, the disease-linked STRs used are sufficiently numerous that most families are found to have at least two or three that are informative and therefore able to provide a diagnosis [14]. Nonetheless, some couples are still excluded because of lack of informative markers within the STR panels and any new or rare condition still requires the development of an additional single cell test. Essentially, therefore, PGD by highly multiplexed fluorescent PCR directly from single cells has reached its practical limits and although well established in clinical practice and accurate, remains specialised, labour intensive and rate limiting, preventing widespread application.

With the development of new methods for WGA by, for example, the use of isothermal multiple displacement amplification (MDA), it is now possible to amplify microgram quantities of DNA from a single cell [15–17]. This has revolutionised prospects for single cell analysis since it allows the amplified DNA to be analysed under conventional conditions and provides enough DNA for microarray-based testing or sequencing. Disappointingly, however, ADO, following either MDA [16] or PCR library-based methods of WGA, remains a significant problem. Nevertheless, WGA methods have been successfully applied for the genetic analysis of oocytes and embryos, especially in conjunction with microarrays. The use of microarray comparative genomic hybridisation (array CGH) has been expanding particularly rapidly over the last few years and is now widely used for PGD of aneuploidy (also known as preimplantation genetic screening—PGS) [18–22]. Microarray-CGH is discussed in detail elsewhere in this book (see Chap. 13). In this chapter we will limit ourselves to reviewing current developments using microarrays for the interrogation of single nucleotide polymorphisms (SNPs) in human embryos and discuss the possibility of employing powerful next generation sequencing technologies for PGD. These provide the potential to move beyond family or disease specific testing, to genome-wide methods which overcome issues related to ADO and provide comprehensive testing for any SGDs combined with molecular cytogenetic analysis.

Single Nucleotide Polymorphisms and SNP Microarrays

SNPs are a common type of genetic variation, in which one of two or more bases may be present at a particular position in the DNA sequence. Over ten million SNPs have been identified in the human genome and allele frequencies studied by genotyping multiple individuals in different populations. Most SNPs occur in noncoding regions and are not known to cause a clinical phenotype. However, SNPs collectively are thought to contribute to variation between individuals and some SNPs are associated with disease haplotypes.

Biallelic SNPs with a relatively high minor allele frequency and heterozygosity ratio represent an important set of DNA markers. By convention, each SNP locus is genotyped as AA or BB if homozygous, or AB, if heterozygous, irrespective of the actual nucleotides (i.e. G, A, T or C) present. Furthermore, microarrays capable of genotyping up to a million or more SNPs, either evenly distributed at high density across the genome or clustered around known genes, provide a rapid and cost-effective tool for genotyping large numbers of samples. The various microarray technologies available for SNP genotyping differ in the methodologies used. For example, some platforms involve affixing oligonucleotide probes of complementary sequence to individual SNP alleles directly to glass slides, whereas another system attaches probes to polystyrene beads. Also, some arrays use the same probe to detect both alleles while others have different probes for each allele and some arrays have multiple features for each SNP locus. All of them, however, use some form of fluorescence-based chemistry, enabling genotyping to be combined with allele-specific measurement of fluorescence intensity, potentially providing a quantification of the amount of DNA from an individual SNP locus. SNP genotyping arrays are used extensively both for genome-wide association studies of common diseases and for high resolution molecular cytogenetics.

The combination of a high density of SNP markers genome-wide, permitting universal linkage-based diagnosis of SGDs, combined with the possibility of allele-specific quantification for chromosome copy number, is of great potential value for preimplantation genetics. STR markers are generally more informative than SNPs since each locus may have multiple alleles of different lengths, often allowing all four parental chromosomes to be distinguished at a specific locus. In contrast, SNPs are almost always only bialleleic and can therefore only identify the presence of a maximum of two different chromosomes at a given locus. However, because of the high density of SNP loci, it is usually possible to find four different SNP loci, each suitable for the detection of a different parental chromosome, all within the close proximity to the gene of interest. Hence it is possible to diagnose the presence of a SGD via linkage analysis, examining informative SNP loci in the region of the affected gene. Furthermore, the ability to measure the fluorescence intensity of signals from both alleles at successive loci across each chromosome allows high resolution molecular cytogenetic analysis which, unlike array CGH, when combined with genotype analysis of DNA from the parents, can identify the parental origin of the abnormality as well as revealing instances of uniparental disomy.

For PGD, high density SNP genotyping arrays have so far mainly been used for detection of chromosome aneuploidy, using four distinct strategies. The first of these strategies, developed by Kearns and colleagues, is simply to optimise the lysis and WGA protocols for single and small numbers of cells to reduce amplification bias and use a large series of WGA products from chromosomally normal single cells to optimise the SNP genotype calls at each locus [23]. This then enables aneuploidy to be detected by analysis of the general features of the SNP data across each chromosome in the same way as would be done for any genomic DNA sample (Fig. 1). So for example, trisomy can be detected by examining the B allele ratio of each SNP locus. In a euploid sample, the B allele ratio of thousands of consecutive SNP loci should fall into three bands corresponding to the genotypes AA (0, B allele ratio), BB (1 B allele ratio) and AB (0.5 B allele ratio). In a trisomic sample, however, the heterozygous band splits into two, corresponding to AAB (0.33 B allele ratio) and BBA (0.67 B allele ratio). Whereas, in a sample with a chromosome monosomy or heterozygous deletion, there should be no heterozygous calls and this loss of heterozygosity (LOH) is then detected by the absence of any heterozygous band in the B allele ratio plot.

In practice, this strategy has been difficult to replicate. Although regions showing LOH are easily and accurately identified, amplification bias occurring during WGA combined with the scatter in the SNP intensity data generally makes detection of the split heterozygous band by analysis of the B allele ratio very difficult. An alternative strategy, developed by Treff and colleagues, is to use copy number assignments for each individual SNP locus and apply statistical methods to examine the copy number distribution of all of the SNPs on a particular chromosome and assign chromosome copy number on the basis of the copy number of the majority (>50 %) of SNP loci [24]. To date, this approach has not been attempted on other SNP microarray platforms. An important consideration when considering the clinical application of SNP microarrays is that the protocol is not easy to fit within a normal working day. This has made it challenging to use SNP microarrays in embryo testing cycles in which a fresh transfer is desired and has led some groups to move towards faster methods such as real-time quantitative PCR (see Chap. 14).

Another strategy developed by Rabinowitz and colleagues, is to use SNP genotyping of both parents to enable the use of advanced bioinformatic algorithms to enhance the accuracy of SNP genotyping in single cell samples and to detect aneuploidy by identifying the presence of specific parental haplotypes [25]. Because the precise

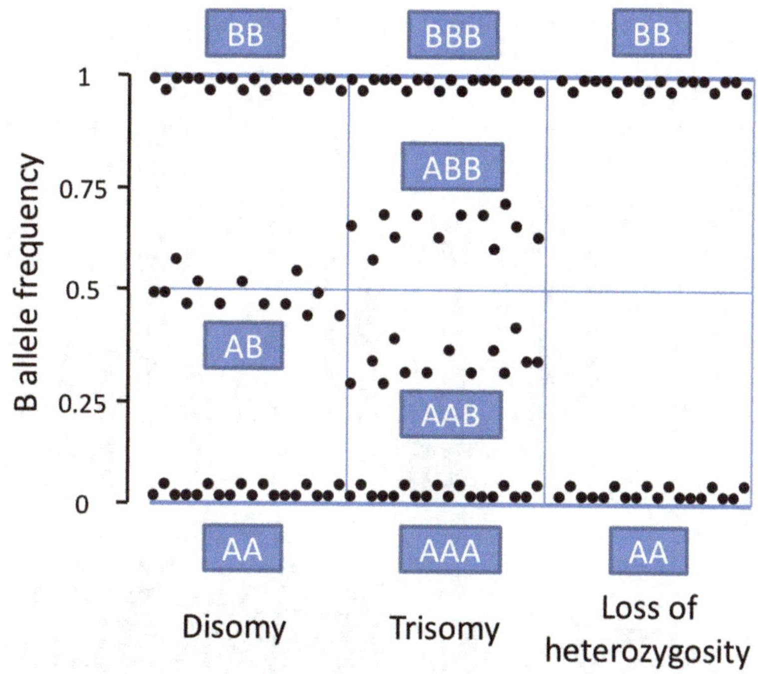

Fig. 12.1 Molecular cytogenetics using high density single nucleotide polymorphism (SNP) arrays. For molecular cytogenetic analysis, the relative intensity of the A and B alleles at each SNP locus (*black dots*) is analysed across each chromosome. In normal genomic DNA, each locus on a pair of homologous chromosomes (disomy) is either homozygous AA or BB, or heterozygous AB with B allele frequencies of 0, 0.5 and 1, respectively (*left panel*). Where there is an extra third copy of a chromosome (trisomy) or a regional duplication, the relative intensity of the A and B alleles at heterozygous loci now separate into two bands corresponding to those loci which are AAB and ABB with B allele frequencies of about 0.33 and 0.66, respectively (*middle panel*). If only a single chromosome is present (monosomy) or there is a heterozygous deletion on one chromosome, all of the SNP loci are genotyped as AA or BB and there is a loss of heterozygosity i.e. no heterozygous AB loci are detected (*right panel*)

algorithms are proprietary and have not been fully disclosed, it is not possible to replicate their results. Furthermore, some unusual features in published data obtained using this approach, specifically concerning the frequency and origin of aneuploidies [25, 26], have led to the methodology being criticised on theoretical grounds [27]. Nevertheless, the results are broadly similar to the patterns of aneuploidy established by other methods such as fluorescence in situ hybridisation (FISH).

Finally, the fourth strategy, karyomapping, uses genome-wide high density SNP genotyping and Mendelian analysis of both parents and a close relative of known disease status (often an existing child) as a universal method for linkage-based analysis of the inheritance of SGDs combined with the detection of a range of cytogenetic abnormalities including meiotic trisomies, monsomies and deletions [28]. The basic principle is simple. At informative SNP loci, in which one parent is homozygous (AA or BB) and the other is heterozygous (AB), the genotype of the biopsied cell(s) from the embryo at that locus enables the identification of which chromosome has been inherited from the heterozygous parent and whether this is the same chromosome as the reference child. So for example, if the genotype of a SNP in the vicinity of a dominant disease gene is AA for the father, AB for the mother and AB for an affected child previously born to the couple, then the conclusion is that the chromosome carrying allele B has been inherited from the mother and is associated with the disorder. If the genotype of an embryo from the same couple is also found to be AB, it is clear that it has

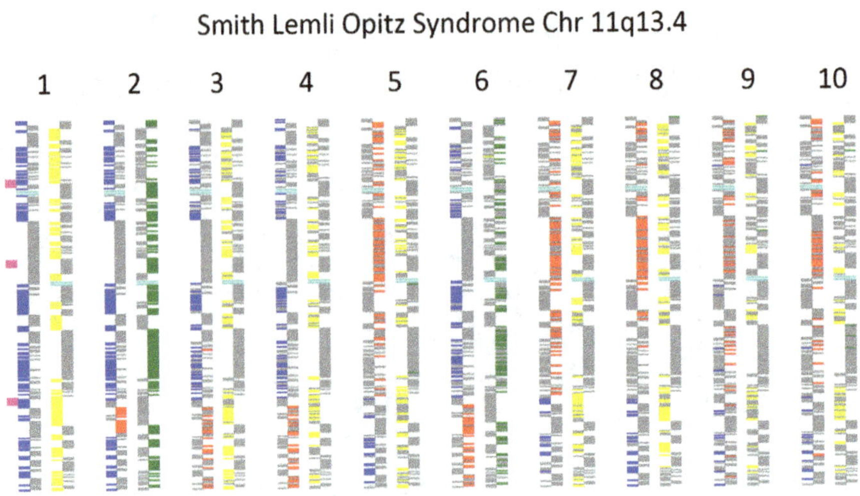

1. Child (reference)	Blue – Yellow	Pat Carrier	6. Embryo 4 Bm#1	Blue – Green	Affected
2. Affected fetus	Blue – Green	Affected	7. Embryo 5 Bm#1	Red – Yellow	Unaffected
3. Embryo 2 Bm#1	Blue – Yellow	Pat Carrier	8. Embryo 3 Bm#2	Red – Yellow	Unaffected
4. Embryo 2 Bm#2	Blue – Yellow	Pat Carrier	9. Embryo 3 Bm#3	Red – Yellow	Unaffected
5. Embryo 3 Bm#1	Red – Yellow	Unaffected	10. Embryo 3 Bm#4	Red - Yellow	Unaffected

Fig. 12.2 Karyomaps of chromosome 11q13.4 in a couple at risk of Smith Lemli Opitz syndrome. The karyomaps of an existing child, known to be a carrier of the paternal mutation (sample 1), an affected foetus from a previous pregnancy (sample 2) and whole genome amplification products of single blastomeres biopsied from four cleavage stage embryos (samples 3–10) for chromosome 11q13.4 are displayed for comparison. Consecutive informative single nucleotide polymorphism (SNP) loci for the four parental chromosomes are represented by two pairs of columns in each case (paternal, *left* and maternal, *right*) in which each segment is an informative SNP. Informative SNP loci which are heterozygous in the sample are coloured indicating the presence of that chromosome (paternal, *blue* and *red* and maternal, *yellow* and *green*). Negative informative SNP loci or those in which genotyping failed are coloured *grey*. The position of 7-dehydrocholesterol reductase (*DHCR7*) relative to the SNP loci is indicated by the *light blue bars*. The position of the three short tandem repeat (STR) markers used for conventional analysis is indicated in *purple* to the *left* of sample 1. The key below the karyomaps indicates the interpretation of the chromosomes present in the critical region flanking *DHCR7*. One embryo is shown to be a carrier of the paternal mutation, two embryos are unaffected (*shaded green*) and one embryo is homozygous affected

inherited the same maternal chromosome as the previous child and has therefore inherited her mutation. Alternatively if the genotype is AA, the embryo has inherited the other maternal chromosome and is therefore unaffected. As the probability that any individual SNP is heterozygous in one of the parents is high and there is a high density of SNP loci, then for most parents, a correspondingly dense set of informative markers for all four distinct parental chromosomes can be identified. Furthermore, the phase of the A and B alleles at successive heterozygous loci in each parent can be established by comparison with the genotype of the reference child or other close relative, allowing the creation of extended haplotypes covering all chromosomes (Fig. 2).

The rate of ADO at SNP loci in single cells following WGA by PCR library-based or MDA methods is relatively high, reaching 30 % in some instances. This remains a significant limitation for any downstream genetic analysis irrespective of the methodology employed. For karyomapping, ADO is potentially a problem since heterozygous SNP loci are needed to identify which parental chromosomes have been inherited. Hence, in the example described above, instead of the single cell genotyping as AB, ADO may occur resulting in the genotype AA (indicative of the other maternal chromosome) or alternatively, if the other allele drops out, BB, which is an impossible combination of alleles at this locus in these parents. In practice, therefore, only informative SNP loci, which are heterozygous in the embryo are used for karyomapping, avoiding ADO errors. Any 'impossible' genotypes are assumed to be heterozygous loci with ADO.

As karyomapping identifies a set of markers for each parental chromosome, it also enables chromosomal abnormalities to be identified in the embryo, independently of any quantitative SNP intensity analysis. Normally the embryo inherits one chromosome of each pair from each parent. However, recombination between the parental chromosomes occurs during the first meiotic division resulting in nonrecombinant and recombinant chromosomes and this is reflected in the karyomap for that chromosome either being identical to one of the parental chromosomes or switching from one to the other at the point of recombination. If an error occurs in meiosis such that two chromosomes with different patterns of recombination are inherited from one parent (as is generally the case), both sets of markers for the two chromosomes from that parent will be present for some or all of that chromosome indicating trisomy for that chromosome in the embryo. Nondisjunction or premature predivision of chromatids in the first meiotic division will be characterised by the presence of both sets of SNP markers in the region of the centromere and then distal to any crossovers. Alternatively, if both parental marker sets are only identified in more distal regions of the chromosome arms, this indicates a trisomy, which may have arisen in the second meiotic division. However, mitotic duplication of a chromosome by, for example nondisjunction cannot be detected because both chromosomes have the same SNP alleles at all loci. These therefore require quantitative analysis to be detected. In contrast, if all markers are found to be derived from a single parent for a particular chromosome or chromosome segment that indicates monosomy or a deletion, respectively.

An advantage of karyomapping over other methods for detecting chromosome copy number in single cells, such as array CGH or real-time PCR, is that the parental origin is identified which can be useful clinically. Furthermore, the high density of SNP markers provides higher resolution analysis than is possible with array CGH which is ideal for detection of chromosome imbalance resulting from structural chromosome abnormalities in one of the parents. Furthermore, SNP microarrays offer some advantages for PGD undertaken for carriers of reciprocal and Robertsonian translocations, since embryos with an entirely normal set of chromosomes, as revealed by their SNP profile, can be distinguished from those that are balanced but have inherited the two derivative, translocated chromosomes.

Next Generation Sequencing

Despite the mounting evidence that microarray-based methods can assist in the identification of viable embryos, leading to significant improvements in IVF outcomes, the relatively high cost of testing has limited the clinical application of these techniques. While technical innovations have allowed the costs associated with microarray analysis to be reduced significantly in recent years, further reductions in the price of genetic testing may be difficult to achieve. As such, the genetic analysis of embryos remains a relatively costly addition to the already expensive procedure of IVF. In order to continue the downward trend in the cost of genetic testing it may be necessary to move away from microarray-based methods, employing entirely new techniques.

Any new method for the analysis of embryos must match or surpass existing techniques in terms of speed and accuracy and should ideally have the capacity to provide data on both chromosomal copy number (i.e. aneuploidy) and DNA sequence (i.e. detection of gene mutations). New techniques should be scalable, permitting the simultaneous analysis of multiple samples, and be of lower cost than current alternatives. A prime candidate for such a method, potentially capable of fulfilling all of these criteria, is next generation sequencing (NGS). There are a number of different NGS strategies, but essentially all have the same purpose—the rapid generation of vast quantities of DNA sequence data at low cost. In most cases, NGS involves extraction of DNA from the sample followed by its fragmentation. The pieces of DNA produced then undergo an amplification step after which sequencing is initiated, simultaneously generating huge numbers of short DNA sequences. A computer compares the sequences produced to the known sequence of the human genome, allowing them to be placed in the correct chromosomal location, orientation and order. The alignment of DNA sequences with respect to a reference genome highlights any differences associated with the presence of mutations and polymorphisms. Additionally, the quantity of sequences derived from individual chromosomes provides an indication of their copy number, trisomic chromosomes presenting more than the expected number of sequences and those affected by monosomy producing too few.

NGS technology is revolutionising clinical genetics and is increasingly widely applied for the detection of mutations in individual genes and for the characterisation of chromosomal abnormalities. At the time of writing this chapter, there has not yet been any publication describing the application of NGS to cells biopsied from human embryos. However, the authors have conducted extensive preliminary work in this area and other groups are also actively involved in optimising and refining NGS techniques for the purposes of embryo diagnosis. We have been able to complete NGS analysis of single blastomeres within 15 h, a rate similar or faster than speeds achieved using the most rapid array CGH methods currently available. Importantly, high sample throughput was easily achieved. More than 30 samples have been successfully assessed in a single experiment and the data obtained indicated that simultaneous analysis of more than 100 samples should be technically feasible. A large number of cells biopsied from preimplantation embryos have now been subjected to NGS and chromosome abnormalities detected with high accuracy. The cost per sample was low, being only two thirds the price of the most cost-effective microarray platform currently available. The potential reduction in the price of genetic testing afforded by NGS has significant implications for the future clinical utilisation of preimplantation aneuploidy screening, potentially making it accessible to much greater numbers of infertile couples. Furthermore, the cost of NGS has been on a rapid downward trajectory and is likely to continue to get cheaper in the coming months and years.

Not only was NGS capable of revealing chromosome abnormalities, but it also provided information concerning the presence of mutations and polymorphisms of the DNA sequence. This was highlighted by the successful detection of the common *CFTR* DF508 mutation, associated with cystic fibrosis, in single cells from an affected cell line. Combining the detection of single gene mutations and aneuploidy screening has been extremely challenging using conventional methods. The ability of NGS to provide both chromosomal and DNA sequence information represents a significant advantage of this approach.

Although there is growing evidence that aneuploidy may be the single most important factor determining the ability of an embryo to implant and form a viable pregnancy, it remains the case that even the transfer of a chromosomally normal, morphologically perfect embryo cannot guarantee that a viable pregnancy will be established (Fig. 3). Clearly, there are other, less well-defined aspects of embryo biology that are also critical for successful development. A prime candidate in this regard is mitochondrial copy number, which previous studies have linked to various aspects of oocyte and embryo competence [29, 30]. Unlike all other methods of chromosome screening currently in use, NGS strategies have the potential to simultaneously provide data on mtDNA copy number and mutations as well as aneuploidy. This may provide an extra dimension to embryo screening. Our preliminary work using NGS has shown that the ratio of mtDNA sequences to nuclear DNA sequences often differs significantly between embryos derived from the same couple. The clinical significance of this finding is not yet known, but it seems likely that variation in this key organelle would have biological and clinical consequences.

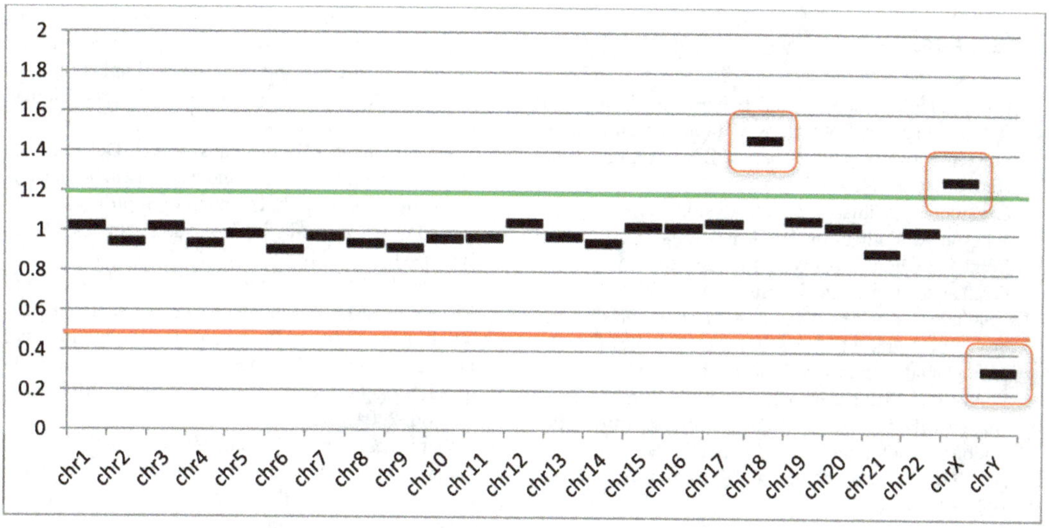

Fig. 12.3 Next generation sequencing-based aneuploidy detection. Next generation sequencing was applied to a WGA product generated from a trophectoderm biopsy. Approximately ten million DNA sequences were produced per sample. The proportion of sequences derived from each chromosome was compared to the proportions obtained from each chromosome in a control sample (known to be euploid). Chromosomes displaying a significant deviation in the expected proportion of sequences were scored as aneuploid. In this example, an excess of chromosome 18 sequences was observed, indicating trisomy 18. Relative to a normal male sample, the proportion of X-chromosome sequences was increased and the proportion of Y-chromosome sequences decreased, indicating that the embryo was female (47,XX,+18)

As well as providing data concerning the relative amount of mtDNA, NGS is also capable of providing a detailed insight into mutations of the mitochondrial genome. Mitochondrial DNA disorders are responsible for a number of devastating conditions for which there is no cure and few treatment options. Affected individuals are heteroplasmic, having a mixture of normal and mutant mitochondria in their cells. The severity of the symptoms is determined by the proportion of organelles that are defective. As many as 1 person in 400 is affected by an mtDNA disorder [31] and the phenomenon of the mitochondrial bottleneck during oogenesis means that the phenotype can swing from mild to severe in a single generation. One possibility for the avoidance of mtDNA disorders is to test cells biopsied from preimplantation embryos, transferring only those with entirely normal mitochondria or with low mutation loads [32–34]. However, accurate quantification of mtDNA mutations has been technically challenging at the single cell level. We have applied NGS to assess single cells isolated from a cell line affected with an mtDNA disorder and found that the method provides accurate mutation detection and quantification of the proportion of mitochondrial genomes affected.

The introduction of new technologies such as SNP microarrays and NGS, hold the promise of streamlined methods for the genetic diagnosis of human embryos, avoiding the need for expensive, time consuming, patient-specific protocols and allowing patients carrying inherited conditions to rapidly proceed to PGD. Both methods allow the possibility of simultaneously testing embryos for aneuploidy and SGDs. Furthermore, they offer the potential to extend genetic analysis further still, revealing other factors that may be of biological and clinical relevance to infertility, embryo viability and human health. Importantly, methods such as NGS will reduce the costs of aneuploidy screening, increasing patient access to this important means of identifying viable embryos.

References

1. Handyside AH, Kontogianni EH, Hardy K, Winston RM. Pregnancies from biopsied human preimplantation embryos sexed by Y-specific DNA amplification. Nature. 1990;344:768–70.
2. Coutelle C, Williams C, Handyside A, Hardy K, Winston R, Williamson R. Genetic analysis of DNA from single human oocytes: a model for preimplantation diagnosis of cystic fibrosis. BMJ. 1989;299:22–4.
3. Holding C, Monk M. Diagnosis of beta-thalassaemia by DNA amplification in single blastomeres from mouse preimplantation embryos. Lancet. 1989;2:532–5.
4. Handyside AH, Lesko JG, Tarin JJ, Winston RM, Hughes MR. Birth of a normal girl after in vitro fertilization and preimplantation diagnostic testing for cystic fibrosis [see comments]. N Engl J Med. 1992;327:905–9.
5. Ray PF, Winston RM, Handyside AH. Reduced allele dropout in single-cell analysis for preimplantation genetic diagnosis of cystic fibrosis. J Assist Reprod Genet. 1996;13:104–6.
6. Piyamongkol W, Bermúdez MG, Harper JC, Wells D. Detailed investigation of factors influencing amplification efficiency and allele drop-out in single cell PCR: implications for preimplantation genetic diagnosis. Mol Hum Reprod. 2003;9:411–20.
7. Ao A, Wells D, Handyside AH, Winston RM, Delhanty JD. Preimplantation genetic diagnosis of inherited cancer: familial adenomatous polyposis coli. J Assist Reprod Genet. 1998;15:140–4.
8. Kuliev A, Rechitsky S, Verlinsky O, Ivakhnenko V, Evsikov S, Wolf G, et al. Preimplantation diagnosis of thalassemias. J Assist Reprod Genet. 1998;15:219–25.
9. Fiorentino F, Biricik A, Nuccitelli A, De Palma R, Kahraman S, Iacobelli M, et al. Strategies and clinical outcome of 250 cycles of Preimplantation Genetic Diagnosis for single gene disorders. Hum Reprod. 2006;21:670–84.
10. Bermudez MG, Piyamongkol W, Tomaz S, Dudman E, Sherlock JK, Wells D. Single-cell sequencing and mini-sequencing for preimplantation genetic diagnosis. Prenat Diagn. 2003;23:669–77.
11. Fiorentino F, Kahraman S, Karadayi H, Biricik A, Sertyel S, Karlikaya G, et al. Short tandem repeats haplotyping of the HLA region in preimplantation HLA matching. Eur J Hum Genet. 2005;13:953–8.
12. Van de Velde H, De Rycke M, De Man C, De Hauwere K, Fiorentino F, Kahraman S, et al. The experience of two European preimplantation genetic diagnosis centres on human leukocyte antigen typing. Hum Reprod. 2009;24:732–40.
13. Fiorentino F, Kokkali G, Biricik A, Stavrou D, Ismailoglu B, De Palma R, et al. Polymerase chain reaction-based detection of chromosomal imbalances on embryos: the evolution of preimplantation genetic diagnosis for chromosomal translocations. Fertil Steril. 2010;94:2001–11, 2011.e1–6.
14. Renwick PJ, Trussler J, Ostad-Saffari E, Fassihi H, Black C, Braude P, et al. Proof of principle and first cases using preimplantation genetic haplotyping—a paradigm shift for embryo diagnosis. Reprod Biomed Online. 2006;13:110–9.
15. Wells D, Sherlock JK, Handyside AH, Delhanty JD. Detailed chromosomal and molecular genetic analysis of single cells by whole genome amplification and comparative genomic hybridisation. Nucleic Acids Res. 1999;27:1214–8.
16. Handyside AH, Robinson MD, Simpson RJ, Omar MB, Shaw MA, Grudzinskas JG, et al. Isothermal whole genome amplification from single and small numbers of cells: a new era for preimplantation genetic diagnosis of inherited disease. Mol Hum Reprod. 2004;10:767–72.
17. Hellani A, Coskun S, Benkhalifa M, Tbakhi A, Sakati N, Al-Odaib A, et al. Multiple displacement amplification on single cell and possible PGD applications. Mol Hum Reprod. 2004;10:847–52.
18. Fishel S, Gordon A, Lynch C, Dowell K, Ndukwe G, Kelada E, et al. Live birth after polar body array comparative genomic hybridization prediction of embryo ploidy-the future of IVF? Fertil Steril. 2010;93:1006.e7–10.
19. Geraedts J, Montag M, Magli MC, Repping S, Handyside A, Staessen C, et al. Polar body array CGH for prediction of the status of the corresponding oocyte. Part I: clinical results. Hum Reprod. 2011;26:3173–80.
20. Schoolcraft WB, Fragouli E, Stevens J, Munne S, Katz-Jaffe MG, Wells D. Clinical application of comprehensive chromosomal screening at the blastocyst stage. Fertil Steril. 2010;94:1700–6.
21. Fragouli E, Katz-Jaffe M, Alfarawati S, Stevens J, Colls P, Goodall NN, et al. Comprehensive chromosome screening of polar bodies and blastocysts from couples experiencing repeated implantation failure. Fertil Steril. 2010;94:875–87.
22. Yang Z, Liu J, Collins GS, Salem SA, Liu X, Lyle SS, et al. Selection of single blastocysts for fresh transfer via standard morphology assessment alone and with array CGH for good prognosis IVF patients: results from a randomized pilot study. Mol Cytogenet. 2012;5:24.
23. Brezina PR, Benner A, Rechitsky S, Kuliev A, Pomerantseva E, Pauling D, et al. Single-gene testing combined with single nucleotide polymorphism microarray preimplantation genetic diagnosis for aneuploidy: a novel approach in optimizing pregnancy outcome. Fertil Steril. 2011;95:1786 e5–8.
24. Treff NR, Su J, Tao X, Levy B, Scott Jr RT. Accurate single cell 24 chromosome aneuploidy screening using whole genome amplification and single nucleotide polymorphism microarrays. Fertil Steril. 2010;94:2017–21.
25. Johnson DS, Cinnioglu C, Ross R, Filby A, Gemelos G, Hill M, et al. Comprehensive analysis of karyotypic mosaicism between trophectoderm and inner cell mass. Mol Hum Reprod. 2010;16:944–9.

26. Rabinowitz M, Ryan A, Gemelos G, Hill M, Baner J, Cinnioglu C, et al. Origins and rates of aneuploidy in human blastomeres. Fertil Steril. 2012;97: 395–401.
27. Bisignano A, Wells D, Harton G, Munne S. PGD and aneuploidy screening for 24 chromosomes: advantages and disadvantages of competing platforms. Reprod Biomed Online. 2011;23(6):677–85.
28. Handyside AH, Harton GL, Mariani B, Thornhill AR, Affara N, Shaw MA, et al. Karyomapping: a universal method for genome wide analysis of genetic disease based on mapping crossovers between parental haplotypes. J Med Genet. 2010;47:651–8.
29. Wai T, Ao A, Zhang X, Cyr D, Dufort D, Shoubridge EA. The role of mitochondrial DNA copy number in mammalian fertility. Biol Reprod. 2010;83:52–62.
30. El Shourbagy SH, Spikings EC, Freitas M, St John JC. Mitochondria directly influence fertilisation outcome in the pig. Reproduction. 2006;131:233–45.
31. Manwaring N, Jones MM, Wang JJ, Rochtchina E, Howard C, Mitchell P, et al. Population prevalence of the MELAS A3243G mutation. Mitochondrion. 2007; 7:230–3.
32. Tajima H, Sueoka K, Moon SY, Nakabayashi A, Sakurai T, Murakoshi Y, et al. The development of novel quantification assay for mitochondrial DNA heteroplasmy aimed at preimplantation genetic diagnosis of Leigh encephalopathy. J Assist Reprod Genet. 2007;24:227–32.
33. Bredenoord AL, Dondorp W, Pennings G, De Die-Smulders CE, De Wert G. PGD to reduce reproductive risk: the case of mitochondrial DNA disorders. Hum Reprod. 2008;23:2392–401.
34. Gigarel N, Hesters L, Samuels DC, Monnot S, Burlet P, Kerbrat V, et al. Poor correlations in the levels of pathogenic mitochondrial DNA mutations in polar bodies versus oocytes and blastomeres in humans. Am J Hum Genet. 2011;88:494–8.

13 Use of Comparative Genomic Hybridisation (CGH) and Microarray-CGH for Preimplantation Genetic Screening

Leeanda Wilton and Dagan Wells

Early Attempts to Assess Chromosomes in Human Embryos

It has been known for many decades that chromosomal aneuploidies are responsible for more than half of all spontaneous miscarriages and still births [1–3], making aneuploidy one of the most lethal genetic conditions. Most commonly miscarriages are associated with trisomy of chromosomes 16, 21 and 22 [1, 4, 5]. Aneuploidy of other chromosomes is rarely seen in prenatal samples or miscarriages possibly because such errors are so lethal that the conceptuses are lost very early in gestation or prior to implantation. The advent of in vitro fertilisation (IVF) technologies and access to early human embryos in the laboratory provided the opportunity to investigate aneuploidy during first few days after conception.

The earliest attempts to look at the chromosomes of a preimplantation human embryo were performed using standard karyotyping techniques [6–9]. Useful information was obtained but the work was arduous as it proved very difficult to obtain informative metaphase spreads from such a small population of cells. Nevertheless these early efforts did indicate that there seemed to be a greater frequency of chromosome abnormalities in preimplantation embryos compared to later stages of development [7].

The development of fluorescent in situ hybridisation (FISH) technology and particularly its application to single cells [10] significantly enhanced cytogenetic research, enabling several chromosomes to be assessed in multiple cells from individual embryos. This revealed two previously unknown phenomena, firstly that a surprisingly high proportion of human embryos contained aneuploidy, or numerical chromosome errors, and secondly that the chromosomal complements often varied between different cells from within the one embryo, an occurrence known as mosaicism.

Even the first applications of FISH, using just one or two chromosome-specific probes, demonstrated that approximately 30 % of human embryos from IVF patients were aneuploid [10–12]. The availability of additional fluorochromes for FISH probes and the ability to perform multiple rounds of FISH soon meant that most laboratories involved in preimplantation genetic diagnosis (PGD) around the world were routinely analysing 8–10 chromosomes in human embryos. Numerous studies over many years have shown that, using multiple chromosome FISH, some 50–60 % of all human cleavage stage embryos contain aneuploid cells [13–16].

L. Wilton (✉)
Preimplantation Genetics, Melbourne IVF, East Melbourne, VIC, Australia
e-mail: leeanda.wilton@mivf.com.au

D. Wells
Nuffield Department of Obstetrics and Gynaecology, University of Oxford, Institute of Reproductive Sciences, Oxford, UK

D.K. Gardner et al. (eds.), *Human Gametes and Preimplantation Embryos: Assessment and Diagnosis*, DOI 10.1007/978-1-4614-6651-2_13, © Springer Science+Business Media New York 2013

Preimplantation Genetic Screening

The high frequency of presumably lethal abnormalities in preimplantation embryos suggests that aneuploidy may be one of the major contributors to failure of patients to become pregnant after IVF treatment. In response to the problem of aneuploidy, it has been proposed that each of the embryos produced during an IVF cycle should undergo genetic testing, allowing chromosomally normal embryos to be identified and given priority for transfer to the uterus [17]. This strategy has become known as PGD of aneuploidy or preimplantation genetic screening (PGS) and has been predominantly applied to the embryos of patients who are thought to be at higher risk of producing aneuploid gametes (e.g. women of advanced age and those patients who have suffered recurrent miscarriage or multiple implantation failures after embryo transfer in IVF).

The underlying principle behind PGS (the transfer of embryos that are more likely to be euploid and viable) would seem to have obvious merit and should increase IVF pregnancy rates, yet the procedure has met with limited clinical success, with randomised controlled trials showing no clear benefit [18–23]. One of the key reasons for this failure is likely to be that FISH can only enumerate a limited number of chromosomes and embryos that are diagnosed as euploid by FISH may have errors of chromosomes that were not tested for.

Comprehensive Assessment of Chromosomes in Embryos Using CGH

Spectral karyotyping (SKY), a methodology related to FISH that utilises probes labelled with a combination of fluorochromes has been successfully employed to analyse all 24 chromosomes. However, its use in single cell analysis is challenging, particularly if it is applied to cells in interphase of the cell cycle, with only about half of all nuclei giving interpretable results [24]. Ultimately, a move towards molecular cytogenetic methods and away from techniques involving the hybridisation of DNA probes to embryo cells fixed on microscope slides (e.g. FISH and SKY) was required in order to achieve reliable comprehensive chromosome assessment of single cells.

Complete molecular karyotyping has been possible for many years now. While many methods exist, the one that has been most widely applied is comparative genomic hybridisation (CGH). The CGH technique involves the labelling of test DNA from the sample under investigation with a fluorochrome (by convention the colour is green) while a reference DNA, known to be normal (euploid), is labelled with a different fluorochrome (by convention red). These DNAs are co-hybridised onto normal metaphase chromosomes that have been spread on a microscope slide (Fig. 1). Image analysis software then analyses the relative green:red fluorescence along the length of each of the chromosomes on the slide [25]. An increase in this ratio for any given chromosome above a certain threshold indicates that there was an excess of this chromosome in the original sample compared to the known normal reference DNA (e.g. trisomy). Conversely, a decreased ratio is indicative of chromosome loss in the sample (e.g. monosomy). In this way chromosome copy number is determined. This CGH methodology, involving hybridisation of labelled test and reference DNA samples to metaphase chromosomes is sometimes referred to as conventional CGH or metaphase CGH (mCGH).

Wells et al. [26], first reported the successful application of CGH to single cells. Critically, it was ascertained that, when starting with such a small amount of DNA, whole genome amplification was essential and that the degenerative oligonucleotide primed PCR (DOP-PCR) proved to be the most reliable method to achieve this [26]. Two reports describing the use of mCGH for the analysis of multiple single blastomeres from cleavage stage embryos soon followed, confirming the high frequency of aneuploidy in early human embryos [27, 28]. These reports also demonstrated that errors of all chromosomes, not just those most commonly seen in spontaneous abortuses and prenatal samples, occurred in early embryos. Additionally, unlike FISH, mCGH provided information along the entire length of

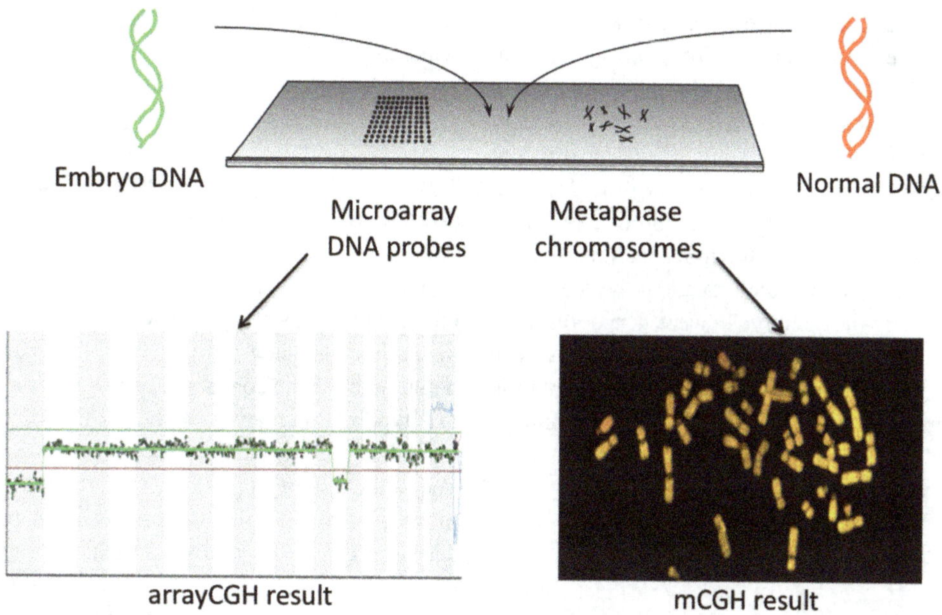

Fig. 13.1 Comparative genomic hybridisation using metaphase chromosomes or microarray. Differentially labelled test (embryo) and reference (normal) DNA samples are simultaneously applied to a slide (usually glass). In the case of mCGH, the surface of the slide is covered with numerous cells in metaphase, their chromosomes readily identifiable using fluorescence microscopy. In the case of arrayCGH, multiple chromosome-specific DNA probes are affixed to the surface of the slide and detected using a microarray scanner. After hybridization of the two labelled DNA samples, their relative fluorescence is compared, revealing any increases (e.g. trisomy) or decreases (e.g. monosomy) in the amount of test DNA derived from individual chromosomes

the chromosome and a significant number of partial aneuploidies, presumably caused by chromosome breakage in earlier cleavage divisions, were reported for the first time in human embryos [27, 28].

These early studies of blastomeres certainly demonstrated the value of investigating all chromosomes in early embryos and confirmed that FISH methods had been failing to detect many aneuploidies. Clinical application however proved somewhat challenging, primarily because the technique was laborious and required several days to obtain results. This was incompatible with standard clinical PGS protocols at the time, where embryos were typically biopsied on day-3 and then transferred on day-3 or -4. To circumvent these difficulties, Wilton et al. [29] opted to cryopreserve embryos while waiting for the results to become available. This resulted in the first birth of a baby that had developed from an embryo that had been fully karyotyped prior to transfer [29]. This was followed with a small clinical trial using mCGH on the embryos from patients with recurrent implantation failure, which led to three more births [30]. Despite these initial successes, it was acknowledged that freezing the embryos could result in some loss of viability. Another approach to the clinical application of mCGH was to karyotype polar bodies, rather than blastomeres [31]. This allowed up to 5 days to complete the mCGH process enabling transfer of fresh embryos. One disadvantage of this approach was that only maternal meiotic errors could be detected and it was well known that many aneuploidies in preimplantation embryos arose post-zygotically. Although recent years have seen the development of accelerated mCGH methods that, combined with improved embryo culture to the blastocyst stage, allow the possibility of day-3 biopsy and fresh embryo transfer [32], the cumbersome and technically demanding nature of the mCGH method has continued to limit its clinical application. Since the initial clinical studies using mCGH were reported a decade ago there have been only a handful of studies reporting application during clinical cycles [32–35]. While mCGH remains extremely challenging and is unlikely to ever be widely applied for this reason, some of the most recent clinical data using this technology provides reassurance that the concept of comprehensive chromosome screening is valid. Indeed, clinical cycles in which biopsy was undertaken at the blastocyst stage and the embryos were cryopreserved (vitrified) while mCGH was carried out have been associated with some remarkable implantation and pregnancy rates, albeit in a non-randomised study [35].

Microarray-CGH (ArrayCGH)

Despite promising results obtained using mCGH, it was clear that a further evolution of the technology, increasing speed and simplifying the procedure, was needed in order for chromosome screening to be offered to larger numbers of patients. Ultimately, this has come in the form of microarray-CGH (arrayCGH). As with conventional CGH, most microarray methods involve the hybridisation of differentially labelled test and reference DNA samples. However, in the case of microarrays the labelled DNAs are hybridised to DNA probes affixed to a microscope slide rather than metaphase chromosomes. Each probe is specific to a different chromosomal region and occupies a discrete spot on the slide. Microarrays are read by scanning using a laser, with chromosomal losses and gains revealed by the colour of each spot (i.e. ratio of fluorescence intensity for the two colours) (Fig. 1).

The principal advantages of microarrays in comparison with mCGH are a decreased length of time needed for hybridisation, some protocols requiring as little as 3 h compared with 48 h for most mCGH protocols, and greatly accelerated interpretation of data. Whereas the analysis of mCGH results typically requires approximately 45 min per sample, diagnosis using microarrays can be completed in less than 5 min. The rapid speed of analysis, coupled with the relative ease with which procedures such as microarray scanning can be automated, greatly increases the scalability of the procedure, allowing hundreds of samples to be tested each day.

Types of Microarray Compatible with CGH

A number of studies, almost a decade ago, demonstrated the feasibility of detecting aneuploidies in single cells using arrayCGH, although at that point there was no consensus concerning the optimal type of microarray or the most appropriate method of whole genome amplification [36–38]. Today, the dominant platform used for arrayCGH in the context of PGD/PGS utilises DNA probes derived from BACs (bacterial artificial chromosomes). The microarrays consist of thousands of individual spots, each of which comprises DNA from relatively large chromosomal regions (typically 150–200 kb). Although the number of distinct probes (BAC clones) used by this type of microarray are fewer than those found on some alternative microarray platforms, there are more than enough to achieve the principal objective of PGS: detection of aneuploidy affecting large chromosomal segments or whole chromosomes.

The sizes of BAC probes are such that many different amplified DNA fragments derived from the region encompassed by the BAC will hybridise to each spot on the microarray. The annealing of multiple distinct DNA fragments, from adjacent regions of the chromosome, reduces the influence of artefacts that can arise during whole genome amplification (e.g. preferential amplification and allele dropout). Amplification artefacts are very common when single cells are used and have the potential to produce false losses and gains of chromosomal material. However, in the case of BAC probes, each spot on the microarray provides an average result for the thousands of amplified fragments that have hybridised to it, diluting the influence of any individual fragments with anomalous amplification characteristics. Additionally, single cell diagnoses are never based upon the result from a single BAC, but depend on the average fluorescence ratio obtained for several neighbouring probes, further reducing the effects of any artefacts of whole genome amplification. The need to combine results from several probes limits the potential resolution of BAC arrays applied to single cells, precluding the detection of submicroscopic abnormalities (e.g. microdeletions).

An alternative type of microarray involves the use of probes composed of short oligonucleotides (25–85 nucleotides in length). Oligonucleotide arrays of this type involve many more unique probes than BAC arrays, typically ranging from 15,000 to more than 100,000, which allows for extremely high-resolution when used to test large DNA samples. However, when applied to single cells, the small size of the individual probes increases the risk that artefactual losses and gains, caused by errors introduced during whole genome amplification, will be observed. It is possible to compensate for this problem by summing together data from a large numbers of probes, but this essentially eliminates any possibility of high-resolution analysis.

Another method utilising the same concept as CGH is to secure chromosome-specific probes (e.g. BACs) to microscopic polystyrene beads rather than affixing them to the surface of a glass slide. As with other CGH technologies, differentially labelled test (e.g. embryo) and reference (normal) DNAs are allowed to hybridise to the probes in ratios that reveal the copy number of individual chromosomes. The beads can be readily suspended in liquid, allowing for more efficient hybridisation kinetics, which improves the speed, throughput and cost-efficiency of cytogenetic analysis. For analysis, the beads are passed in single-file through a pair of lasers, the first of which classifies the type of bead (based on the quantity of two dyes with which the bead was stained at the time of manufacture) and thereby identifies the probes being tested, the second laser measures the fluorescence ratio of the two hybridised DNA samples, thus providing the actual CGH result. No publications concerning clinical application of this socalled BACs-on-Beads (Perkin Elmer) approach have as yet been published, but it appears to be a promising methodology that may help to reduce the costs of comprehensive chromosome screening.

Clinical Application of ArrayCGH to Detect Aneuploidy in Embryos

The first report of the successful clinical application of arrayCGH in the context of PGS was by Hellani et al. [39], who used a 60mer oligo-array produced by Agilent Technologies to detect the aneuploidy in blastomeres from >8-cell embryos from 8 patients who had been unsuccessful in previous IVF cycles. A cautious approach was taken and two cells were tested from each embryo. Approximately 60 % of embryos had a chromosomal error but despite this, 6 of the patients had at least one euploid embryo for transfer and 5 of these had a positive pregnancy test [39].

In the past 5 years there have been numerous abstracts and conference presentations describing the clinical application of microarray technology to PGS of embryos suggesting positive outcomes. These have predominantly focussed on patients with an apparent indication, including couples where the woman is of advanced age, or those who have experienced multiple implantation failures or recurrent miscarriage. To date, very few of these studies have appeared in the peer-reviewed scientific literature.

Only rarely has PGS been offered to patients who have no apparent increased risk of aneuploidy in their embryos. However, recent research carried out by Yang et al. [40], investigated whether PGS using arrayCGH could improve outcomes for young patients on their first cycle of IVF with the transfer of just a single embryo. The rationale for this was to promote single embryo transfer, reducing the incidence of multiple pregnancy and its associated risks, while maximising pregnancy rate. In this study, the first randomised controlled trial involving arrayCGH, blastocysts were biopsied on day-5 and the trophectoderm sample obtained was subjected to arrayCGH using the BlueGnome 24sure system. Single, euploid blastocysts were transferred on day-6 and the outcomes compared to a control group of patients whose best embryo was selected on day-6 on the basis of morphology alone. This demonstrated a significantly higher clinical pregnancy rate and ongoing pregnancy rate [40].

The improvement in outcomes is consistent with recent studies using mCGH and arrayCGH that have indicated that even good quality blastocysts from young IVF patients are often aneuploid [41, 42].

Further studies need to be done, but based on the results of Yang and colleagues it is tempting to suggest that the application of PGS with 24-chromosome screening should be broadened to include all patients who have sufficient, good quality embryos. Indeed, it may be that 'good prognosis' patients will benefit from this technology more than the groups of patient traditionally offered PGS, at least in terms of enhanced pregnancy rate. In theory, the use of an embryo selection technique that reveals non-viable embryos would improve the success rates achieved in single embryo transfer cycles, providing more singleton pregnancies and leading to a significant reduction in the number of cryopreserved embryos. This would provide an economic benefit to clinics as well as patients. Additionally, it should reduce the time to pregnancy for many patients as they would not be undergoing repeated transfers of thawed embryos which were affected with an aneuploidy that made them non-viable.

The Use of ArrayCGH to Detect Imbalances Due to Chromosomal Rearrangement

ArrayCGH can also be applied to PGD of the embryos of Robertsonian and reciprocal translocation carriers. Unbalanced forms of Robertsonian translocations result in what is effectively whole chromosome aneuploidy and so this can be detected using the same methodology as for PGS [43, 44]. Unbalanced embryos from reciprocal translocation carriers will have excess or missing segments of chromosomes equivalent to partial aneuploidy. ArrayCGH provides information along the entire length of the chromosome so imbalance of large segments is also readily detectable. Currently, one commercial provider of arrays has developed a BAC array (24sure+, BlueGnome, UK) where additional clones are concentrated in the telomeric regions of all chromosomes. This enables smaller imbalances to be detected and provides extra confidence in the detection of all imbalances. These arrays have been used in clinical practice and demonstrated that embryos from translocation carriers were often affected with aneuploidy of other chromosomes in addition to those involved in the translocation [43, 44]. This approach represents a significant advance on detecting imbalance in the embryos of translocation carriers using FISH where, in most cases, only the chromosomes involved in the translocation were analysed.

Aneuploidy Detection in Oocytes Via ArrayCGH Analysis of Polar Bodies

The data now emerging from clinical studies using arrayCGH for embryo selection at the cleavage and blastocyst stages is extremely encouraging. However, despite these promising results, concerns remain over the impact of chromosomal mosaicism on the efficacy of PGS. Mosaicism, where cells within the same embryo have different chromosome complements, was originally identified in FISH studies and has long been a concern in terms of the accurate diagnosis of aneuploidy in human embryos. Research using FISH to detect limited numbers of chromosomes suggested that between 25 and 60 % of cleavage stage embryos were mosaic [45–50]. This was confirmed by comprehensive cytogenetic studies using mCGH, which indicated that approximately two-thirds of embryos are mosaic on day-3 [27, 28]. Mosaicism can be broadly separated into two categories: aneuploid/aneuploid mosaicism where all cells in the embryo are aneuploid but different chromosomes are affected in different cells and diploid/aneuploid mosaicism where some cells are aneuploid and others are diploid. The latter of these two possibilities is the more troubling diagnostically, since the diagnosis assigned to the biopsied cell(s) (normal or aneuploid) might not be representative of the remaining cells of the embryo. Reassuringly however, most mosaic embryos are found to be devoid of any normal cells (i.e. aneuploid/aneuploid), in which case any cell chosen for biopsy will yield a correct (abnormal) result.

Anxiety over the diagnostic impact of mosaicism has led some clinics to pursue a strategy of assessing oocytes rather than embryos. In theory, any aneuploidy affecting the oocyte should be present in all cells of the embryo it produces and consequently mosaicism should not be an issue. Oocyte analysis is accomplished by testing the polar bodies extruded at the end of each meiotic division. The two polar bodies are bi-products of female meiosis, containing the chromosomes discarded as the oocyte becomes haploid. In theory, the detection of extra chromosomal material in a polar body means that the oocyte is at risk of deficiency for the chromosome concerned and that any resulting embryo will be monosomic. Conversely, the detection of loss of a chromosomal material in one of the polar bodies indicates that the oocyte has retained an extra copy of the chromosome or chromatid involved, leading to a high risk of trisomy after fertilisation.

As well as avoiding problems associated with chromosomal mosaicism, polar body analysis has the advantage that it does not lead to a reduction in the mass of the embryo. Consequently, it is likely to have little if any negative impact on implantation potential. Furthermore, in some countries that have restrictive laws governing embryo testing, analysis of polar bodies may be the only form of PGS permitted. A number of studies have suggested that mCGH and array-CGH applied to polar bodies is accurate and have demonstrated that this form of screening can be used in a clinical context [51–53]. The European Society of Human Reproduction and Embryology (ESHRE) are sponsoring a randomised trial, underway at the time of writing, to assess the clinical utility of embryo selection based upon polar body testing using arrayCGH.

While polar body testing seems to have a number of advantages compared with analysis at later embryonic stages, it is important to note that this approach cannot detect any aneuploidies contributed by the sperm and is incapable of revealing mitotic errors occurring after fertilisation. Additionally, a recent study involving arrayCGH analysis of blastocysts, derived from oocytes that had previously undergone polar body biopsy and testing (again using arrayCGH), has indicated that polar body analysis may be considerably less predictive of embryo aneuploidy that previously thought [54]. These findings are yet to be verified, but suggest that polar body testing should be approached with caution, at least until the results of the ESHRE trial are available.

Conclusion

The use of mCGH and arrayCGH has provided an unprecedented amount of information concerning the cytogenetics of human oocytes and embryos, indicating the true extent of aneuploidy during the first few days of life and shedding light on phenomena such as mosaicism and chromosome breakage. Results obtained using these techniques have strengthened the argument for PGS, confirming that a high frequency of abnormalities exist even amongst embryos of excellent morphology. The clinical use of mCGH and arrayCGH has been associated with excellent outcomes in case controlled studies and prospective trials, but more data from well-designed randomised trials are needed in order to more accurately quantify the extent of improvements in IVF outcome conveyed by PGS and to define exactly which categories of patient are likely to benefit the most. This information is vital for the appropriate selection of patients and for their counselling. One randomised trial has already reported data, demonstrating significantly improved pregnancy rates for good prognosis patients, and others are already underway applying arrayCGH to patients with various indications and utilising testing at different stages of preimplantation development. The results of these key studies are eagerly anticipated.

References

1. Hassold T, Chen J, Funkhouser J, Jooss T, Manuel B, Matsuura J, et al. A cytogenetic study of 1000 spontaneous abortions. Ann Hum Genet. 1980;44:151–78.
2. Chandley AC. Infertility and chromosome abnormality. Oxf Rev Reprod Biol. 1984;6:1–46.
3. Jacobs PA. The chromosome complement of human gametes. Oxf Rev Reprod Biol. 1992;14:47–72.
4. Kalousek D. Anatomic and chromosome anomalies in specimens of early spontaneous abortion; seven-year

experience. Birth Defects Orig Artic Ser. 1987; 23:153–68.
5. Griffin DK, Millie EA, Redline RW, Hassold TJ, Zaragoza MV. Cytogenetic analysis of spontaneous abortions: comparison of techniques and assessment of confined placental mosaicism. Am J Med Genet. 1997;72:297–301.
6. Wilton L. In vitro culture of biopsied blastomeres and diagnosis of aneuploidy. In Gamete and embryo micromanipulation in human reproduction. London, UK: Edward Arnold; 1993. p. 187–193.
7. Jamieson ME, Coutts JRT, Connor JM. The chromosome constitution of human preimplantation embryos fertilized in vitro. Hum Reprod. 1994;9:709–15.
8. Santalo J, Veiga A, Calafell JM, Calderon G, Vidal F, Barri PN, et al. Evaluation of cytogenetic analysis for clinical preimplantation diagnosis. Fertil Steril. 1995; 64:44–50.
9. Clouston HJ, Fenwick J, Webb AL, Herbert M, Murdoch A, Wolstenholme J. Detection of mosaic and non-mosaic chromosome abnormalities in 6- to 8-day old human blastocysts. Hum Genet. 1997;101:30–6.
10. Griffin DK, Wilton LJ, Handyside AH, Winston RML, Delhanty JDA. Dual fluorescent in situ hybridisation for simultaneous detection of X and Y chromosome-specific probes for the sexing of human preimplantation embryonic nuclei. Hum Genet. 1992;89:18–22.
11. Benkhalifa M, Janny L, Vye P, Malet P, Boucher D, Menezo Y. Assessment of polyploidy in human morulae and blastocysts using co-culture and fluorescent in-situ hybridization. Hum Reprod. 1993;8:895–902.
12. Schrurs B, Winston RML, Handyside AH. Preimplantation diagnosis of aneuploidy using fluorescent in-situ hybridization: evaluation using a chromosome 18-specific probe. Hum Reprod. 1993; 8:296–301.
13. Munné S, Alikani M, Tomkin G, Grifo J, Cohen J. Embryo morphology, developmental rates and maternal age are correlated with chromosome abnormalities. Fertil Steril. 1995;64:382–91.
14. Bielanska M, Tan SL, Ao A. Chromosomal mosaicism throughout human preimplantation development in vitro: incidence, type and relevance to embryo outcome. Hum Reprod. 2002;17:413–9.
15. Munné S, Chen S, Colls P, Garrisi J, Zheng X, Cekleniak N, et al. Maternal age, morphology, development and chromosome abnormalities in over 6000 cleavage-stage embryos. Reprod Biomed Online. 2007;14:628–34.
16. Magli MC, Gianaroli L, Ferraretti AP, Lappi M, Ruberti A, Farfalli V. Embryo morphology and development are dependent on the chromosomal complement. Fertil Steril. 2007;87:534–41.
17. Munné S, Lee A, Rosenwaks Z, Grifo J, Cohen J. Diagnosis of major chromosome aneuploidies in human preimplantation embryos. Hum Reprod. 1993;8:2185–91.
18. Staessen C, Platteau P, Van Assche E, Michiels A, Tournaye H, Camus M, et al. Comparison of blastocyst transfer with or without preimplantation genetic diagnosis for aneuploidy screening in couples with advanced maternal age: a prospective randomised trial. Hum Reprod. 2004;19:2849–58.
19. Mastenbroek S, Twisk M, van-Echten-Arends J, Sikkema-Raddatz B, Korevaar JC, Verhoever HR. In vitro fertilization with preimplantation genetic screening. N Engl J Med. 2007;357:9–17.
20. Hardarson T, Hanson C, Lundin K, Hillensjö T, Nilsson L, Stevic J, et al. Preimplantation genetic screening in women of advanced maternal age caused a decrease in clinical pregnancy rate: a randomized controlled trial. Hum Reprod. 2008;23:2806–12.
21. Jansen RP, Bowman MC, de Boer KA, Leigh DA, Lieverman DB, McArthur SJ. What next for preimplantation screening (PGS). Experience with blastocyst biopsy and testing for aneuploidy. Hum Reprod. 2008;23:1476–8.
22. Debrock S, Melotte C, Spiessens C, Peeraer K, Vanneste E, Meeuwis L, et al. Preimplantation genetic screening for aneuploidy of embryos after in vitro fertilization in women aged at least 35 years: a prospective randomised trial. Fertil Steril. 2010;93:364–73.
23. Schoolcraft WB, Katz-Jaffe MG, Stevens J, Rawlins M, Munné S. Preimplantation aneuploidy testing for infertile patients of advanced maternal age: a randomized prospective trial. Fertil Steril. 2009;92:157–62.
24. Weier HU-G, Munné S, Lersch RA, Ben Hsieh H, Smida J, Chen X-N, et al. Towards a full karyotype screening of interphase cells: 'FISH and chip' technology. Mol Cell Endocrinol. 2001;183:S41–5.
25. Kallionemi A, Kallionemi O-P, Sudar D, Rutovitz D, Gray JW, Waldman F, et al. Comparative genomic hybridization for molecular cytogenetic analysis of solid tumours. Science. 1992;258:818–21.
26. Wells D, Sherlock JK, Handyside AH, Delhanty JDA. Detailed chromosomal and molecular genetic analysis of single cells by whole genome amplification and comparative genomic hybridisation. Nucleic Acids Res. 1999;27:1214–8.
27. Wells D, Delhanty JD. Comprehensive chromosomal analysis of human preimplantation embryos using whole genome amplification and single cell comparative genomic hybridization. Mol Hum Reprod. 2000;6:1055–62.
28. Voullaire L, Slater H, Williamson R, Wilton L. Chromosome analysis of blastomeres from human embryos by using comparative genomic hybridization. Hum Genet. 2000;106:210–7.
29. Wilton L, Williamson R, McBain J, Edgar D, Voullaire L. Birth of a healthy infant after preimplantation confirmation of euploidy by comparative genomic hybridisation. N Engl J Med. 2001;345:1537–41.
30. Wilton L, Voullaire L, Sargeant P, Williamson R, McBain J. Preimplantation aneuploidy screening using comparative genomic hybridisation or fluorescent in situ hybridisation of embryos from patients with recurrent implantation failure. Fertil Steril. 2003;80:860–8.
31. Wells D, Escudero T, Levy B, Hirschhorn K, Delhanty JDA, Munné S. First clinical application of compara-

tive genomic hybridisation and polar body testing for preimplantation genetic diagnosis of aneuploidy. Fertil Steril. 2002;78:543–9.
32. Rius M, Obradors A, Daina G, Ramos L, Pujol A, Martínez-Passarell O, et al. Detection of unbalanced chromosome segregations in preimplantation genetic diagnosis of translocations by short comparative genomic hybridization. Fertil Steril. 2011;96:134–42.
33. Obradors A, Fernández E, Oliver-Bonet M, Rius M, de la Fuente A, Wells D, et al. Birth of a healthy boy after a double factor PGD in a couple carrying a genetic disease and at risk for aneuploidy: case report. Hum Reprod. 2008;23:1949–56.
34. Sher G, Keskintepe L, Keskintepe M, Maassarani G, Tortoriello D, Brody S. Genetic analysis of human embryos by metaphase comparative genomic hybridization (mCGH) improves efficiency of IVF by increasing embryo implantation rate and reducing multiple pregnancies and spontaneous miscarriages. Fertil Steril. 2009;92:1886–94.
35. Schoolcraft WB, Fragouli E, Stevens J, Munné S, Katz-Jaffe MG, Wells D. Clinical application of comprehensive chromosomal screening at the blastocyst stage. Fertil Steril. 2010;94:1700–6.
36. Hu DG, Webb G, Hussey N. Aneuploidy detection in single cells using DNA array-based comparative genomic hybridization. Mol Hum Reprod. 2004;10: 283–9.
37. Wells D, Bermudez MG, Steuerwald N, Chu L, Weier U, Cohen J, et al. Microarrays for analysis and diagnosis of human embryos. In: Papp Z, Rodeck C, editors. Recent advances in prenatal genetic diagnosis. Italy: Medimond; 2004. p. 9–17.
38. Le Caignec C, Spits C, Sermon K, De Rycke M, Thienpont B, Debrock S, et al. Single-cell chromosomal imbalances detection by array CGH. Nucleic Acids Res. 2006;34:e68.
39. Hellani A, Abu-Amero K, Azouri J, El-Akoum S. Successful pregnancies after application of array-comparative genomic hybridization in PGS-aneuploidy screening. Reprod Biomed Online. 2008;17:814–7.
40. Yang Z, Lui J, Collins GS, Salem SA, Liu X, Lyle SS, et al. Selection of single blastocysts for fresh transfer via standard morphology assessment alone and with array CGH for good prognosis IVF patients: results from a randomized pilot study. Mol Cytogenet. 2012; 5:24–9.
41. Fragouli E, Alfarawati S, Daphnis DD, Goodall NN, Mania A, Griffiths T, et al. Cytogenetic analysis of human blastocysts with the use of FISH, CGH and aCGH: scientific data and technical evaluation. Hum Reprod. 2011;26:480–90.
42. Alfarawati S, Fragouli E, Colls P, Stevens J, Gutiérrez-Mateo C, Schoolcraft WB, et al. The relationship between blastocyst morphology, chromosomal abnormality, and embryo gender. Fertil Steril. 2011;95:520–4.
43. Alfarawati S, Fragouli E, Colls P, Wells D. First births after preimplantation genetic diagnosis of structural chromosome abnormalities using comparative genomic hybridization and microarray analysis. Hum Reprod. 2011;26:1560–74.
44. Fiorentino F, Spizzichino L, Bono S, Biricik A, Kokkali G, Rienzi L, et al. PGD for reciprocal and Robertsonian translocations using array comparative genomic hybridization. Hum Reprod. 2011;26:1925–35.
45. Delhanty J, Griffin D, Handyside AH, Harper JC, Atkinson G, Pieters MHEC, et al. Detection of aneuploidy and chromosomal mosaicism in human embryos during preimplantation sex determination by fluorescent in situ hybridisation. Hum Mol Genet. 1993;2:1183–5.
46. Delhanty JDA, Harper JC, Ao A, Handyside AH, Winston RML. Multicolour FISH detects frequent chromosomal mosaicism and chaotic division in normal preimplantation embryos from fertile patients. Hum Genet. 1997;99:755–60.
47. Munné S, Weier H-UG, Cohen J. Chromosome mosaicism in human embryos. Biol Reprod. 1994;51:373–9.
48. Munné S, Magli C, Adler A, Wright G, deBoer K, Mortimer D, et al. Treatment-related chromosome abnormalities in human embryos. Hum Reprod. 1997; 12:780–4.
49. Benadiva CA, Kligman I, Munné S. Aneuploidy 16 in human embryos increases significantly with maternal age. Fertil Steril. 1996;66:248–55.
50. Daphnis DD, Delhanty JD, Jerkovic S, Geyer J, Craft I, Harper JC. Detailed FISH analysis of day 5 human embryos reveals the mechanisms leading to mosaic aneuploidy. Hum Reprod. 2005;20:129–37.
51. Fragouli E, Katz-Jaffe M, Alfarawati S, Stevens J, Colls P, Goodall NN, et al. Comprehensive chromosome screening of polar bodies and blastocysts from couples experiencing repeated implantation failure. Fertil Steril. 2010;94:875–87.
52. Geraedts J, Montag M, Magli MC, Repping S, Handyside A, Staessen C, et al. Polar body array CGH for prediction of the status of the corresponding oocyte. Part I: clinical results. Hum Reprod. 2011;26:3173–80.
53. Fishel S, Gordon A, Lynch C, Dowell K, Ndukwe G, Kelada E, et al. Live birth after polar body array comparative genomic hybridization prediction of embryo ploidy-the future of IVF? Fertil Steril. 2010;93:1006. e7–e10.
54. Wells D, Alfarawati S, Konstantinidis M, Jaroudi S, Fragouli E. Characterisation of mechanisms causing oocyte aneuploidy reveals a flaw in embryo selection strategies based upon polar body chromosome screening. Hum Reprod. 2012;27 Suppl 2:ii106–8.

14 Quantitative SNP Array and Real-Time PCR-Based Human Preimplantation Embryo Aneuploidy Screening

Nathan R. Treff

Chromosome imbalance (aneuploidy) is the most common genetic abnormality found in human embryos, and the leading genetic cause of implantation failure and miscarriage. Screening embryos for aneuploidy prior to their transfer during IVF should therefore provide a substantial benefit to many patients with infertility. Indeed, preimplantation genetic screening (PGS) is currently the subject of exciting advancements that may result in finally realizing the potential to improve the success of IVF and revolutionize the standard of care in reproductive medicine. The ideal of routine elective single embryo transfer may soon become a reality with the incorporation of valid comprehensive chromosome screening (CCS) technology. Furthermore, selective transfer of embryos predicted to possess a normal complement of 23 pairs of chromosomes not only represents an important clinical application but also a unique opportunity to conduct more well-controlled research to develop additional prognostic markers of embryonic reproductive potential. While there are a large number of unique methodologies for CCS, this chapter will focus on results of research and development of two specific technologies.

N.R. Treff (✉)
Reproductive Medicine Associates of New Jersey, Basking Ridge, NJ, USA

Department of Obstetrics, Gynecology, and Reproductive Sciences, UMDNJ-Robert Wood Johnson Medical School, New Brunswick, NJ, USA
e-mail: ntreff@rmanj.com

Quantitative SNP Microarray-Based CCS

Although one initial intended IVF-specific application of Affymetrix SNP microarrays was to perform DNA fingerprinting [1], the ability of SNP arrays to produce accurate copy number analyses in single cells soon followed. In 2007, preliminary results of research and development directed at validation of a new CCS technology were presented at the American Society for Reproductive Medicine (ASRM) Annual Meeting [2]. The methodology involves PCR-based whole genome amplification (WGA) and copy number analysis using the Affyemtrix NspI SNP microarray (Affymetrix Inc., Santa Clara, CA). Results indicated a 98.6 % diagnostic accuracy when applied to single cells from established and karyotypically defined cell lines, and high levels of concordance within blastomeres from cleavage stage embryos [3]. This success led to the development of a series of preclinical research projects and clinical trials.

First, to address the potential differential performance of alternative methodologies of whole genome amplification (WGA), a comparative study was conducted [4]. Four cell lines with varying X chromosome copy number were used as the source of single cells subject to three different WGA procedures [5–7]. Results indicated that multiple displacement amplification provided the greatest genotyping accuracy, while PCR-based WGA provided the greatest copy

D.K. Gardner et al. (eds.), *Human Gametes and Preimplantation Embryos: Assessment and Diagnosis*, DOI 10.1007/978-1-4614-6651-2_14, © Springer Science+Business Media New York 2013

number accuracy. The performance of the Affyemtrix SNP array was also compared to a 32K comparative genomic hybridization (CGH) array from the University of California at San Francisco, where CGH array technology was pioneered. Results indicated significant underperformance by array CGH despite hybridization for more than 48 h [8].

Since fluorescence in situ hybridization (FISH)-based methods have been predominating in PGS, comparative studies with SNP microarrays were performed. The first study involved randomization of dispersed blastomeres from arrested cleavage stage embryos so that half the blastomeres from each embryo were evaluated by SNP arrays and half by FISH [9]. Since the blastomeres were randomized, the prevalence of mosaicism could be expected to be equivalent by the two methods unless one was less consistent. Indeed, FISH resulted in finding 100 % mosaicism in the 13 embryos evaluated, significantly more than the 31 % found by SNP array analysis, despite evaluating fewer chromosomes (9 instead of 24) and fewer cells (due to lower reliability of obtaining a result). These results not only demonstrated significant technical inconsistency by FISH, but also overdiagnosis of mitotic aneuploidy. The second study evaluated multiple biopsies of 50 blastocysts that developed from embryos diagnosed as aneuploid by cleavage stage FISH [10]. Results demonstrated that nearly 60 % were euploid for all 24 chromosomes and in four different segments of the embryo, indicating that cleavage stage FISH is poorly predictive of aneuploidy. In addition, putative self-correction mechanisms, such as chromosome duplication or extrusion, and mosaicism, were eliminated as possible explanations for the failure of FISH to correctly predict aneuploidy.

With these preclinical studies completed, a unique study design was employed to investigate the clinical predictive value of SNP array-based CCS [11]. This was particularly important given the apparent lack of negative predictive value of cleavage stage FISH. That is, despite predicting aneuploidy at the cleavage stage, ~60 % of the blastocysts were euploid, suggesting that FISH-based aneuploidy screening has resulted in the erroneous disposal of euploid embryos with reproductive potential. To address this issue more directly, embryos were biopsied for SNP array-based CCS, and transferred based only on morphology (CCS was intentionally not used for selection). Pregnancies were evaluated by DNA fingerprinting to determine which embryos implanted. Results indicated a 96 % predictive value of an aneuploid SNP array CCS diagnosis for a negative clinical outcome (failure to sustain implantation).

Interestingly, the positive predictive value of trophectoderm-based CCS was significantly better than blastomere-based CCS. This led to specific investigation of the impact of biopsy at the cleavage and blastocyst stage of development [12]. Indeed, blastomere biopsy resulted in a 39 % reduction in reproductive potential, while blastocyst biopsy did not significantly influence implantation rates. This result in turn led to the development of methodologies for trophectoderm-based CCS. The first of these incorporated the use of blastocyst vitrification in order to accommodate the time needed for SNP array-based CCS [13]. Application in patients carrying balanced translocations was also developed and demonstrated excellent clinical outcomes and resolution of analysis [14]. In parallel, more rapid methods of SNP array-based methods were developed [15], but remained insufficient to maintain putative blastocyst and endometrial synchrony.

An alternative to blastomere or trophectoderm biopsy involving polar body-based screening has been proposed as a means to avoid issues with mosaicism. The main argument relates to the observation that aneuploidy found in products of conception primarily originates from maternal meiosis. However, the predictive value of polar body-based screening has yet to be established. Recent data indicates that there is a 6 % false positive aneuploidy diagnosis based upon identification of euploid embryos derived from oocytes with aneuploid polar bodies [16]. This reduction in the negative predictive value, which may be technical in nature, does not account for an additional biological contribution to reduced predictive value that can result from premature separation of sister chromatids (PSSC). Indeed, PSSC is thought to represent more than 90 % of the meiosis I errors observed in human oocytes [17, 18]. Since the abnormalities derived from PSSC could be resolved through segregation during meiosis II, it is possible that oocytes with reciprocal aneuploid polar bodies can develop into euploid reproductively competent embryos. In fact this has been observed previously [18], indicating that it may result in erroneous disposal of as many as 7 % of embryos with aneuploid polar bodies. Together, the technical and biological error associated with polar body screening may hinder its routine application and ability to demonstrate clinical efficacy in ongoing randomized controlled trials.

Quantitative Real-Time PCR-Based CCS

With the desire for more rapid analysis of trophectoderm, a methodology involving quantitative real-time (q)PCR was established [19]. The initial concept was based on the Mendelian inheritance of SNPs from parents homozygous for opposite alleles. Since all euploid embryos should inherit a heterozygous genotype, identification of homozygosity would indicate monosomy, and identification of 1:2 or 2:1 allele ratios would indicate the presence of trisomy. The ability to perform high throughput and rapid evaluation of informative SNPs with qPCR provided a unique opportunity to obtain CCS results within the window of synchrony without cryopreservation. However, the need to evaluate parental genotypes and the low frequency of SNPs in which the parents are homozygous for opposite alleles made routine application difficult.

Instead, a method of relative quantitation by qPCR was developed such that parental information was not necessary [20]. This methodology employs a modification of a previously described comparative CT method [21] which avoids the requirement of evaluating polymorphic genomic loci. This modified qPCR protocol demonstrated 98–100 % accuracy on cells from cell lines and 99 % consistency with SNP arrays on trophectoderm from blastocysts. An important feature of this particular study was the emphasis on preventing mosaicism from impacting the estimate of accuracy. This was accomplished by limiting qPCR evaluation of embryos to those which had two consistent results when testing was performed with SNP arrays. Cell lines with little to know mosaicism for the whole chromosome aneuploidies were also utilized.

Given the high level of consistency between qPCR and SNP array-based CCS, the same negative predictive value can be expected from qPCR. As such, a randomized controlled trial (RCT) was initiated to determine the clinical efficacy of qPCR-based CCS [22]. Patients of all ages and with no more than one prior failed IVF cycle were included and randomized on day 5 of embryo development. In the patients randomized to CCS, a trophectoderm biopsy was performed, qPCR was conducted, and 1–2 euploid embryos were selected for transfer. In the control arm, patients had two unscreened blastocysts transferred. Results indicated a significant increase in ongoing pregnancy rates and a significant decrease in miscarriage rates. Patients of advanced maternal age (>35) benefited the most from the use of CCS.

With the observed improved success of IVF with CCS, a retrospective evaluation of single embryo transfer outcomes with and without CCS was conducted [23]. Again, results demonstrated significantly improved ongoing pregnancy rates and reduced miscarriage rates. This led to the development of a second RCT involving the comparison of single euploid blastocyst transfers (case) to two unscreened embryo transfers (control). This study is currently ongoing but could represent critical data to support a paradigm shift in IVF, routine elective single euploid blastocyst transfer.

Future Applications of CCS

While CCS clinical applications should dramatically change the standard of care in reproductive medicine, new powerful approaches to research and development have also been made possible from the introduction of CCS technology. Great effort in the development of other markers of reproductive potential has been made, particularly in the areas of metabolomics, proteomics, and additional genomics (i.e. mitochondrial, telomeric DNA content). These areas of research stand to benefit dramatically from the simultaneous incorporation of CCS to eliminate aneuploidy from the variables affecting clinical outcomes. This should provide greater control over evaluating putative markers of or interventions that may influence reproductive potential of human embryos. Examples of applying CCS to control for aneuploidy during the evaluation of putative markers have already emerged [24–26] and there are likely to be more in the near future.

These and other CCS methodologies have also been applied in a research setting to better understand the origins of aneuploidy. For example, the origin of maternal meiotic aneuploidy appears to be primarily from premature separation of sister chromatids rather than classic non-disjunction [18, 27]. In addition, SNP array-based analysis of heterozygosity has revealed that polar body morphology is not predictive of its cell division origin [28]. This result indicates that studies of the origin of maternal aneuploidy which rely upon polar body morphology to assign errors as originating from meiosis I or meiosis II may be inaccurate [29, 30]. SNP arrays have also been used in their more conventional capacity for genome wide association studies to understand whether there are specific genes which predispose patients to higher rates of aneuploidy in their embryos [31]. An exciting outcome may be a diagnostic test to help patients understand their risk of producing an aneuploid conception without having to first perform IVF-related procedures.

References

1. Treff NR, Su J, Bergh EP, Levy B, Miller KA, Scott J. Single-blastomere whole-genome DNA fingerprinting results in unequivocal embryo identification – a powerful new clinical and diagnostic tool. Fertil Steril. 2007;88:S3–4.
2. Treff NR, Su J, Mavrianos J, Bergh PA, Miller KA, Scott J. Accurate 23 chromosome aneuploidy screening in human blastomeres using single nucleotide polymorphism (SNP) microarrays. Fertil Steril. 2007; 88:S1.
3. Treff NR, Su J, Tao X, Levy B, Scott Jr RT. Accurate single cell 24 chromosome aneuploidy screening using whole genome amplification and single nucleotide polymorphism microarrays. Fertil Steril. 2010;94:2017–21.
4. Treff NR, Su J, Tao X, Northrop LE, Scott Jr RT. Single-cell whole-genome amplification technique impacts the accuracy of SNP microarray-based genotyping and copy number analyses. Mol Hum Reprod. 2011;17:335–43.
5. Fiegler H, Geigl JB, Langer S, Rigler D, Porter K, Unger K, et al. High resolution array-CGH analysis of single cells. Nucleic Acids Res. 2007;35:1–10.
6. Handyside AH, Robinson MD, Simpson RJ, Omar MB, Shaw MA, Grudzinskas JG, et al. Isothermal whole genome amplification from single and small numbers of cells: a new era for preimplantation genetic diagnosis of inherited disease. Mol Hum Reprod. 2004;10:767–72.
7. Le Caignec C, Spits C, Sermon K, De Rycke M, Thienpont B, Debrock S, et al. Single-cell chromosomal imbalances detection by array CGH. Nucleic Acids Res. 2006;34:e68.
8. Treff NR, Scott Jr RT. Genome-wide chromosome aneuploidy assessment on single cells using two types of arrays – SNP based arrays are more accurate and less variable than BAC arrays. Fertil Steril. 2007;88:S87–8.
9. Treff NR, Levy B, Su J, Northrop LE, Tao X, Scott Jr RT. SNP microarray-based 24 chromosome aneuploidy screening is significantly more consistent than FISH. Mol Hum Reprod. 2010;16:583–9.
10. Northrop LE, Treff NR, Levy B, Scott Jr RT. SNP microarray-based 24 chromosome aneuploidy screening demonstrates that cleavage-stage FISH poorly predicts aneuploidy in embryos that develop to morphologically normal blastocysts. Mol Hum Reprod. 2010;16:590–600.
11. Scott Jr RT, Ferry K, Su J, Tao X, Scott K, Treff NR. Comprehensive chromosome screening is highly predictive of the reproductive potential of human embryos: a prospective, blinded, nonselection study. Fertil Steril. 2012;97(4):870–5.
12. Treff NR, Ferry KM, Zhao T, Su J, Forman EJ, Scott RT. Cleavage stage embryo biopsy significantly impairs embryonic reproductive potential while blastocyst biopsy does not: a novel paired analysis of cotransferred biopsied and non-biopsied sibling embryos. Fertil Steril. 2011;96:S2.
13. Schoolcraft WB, Treff NR, Stevens JM, Ferry K, Katz-Jaffe M, Scott Jr RT. Live birth outcome with trophectoderm biopsy, blastocyst vitrification, and single-nucleotide polymorphism microarray-based comprehensive chromosome screening in infertile patients. Fertil Steril. 2011;96:638–40.
14. Treff NR, Northrop LE, Kasabwala K, Su J, Levy B, Scott Jr RT. Single nucleotide polymorphism microarray-based concurrent screening of 24 chromosome aneuploidy and unbalanced translocations in preimplantation human embryos. Fertil Steril. 2010;95: 1606–12. e1–2.

15. Treff N, Su J, Tao X, Miller K, Scott Jr RT. First IVF babies born after rapid 24 chromosome embryo aneuploidy screening and fresh embryo transfer. Fertil Steril. 2009;92:S49.
16. Geraedts J, Montag M, Magli MC, Repping S, Handyside A, Staessen C, et al. Polar body array CGH for prediction of the status of the corresponding oocyte. Part I: clinical results. Hum Reprod. 2011; 26(11):3173–80.
17. Gabriel AS, Thornhill AR, Ottolini CS, Gordon A, Brown AP, Taylor J, et al. Array comparative genomic hybridisation on first polar bodies suggests that non-disjunction is not the predominant mechanism leading to aneuploidy in humans. J Med Genet. 2011;48(7): 433–7.
18. Treff NR, Su J, Tao X, Katz-Jaffe M, Schoolcraft WB, Scott Jr RT. Characterizing the nature of meiotic errors: PSSC is the principal meiotic error in human oocytes and may correct during the 2nd meiotic division and result in the birth of a healthy infant. Fertil Steril. 2009;92:S25.
19. Treff NR, Tao X, Lonczak A, Su J, Taylor D, Scott Jr RT. Four hour 24 chromosome aneuploidy screening using high throughput PCR SNP allele ratio analyses. Fertil Steril. 2009;92:S49–50.
20. Treff NR, Tao X, Ferry KM, Su J, Taylor D, Scott Jr RT. Development and validation of an accurate quantitative real-time PCR based assay for human blastocyst comprehensive chromosomal aneuploidy screening. Fertil Steril. 2012;97(4):819–24.
21. Schmittgen TD, Livak KJ. Analyzing real-time PCR data by the comparative CT method. Nat Protoc. 2008;3:1101–8.
22. Scott Jr RT, Tao X, Taylor D, Ferry K, Treff N. A prospective randomized controlled trial demonstrating significantly increased clinical pregnancy rates following 24 chromosome aneuploidy screening: biopsy and analysis on day 5 with fresh transfer. Fertil Steril. 2010;94:S2.
23. Forman EJ, Tao X, Ferry KM, Taylor D, Treff NR, Scoott Jr RT. Single embryo transfer with comprehensive chromosome screening results in improved ongoing pregnancy rates and decreased miscarriage rates. Hum Reprod. 2012;27(4):1217–22.
24. Treff NR, Su J, Taylor D, Scott Jr RT. Telomere DNA deficiency is associated with development of human embryonic aneuploidy. PLoS Genet. 2011;7:e1002161.
25. Treff NR, Su J, Lonczak A, Taylor D, Scott Jr RT. A subset of the cumulus cell transcriptome is predictive of euploid human oocyte reproductive potential. Fertil Steril. 2010;94:S34–5.
26. Su J, Tao X, Baglione G, Treff NR, Scott RT. Mitochondrial DNA is significantly increased in aneuploid human embryos. Fertil Steril. 2010;94:S88–9.
27. Treff NR, Su J, Tao X, Frattarelli JL, Miller KA, Scott RT. Characterization of the source of human embryonic aneuploidy using microarray-based 24 chromosome preimplantation genetic diagnosis (mPGD) and aneuploid chromosome fingerprinting. Fertil Steril. 2008;90:S37.
28. Treff NR, Scott Jr RT, Su J, Campos J, Stevens J, Schoolcraft W, et al. Polar body morphology is not predictive of its cell division origin. J Assist Reprod Genet. 2012;29(2):137–9.
29. Fragouli E, Alfarawati S, Goodall NN, Sanchez-Garcia JF, Colls P, Wells D. The cytogenetics of polar bodies: insights into female meiosis and the diagnosis of aneuploidy. Mol Hum Reprod. 2011;17:286–95.
30. Handyside AH, Montag M, Magli MC, Repping S, Harper J, Schmutzler A, et al. Multiple meiotic errors caused by predivision of chromatids in women of advanced maternal age undergoing in vitro fertilisation. Eur J Hum Genet. 2012;20:1–6.
31. Taylor D, Pike JW, Kasabwala K, Northrop LE, Treff NR, Scott RT. A genome-wide association scan identifies several maternal susceptibility loci for embryo aneuploidy. Fertil Steril. 2010;94:S183.

Regulation of Gene Expression in the Oocyte and Early Embryo: Implications for Transcriptomic and Proteomic Embryo Assessment

15

Helena Kristiansson and Emre Seli

Reproduction requires the accurate transfer of genetic information from one generation to the next using highly controlled mechanisms that are conserved among evolutionarily distant species. Metazoa is the large division of the animal kingdom, which includes all multicellular animals whose cells become differentiated into tissues. Independent of their complexity, sexually reproducing metazoan are formed by the union of two distinct gametes, an egg and a sperm. Importantly, control of gene expression in the gametes or the early embryo significantly differs from that in other, somatic, cells within an organism. In addition, while the zygote results from the union of the egg and the sperm, each contributing equal amounts of genetic material, the precise cellular machinery that mediates early embryonic development is largely derived from the egg.

In order to better interpret novel technologies utilizing global analysis of transcripts, proteins, and metabolites to predict embryo viability, it is essential to develop a detailed understanding of the unique mechanisms of gene expression in gametes and early embryos. In this chapter, we will first review the key aspects of mRNA and protein production in somatic cells. Then, we will delineate oocyte and embryo-specific mechanisms and their implications for diagnostic approaches in assisted reproduction.

H. Kristiansson, PhD • E. Seli, MD(✉)
Department of Obstetrics, Gynecology
and Reproductive Sciences, Yale School of Medicine,
310 Cedar Street, LSOG 304D,
New Haven, CT 06520-8063, USA
e-mail: emre.seli@yale.edu

Transcription and Translation in Somatic Cells

Transcription and Processing of Pre-mRNAs in Somatic Cells

The first step in the process of producing proteins from the genetic material is the transcription of DNA into messenger RNA (mRNA). In eukaryotes, transcription takes place in the nucleus of the cell. A key mediator of this process is RNA polymerase II, which produces unprocessed pre-mRNA from the DNA (Fig. 1). The pre-mRNA is processed within the nucleus through three key steps: capping, splicing, and cleavage/polyadenylation. The final transcript (mRNA) is then transported into the cytoplasm.

Capping

As the RNA polymerase moves in the 5′–3′ direction on the DNA strand to be transcribed, the 5′ end of the newly produced pre-mRNA becomes exposed. To protect the pre-mRNA from degradation, a 7-methylguanosine cap (m^7Gppp) becomes covalently attached to the exposed 5′ end (Fig. 1) [1, 2].

Splicing

While the RNA polymerase moves along the DNA sequence to be transcribed, preparations are

D.K. Gardner et al. (eds.), *Human Gametes and Preimplantation Embryos: Assessment and Diagnosis*, DOI 10.1007/978-1-4614-6651-2_15, © Springer Science+Business Media New York 2013

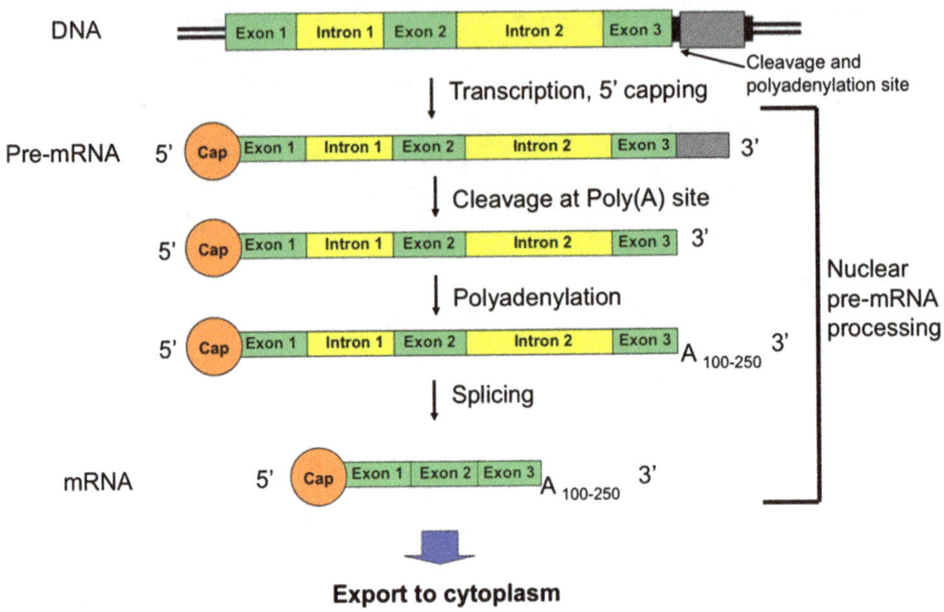

Fig. 15.1 Pre-mRNA processing in the eukaryotes. Follow-ing the initiation of transcription by RNA polymerase II, the 5′-end of the nascent RNA is capped with 7-methylguanylate. Next, the pre-mRNA transcript is cleaved at the poly(A) site, and adenosine (A) residues added to the 3′-end. The poly(A) tail consists of approximately 250 A residues in mammals. Splicing may occur following cleavage/polyadenylation or during transcription

made for the removal of introns in order to produce the correct transcript. This step is called RNA splicing (Fig. 1). RNA splicing consists of a series of very complex reactions that require over 50 additional proteins, including the 5′-cap and will not be described here (Fig. 1) [2].

Cleavage and Polyadenylation

Within the 3′ UTR of the newly transcribed pre-mRNA there is an AAUAAA hexamer consensus sequence where a cleavage and polyadenylation specificity factor (CPSF) binds. The CPSF travels with the RNA polymerase and binds to this 3′-end processing sequence while the RNA polymerase continues along the DNA molecule, transcribing several hundred additional nucleotides. CPSF will then remove these additional nucleotides, making it possible for a poly(A) polymerase to bind to the same site and mediate the addition of approximately 250 adenosines to produce a poly(A) tail at the 3′ end of the pre-mRNA (Fig. 1) [3, 4]. This poly(A) tail protects the pre-mRNA from degradation and mediates its translation [1]. As the poly(A) tail is being synthesized, a nuclear poly(A) binding protein (PABPN1) attaches to the rapidly growing poly(A) tail and not only enhances the polyadenylation reaction but also acts as protection from exonucleases. Once the processing of the pre-mRNA is complete, the 5′ cap, with the help of mRNA transport proteins, safely guides the mRNA through the nuclear pores and into the cytoplasm [2].

Translation in Somatic Cells

In eukaryotic cells, once a pre-mRNA is processed into mRNA, it is transported into the cytoplasm, where it gets access to the ribosomes in order to be translated into a protein. Once the mRNA is in the cytoplasm, the PABPN1 is replaced by a cytoplasmic poly(A) binding protein, PABPC1. PABPC1 is significantly larger (70.2 kDa) than PABPN1 (32.8 kDa) and contains four RNA-recognition motifs (RRMs) and a poly(A) binding domain [5]. PABPC1's main function is to protect the mRNA from deadenylation and facilitate its translation.

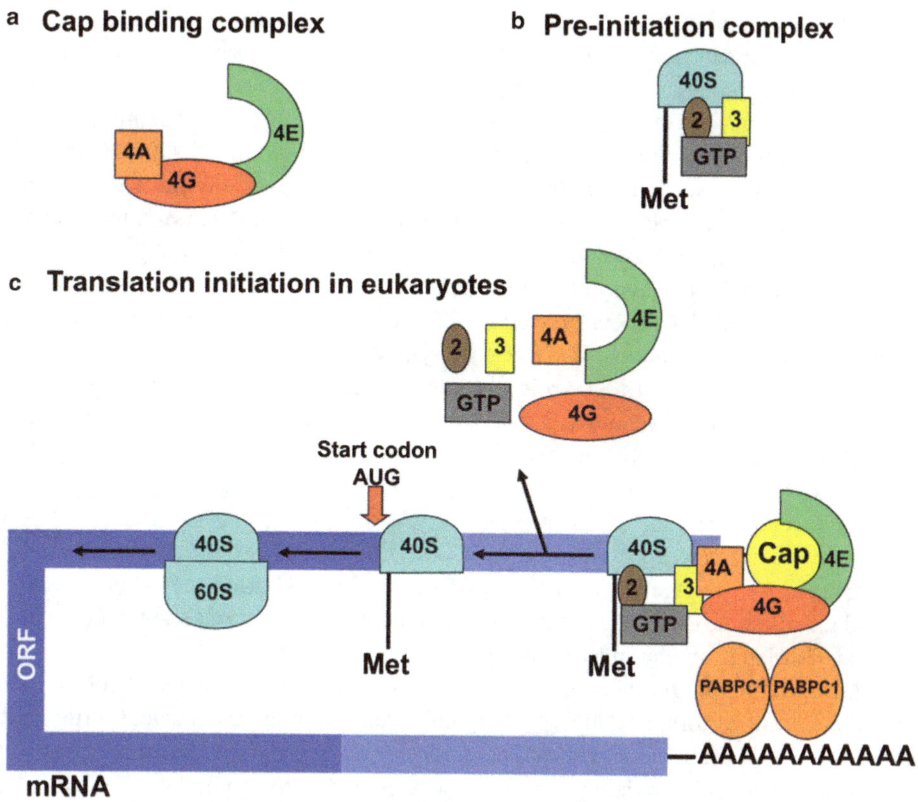

Fig. 15.2 Control of translation in somatic cells of eukaryotes. (**a**) Cap-binding complex consists of three eukaryotic initiation factors (eIF): eIF4E (the cap-binding protein), eIF4A (an RNA helicase), and eIF4G (a scaffolding protein). 4E: eIF4E; 4A: eIF4A; 4G: eIF4G. (**b**) Translation pre-initiation complex consists of a 40S ribosomal subunit-eIF3 complex bound by eIF1A and the ternary complex (Met-tRNA$_i$, eIF2, and GTP). 40S: 40S ribosomal subunit; 3: eIF3, Met: Met-tRNA$_i$; 2: eIF2. (**c**) The 48S translation initiation complex is formed when the translation pre-initiation complex becomes associated with the cap-binding complex and the mRNA. Within the 48S initiation complex, eIF4G binds eIF4E and eIF4A, forming a bridge between the ribosome and the mRNA, and also binds the PABPC1 to facilitate the translation. Once bound to the cap structure, the 40S ribosomal subunit with associated proteins scans the mRNA toward the 3′ end until it reaches the initiation codon (AUG). When the initiation codon is reached, initiation factors become released and the 60S ribosomal subunit is recruited, initiating translation. This model is simplified for clarity and not all the initiation factors are depicted. 60S: 60S ribosomal subunit; PABPC1: poly(A) binding protein cytoplasmic 1 (Modified from Friend K, Seli E. Molecular biology of the gamete. In: Pellicer A, Simon C, editors. Stem cells in human reproduction. 2nd ed. New York: Springer Science + Business Media; 2009. p. 22–34, with permission)

At this stage, another role of the 5′-cap comes into play as it helps the cell to distinguish between different types of RNAs, channelling mRNAs into the translational machinery [2]. Indeed, unlike mRNAs produced by RNA polymerase II, ribosomal RNAs (rRNAs, used in the building of ribosomes) or tRNAs (that carry amino acids to the growing polypeptides during translation), produced by RNA polymerase I, or III, respectively, do not have a 5′-cap.

When the mRNA enters the cytosol, additional proteins bind to the 5′-cap, forming the cap-binding complex. Importantly, this complex includes three translational initiation factors; eIF4A (a RNA helicase), eIF4E (cap-binding protein), and eIF4G (a scaffolding protein) (Fig. 2) [6].

In order for the translation to begin, another complex needs to form and attach to the cap-binding complex (Fig. 2). The 43S translation pre-initiation complex consists of the two eukaryotic initiation factors eIF2 and eIF3, a GTP and a met-tRNA attached to the 40S small ribosomal subunit. The binding of the 43S translation pre-initiation complex to the mRNA bound cap-binding complex produces the 48S initiation complex. The 48S subunit scans the mRNA to locate the AUG start codon. Once the 48S subunit reaches the start signal, a subset of the initiation factors are released, and the 60S large ribosomal subunit is recruited to produce the 80S ribosome, which can start translation of the RNA message [6]. It is noteworthy that a key role of the poly(A) tail is to help the 5′-end and 3′-end of the mRNA to interact, thereby enhancing translation [7].

The elongation of the amino acid sequence halts when the ribosome comes upon one of three possible stop codons. At this stage the polypeptide is released and the ribosome dissociates so it may start over again, translating another mRNA into a protein [8, 9]. Depending on the function of the protein and where it will perform its duties, it may be subjected to post-translational modifications such as phosphorylation or glycosylation.

Regulation of Gene Expression in the Oocyte and the Early Embryo

In most metazoan, oocytes differentiate from primordial germ cells (PGCs) that arise at a distant site and migrate to the somatic gonad [10]. Oocytes enter meiosis; however, they become arrested at the prophase of the first meiotic division [11, 12]. The length of this first meiotic arrest differs between species and may last up to a few years in *Xenopus* and mouse and several decades in humans. Large quantities of dormant mRNA are synthesized and stored within the oocyte during this period [13, 14]. The resumption of meiosis, stimulated by gonadotropins in mouse and human, marks the onset of oocyte maturation.

Oocyte maturation is associated with suppression of transcription and by a complex network of translational activation and repression that regulate gene expression [15–18]. The maternally derived mRNAs stored in the oocyte drive its re-entry into meiosis and control the rate of mitosis during the early cleavage divisions. The transcriptional silencing that begins with oocyte maturation persists during the initial mitotic divisions of the embryonic cells. In *Xenopus*, after 12 rapid embryonic cell divisions generating more than 4,000 cells, initiation of transcription in the embryo, called the zygotic genome activation (ZGA), occurs [19, 20]. In mouse and human, ZGA occurs at the 2-cell, and 4- to 8-cell stages, respectively [21–24]. Despite the earlier occurrence of ZGA in mammals compared to *Xenopus*, translational activation of maternally inherited mRNAs appears to utilize similar mechanisms.

Translational Control of Gene Expression in the Oocyte by Cytoplasmic Polyadenylation

As described above, virtually all mRNAs undergo polyadenylation in the nucleus prior to being transported into the cytoplasm for translation. In oocytes and early embryos, in addition to the nucleus, polyadenylation also takes place in the cytoplasm and constitutes the central pathway for translational regulation of gene expression following suppression of transcription (Fig. 3).

Cytoplasmic polyadenylation requires cytoplasmic polyadenylation element binding protein 1 (CPEB1), which mediates the cytoplasmic elongation of poly(A)-tails on mRNAs that contain an RNA motif called the cytoplasmic polyadenylation element (CPE) [25, 26]. Indeed, oocyte mRNAs that are translationally activated by cytoplasmic polyadenylation contain the CPE (consensus sequence: $UUUUA_{1\text{-}2}U$) in their 3′-UTR, which is localized approximately 20–30 nucleotides upstream from the previously mentioned hexameric signal (AAUAAA) necessary for cleavage and polyadenylation in the nucleus.

CPEB1 functions in coordination with Symplekin (SYMPK), poly(A)-specific ribonuclease (PARN), CPSF and GLD2, an atypical poly(A)-polymerase, and an embryonic poly(A) binding protein (EPAB) [15, 25, 27, 28] (Fig. 3). As studied in detail in *Xenopus*, upon stimulation of oocyte maturation, Eg2, a serine/threonine

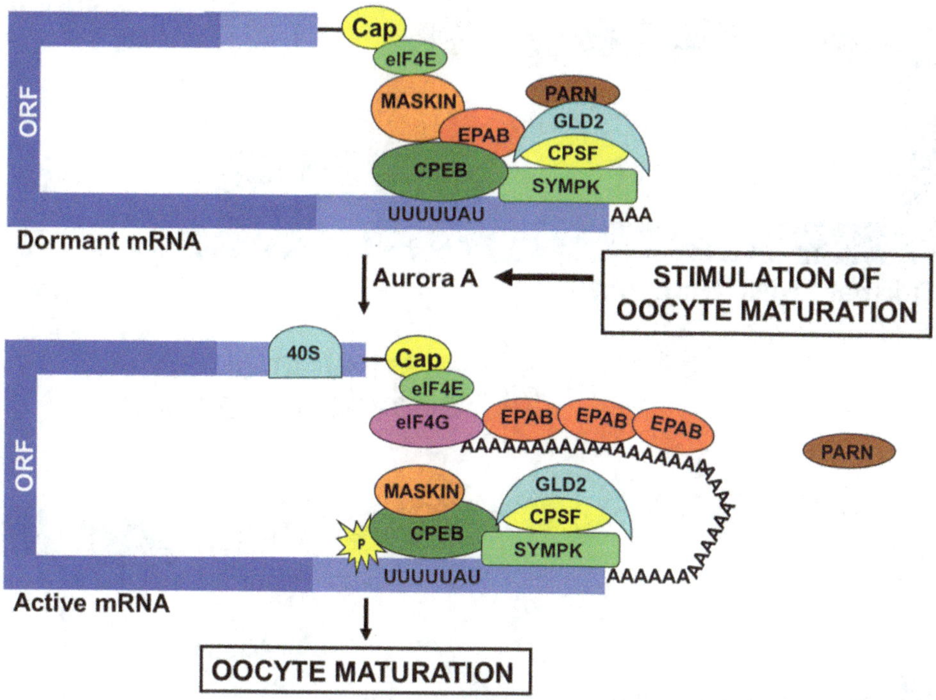

Fig. 15.3 Model for cytoplasmic polyadenylation-dependent control of translation in oocytes. Dormant CPE-containing mRNAs in immature oocytes are bound by CPEB, which in turn is bound to MASKIN, which in turn is bound to eIF4E, the cap-binding factor. The binding of MASKIN to eIF4E precludes the binding of eIF4G to eIF4E, thus inhibiting the formation of the translation initiation complex. Following stimulation of oocyte maturation, the kinase aurora A is activated and phosphorylates CPEB. This leads to dissociation of PARN from the complex and extension of the poly(A) tail by GLD2. The newly elongated poly(A) tail is then bound by EPAB, which in turn associates with eIF4G. eIF4G, when associated with EPAB, then displaces MASKIN from and binds to, eIF4E, thereby initiating translation. The open reading frame (ORF) is shown in *dark blue*. The 5′ UTR and 3′ UTR regions are shown in *light blue*. *ORF* open reading frame, *CPEB1* cytoplasmic polyadenylation element binding protein 1, *SYMPK* Symplekin, a scaffolding protein, *PARN* a poly(A)-specific ribonuclease, *GLD2* an atypical poly(A)-polymerase, *EPAB* embryonic poly(A) binding protein (Modified from Friend K, Seli E. Molecular biology of the gamete. In: Pellicer A, Simon C, editors. Stem cells in human reproduction. 2nd ed. New York: Springer Science + Business Media; 2009. p. 22–34, with permission)

protein kinase from the Aurora A family, becomes activated and phosphorylates CPEB. CPEB phosphorylation results in the displacement of PARN, and elongation of the mRNA poly(A) tail by GLD2. Phosphorylation of CPEB also displaces MASKIN (a translational repressor), allowing the binding of eukaryotic translation initiation factor eIF4G, to eIF4E, thereby initiating translation (Fig. 3). CPEB-mediated cytoplasmic polyadenylation regulates translational activation of important mRNAs that play a key role in the regulation of oocyte maturation (c-MOS and Cyclin B1). While many of the functions of the CPEB have been investigated in the *Xenopus* model, the key role of CPEB in translational regulation of gene expression is conserved in mammals and CPEB knockout female mice are infertile [29, 30].

In the oocyte, translational activation by cytoplasmic polyadenylation requires the presence of a poly(A) binding protein. Interestingly, instead of PABPC1, the oocyte contains a specific embryonic poly(A) binding protein (EPAB) [27, 31–33], which differs from PABPC1 primarily in the region between its conserved RRMs and the PABC (C-terminal) domain. EPAB is the predominant poly(A) binding protein in oocytes and early embryos [27, 31–33]. In *Xenopus* oocytes,

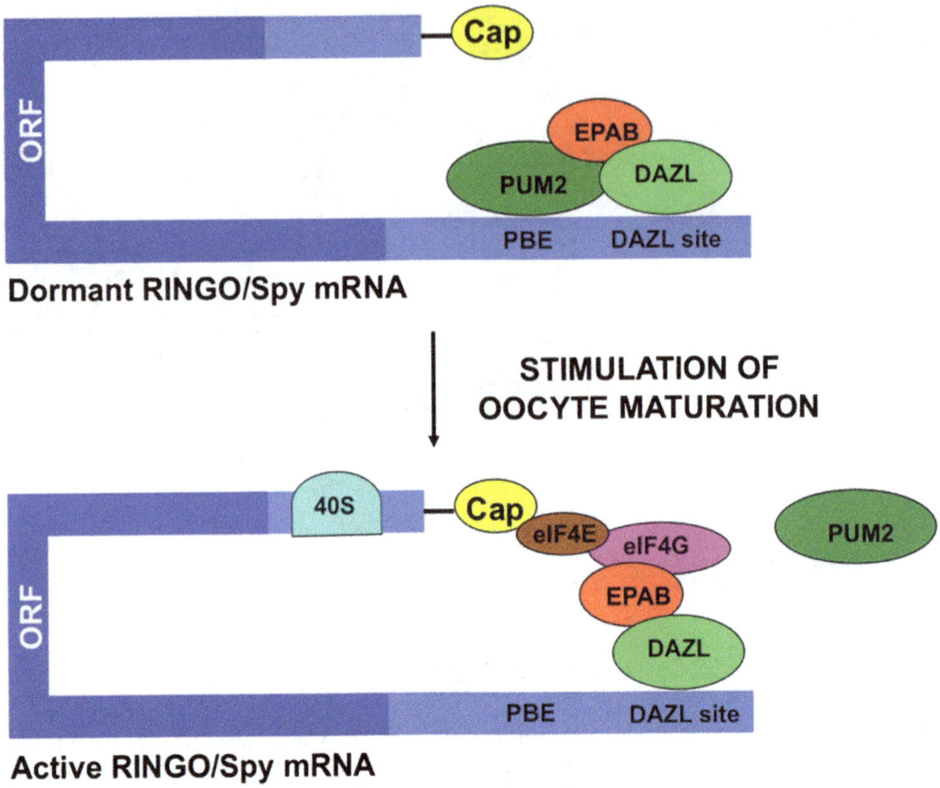

Fig. 15.4 Model for polyadenylation-independent translational control. In immature oocytes, Pumilio-2 (PUM2) binds the Pumilo binding element (PBE) in the 3′ UTR of RINGO/Spy mRNA, and also interacts with DAZL and EPAB. Following stimulation of oocyte maturation, PUM2 dissociates from the RINGO/Spy mRNA thereby allowing recruitment of eukaryotic initiation factors and translation of RINGO/Spy protein. The open reading frame (ORF) is shown in *dark blue*. The 5′ UTR and 3′ UTR regions are shown in *light blue*. *eIF4E* eukaryotic initiation factor 4E, the cap-binding protein; *eIF4A* eukaryotic initiation factor 4A, an RNA helicase; *PUM2* Pumilio-2; *DAZL* deleted in azoospermia like; *EPAB* embryonic poly(A) binding protein (Adapted from Padmanabhan K, Richter JD. Regulated Pumilio-2 binding controls RINGO/Spy mRNA translation and CPEB activation. Genes Dev. 2006;20:199–209, with permission)

EPAB interacts with the CPEB1/SYMPK/CPSF [34] and DAZL/Pumilio [35] complexes, prevents deadenylation of mRNAs [27], enhances translation initiation [32], and promotes cytoplasmic polyadenylation in vitro [34].

Translation Regulatory Cascades in the Oocyte

Cytoplasmic polyadenylation appears to be the predominant translational regulator of maternally stored mRNAs within the oocyte. However, to achieve timely expression of distinct genes necessary for specific steps of meiotic reactivation, oocyte maturation, and embryonic cleavage divisions, the presence of additional control mechanisms seems necessary [36].

One such mechanism has recently been described and regulates translational activation of the rapid inducer of G2/M progression in oocytes/Speedy (RINGO/Spy), one of the first mRNAs to be translated when the G2-arrested oocyte reenters meiosis [6, 37–39].

In the prophase-I-arrested oocyte, the translation of RINGO/Spy mRNA is repressed by Pumilio-2 which is bound to a pumilio-binding element (PBE) in the 3′-UTR (Fig. 4). Acting as translational co-repressors are the DAZL (Deleted in Azoospermia-Like protein) and EPAB proteins, which are also bound to the 3′-UTR of the same mRNA.

When the oocyte receives the hormonal signal to re-enter meiosis, PUM2 dissociates from the 3′-UTR of RINGO/Spy. Translation initiation factors are then recruited and translation of the RINGO/Spy protein can commence (Fig. 4). Once translated, RINGO/Spy activates the cyclin-dependent kinase Cdk2, which in turn activates another protein kinase—Eg2 from the Aurora family by phosphorylation [37, 39–42]. It is noteworthy that the translational activation of RINGO/Spy is independent of and precedes the polyadenylation-dependent translational regulation mediated by the CPEB/SYMPK/CPSF complex.

A central role for DAZL in mammalian oocyte translational regulation has recently been shown in the mouse, where CPEB acts as a regulator of DAZL translation by activating polyadenylation of the Dazl mRNA [43]. Subsequently, the high concentration of DAZL in the cytoplasm will act as a positive feedback loop, thereby promoting translation of its own mRNA and producing more DAZL. DAZL in turn activates a translational cascade of several mRNAs that are needed at later stages during fertilization and embryonic cleavage. DAZL does not only act as a translational control mechanism, but is also important during meiosis as a lack of the DAZL protein disrupts the formation of the meiotic spindle [43].

Summary and Discussion of Implications for Embryo Assessment in IVF

Timely expression and degradation of distinct mRNAs and proteins is required for specific steps of meiotic reactivation, oocyte maturation, and embryonic cleavage divisions [36]. Novel approaches utilizing global analysis of transcriptome or proteome have been proposed as technologies that may help improve embryo viability assessment in the IVF laboratory.

Potential sources for transcriptomic analysis are cumulus and/or granulosa cells that surround the oocyte, or the blastomeres removed from an embryo (reviewed in Chaps. 16 and 17). To interpret the findings of studies that perform transcriptomic analysis, it is crucial to make the distinction between somatic and gametogenic sources of mRNAs and to remember the differences between these cell types in regulating gene expression.

As cumulus and granulosa cells are somatic cells, their transcriptome may be interpreted as an accurate reflection of gene expression. Conversely, oocytes and early embryos until ZGA (which occurs at 4- to 8-cell stage in human) mainly regulate gene expression through translational control. Therefore, a simple analysis of mRNA content in an oocyte or a blastomere using a microarray will not be a true reflection of gene expression. To identify mRNAs that are being translated in an oocyte or a blastomere obtained from an early embryo, mRNAs with a long poly(A) tail, or bound to polysomes (collection of ribosomes), need to be selectively measured [43]. Unfortunately, this would require significant expertise and higher amount of sample than would be available in a single oocyte or blastomere.

Analysis of the proteome (reviewed in Chaps. 18, 19, and 20) may also be performed in oocytes, blastomeres, granulosa, or cumulus cells. However, the most important advantage of a proteomic approach is that it can be used to noninvasively assess the secretome of the oocyte or the embryo by the analysis of the culture media in which they are grown. Another key aspect of proteomic analysis is that its results are not biased by activation/repression status of existing mRNAs and it reflects the final protein outcome of gene expression, determined by the balance between protein synthesis and degradation.

References

1. Izaurralde E, Lewis J, McGuigan C, Jankowska M, Darzynkiewicz E, Mattaj IW. A nuclear cap binding protein complex involved in pre-mRNA splicing. Cell. 1994;78(4):657–68.
2. Flaherty SM, Fortes P, Izaurralde E, Mattaj IW, Gilmartin GM. Participation of the nuclear cap binding complex in pre-mRNA 3′ processing. Proc Natl Acad Sci USA. 1997;94(22):11893–8.

3. Zhao J, Hyman L, Moore C. Formation of mRNA 3′ends in eukaryotes: mechanism regulation and interrelationships with other steps in mRNA synthesis. Microbiol Mol Biol Rev. 1999;63:405–45.
4. Proudfoot N. New perspectives on connecting messenger RNA 3′ end formation to transcription. Curr Opin Cell Biol. 2004;16(3):272–8.
5. Kuhn U, Wahle E. Structure and function of poly(A) binding proteins. Biochim Biophys Acta – Gene Structure and Expression. 2004;1678(2/3):67–84.
6. Mendez R, Richter JD. Translational control by CPEB: a means to the end. Nat Rev Mol Cell Biol. 2001;2(7):521–9.
7. Wells S, Hillner P, Vale R, Sachs A. Circularization of mRNA by eukaryotic translation initiation factors. Mol Cell. 1998;2:135–40.
8. Mazumder B, Seshadri V, Fox PL. Translational control by the 3′-UTR: the ends specify the means. Trends Biochem Sci. 2003;28(2):91–8.
9. Huang YS, Richter JD. Regulation of local mRNA translation. Curr Opin Cell Biol. 2004;16:308–13.
10. Matova N, Cooley L. Comparative aspects of animal oogenesis. Dev Biol. 2001;231(2):291–320.
11. Sagata N. Meiotic metaphase arrest in animal oocytes: its mechanisms and biological significance. Trends Cell Biol. 1996;6:22–8.
12. Page AW, Orr-Weaver TL. Stopping and starting the meiotic cell cycle. Curr Opin Genet Dev. 1997;7(1):23–31.
13. LaMarca MJ, Smith LD, Strobel MC. Quantitative and qualitative analysis of RNA synthesis in stage 6 and stage 4 oocytes of Xenopus laevis. Dev Biol. 1973;34(1):106–18.
14. Rodman TC, Bachvarova R. RNA synthesis in preovulatory mouse oocytes. J Cell Biol. 1976;70(1):251–7.
15. Stebbins-Boaz B, Hake LE, Richter JD. CPEB controls the cytoplasmic polyadenylation of cyclin, Cdk2 and c-mos mRNAs and is necessary for oocyte maturation in Xenopus. EMBO J. 1996;15(10):2582–92.
16. Mendez R, Hake LE, Andresson T, Littlepage LE, Ruderman JV, Richter JD. Phosphorylation of CPE binding factor by Eg2 regulates translation of c-mos mRNA. Nature. 2000;404(6775):302–7.
17. Gebauer F, Xu W, Cooper GM, Richter JD. Translational control by cytoplasmic polyadenylation of c-mos mRNA is necessary for oocyte maturation in the mouse. EMBO J. 1994;13(23):5712.
18. Oh B, Hwang S, McLaughlin J, Solter D, Knowles BB. Timely translation during the mouse oocyte-to-embryo transition. Development. 2000;127(17):3795–803.
19. Newport J, Kirschner M. A major developmental transition in early Xenopus embryos: II. Control of the onset of transcription. Cell. 1982;30:687–96.
20. Newport J, Kirschner M. A major developmental transition in early Xenopus embryos: I. Characterization and timing of cellular changes at the midblastula stage. Cell. 1982;30:675–86.
21. Radford HE, Meijer H, de Moor C. Translational control by cytoplasmic polyadenylation in Xenopus oocytes. Biochim Biophys Acta (BBA) – Gene Regulatory Mechanisms. 2008;1779(4):217–29.
22. Clegg KB, Piko L. RNA synthesis and cytoplasmic polyadenylation in the one-cell mouse embryo. Nature. 1982;295(5847):343–4.
23. Flach G, Johnson MH, Braude PR, Taylor RA, Bolton VN. The transition from maternal to embryonic control in the 2-cell mouse embryo. EMBO J. 1982;1(6):681–6.
24. Braude P, Bolton V, Moore S. Human gene expression first occurs between the four- and eight-cell stages of preimplantation development. Nature. 1988;332(6163):459–61.
25. Hake LE, Richter JD. CPEB is a specificity factor that mediates cytoplasmic polyadenylation during Xenopus oocyte maturation. Cell. 1994;79(4):617–27.
26. Gebauer F, Richter JD. Mouse cytoplasmic polyadenylation element binding protein: an evolutionarily conserved protein that interacts with the cytoplasmic polyadenylation elements of c-mos mRNA. Proc Natl Acad Sci USA. 1996;93(25):14602–7.
27. Voeltz GK, Ongkasuwan J, Standart N, Steitz JA. A novel embryonic poly(A) binding protein, ePAB, regulates mRNA deadenylation in Xenopus egg extracts. Genes Dev. 2001;15(6):774–88.
28. Barnard D, Ryan K, Manley J, Richter J. Symplekin and xGLD-2 are required for CPEB-mediated cytoplasmic polyadenylation. Cell. 2004;119(5):641–51.
29. Racki WJ, Richter JD. CPEB controls oocyte growth and follicle development in the mouse. Development. 2006;133:4527–37.
30. Tay J, Richter JD. Germ cell differentiation and synaptonemal complex formation are disrupted in CPEB knockout mice. Dev Cell. 2001;1(2):201–13.
31. Seli E, Lalioti MD, Flaherty SM, Sakkas D, Terzi N, Steitz JA. An embryonic poly(A)-binding protein (ePAB) is expressed in mouse oocytes and early preimplantation embryos. Proc Natl Acad Sci USA. 2005;102(2):367–72.
32. Wilkie GS, Gautier P, Lawson D, Gray NK. Embryonic poly(A)-binding protein stimulates translation in germ cells. Mol Cell Biol. 2005;25:2060–71.
33. Guzeloglu-Kayisli O, Pauli SA, Demir H, Lalioti MD, Sakkas D, Seli E. Identification and characterization of human embryonic poly(A) binding protein (ePAB). Mol Hum Reprod. 2008;14:581–8.
34. Kim JH, Richter JD. RINGO/cdk1 and CPEB mediate poly(A) tail stabilization and translational regulation by ePAB. Genes Dev. 2007;21:2571–9.
35. Padmanabhan K, Richter JD. Regulated Pumilio-2 binding controls RINGO/Spy mRNA translation and CPEB activation. Genes Dev. 2006;20:199–209.
36. Vasudevan S, Seli E, Steitz JA. Metazoan oocyte and early embryo development program: a progression through translation regulatory cascades. Genes Dev. 2006;20(2):138–46.
37. Ferby I, Blazquez M, Palmer A, Eritja R, Nebreda AR. A novel p34(cdc2)-binding and activating protein that is necessary and sufficient to trigger G(2)/M

progression in Xenopus oocytes. Genes Dev. 1999;13:2177–89.

38. Eichenlaub-Ritter U, Peschke M. Expression in in-vivo and in-vitro growing and maturing oocytes: focus on regulation of expression at the translational level. Hum Reprod Update. 2002;8(1):21–41.
39. Dekel N. Cellular, biochemical and molecular mechanisms regulating oocyte maturation. Mol Cell Endocrinol. 2005;234:19–25.
40. Lenormand JL, Dellinger RW, Knudsen KE, Subramani S. Speedy: a novel cell cycle regulator of the G2/M transition. EMBO J. 1999;18:1869–77.
41. Terret TE, Ferby I, Nebreda AR, Verlhac MH. RINGO efficiently triggers meiosis resumption in mouse oocytes and induces cell cycle arrest in embryos. Biol Cell. 2001;93:89–97.
42. Cheng A, Xiong W, Ferrell JE, Solomon MJ. Identification and comparative analysis of multiple mamalian Spedy/Ringo proteins. Cell Cycle. 2005;4:155–65.
43. Chen J, Melton C, Suh N, Oh JS, Horner K, Xie F, et al. Genome-wide analysis of translation reveals a critical role for deleted in azoospermia-like (Dazl) at the oocyte-to-zygote transition. Genes Dev. 2011;25:755–66.

Transcriptomics Technology: Promise and Potential Pitfalls

16

Can Bruce and Asli Uyar

The developmental program of an embryo rests on the outcome of the complex interactions of gene products of the embryonic cell. As information flows from DNA to RNA and to protein, each step is potentially a predictor of the physiologic state of the cell. While protein content is more closely related to cellular phenotype than RNA content, current technology is much more sensitive for characterization of all RNA molecules of the cell (the transcriptome) than protein content. Taking RNA expression levels as a proxy for the expression levels of corresponding proteins, one can approximate the molecular composition of the cell and attempt to correlate it with its physiologic state. In the context of assisted reproductive technologies (ART), transcriptome analysis is a powerful tool that can be used to identify genes whose expressions are predictive of implantation and developmental success. At a more practical level, RNA expression profiles of blastocyst biopsies might be used for pre-implantation embryo screening.

We review here the current state of the technology for characterizing the transcriptome of a single or a small number of cells as it relates to ART. While small numbers of genes can be assayed by quantitative reverse transcriptase polymerase chain reaction (qRT-PCR), the comprehensive characterization of the transcriptome has been possible with DNA microarray chips. Recently, high-throughput sequencing technologies have been applied to transcriptomics in an approach generally referred to as RNA-seq. The large amount of data produced by both methods carries computational challenges and there are potential pitfalls in the proper analysis of the resultant data. RNA-seq is the method of choice for achieving high sensitivity and discovery of new transcripts, while microarrays are still quicker to perform, less costly, and may well be adequate for simple applications.

Sample Preparation

Some aspects of sample preparation are common to microarray and RNA-seq. Because RNA can be rapidly degraded by RNase released by the homogenized cells, the use of RNase inhibitors is critical. An amplification step, either by PCR or in vitro transcription-based linear amplification, is needed to convert the picogram quantities of RNA to the microgram amounts needed for microarray hybridization or sequencing. To ensure that the same amplification is achieved for all transcripts regardless of abundance, appropriate controls are needed. It is often useful to introduce a known quantity of exogenous RNA before the extraction

C. Bruce (✉)
Department of Molecular Biochemistry and Biophysics, W. M. Keck Foundation Biotechnology Resource Laboratory, Yale School of Medicine, 300 George Street, Suite 501, New Haven, CT, 06511, USA
e-mail: can.bruce@yale.edu

A. Uyar
Department of Obstetrics and Gynecology, Yale School of Medicine, New Haven, CT, USA

D.K. Gardner et al. (eds.), *Human Gametes and Preimplantation Embryos: Assessment and Diagnosis*, DOI 10.1007/978-1-4614-6651-2_16, © Springer Science+Business Media New York 2013

process to validate the extraction efficiency and ensure the linearity of amplification [1].

Protocols for sample preparation for microarray analysis [2] and RNA-seq analysis [3] from single blastomeres have been published. In brief, a fragment is cut from a blastocyst using a glass knife, the cells are dissociated in trypsin-EDTA buffer, a single cell is transferred into a PCR tube containing cell lysis buffer. The released RNA is then reverse-transcribed and poly(dA)-tailed. Then, the cDNA is PCR-amplified. Later steps are distinct for microarray and RNA-seq analysis. As data generation and its analysis takes several days for microarrays or 1–2 weeks for RNA-seq, the biopsied blastocyst needs to be frozen until implantation.

Microarray Technology

A DNA microarray consists of hundreds of thousands of distinct single-stranded oligonucleotides that are synthesized as a dense array on a solid surface (in the case of microarrays from companies such as Affymetrix, Agilent, ABI, etc.) or on microscopic beads that are spread on a silica surface (in the case of BeadArray technology from Illumina). Such chips are typically a few square centimeters in size and the individual spots on them are visualized by a microscope-coupled camera. After being fluorescently labeled, sample DNA molecules are placed on this chip so that they hybridize with the probe molecules on the surface. The fluorescent signal associated with each spot can be detected with a scanner, providing a concentration value for each DNA probe. Microarrays are produced by a number of commercial companies and regarding the sequence on the probes, various designs are available depending on the experimental objective. For transcript analysis, DNA that is hybridized to the microarray is complementary in sequence to the RNA molecules to be detected, i.e., cDNA. Exon arrays are microarrays with probes corresponding only to the exonic sequences of genes. When probes corresponding to the exons of a given transcript are all detected, the total signal from this probe set is taken as a value of its expression level.

Most transcriptomic analyses are done with microarrays containing probes specific to exons. The design of these microarrays is based on the known exon structures of genes and cannot be used to detect previously unknown transcript isoforms. There are also microarrays designed to detect exon junctions (for alternative splicing detection and microRNAs). Another type of microarray, tiling arrays, consists of overlapping probes that cover the whole length of the genome and are used to detect expression of all transcripts.

The purified cellular RNA is used to synthesize single-stranded cDNA by reverse transcription. Then, the cDNAs are labeled with a fluorescent dye and incubated over the microarray. The labeled targets bind to the complementary probes on the array. Then the array is washed to exclude the targets that have not been hybridized. The target cDNA molecules bind the probes at an amount proportional to their concentration. Typically, the slide is illuminated with a laser light which causes fluorescence from each spot, and the image of the microarray is captured for data analysis (Fig. 1).

The data from this image file is processed by software provided by the instrument vendors to correct for various artifacts and to produce an expression level at the exon level. In the case of Affymetrix, the data are further summarized as probe sets, that is, a number of probes whose expression corresponds to an mRNA containing all of them. The data quality is assessed by the use of spiked-in control RNAs that are not encoded by the organism being studied. The External RNA Control Consortium (ERCC) [4] and Microarray Quality Control (MAQC) Consortium [5] provide resources to assess the performance of microarray platforms using external RNA controls.

Statistical Analysis

The data produced by microarrays requires significant processing to correct bias due to systematic effects and to make data from separate microarrays comparable. Robust Multichip Average (RMA) is considered the most efficient analysis procedure. It consists of background adjustment, quantile normalization, and probe set

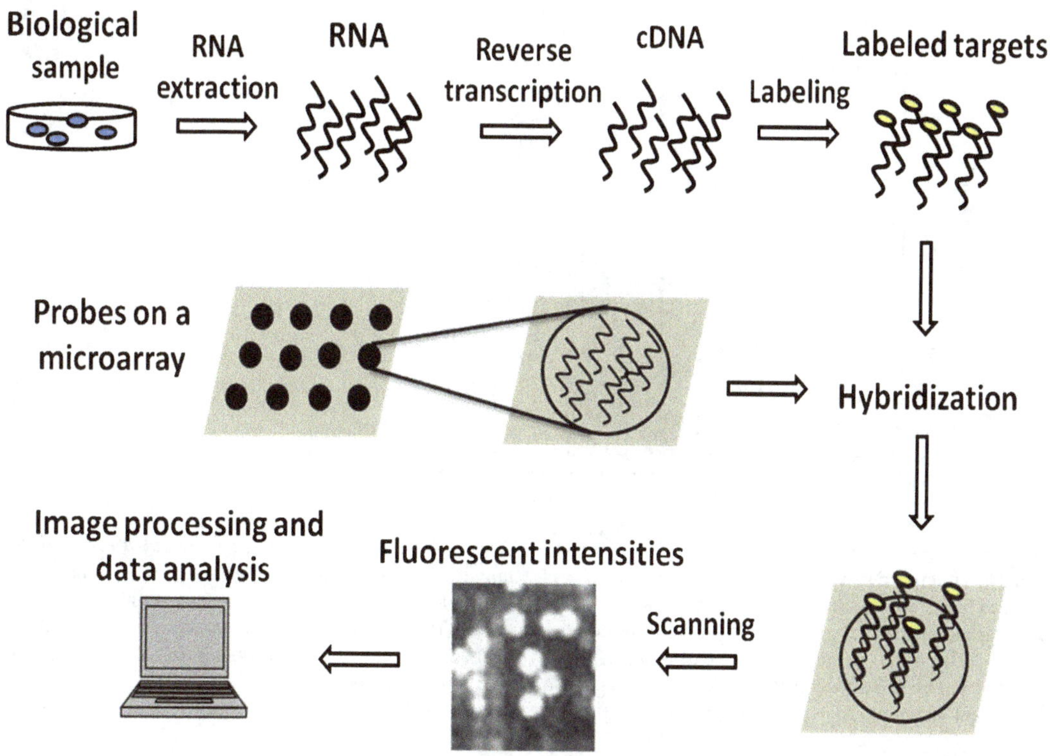

Fig. 16.1 Major steps of a typical microarray experiment. Total RNA is extracted from the biological sample and mRNA is reverse-transcribed to cDNA. Resulting cDNA is fluorescent-labeled and hybridized to microarray. Labeled targets bind to their complementary oligonucleotides attached in the microscopic probes. The array is then washed and scanned to obtain the fluorescent image which is further processed to get the intensity values for data analysis

summarization [6–8]. The intensity distribution of a microarray is shown to be log-normal, the expression values are converted to log base 2 and processed afterwards. In most protocols, each microarray corresponds to one sample, so it is important to ensure that any technical variability due to sample preparation, hybridization efficiency, array scanning, etc. are normalized in order to make the data comparable. Among various normalization methods, the well-accepted quantile normalization [7] is based on the assumption that the intensity data have identical intensity distributions, and that a treatment would cause only small fraction of the genes to be differentially regulated.

In Affymetrix GeneChip arrays, probes consist of 25 base oligomers and a gene is represented by a set of probes (~27). Each probe maps to annotated exons of known genes. After background adjustment and quantile normalization at probe level, the intensities of probes within a probe set are summarized to a single value using median polish method [8]. The resulting intensity value is assigned to the gene represented with that probe set. Differential expression analysis is performed on the background adjusted, normalized, and summarized intensities.

Because microarray analysis often involves two groups (control vs. treatment) with a few replicates, for thousands of genes, statistical correction for multiple comparisons is needed. When thousands of hypotheses are tested simultaneously for each gene with a specified Type I (false positive) error probability (e.g. 0.05), the chance of such errors increases with the number of hypotheses. Adjustment of the threshold p-value using the Bonferroni method is generally considered to be too conservative. A preferred way to

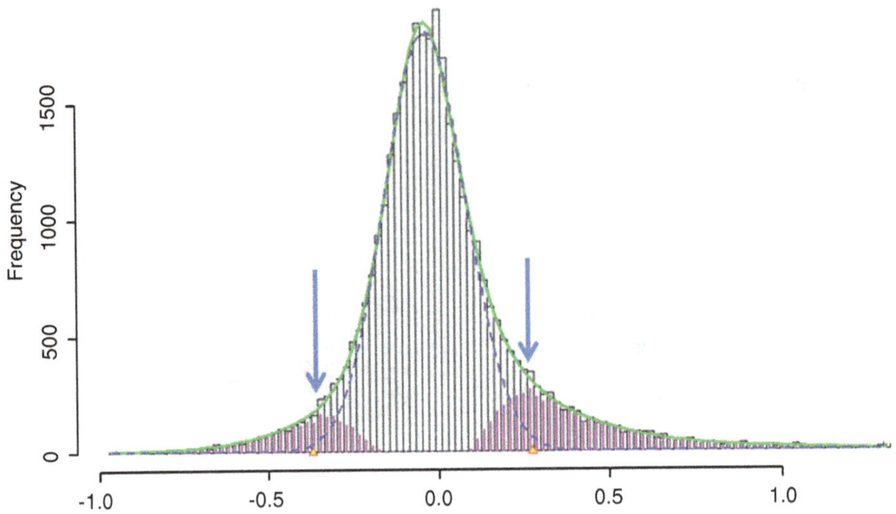

Fig. 16.2 False discovery rate thresholding of expression ratios in a microarray experiment. The distribution of normalized log(2) expression ratios is shown as a histogram. The background signal has been drawn here by fitting a normal distribution (*dashed line*) to the central part of the histogram. The difference between the background and the signal distribution represents the distribution of differentially expressed transcripts (*shaded areas* in the tails of the histogram). The *vertical arrows* indicate the threshold for expression change values with a false discovery rate (FDR) of 0.05. From the position of these arrows to the end of the nearest tail, the ratio of the signal area to the signal+background area is 0.95 (figure generated using the locfdr package [44])

identify significantly differentially regulated genes is to rank the transcripts according to the deviation of their expression level from the mean expression level of the control group, and then determine the false discovery rate (FDR) for each gene [9] (Fig. 2). The false discovery rate (FDR) is the expected proportion of Type I errors among the rejected hypotheses. In routine microarray data analysis, the expression levels are investigated in terms of biological significance in addition to statistical significance. Although an FDR threshold may identify a number of genes whose change is statistically significant, practitioners often also use an arbitrary fold-change threshold, like two-fold, to select genes that show a biologically interesting level of change.

RNA-Seq

The development of high-throughput sequencing technologies has made possible a novel approach to transcriptome analysis. These enable the characterization of the transcriptome by sequencing it many times over, an approach generally called "RNA-seq." While microarray technology is still used for transcriptome analysis when time and cost are of concern, RNA-seq is preferred for more detailed and accurate studies.

RNA-seq is the high-throughput sequencing of cDNA in order to characterize the RNA in a sample. Currently the most commonly used platforms for RNA-seq are the Genome Analyzer (Illumina), SOLiD (ABI) and 454 Sequencing (Life Technologies) for sequencing of DNA, and DRS (Helicos) for direct RNA sequencing. This is a very dynamic field, as many other companies and academic groups are actively working to develop alternative technologies to improve the number, quality, and length of sequences produced in one sequencing run and making it cheaper per nucleotide sequenced. The cost per nucleotide sequenced for all these technologies is at least three-orders of magnitude lower than the classical Sanger sequencing technique.

The low cost per nucleotide sequenced for the new sequencing technologies comes at the expense of sequence length and a higher error rate, especially in the case of Illumina. The error rate is compensated by the number of times each nucleotide is sequenced. Currently, Illumina Genome Analyzer has a read length of 50–150 nucleotides, and SOLiD of 35–75 nucleotides, depending on the instrument model. The short sequence lengths make the de novo assembly of a transcriptome difficult, because the amount of sequence overlap between different reads is limited. However, if the transcriptome belongs to an organism whose genome is known, then the reads can be aligned to the genome for assembling the transcriptome of the sample. The 454 system can produce reads of about 500 nucleotides, a length which is useful for de novo assembly, but because its cost per nucleotide is currently around a hundred times higher than Illumina and SOLiD, it is generally not used for transcriptome analysis [10].

High-throughput sequencing technologies produce many millions of sequence reads in one batch, and while the cost per base sequenced is quite low, the total amount cannot be decreased if fewer sequences are desired. However, multiple samples can be processed simultaneously by attaching sequence tags ("barcodes") to the DNA molecules being sequenced, to distinguish their reads from each other.

RNA-seq is superior to microarrays in not requiring prior knowledge of the transcript isoforms of the organism being studied. In fact, knowing the genome sequence is not required to assemble the transcriptome of an organism whose genome has not been sequenced. While the probes of a microarray rely on genome annotation, RNA-seq produces data that can lead to detailed characterization of each transcript species, both quantitatively and qualitatively.

The alignment of short reads to the genomic sequences can help assemble sequences into exons, but in order to assemble complete transcripts, it is necessary to find short reads that span two exons. Such reads can be aligned to a reference transcriptome sequence in which intronic sequences are removed. A more powerful approach is the "paired-end" sequencing method, in which the cDNA is fragmented; approximately 200–300 bp-long pieces are isolated and then partially sequenced from both ends. If one of the short reads is in one and another is in another exon, this is evidence that the two exons are connected. If one of the short reads cannot be reliably localized (due to similarities to evolutionarily related genes, or because its sequence is split by an exon junction), the sequence of the second member of the pair can provide a distance constraint that helps resolve the ambiguity (Fig. 3).

The use of RNA-seq for measuring gene expression levels relies on the principle that the number of sequence reads that map to a particular transcript is proportional to its expression level. Because alternatively spliced genes can produce multiple RNA isoforms, there are computational tools such as Cufflinks [11] or MISO [12] to assign probabilistically the expression level of each exon to each of the transcript isoforms it may belong and estimate the overall expression level of these transcripts.

Using the annotation file for the genome, it is thus possible to group the sequence reads into transcripts that (1) belong to the same gene, (2) share the same transcription start site (TSS), (3) that code the same protein sequence, and (4) are not grouped at all (Fig. 4). Each grouping can be evaluated separately for differential expression to uncover potentially a great level of regulatory complexity. Differentially expressed transcripts having the same TSS are presumably regulated by the same transcription factors, while two transcripts having the same TSS but different protein products that are differentially expressed are presumably regulated at the splicing level.

Protocol

RNA-seq is usually done on cDNA libraries from which ribosomal RNA sequences have been removed. If long RNA molecules such as mRNA are to be analyzed, it needs to be fragmented into smaller pieces first, but small RNA molecules like microRNA do not need to be fragmented. RNA is fragmented by hydrolysis or nebulization. Alternatively, RNA is first reverse-transcribed to cDNA, using either random hexamers or oligo(dT), then the cDNA is fragmented by DNAse I treatment or sonication. The cDNA is

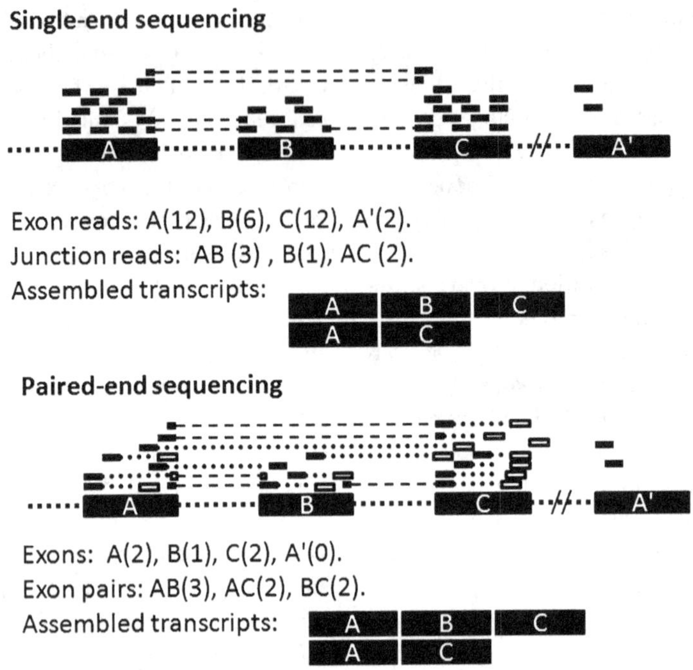

Fig. 16.3 Single-end and paired-end sequencing in RNA-seq. *Upper panel* shows how mapping of short sequence reads to exons (A, B, and C) can be used to assemble alternatively spliced transcripts from a gene. The *short filled rectangles* represent sequence reads, some of which may be interrupted (shown as *dashed lines*) by exon boundaries. Such junction reads quantify the relative amounts of transcript isoforms having that particular junction. Exon A′ is a paralog of exon A and belongs to another gene. As some sequences are present in both A and A′, this many lead to an uncertainty to the correct mapping of some of the reads. *Lower panel* shows how sequences from two ends of cDNA fragments selected to be of a fixed length (shown by a *filled and empty rectangle* connected by a *dotted line*) can impose a distance constraint in localizing the short reads. In this case the homologous reads mapping to A′ are not used in the assembly because they are not at the right distance from their paired-end sequence

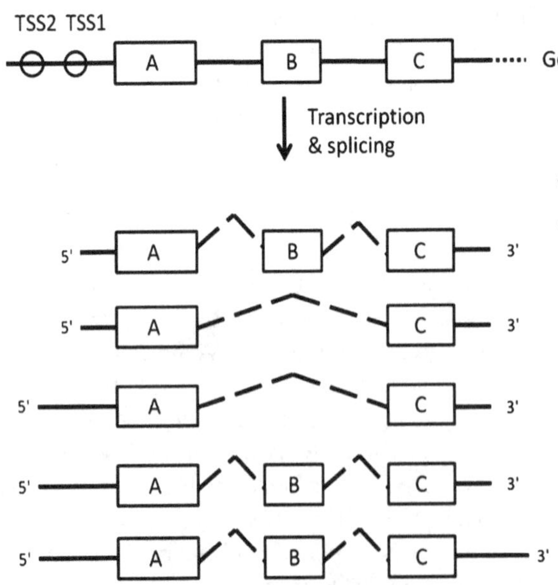

Gene	TSS	Protein -coding	transcript isoform
1	1	1	1
1	1	2	2
1	2	2	3
1	2	1	4
1	2	2	5

Fig. 16.4 Alternative groupings of sequence reads in RNA-seq. Five transcript isoforms (1–5) from a hypothetical gene "1" having two alternative transcription start sites (TSS 1 and 2) and coding for two protein-coding sequences (proteins 1 and 2) are shown. RNA-seq data can be summarized separately for each of these expression levels to reveal potentially different forms of differential expression

typically cut out of a gel to constrain its size distribution to about 250 nt. Strandedness of the mRNA may be preserved if needed, as there are protocols for this that introduce additional steps to the procedure [13–15]. Details of the different platforms used in RNA-seq can be found elsewhere [16].

A protocol for performing RNA-seq on single cells has been published [3]. For single cell RNA-seq analysis, mRNA is isolated from the cell lysate using oligo(dT)-coated magnetic beads. The mRNA is reverse-transcribed and tailed, then amplified by either PCR or in vitro fertilization (IVT). However, this protocol is limited to the purification of poly(A)+ mRNA and to the amplification of its 3′ end of up to 3 kb size; furthermore, the strandedness of the mRNA is lost.

Limitations of RNA-Seq

RNA-seq carries many of the bioinformatics challenges associated with high-throughput sequencing in general [17]. The large amount of data that this technology generates requires plenty of data storage and powerful computing facilities, often multiple computers doing parallel processing. RNA-seq is the preferred method for discovering new transcripts and annotating genomes. For well-characterized genomes, microarray technology is cheaper when analyzing large numbers of samples.

RNA-seq sample preparation has several steps that can potentially introduce biases to the sequence distribution. Sequencing of large RNA species needs to be fragmented into smaller pieces of 200–500 nt. Fragmentation of RNA has been shown to produce a loss of end fragments, while fragmentation of cDNA favors the preservation of sequences toward the 3′ end of the transcript. PCR artifact can cause the overrepresentation of certain sequences (the Helicos tSMS system sequences RNA directly, and so does not have this shortcoming). Strand-specific libraries are more informative, but require several additional manipulations that can incorporate further biases [18].

A number of pitfalls have been identified in RNA-seq technology [19]. Illumina sequencing has a bias toward GC-rich regions compared with AT-rich regions [20] due to biases at the PCR amplification and reverse transcription. Each short sequence is primed from a random hexamer, but the binding affinities of these hexamers are not identical, resulting in uneven reads at different positions. Also, chemical fragmentation can occur unevenly along the RNA being sequenced, leading to "read pileups." Secondary structure formation on the RNA can affect reverse transcription and PCR. Some of these biases can be expected to average out, but not all. Thus, the reads are not evenly distributed along transcript. These biases can be computationally predicted to correct the position-specific count values. As implemented in the Cufflinks program, depending on the experimental protocol, expression values can change around 1.5× after correcting for these biases [21].

Another consideration is that the reference genome used to map sequence reads may not correspond exactly to the genome of the tissue/cell line being analyzed. Constructing a reference genome incorporating information on polymorphic loci has been shown to improve the number of sequence reads by 15 % [22].

Statistical Design

As in microarray experiments, proper design of RNA-seq experiments can lower the variability in the data and improve the accuracy of exon detection and expression change. Biological replicates are needed to establish variability at the biological level and identify features that correlate with biological process of interest. However, RNA-seq data also show significant variability for technical replicates obtained from the same biological sample. Among the sources of these variations are the flow cell, the lane of the flow cell, and the sequence library batch. It is possible to do a randomized block design to control for these sources of variation. By using sequence tags to label different samples that are processed simultaneously (i.e., "multiplexed"), one can even out the effect of these technical variables on the variance of counts. Thus, instead of running one sample in each lane of a flow cell, one would run a mixture of all the samples in all the lanes, and then separate the results according to the sequence tags present within the short reads [23, 24].

Statistical Analysis

RNA-Seq data is often expressed in terms of reads per kilobase length per million read (RPKM), or in the case of paired-end sequences, fragments per kilobase length per million read (FPKM). The reason for this unit is that the longer the transcript is, the more "hits" there will be in it, and multiple samples are often normalized by expressing each read number as a fraction of the total number of hits. Because longer transcripts have more counts than shorter genes, longer genes are more likely to be found differentially expressed. Normalizing counts by transcript length does not remove this bias; however, normalizing by the inverse square root of transcript length has been found empirically to remove the length bias [25].

RNA-seq methodology has a number of aspects that introduce bias to the read count data. The lanes of the Illumina flow cell have different total number of sequences, so counts in each lane is usually normalized to the total number of counts in each lane. However, this approach is not ideal as the total number in each lane is dominated by a small number of abundantly expressed genes; so if these genes are differentially expressed, the normalization may skew the results. Using a housekeeping gene known not to be differentially expressed can be one solution of this problem, but it may be difficult to justify why the chosen gene should not be differentially expressed. A better method of count normalization is to remove the data for transcripts having zero counts across all lanes, then using the 75th percentile of the remaining transcripts as a normalization factor [25] or to use a weighted trimmed mean of the log expression ratios [26]. These normalization methods perform similarly [27]. Quantile normalization is another normalization method, often used in microarray data analysis, but it is computationally more demanding and does not produce an appreciable decrease in variability [25].

Estimating the statistical significance of differential expression between two groups can be done by a number of tests. The *t*-test and its variants are generally insensitive for low count numbers and become equivalent to more sensitive tests such as Fisher's Exact Test (FET) only if transcripts with less than 20 counts are discarded [25]. Because a generalized linear model can consider sample type as one of its parameters, it is more suited for comparison of more than two groups, compared to FET or the *t*-test. Programs modeling the data using a negative binomial distribution (edgeR, DESeq, baySeq) or using a non-parametric approach implemented in the program NOISeq were found to perform better than other alternatives tested [27, 28]. The Cuffdiff program also uses a negative binomial model for assessing differential expression, but its results are not directly comparable with the other programs because it uses a complex algorithm to estimate the expression levels of different isoforms, while the other programs assume that the length of a transcript does not change between two conditions. This assumption may be invalid in the case of differential alternative splicing. On the other hand, with EdgeR and DESeq, one can create generalized linear models which may provide greater sensitivity when it is necessary to tease out multiple factors that may affect gene expression.

Normalization of RNA-seq data for small RNA molecules (miRNA, snoRNA, etc.) has been found to be more complex than normalization for mRNA [29]. There are biases for specific small RNA molecules, making comparison between different RNA molecules difficult. While library size normalization similar to that used for mRNA with the RPKM unit can be used, the validity of this approach has been discussed, because the composition of the RNA population is unknown. Lowess normalization and quantile normalization have been suggested to remove RNA composition bias [30]. Because of the bias of RNA-seq for short RNA sequences, microarrays have been suggested to be superior to RNA-seq for small RNA quantitation, if novel microRNA discovery is not the primary aim [29].

Comparison of Microarray and RNA-Seq

RNA-seq correlates well with microarray data for genes expressing at medium levels, and not so for genes expressing at low and high levels, due to the narrower dynamic range (the ratio between the largest and smallest values that are measurable) of microarrays. When validated with the "gold-standard" technique of qRT-PCR, RNA-seq data reveal better accuracy than microarray data [31].

In terms of quantitation, microarray measurements suffer from nonlinearities at very low and very high expression values. At very low levels, signal is indistinguishable from noise due to non-specific binding of the cDNA to the probes, while at high levels there is signal saturation. With RNA-seq, there is no non-specific sequence generation at the low end and no saturation. However, sequencing errors may cause some reads to be mapped to the wrong region. Computational treatment of the data can be used to filter low quality sequences. A dynamic range of five-orders of magnitude has been reported with RNA-seq, while with microarrays it is less than 3 orders of magnitude. RNA-seq has been shown to be highly accurate by comparison with qRT-PCR. The downside of the high sensitivity of RNA-seq is that, to detect very low abundance transcripts, much greater coverage is needed. A typical Illumina run produces around 30 million 50 nucleotide-long sequences. As more and more sequences are obtained fewer and fewer new transcripts are discovered, but the diminishing returns on the effort means that an exhaustive enumeration of all transcripts may not be practical. A study of mouse embryonic stem cells found the number of unique TSSs to reach a plateau at 80 million reads, although at this point the number of unique transcripts discovered was still increasing monotonously relative to read number [32]. Experimental removal of abundantly expressed sequences by sequence normalization methods has been shown to increase detection sensitivity of rare transcripts without altering the number of genes found to be differentially expressed [33]. However, one should be aware that the lowest abundance transcripts in the cell, averaging less than one mRNA molecule per cell, may be a stochastic phenomenon caused by "leaky" gene expression and may not be representative of all cells in the sample [34].

Microarray technology requires the transcriptome to be annotated, because probe sets are designed specifically to measure the level of a known transcript. Tiling arrays with base-pair resolution can measure expression levels of individual exons, but cannot assemble transcript isoforms as reliably as RNA-seq. In contrast, RNA-seq can be used to discover previously unknown transcripts, map their splice sites with base-pair resolution, and using appropriate methodologies to map the 5′ and 3′ ends of the transcripts.

The depth of sequencing allows heterozygotic alleles to be quantified and their transcripts to be assembled separately from each other, resulting in allele-specific analysis of gene expression. Furthermore, RNA-seq can be used to detect the occurrence of RNA editing, where a base on an RNA molecule is different from what would be predicted based on the genomic sequence.

Currently, the cost of analyzing one sample by microarray is roughly tenfold less than the cost of running a (possibly multiplexed) sample through one lane of a flow cell for RNA-seq. Considering that separate microarrays would be needed for multiple samples with replicates, the costs of the two techniques can become comparable.

Biological Applications

Transcriptomics can be used for various applications of relevance to in vitro fertilization (IVF). From an analytic perspective, it enables the comparison of different tissues or stages of embryo, in order to better understand embryologic development. By looking at differences between individuals or populations, relevant candidate genes may be identified. From a clinical perspective, one can envision the identification of embryos expressing non-deleterious alleles or biomarkers predictive of successful implantation.

The objective of some transcriptomics studies is simply to identify biomarkers that correlate with a physiologic state such as developmental potential for a blastocyst. Other lines of investigation may approach the problem of blastocyst screening more indirectly, by understanding the molecular interactions that lead to a particular process. For such studies, using network or enrichment analysis of genes that show differential expression can yield useful biological insight. Programs such as IPA (Ingenuity), Pathway Studio (Ariadne), or MetaCore (GeneGo) generate networks of interactions that are significantly enriched with members of a gene list. The proteins that constitute such a network are presumably all involved in the biological process being investigated. Their presence is therefore suggestive of other gene products that were not detected at the mRNA level, but may still be involved through other mechanisms (protein-protein binding, phosphorylation, etc.). Another method of analyzing differentially expressed genes is to identify transcription factors whose targets are significantly enriched among members of the list. Observing such enrichment may help form the hypothesis that those transcription factors are important to the process being investigated. Understanding the biological context of the data from a transcriptomics analysis could possibly help guide further research for biomarkers detection using alternative methods, such as immuno-detection techniques.

A number of genes have been shown through hypothesis-driven studies on trophectoderm biopsies of mouse oocytes to be associated with success of implantation [35]. Transcriptomics studies are likely to identify many more such genes. Microarray analysis has been applied to embryo assessment. Transcript levels of the certain genes in cumulus cells have been found to be associated with embryo quality [36] or pregnancy outcome [37, 38]. A study on follicular cells has also identified genes whose expression correlate with pregnancy outcome [39]. In cattle, a number of transcripts in the granulosa cell were found to be associated with developmental competence of the oocyte [40]. cDNA can be amplified from a single blastomere to study this cell's transcriptome by microarray [2], so blastocyst screening by microarray is currently feasible.

Similar studies have been performed using RNA-seq technology. RNA-seq has been performed on pools of Day-8 bovine blastocysts that were produced either naturally or by IVF, and many genes were found to be differentially expressed or showing alternative splicing between the two groups [41]. Such differences are likely at the origin for the low implantation success of IVF embryos. RNA-seq has also been applied to single Day-7 blastocysts [42, 43] and even to single blastomeres in a blastocyst [3]. This methodology has also been used at the single cell level to characterize the derivation of pluripotent embryonic stem cells from the inner cell mass of blastocysts [43]. An interesting finding of such single cell studies has been that when pairs of cells from the same blastocysts are compared, most RNA species carrying the same allele have the same expression level, but a small minority's expression level shows stochastic differences. The proportion of transcripts that show stochastic expression increases over time and for 8-cell blastocysts has a proportion of about 12 % [3]. This would imply that the transcriptome of more than one cell may need to be characterized in order to compensate for the variability between cells.

Perspectives

Transcriptomics technologies have made immense strides in recent years. Measuring the expression of most RNA species has become feasible, not only for populations of cells but even for individual cells. The availability of these methods is surely going to be applied to embryo screening in the near future. As of this writing there are still certain limitations in terms of the ability to identify all RNA molecules of the cell, but even at this stage of the technology, it is reasonable to expect that studies will soon be performed on the RNA content of oocyte biopsy samples, and relate it to its capacity for a normal embryonic development. It can be hypothesized that the transcript profile of cells from oocytes with high likelihood of successful pregnancy will be distinguishable from that of oocytes with a low likelihood. The finding that oocytes produced naturally have a distinct transcript composition from oocytes produced by

IVF suggests that the oocyte transcripts can vary significantly and some oocytes are likely to be have an RNA expression profile that is closer to the "natural" profile. Also, the fact that there is cell-to-cell variability in embryo cells will mean that the number of cells to be biopsied should be high enough to give statistical power to the expression values, and still be low enough to not harm the embryo. Finally, we should be mindful of the fact that the physiology of the cell is the result of the structure and function of proteins, and only indirectly that of the RNA. Insignificant changes in certain RNA species may result in significant changes in post-translational modification of proteins with significant changes in their functionality. Despite these caveats, transcriptomic technologies offer great promise for understanding embryonic development and the assessment of cultured embryos.

Acknowledgments This work was supported in part with federal funds from NIH grants DA018343, DK090744 and UL1 RR024139.

References

1. Gilbert I, Scantland S, Dufort I, et al. Real-time monitoring of aRNA production during T7 amplification to prevent the loss of sample representation during microarray hybridization sample preparation. Nucleic Acids Res. 2009;37(8):e65.
2. Kurimoto K, Yabuta Y, Ohinata Y, Saitou M. Global single-cell cDNA amplification to provide a template for representative high-density oligonucleotide microarray analysis. Nat Protoc. 2007;2(3):739–52.
3. Tang F, Lao K, Surani MA. Development and applications of single-cell transcriptome analysis. Nat Methods. 2011;8(4 Suppl):S6–11.
4. External RNA Controls Consortium. Proposed methods for testing and selecting the ERCC external RNA controls. BMC Genomics. 2005;6:150.
5. Shi L, Reid LH, Jones WD, et al. The MicroArray Quality Control (MAQC) project shows inter- and intraplatform reproducibility of gene expression measurements. Nat Biotechnol. 2006;24(9):1151–61.
6. Irizarry RA, Hobbs B, Collin F, et al. Exploration, normalization, and summaries of high density oligonucleotide array probe level data. Biostatistics. 2003;4(2):249–64.
7. Bolstad BM, Irizarry RA, Astrand M, Speed TP. A comparison of normalization methods for high density oligonucleotide array data based on variance and bias. Bioinformatics. 2003;19(2):185–93.
8. Irizarry RA, Bolstad BM, Collin F, Cope LM, Hobbs B, Speed TP. Summaries of Affymetrix GeneChip probe level data. Nucleic Acids Res. 2003; 31(4):e15.
9. Benjamini Y, Hochberg Y. Controlling the false discovery rate—a practical and powerful approach to multiple testing. J R Stat Soc B Met. 1995;57(1): 289–300.
10. Glenn TC. Field guide to next-generation DNA sequencers. Mol Ecol Resour. 2011;11(5):759–69.
11. Trapnell C, Roberts A, Goff L, et al. Differential gene and transcript expression analysis of RNA-seq experiments with TopHat and Cufflinks. Nat Protoc. 2012; 7(3):562–78.
12. Katz Y, Wang ET, Airoldi EM, Burge CB. Analysis and design of RNA sequencing experiments for identifying isoform regulation. Nat Methods. 2010;7(12): 1009–15.
13. He Y, Vogelstein B, Velculescu VE, Papadopoulos N, Kinzler KW. The antisense transcriptomes of human cells. Science. 2008;322(5909):1855–7.
14. Core LJ, Waterfall JJ, Lis JT. Nascent RNA sequencing reveals widespread pausing and divergent initiation at human promoters. Science. 2008;322(5909):1845–8.
15. Parkhomchuk D, Borodina T, Amstislavskiy V, et al. Transcriptome analysis by strand-specific sequencing of complementary DNA. Nucleic Acids Res. 2009; 37(18):e123.
16. Ansorge WJ. Next-generation DNA sequencing techniques. N Biotechnol. 2009;25(4):195–203.
17. Pop M, Salzberg SL. Bioinformatics challenges of new sequencing technology. Trends Genet. 2008; 24(3):142–9.
18. Wang Z, Gerstein M, Snyder M. RNA-Seq: a revolutionary tool for transcriptomics. Nat Rev Genet. 2009;10(1):57–63.
19. Sendler E, Johnson GD, Krawetz SA. Local and global factors affecting RNA sequencing analysis. Anal Biochem. 2011;419(2):317–22.
20. Dohm JC, Lottaz C, Borodina T, Himmelbauer H. Substantial biases in ultra-short read data sets from high-throughput DNA sequencing. Nucleic Acids Res. 2008;36(16):e105.
21. Roberts A, Trapnell C, Donaghey J, Rinn JL, Pachter L. Improving RNA-Seq expression estimates by correcting for fragment bias. Genome Biol. 2011;12(3):R22.
22. Vijaya Satya R, Zavaljevski N, Reifman J. A new strategy to reduce allelic bias in RNA-Seq readmapping. Nucleic Acids Res. 2012;40(16):e127.
23. McIntyre LM, Lopiano KK, Morse AM, et al. RNA-seq: technical variability and sampling. BMC Genomics. 2011;12:293.
24. Auer PL, Doerge RW. Statistical design and analysis of RNA sequencing data. Genetics. 2010;185(2):405–16.
25. Bullard JH, Purdom E, Hansen KD, Dudoit S. Evaluation of statistical methods for normalization and differential expression in mRNA-Seq experiments. BMC Bioinformatics. 2010;11:94.
26. Robinson MD, Oshlack A. A scaling normalization method for differential expression analysis of RNA-seq data. Genome Biol. 2010;11(3):R25.

27. Kvam VM, Liu P, Si Y. A comparison of statistical methods for detecting differentially expressed genes from RNA-seq data. Am J Bot. 2012;99(2):248–56.
28. Tarazona S, Garcia-Alcalde F, Dopazo J, Ferrer A, Conesa A. Differential expression in RNA-seq: a matter of depth. Genome Res. 2011;21(12):2213–23.
29. Meyer SU, Pfaffl MW, Ulbrich SE. Normalization strategies for microRNA profiling experiments: a 'normal' way to a hidden layer of complexity? Biotechnol Lett. 2010;32(12):1777–88.
30. Garmire LX, Subramaniam S. Evaluation of normalization methods in mammalian microRNA-Seq data. RNA. 2012;18(6):1279–88.
31. Marioni JC, Mason CE, Mane SM, Stephens M, Gilad Y. RNA-seq: an assessment of technical reproducibility and comparison with gene expression arrays. Genome Res. 2008;18(9):1509–17.
32. Cloonan N, Forrest AR, Kolle G, et al. Stem cell transcriptome profiling via massive-scale mRNA sequencing. Nat Methods. 2008;5(7):613–9.
33. Ekblom R, Slate J, Horsburgh GJ, Birkhead T, Burke T. Comparison between normalised and unnormalised 454-sequencing libraries for small-scale RNA-Seq studies. Comp Funct Genomics. 2012;2012:281693.
34. Hebenstreit D, Fang M, Gu M, Charoensawan V, van Oudenaarden A, Teichmann SA. RNA sequencing reveals two major classes of gene expression levels in metazoan cells. Mol Syst Biol. 2011;7:497.
35. Parks JC, McCallie BR, Janesch AM, Schoolcraft WB, Katz-Jaffe MG. Blastocyst gene expression correlates with implantation potential. Fertil Steril. 2011;95(4):1367–72.
36. Cillo F, Brevini TA, Antonini S, Paffoni A, Ragni G, Gandolfi F. Association between human oocyte developmental competence and expression levels of some cumulus genes. Reproduction. 2007;134(5):645–50.
37. Assou S, Haouzi D, Mahmoud K, et al. A non-invasive test for assessing embryo potential by gene expression profiles of human cumulus cells: a proof of concept study. Mol Hum Reprod. 2008;14(12):711–9.
38. Assidi M, Montag M, Van der Ven K, Sirard MA. Biomarkers of human oocyte developmental competence expressed in cumulus cells before ICSI: a preliminary study. J Assist Reprod Genet. 2011;28(2): 173–88.
39. Hamel M, Dufort I, Robert C, Leveille MC, Leader A, Sirard MA. Identification of follicular marker genes as pregnancy predictors for human IVF: new evidence for the involvement of luteinization process. Mol Hum Reprod. 2010;16(8):548–56.
40. Gilbert I, Robert C, Vigneault C, Blondin P, Sirard MA. Impact of the LH surge on granulosa cell trancript levels as markers of oocyte developmental competence in cattle. Reproduction. 2012;143(6): 735–47.
41. Driver AM, Penagaricano F, Huang W, et al. RNA-Seq analysis uncovers transcriptomic variations between morphologically similar in vivo- and in vitro-derived bovine blastocysts. BMC Genomics. 2012;13(1):118.
42. Ross PJ, Chitwood JL. Transcriptome analysis of single bovine embryos by Rna-Seq. Reprod Fertil Dev. 2012;24(1):182.
43. Tang F, Barbacioru C, Bao S, et al. Tracing the derivation of embryonic stem cells from the inner cell mass by single-cell RNA-Seq analysis. Cell Stem Cell. 2010;6(5):468–78.
44. Efron B. Local false discovery rates. Stanford, CA: Department of Statistics, Stanford University; 2005.

17 Transcriptomic Analysis of Cumulus and Granulosa Cells as a Marker of Embryo Viability

Elpida Fragouli and Dagan Wells

As well as contributing the female genetic component to the developing embryo, oocytes also provide a store of mRNAs, proteins and other resources needed to sustain the embryo through the first few mitoses, until activation of its own genome takes place at the 4–8 cell stage. The build up of essential molecules in the oocyte is dependent not only on the oocyte itself but also on other cells within the ovary. Maturing oocytes are enclosed in follicles and are surrounded by multiple layers of somatic cells. These cells protect and support the oocyte and participate in events that regulate its nuclear and cytoplasmic maturation and subsequent ovulation. The cells associated with the oocyte can be divided into two groups, the mural granulosa cells (GCs), which line the wall of the follicle, and the cumulus cells (CCs). The CCs are differentiated GCs that enclose the oocyte, creating what is known as the cumulus-oocyte-complex (COC). The CCs and oocyte have a particularly intimate association, establishing a bi-directional communication involving, but not limited to, exchange of proteins and metabolites through gap junctions that link the two types of cells [1]. These connections allow the CCs to fulfil vital roles in the support and resourcing of the maturing oocyte.

During assisted reproductive technology (ART) procedures, the surrounding CCs are removed and discarded either following oocyte retrieval in cases where intracytoplasmic sperm injection (ICSI) is used for fertilisation, or after fertilisation in cases involving conventional in vitro fertilisation (IVF). However, several research teams have been interested in the possibility that these cells might harbour significant information about the quality of the oocyte with which they were associated and could be utilised for oocyte evaluation rather than discarded. This has led to a growing number of investigations focusing on analyses of the CC and/or GC transcriptomes, and aiming to identifying markers of oocyte and embryo viability. Results from such studies will be summarised in the following sections.

Oogenesis and Follicle Formation

Oogenesis consists of two separate meiotic divisions, meiosis I (MI) and II (MII), and two different stages when the developing oocyte pauses in the cell cycle. The first meiotic division begins during foetal life, at 11–12 weeks of gestation [2]. It is during this time that the newly formed immature diploid oocytes enter prophase of MI. Synapsis (pairing) of homologous chromosomes takes place, followed by the formation

E. Fragouli
Nuffield Department of Obstetrics and Gynaecology, University of Oxford, Oxford, UK

Reprogenetics UK, Oxford, UK

D. Wells (✉)
Nuffield Department of Obstetrics and Gynaecology, University of Oxford, Oxford, UK

Institute of Reproductive Sciences, Oxford, UK
e-mail: dagan.wells@obs-gyn.ox.ac.uk

D.K. Gardner et al. (eds.), *Human Gametes and Preimplantation Embryos: Assessment and Diagnosis*, DOI 10.1007/978-1-4614-6651-2_17, © Springer Science+Business Media New York 2013

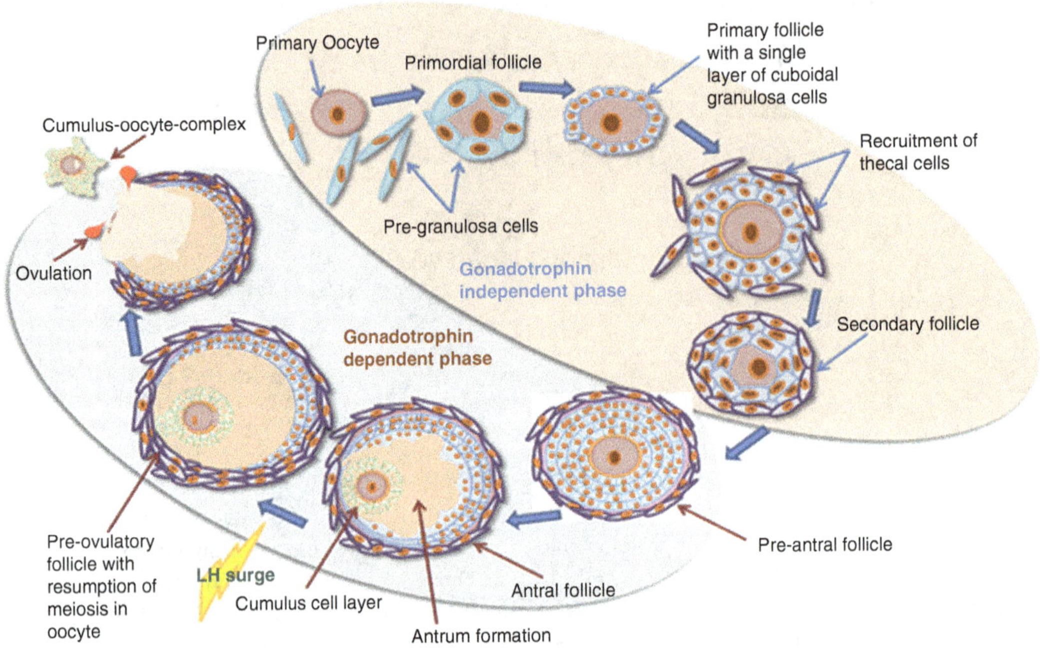

Fig. 17.1 Ovarian folliculogenesis: Follicular development is separated into two individual phases. One of them is gonadotrophin-independent and the other is gonadotrophin-dependent. During the gonadotrophin-independent phase the primordial follicle changes into the secondary follicle, as the surrounding layers of granulosa and theca cells proliferate. The gonadotrophin-dependent phase takes place under the influence of FSH, which causes the follicle to further mature to pre-antral and then antral. The formation of the antral follicle is indicated by the differentiation of the granulosa cells into the mural granulosa cells, which line its walls and the cumulus cells which surround the oocyte. Meiosis resumes under the influence of LH, resulting in the formation of the preovulatory follicle. Ovulation occurs 30–36 h later (figure courtesy of Zhongwei Huang.)

of chiasmata and the exchange of genetic material. The oocytes then begin a protracted arrest stage known as dictyate and remain there, until the onset of puberty and the initiation of the menstrual cycle, taking place under hormonal influence [follicle stimulating hormone (FSH) and the luteinising hormone (LH)]. Usually one oocyte completes maturation each month, resuming MI and arresting again at the metaphase stage of MII (reviewed in Huang et al. [3]). MII is not completed until the oocyte is fertilised.

The proliferation, differentiation and maturation of the somatic follicular cells occur in synchrony with the developing oocyte. The GCs represent the primary cell type in the ovarian follicle and are capable of changing their morphology and modifying their function in response to hormonal fluctuations or to signals coming from the developing oocyte. These changes are described in Fig. 1. At the end of the oocyte growth phase and with the formation of the follicular antrum, GCs differentiate into two anatomically different cell lineages, the mural GCs which have a steroidogenic role and line the follicular wall and the CCs which encircle the oocyte [4, 5].

Of the numerous events involved in oocyte maturation, those taking place at the stage just before ovulation within the COC are of particular significance for the fertilisation potential and developmental competence of the oocyte [6]. Specifically, during the LH surge an oocyte maturation signal is transmitted from the extra-follicular environment via the CCs. This is followed by resumption of MI [7]. Additionally, it has been demonstrated in a mouse animal model that appropriate spindle positioning, which is crucial for the correct segregation of chromosomes during meiosis, is regulated via the bi-directional communication established between the oocyte and its surrounding CCs [8].

Effect of the Follicular Environment on Oocyte Maturation

The mural granulosa cells are the first to receive the external hormone signals responsible for stimulating the oocyte to resume MI. Specifically, it has been shown that LH leads to the production of epidermal growth factor (EGF)-like molecules such as amphiregulin, epiregulin and betacellulin [9]. Not only do these growth factors activate oocyte maturation, but also induce expression of specific genes responsible for CC proliferation and expansion, such as HAS-2, PTGS-2 and TNFAIP6 [10].

Moreover, in a study involving a systematic review of factors influencing oocyte maturation, it was demonstrated that LH activates expression of the progesterone receptor (PGR) in the GCs surrounding oocytes that are destined to ovulate [11]. PGR is a nuclear receptor transcription factor which is actively involved in the regulation of ovulation, and its inactivation leading to a complete ovulation block [11].

Another factor which is crucial for the successful maturation of the oocyte is glucose. The COC requires glucose for a variety of metabolic processes, including energy production, nucleic acid and purine synthesis, mucification and cellular homeostasis [12]. As the oocyte is a poor glucose metaboliser and cannot generate any of the amino acids necessary for energy production, the surrounding CCs must provide this nutritional support [13, 14]. This is thought to take place via an oocyte-CC regulatory loop. Data obtained from a mouse model demonstrated that two oocyte secreted factors, growth differentiation factor 9 (GFD9) and bone morphogenetic factor 15 (BMP15), are responsible for the regulation of key CC metabolic processes such as glycolysis and cholesterol biosynthesis, occurring prior to the LH surge [13]. Additionally, a trancriptomic analysis of CCs removed from human oocytes which went on to produce live births suggested that an active CC metabolism is essential for oocyte maturation and competence [14].

Apart from nutritionally supporting the oocyte, the surrounding CCs are able to protect it from oxidative stress caused by reactive oxygen species via the production of enzymes with antioxidant actions, such as superoxide dismutases (SOD). A study investigating the antioxidant protection of CCs showed that increased SOD activity was associated with the establishment of clinical pregnancies in IVF cycles [15]. Interestingly, a decline in SOD activity was seen to be associated with advancing female age. Advancing female age is the single most important and consistent factor affecting the probability of a healthy birth. The increasing risks of aneuploidy, poor embryo development and failure to implant in the uterus have all been well documented for women aged 35 years and onwards. The data obtained from the above-mentioned investigation suggest that CCs continuously monitor the follicular environment and regulate the production of antioxidants and other molecules in an attempt to provide the optimal conditions for oocyte development. Additionally, it is possible that SOD or other molecules of similar function could be useful biomarkers, assisting in the identification of competent oocytes capable of supporting preimplantation embryo development and producing a healthy live birth.

Another factor which could be indicative of the health of a follicle and the oocyte it contains is anti-müllerian hormone (AMH). It is thought that AMH attenuates the effects of FSH on the recruitment and growth of follicles and in this way regulates their development [16]. Analysis of AMH expression showed that it was higher in CCs of mature human follicles, compared to GCs [17]. This study suggested that as AMH was correlated with the expression of FSH receptor, androgen receptor and the AMH receptor, it may have an intrafollicular function, especially before ovulation [17].

Transmission of molecular signals to and from the maturing oocyte is essential for it to acquire the ability to be fertilised, activated and in order for it to be able to support the embryo during its first few days of life. The crucial function of CCs in mediating these signals makes it likely that pathways regulating their proliferation and apoptosis are prognostic of the corresponding oocyte's health. A high incidence of CC apoptosis has been correlated with poor oocyte quality as well as inferior embryo development [18, 19]. Interestingly, it has recently been shown, that the oocyte secreted factors BMP15 and BMP6 act to protect the surrounding CCs from apoptosis, by establishing a morphogenic paracrine gradient of BMPs [20].

Identification of Novel Biomarkers for Oocyte and Embryo Selection

The fact that CCs share the same follicular environment as the oocyte and are in close communication with it has led to the idea that their analysis may serve as a surrogate for direct analysis of the oocyte itself. In addition, the fact that GCs and CCs can easily be collected without compromising the oocyte makes them attractive targets for the development of noninvasive assays for the selection of the most competent oocytes and embryos. For this reason an increasing number of research laboratories are focusing on the examination of these cells in an attempt to identify novel biomarkers of implantation/pregnancy potential. Particular attention has been paid to transcriptomic analysis of GCs and CCs. Patterns of gene expression reflect the processes active within a cell at a given moment in time, including its responses to environmental challenges. The analysis of the GC or CC transcriptome may therefore provide important information concerning the conditions within the follicle in which the oocyte completed maturation.

A potentially useful biomarker, providing information on the fertilisation ability of oocytes, is the ovulatory gene ADAM-metallopeptidase with thrombospondin type 1 motifs-1 (ADAMTS-1). A null mutation of this gene has been associated with impaired follicular and ovulatory processes in a mouse animal model [21]. It was also shown in humans that ADAMTS-1 is induced by LH, and its GC expression correlated with antral follicular growth [22]. More importantly, it has been reported that the expression of ADAMTS-1 in CCs is indicative of the fertilisation capacity of the corresponding oocyte [22].

Assou et al. [14] employed a combination of microarray and real-time PCR technology is order to try and elucidate specific patterns of CC gene expression in relation to embryonic morphology (a key viability indicator) and pregnancy outcome. A total of three genes were identified as potentially useful biomarkers during this study. The up-regulation in CCs of BCL2L11 involved in apoptosis and PCK1 involved in gluconeogenesis and the down-regulation of the transcription factor NFIB were associated with the generation of embryos able to implant and lead to live births [14].

Unlike Assou's study which involved a preliminary gene expression microarray step to reveal potential candidate genes, Feuerstein et al. [1] chose to examine six specific genes in CCs removed from preovulatory follicles with the use of real-time PCR. These genes were STAR, COX2, AREG, SCD1, SCD5 and Cx43 and they were selected because some are induced by the LH surge, while others have roles in oocyte lipid metabolism, or in the regulation of gap junction formation, all important processes for appropriate CC function. Data obtained from this study showed that five of the six genes (all except Cx43) under investigation increased their expression once MI was resumed. The transcript levels of these genes were also assessed in CCs removed from oocytes capable of forming blastocysts and compared to CCs taken from oocytes whose embryos were considered to be of poor development. Results suggested that mRNA transcripts of these genes were distributed over a narrower range in CCs enclosing oocytes achieving blastocyst development compared with those enclosing oocytes that failed to develop. These results provide evidence for a relationship between CC gene expression patterns and developmental ability [1].

Another investigation correlating CC gene expression with the ability of the corresponding oocyte to produce an embryo capable of reaching the blastocyst stage and leading to a viable pregnancy studied eight genes (SDC4, PTGS2,

VCAN, ALCAM, GREM1, TRPM7, CALM2 and ITPKA) using quantitative real-time PCR [23]. Seven of the examined genes (all apart from VCAN) seemed to be capable of predicting an embryo's ability to form a blastocyst of good morphology, while expression of VCAN and SDC4 in CCs was predictive of pregnancy. This research group created specific multivariate models of gene expression and claimed to be able to predict pregnancy with a sensitivity of >70 % and a specificity of >90 % [23].

Gebhardt et al. [24] followed a similar approach in their examination of 13 genes in CC samples. The genes selected for analysis are involved in regulation of metabolism, signalling and extracellular matrix formation. The aim of the study was to identify possible expression patterns associated with the oocyte's ability to lead to a live birth, after elective single embryo transfer. A general up-regulation of all 13 genes was evident in CCs removed from developmentally competent oocytes. In addition, among the 13 genes, VCAN, PTGS2, GREM1 and PFKP were highlighted as having expression profiles indicative of good quality oocytes [24].

All the above-mentioned investigations had similar aims, measuring specific mRNA transcripts in GCs or CCs and identifying genes whose expression was indicative of oocyte/embryo quality and viability. However, another important aspect of oocyte and embryo competence, not considered by these studies, is the presence of chromosome abnormalities (aneuploidy). Aneuploidy is extremely common in human oocytes and is almost always lethal to the developing embryo or foetus. The vulnerability to chromosome malsegregation increases dramatically with advancing female age, affecting more than half of all oocytes from women over 40 years of age [25]. Methods for testing oocytes for aneuploidy are already well established, based upon biopsy of the polar bodies followed by testing using methods such as microarray comparative genomic hybridisation (aCGH). However, such methods are labour intensive, expensive and somewhat invasive, involving the breach of the zona pellucida, the protective envelope covering the oocyte. Noninvasive methods for testing oocyte aneuploidy are highly desirable.

It is possible that the presence of chromosome abnormalities in an oocyte could alter signalling pathways and disrupt intercellular communication with the surrounding CCs, causing changes in their gene expression patterns. It is also possible that an oocyte maturing in an inappropriate follicular environment (e.g. hypoxic, or otherwise poorly resourced) may be at increased risk of chromosome malsegregation after the resumption of meiosis. A poor microenvironment would be very likely to affect not only the oocyte but also the somatic cells of the follicle, inevitably inducing changes in their gene expression. In order to gain an insight into the follicular environment of aneuploid oocytes and potentially identify cumulus cell markers of oocyte aneuploidy, our group compared the gene expression of CCs associated with chromosomally normal and abnormal oocytes. Similar to previous investigations of CCs, a combination of gene expression microarray analysis and real-time PCR was employed. Interestingly, we observed that CCs enclosing chromosomally abnormal oocytes were less transcriptionally active. This is reminiscent of some of the studies discussed above, in which a general reduction in transcript levels in CCs was associated with poor outcomes. The data obtained showed that 14 genes had highly statistically significant expression differences ($P<0.01$) between the CCs of normal and aneuploid oocytes, all of which were underexpressed in CCs associated with abnormal oocytes. Various biological processes were affected, including metabolism, signalling pathways, apoptosis and transport. Among these genes was SPSB2, the expression of which seemed to correlate both with the chromosome status of the oocyte and also with its ability to lead to a live birth. SPSB2 is involved in proteasomal degradation. Its down-regulation in the CCs of aneuploid oocytes may result in the accumulation of excessive levels of abnormal/redundant proteins. This gene could be a particularly useful biomarker, as it may potentially identify oocytes free of chromosome errors and of superior quality, able to lead to the establishment of a successful pregnancy. The findings of all the above-mentioned studies are summarised in Table 1.

Table 17.1 Candidate biomarkers for the selection of competent oocytes and embryos with high implantation potential

Study	Type of follicular cells examined	Methodology used	Selection measure	Candidate genes	Functions
Feuerstein et al. [1]	CCs	Real-time PCR	Development to the blastocyst stage	STAR, COX2, AREG	Induced by LH surge
				SCD1, SCD5	Regulate oocyte lipid metabolism
				Cx43	Involved in gap junction formation
Assou et al. [14]	CCs	Gene expression microarray and real-time PCR	Embryonic morphology and pregnancy outcome	BCL2L11	Regulates apoptosis
				PCK1	Involved in gluconeogenesis
				NFIB	Transcription factor
Matos et al. [15]	CCs	Immunodetection	Female age	SOD	Antioxidant action
Robker et al. [11]	GCs	Review of literature	Ovulation	PGR	Induced by LH surge, regulates ovulation
Yung et al. [22]	GCs/CCs	Real-time PCR	Oocyte fertilisation ability	ADAMTS-1	Induced by LH surge, indicative of oocyte fertilisation ability
Gebhardt et al. [24]	CCs	Real-time PCR	Live birth after elective single embryo transfer	VCAN	Regulation of extracellular matrix formation
				PTGS2, GREM1	Signalling
				PFKP	Metabolism
Grøndahl et al. [17]	GCs/CCs	Gene expression microarray and real-time PCR	Oocyte maturity/ ovulation	AMH	Indicative of follicle health
Wathlet et al. [23]	CCs	Real-time PCR	Development to the blastocyst stage/ pregnancy	VCAN	Regulation of extracellular matrix formation
				SDC4	(Co)receptor for TGFB
Fragouli and Wells unpublished	CCs	Expression microarray and real-time PCR	Oocyte chromosome status/pregnancy	SPSB2	Involved in proteasomal degradation

Conclusion: The Development of Noninvasive Assays of Oocyte Assessment and Embryo Selection

At the time of oocyte retrieval the CCs can be removed and subjected to analysis. These cells have experienced the same environment as the oocyte during the critical final stages of nuclear and cytoplasmic maturation. It is likely that a footprint of the follicular microenvironment persists in the transcriptome of the CCs, leading to the suggestion that it might be possible to define a specific gene expression 'signature' indicative of a competent oocyte. The development of a noninvasive test, based on the assessment of gene expression in follicular somatic cells, could prove to be very beneficial both clinically and scientifically. Clinically such a test could lead to a significant increase to IVF success rates. Additionally, if oocytes at high risk of chromosome abnormality could be identified, a decrease in the incidence of spontaneous pregnancy losses and aneuploid syndromes (e.g., Down's syndrome) would be expected. Scientifically, the examination of GCs and CCs could provide an insight into events taking place in healthy as well as sub-optimal follicles. Important biological pathways could be highlighted in this way, leading to an increased understanding of the key intrinsic and extrinsic factors influencing oocyte development. This could in turn result in improvements in oocyte in vitro maturation protocols and the optimization of gonadotrophin dosing during IVF cycles, maximising the availability of high quality euploid oocytes.

Even though the data obtained from various different studies are encouraging, a significant amount of work is still necessary before noninvasive tests based upon CCs are widely applied. One obstacle that must be overcome is the definition of how viability is measured. In almost all IVF laboratories worldwide morphological assessment is still the main guide for embryo selection. However, morphology is a relatively poor guide to viability and provides no useful information concerning aneuploidy. A better measure of viability would therefore be the establishment of a sustained clinical pregnancy. Moreover, there is relatively little concordance between the transcriptomic studies of CCs carried out to date. Most investigations have identified different candidate genes. This lack of uniformity between different studies may simply indicate that there are many clinically relevant genes expressed by CCs, with different studies happening upon different genes. Alternatively it may be a consequence of variation in the way that viability has been defined in different studies. However, it might also be a warning that CC gene expression is affected by multiple variables, which could be patient-, clinic-, treatment- or aetiology-specific. The characterization of a universally applicable CC-based test for oocyte competence may prove to be a challenge, but the potential benefits make it a goal well worth pursuing.

References

1. Feuerstein P, Cadoret V, Dalbies-Tran R, Guerif F, et al. Gene expression in human cumulus cells: one approach to oocyte competence. Hum Reprod. 2007; 22:3069–77.
2. Gondos B, Westergaard L, Byskov AG. Initiation of oogenesis in the human fetal ovary: ultrastructural and squash preparation study. Am J Obstet Gynecol. 1986;155:189–95.
3. Huang Z, Fragouli E, Wells D. Biomolecules of human female fertility—potential therapeutic targets for pharmaceutical design. Curr Pharm Des. 2012; 18:310–24.
4. Chian RC, Lim JH, Tan SL. State of the art in vitro oocyte maturation. Curr Opin Obstet Gynecol. 2004; 16:211–9.
5. Gilchrist RB, Lane M, Thompson JG. Oocyte-secreted factors: regulators of cumulus cell function and oocyte quality. Hum Reprod Update. 2008;14:159–77.
6. Russell DL, Robker RL. Molecular mechanisms of ovulation: co-ordination through the cumulus complex. Hum Reprod Update. 2007;13:289–312.
7. Hillier SG. Current concepts of the roles of follicle stimulating hormone and luteinizing hormone in folliculogenesis. Hum Reprod. 1994;9:188–91.
8. Barrett SL, Albertini DF. Cumulus cell contact during oocyte maturation in mice regulates meiotic spindle positioning and enhances developmental competence. J Assist Reprod Genet. 2010;27:29–39.
9. Park JY, Su YQ, Ariga M, et al. EGF-like growth factors as mediators of LH action in the ovulatory follicle. Science. 2004;303:682–4.
10. Hsieh M, Zamah AM, Conti M. Epidermal growth factor-like growth factors in the follicular fluid: role in

oocyte development and maturation. Semin Reprod Med. 2009;27:52–61.
11. Robker RL, Akison LK, Russell DL. Control of oocyte release by progesterone receptor—regulated 1165 gene expression. Nucl Recept Signal. 2009;7:e012.
12. Sutton ML, Gilchrist RB, Thompson JG. Effects of in-vivo and invitro environments on the metabolism of the cumulus-oocyte complex and its influence on oocyte developmental capacity. Hum Reprod Update. 2003;9:35–48.
13. Su YQ, Sugiura K, Wigglesworth K, et al. Oocyte regulation of metabolic cooperativity between mouse cumulus cells and oocytes: BMP15 and GDF9 control cholesterol biosynthesis in cumulus cells. Development. 2008;135:111–21.
14. Assou S, Haouzi D, Mahmoud K, et al. A non-invasive test for assessing embryo potential by gene expression profiles of human cumulus cells: a proof of concept study. Mol Hum Reprod. 2008;14:711–9.
15. Matos L, Stevenson D, Gomes F, et al. Superoxide dismutase expression in human cumulus oophorus cells. Mol Hum Reprod. 2009;15:411–9.
16. Salmon NA, Handyside AH, Joyce IM. Oocyte regulation of anti Mullerian hormone expression in granulosa cells during ovarian follicle stimulation in mice. Dev Biol. 2004;266:201–8.
17. Grøndahl ML, Eilsø Nielsen M, Dal Canto MB, et al. Anti-Mullerian hormone remains highly expressed in human cumulus cells during the final stages of folliculogenesis. Reprod Biomed Online. 2011;22:389–98.
18. Host E, Gabrielsen A, Lindenberg S, et al. Apoptosis in human cumulus cells in relation to zona pellucida thickness variation, maturation stage and cleavage of the corresponding oocyte after intracytoplasmic sperm injection. Fertil Steril. 2002;77:511–5.
19. Corn CM, Hauser-Kronberger C, Moser M, et al. Predictive value of cumulus cells apoptosis with regard to blastocyst development of corresponding gametes. Fertil Steril. 2005;84:627–33.
20. Hussein TS, Froiland DA, Amato F, et al. Oocytes prevent cumulus cell apoptosis by maintaining a morphogenic paracrine gradient of bone morphogenetic proteins. J Cell Sci. 2005;118:5257–68.
21. Shozu M, Minami N, Yokoyama H, et al. ADAMTS-1 is involved in normal follicular development, ovulatory process and organization of the medullary vascular network in the ovary. J Mol Endocrinol. 2005;35:343–55.
22. Yung Y, Maman E, Konopnicki S, et al. ADAMTS-1: a new human ovulatory gene and a cumulus marker for fertilization capacity. Mol Cell Endocrinol. 2010;328:104–8.
23. Wathlet S, Adriaenssens T, Segers I, et al. Cumulus cell gene expression in ICSI patients predicts better cleavage-stage embryo or blastocyst development and pregnancy. Hum Reprod. 2011;26:1035–51.
24. Gebhardt KM, Feil DK, Dunning KR, et al. Human cumulus cell gene expression as a biomarker of pregnancy outcome after single embryo transfer. Fertil Steril. 2011;96:47.e2–52.e2.
25. Fragouli E, Alfarawati S, Goodall NN, et al. The cytogenetics of polar bodies: insights into female meiosis and the diagnosis of aneuploidy. Mol Hum Reprod. 2011;17:286–95.

Mass Spectrometry, Proteomics, and the Study of Sperm Cell Biology

18

Mark A. Baker and R. John Aitken

In the recent past, we have witnessed a sudden explosion of information in the biological sciences triggered by the 'omics' revolution. A new generation scientists, largely unconcerned with hypothesis driven-based research, are using a range of specialized instruments to generate inventories of data on the mRNA, miRNA, protein, lipid, and carbohydrate composition of cells and, in the wake of this information, retrospectively generating concepts about the molecular mechanisms that regulate cell function and fate. While transcriptomics has certainly led the way, the poor correlation between changes in mRNA profile and protein abundance has encouraged many researchers to look directly at the protein composition of cells [1]. In doing so, we are now gaining an understanding of biological systems at a rate that would have been unbelievable, even a decade ago. The reasons for this sudden change can be put down to improvements in equipment sensitivity and accuracy, particularly in the field of mass spectrometry. Furthermore, new protocols for undertaking the pre-fractionation of specific populations of proteins, according to specific post-translational modifications (phosphorylation, glycosylation) or cellular localization, have allowed scientists to generate unprecedented insights into cell biochemistry.

M.A. Baker • R.J. Aitken (✉)
Discipline of Biological Sciences, Faculty of Science and IT, University of Newcastle, Callaghan, NSW, Australia
e-mail: john.aitken@newcastle.edu.au

In the specific context of proteomics, the technology for undertaking such analyses is changing at a bewildering pace. As a result, many biological systems amenable to mass spectrometry are being overlooked. Here we shall review some recent advances in mass spectrometry and consider their application to biological systems with particular emphasis on the cell biology of spermatozoa.

Mass Spectrometers: The Technologies Available?

The marketplace is flooded with an ever-appealing range of mass spectrometers available to researchers, with an estimated "new" machine being released into the marketplace every 1–4 months. Typically, however, such instruments are simply incremental improvements of pre-existing platforms, designed to increase sensitivity, resolution, or mass accuracy. In terms of proteomics, many studies use what is known as a "bottom-up" approach. That is, you take a protein mixture of interest, digest with an enzyme (usually trypsin), and measure the mass of the peptides present (MS). If required, a specific peptide can then be isolated, fragmented, and the daughter ions measured (MS/MS) in order to generate a protein identification [2, 3]. When it comes to the analysis of biological systems no less than five different types of mass spectrometer need to be understood in terms of their technical capabilities. The advantages, disadvantages, and specific niches occupied by each type of instrument are outlined below.

D.K. Gardner et al. (eds.), *Human Gametes and Preimplantation Embryos: Assessment and Diagnosis*, DOI 10.1007/978-1-4614-6651-2_18, © Springer Science+Business Media New York 2013

Quadrupole Time-of-Flight Mass Spectrometer

Typically designed to be used with a liquid chromatography (LC) front end, the quadrupole time-of-flight (Q-ToF) (and all ToF-like instruments) could be considered in terms of a large stop-watch. Ions or peptides enter into one end of the instrument and the time it takes to reach the detector is related to the mass. The advantages of the Q-ToF platform are fourfold. Firstly, apart from Fourier transform (FT) instruments, it possesses the greatest mass accuracy being competent to determine 2 ppm mass error in both MS and MS/MS-mode. Mass accuracy gives greater confidence in peptide or compound identification. While other bench-top instruments can match 2 ppm at the MS level, none (beside FT) can do this at the MS/MS level. Secondly, the Q-ToF is extremely sensitive at the MS level (i.e., will detect very low amounts of peptide). This is important when looking at low abundance proteins, or samples with a high dynamic range (Dynamic range is the term used to describe the difference between the most abundant protein in the sample and the least abundant protein. In blood, the concentration of the most abundant protein, albumin, is 10^{12} times higher than one of the lowest, interferon). Thirdly, the Q-ToF has great resolution; in proteomic terms, it can detect higher charged state peptides, (+4, +5, +6), which is often necessary to secure the molecular weight of the compound. Finally, the Q-ToF has an extremely good mass range. For this reason, the Q-ToF is heavily used for quantification of samples, especially with (i) tags, such as isotope-coded protein labeling (ICPL), (ii) isobaric tagging for relative and absolute quantification (iTRAQ), or (iii) enzyme-catalyzed reactions leading to $^{16}O/^{18}O$ exchange in terminal carboxylic groups conferred by trypsin or other proteases. The Q-ToF is also the instrument of choice for quantitation at the MS level (label-free MS-based and stable isotope labeling by amino acids in cell culture or SILAC). The disadvantage of the Q-ToF, in terms of proteomics research, is the amount of time it takes to perform the MS-scans events and the amount of peptide needed. Often referred to as the "duty cycle", in a typical run, MS/MS fragmentation can take up to 1–2 s, depending on the machine settings. Thus, although a higher confidence of peptide identification is found on the Q-ToF, fewer proteins are often identified (compared to say an ion-trap instrument), due to the slow duty cycle or relative amount of peptide present.

Ion-Trap Mass Spectrometer

This is often the instrument of choice for proteomics, without doubt the greatest asset being the extremely quick duty cycle (~0.3 s) and instrument sensitivity in MS/MS-mode. While the Q-ToF requires a certain amount of peptide to be present before daughter ions will be detected, ion-trap instruments can give fragment ions on parent peptides that cannot be detected from the background noise (referred to as orphan peptides) [4]. The sensitivity and speed of the ion-trap often outweighs the disadvantages associated with the machine, which are the mass range (low mass information is very limited), the mass accuracy (about 100 ppm in MS and MS/MS-mode, with the exception of the Orbitrap which can achieve around 2 ppm in MS-mode only), and resolution (can only detect up to 4+ charge, again with the exception of the Orbitrap which can easily rival a Q-ToF instrument in MS-mode for resolution). As such, ion-traps are effective at generating protein inventories and are extremely sensitive, but cannot but used for quantification when using tag or isobaric-related approaches.

MALDI-ToF-ToF Mass Spectrometer

In terms of mass measurements, the MALDI-ToF-ToF sits in between a Q-ToF and an Ion-Trap. The latest MALDI-ToF-ToF machines match the specifications of a Q-ToF in MS-mode, but an ion-trap in MS/MS-mode. The MALDI is unique among mass spectrometers, in that the sample is spotted onto a target plate and a laser is used to "plume" the peptides into the machine (instead of being sprayed). It should be appreciated that this machine will often detect different peptides in the same sample compared to Q-ToF or Ion-trap instruments, and as such, will generate complementary proteomic data [5, 6]. The MALDI can be used for quantification, but only with isobarically labeled peptides. A major advantage of the MALDI-ToF-ToF is that samples can be re-analyzed time and time again.

Triple Quadrupole Mass Spectrometer

This is the most sensitive mass spectrometer, due to the ability of the first quadrupole to isolate a selected mass and decrease the "noise" that would be seen in other mass spectrometers. For typical applications, however, a researcher must know the identity of the peptide they are looking for, before a triple-quadrupole mass spectrometer can be used. Thus, although biomarker discovery can be performed on any machine, the triple quadrupole is the only instrument currently approved for validation. The triple quadrupole is also unique in that it can detect a mass-offset in real time (other machines do this post-hoc). Hence, if researchers are looking for phosphorylation or glycosylation changes, a neutral-loss scanning event (loss of the phosphate or sugar group) can best be analyzed on a triple quadrupole-MS. However, the duty cycle of the triple quadrupole is extremely slow and it is therefore not used for the creation of lists of proteins.

Induction-Coupled Plasma Mass Spectrometer

In the context of proteomic research, the induction-coupled plasma mass spectrometer (ICP) is primarily used for metal species characterization, although technically such instruments can detect any cation. These machines can be made extremely sensitive (1 part per trillion) and they have excellent low mass sensitivity and accuracy. As an example relevant to biological systems, zinc and iron containing proteins can be identified, however not directly with the ICP. A combination of fractionation, SDS-PAGE and ICP, must be used in order to correlate the metal-containing fractions with the protein of interest.

Gas Chromatography

Gas chromatography (GC) is often used to look into biological samples for compounds with a very low mass range, typically metabolites. The sensitivity of GC-MS is always increasing, and such machines are excellent tools for another 'omics' technology, namely metabolomics. The disadvantage of GC-MS is that samples must be derivatized (so there is sample handling error) and only samples that can be vaporized in an oven will be detected. Finally, identification of the compound using a GC is based upon a known "pattern" or fragmentation profile of a standard. If a standard has never been run, identification is made extremely difficult.

Quantification on a Mass Spectrometer, MS or MS/MS

One often misunderstood aspect of mass spectrometry is in the area of quantification. Many researches are interested in comparing their pathological and normal samples in order to find consistent differences. Although this has been done on a large scale using mRNA, proteomic comparisons are only just beginning to be undertaken. Depending on the procedure being used, peptides can be compared either at the MS (intact, full-length peptides) or the MS/MS levels (daughter ions).

MS Quantification

MS-based quantification includes label-free (MS-based) analysis, SILAC, $^{16}O/^{18}O$ exchange, and the recently established OxICAT protocol. Essentially, the intensity of one full-length peptide is compared to another, either within the same run (SILAC, $^{16}O/^{18}O$ and OxICAT) or between runs (label free). An example of an MS-based quantification is given in Fig. 1. Herein, peptides from a WT and knockout mouse have been digested and run through nano-flow LC with direct injection into a mass spectrometer. The black "streaks" are actually a visual representation of the peptides achieved by plotting their mass:charge ratio (*m/z*; *y*-axis) against the time they elute (*x*-axis). The intensity of the

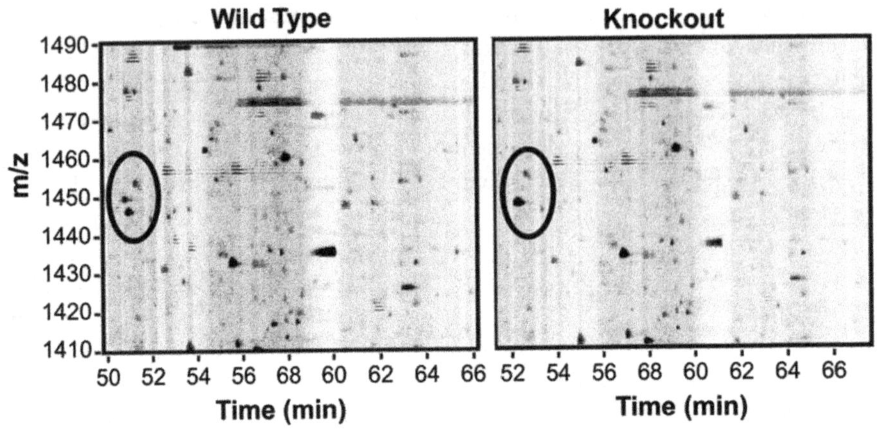

Fig. 18.1 Survey scan generated in silico by plotting the mass-to-charge ratio of each peptide against its elution profile on an MDLC system. Each spot is a peptide and the striated pattern reflects the presence of numerous peptide isoforms varying according to the number of atoms of carbon-13 each contains. Adjacent isoforms therefore have a mass difference of I neutron. *Left hand panel* demonstrates peptides derived from wild type spermatozoa; *right hand side* illustrates the same region of the survey scan for a knock-out mouse. Note missing peptide in the latter (*circled*)

streak is an indication of the abundance of the peptide. In the example shown (Fig. 1), three peptides are present in the left hand side (black circle) from a WT mouse, however one peptide is clearly missing in the knockout mouse, depicted on the right hand side. When biological replicates are performed, statistical information can be obtained on not just one, but all of the peptides detected in the survey scan. A final run is then required in which only those peptides that change are "targeted" for MS/MS analysis in order to obtain sequence (amino acid) information.

MS/MS Quantification

It comes in many forms, including, but not limited to, iCAT, ITRAQ, and ICPL, but always operates on the basic principle that one sample of peptide is labeled with a "light" isotope of some form, while the second sample is labeled with a "heavy" isotope. As an example, iTRAQ reagents have a reactive ester moiety, a "balance" group, and an isobaric tag. Although up to eight different isobaric "tags" can be purchased, every one of the tags has an overall mass of 305 Da. This is achieved through the balance group, which compensates for the increased masses of the radiolabelled tags. Importantly, however, the chemical-isotope should not affect the elution pattern observed following LC-chromatography [7]. Samples are labeled (typically using an ester or iodoacetamide reactive group) then mixed together and analyzed by LC-MS. As peptides elute they are either ionized (Q-ToF) or spotted (MALDI) for mass spectrometry analysis. Isobaric labels are quantified during MS/MS analysis. In the collision cell, the peptide plus the tag undergoes fragmentation, which, apart from breaking up the peptide itself, causes the "isobaric" part of the tag to fragment. Although all the tags are equal in total mass, the isobaric part has differential mass. This is therefore used as the "reported ion". In the case of iTRAQ, increases in 1 Da increments (from 113 to 119 Da, and 121 Da) have been made. These individual masses and their intensities in the MS/MS scan are then compared directly with each other and, in the process, the samples are quantified.

Proteomics Strategies Used in Reproductive Biology

Early investigations into sperm proteomics actually began with studies that documented the major proteins phosphorylated within spermatozoa using phospho-specific antibodies [8]. Such characterizations included the size and isoelectric point of the proteins seen in 2D-gels. The studies performed at that time recognized that certain proteins such as axokinin needed to be phosphorylated in order for the flagella to begin beating [9]. Other identified proteins soon began to surface, including 21S-dynein, which was shown to be present in the sperm tail [10] and the heat shock protein 70 family members [11]. This was not surprising given the relative abundance of both of these proteins. What is not appreciated today is that even as late as 2002, characterization of proteins within 2D gels was still on the basis of the protein size and isoelectric point [12] rather than a mass spec-related identification. The first truly "global" attempt to identify sperm proteins was achieved when 1,000 protein spots were shown to be present in ejaculated human spermatozoa. Of these, 98 unique proteins were identified by MALDI-ToF-MS [13, 14]. Despite these advances, proteomic mapping and protein identification using 2D gels is hindered by the presence of super-abundant proteins that dominate the composition of spermatozoa. In this context, subcellular fractionation can help focus the protein analysis, as when 50 proteins were identified in isolated mouse sperm flagella using 2D PAGE, including glycolytic enzymes that were abundant along the sperm tail [15] and evidently play a major role in the generation of ATP to support flagellar movement [16]. In addition to flagellar proteomics, 2D and 1D gels followed by LC-MS/MS have been performed on purified human sperm nuclei [17]. This approach was indeed worthwhile and informative, since 52.6 % of the 404 proteins had not been previously identified in any large scale sperm proteomic analysis [2, 18, 19], demonstrating the power of this approach. Interestingly, while histone isoforms dominated the makeup of the sperm nucleus, ribosomal proteins composed the second largest family of enzymes present in this organelle [17]. We have argued elsewhere that spermatozoa do not undergo nuclear protein synthesis although they will produce proteins in their mitochondria [20]; so it is uncertain as to why sperm cells maintain nuclear ribosomal proteins. Furthermore, ribosomal proteins are generally localized to the cytoplasm. However, immunofluorescence studies have confirmed the presence of these proteins in the sperm nucleus [17], suggesting that either ribosomal proteins from spermatozoa contribute to embryonic development, or they are simply vestiges of the spermatogenic process [17].

2D Comparative Proteomics: Epididymal Maturation

The third type of 2D-gel approach, and arguably the one that produces the greatest insight into sperm function, is to quantify protein changes occurring within these transcriptionally silent cells as they change their physiological status; for example, as they engage the process of epididymal maturation. The first attempt of this kind that included mass spectrometry identification was based on 2D-DIGE (Difference in Gel Electrophoresis) and revealed several protein changes [3]. This study implied that the metabolic profile of the spermatozoa was altering during epididymal maturation with changes to enolase, F1 ATPase, and lactate dehydrogenase. These results were consistent with existing evidence suggesting metabolic down-regulation during epididymal maturation [21–25]. However, given that only a MALDI-ToF instrument was used for identification purposes in this study, many other proteins were not identified. A follow-up analysis, again using DIGE technology, identified 388 statistically significant changes when comparing the caput and cauda-derived spermatozoa. Of these, 26 spots were excised and sent for MALDI-ToF-ToF sequencing, which identified 23 proteins. Several heat shock family members (HSP 2,5,9), actins, equatorial segment protein, A-kinase anchoring proteins (AKAP), and metabolic enzymes (aldolase, ATPase, NADH-dehydrogenase) were found to have changed their relative abundance during epididymal maturation [26]. This study supports the notion that epididymal transit appears to involve a change in the metabolic status of spermatozoa. Many of the proteins identified, including HSP, actin, and equatorial segment protein, are involved in a secondary sperm maturation process known as capacitation that prepares the sperm for fertilization. Thus, epididymal transit may regulate sperm metabolism, switching off certain pathways in preparation for storage in the cauda, while simultaneously preparing these cells for capacitation. Indeed, in a final study that quantified differences in protein expression from the caput, corpus, and cauda rat epididymis using 2D gels, 28 protein differences were noted [27]. Clustering of the proteins demonstrated enzymes involved in primary metabolism, amino acid metabolism and the antioxidant system, among others [27]. These findings are consistent with the notion that capacitation is a metabolically active, redox sensitive process that involves the reversal of some of changes induced during epididymal maturation [28].

2D Comparative Proteomics: Fertile Versus Infertile Men

Many infertile men are healthy in every other respect and as such could be used as models for the development of male contraceptives if we understood the etiology of their phenotype. By taking 47 sperm samples from infertile patients and comparing these with 10 normozoospermic donors, 67 spots were found to either increase or decrease in intensity, often in a synchronized manner [29]. For example, outer dense fiber 2 (ODF) and cyclin-dependent kinase 5 (Cdk5) consistently went up or down in the infertile samples ($r=0.652$). Interestingly, ODF appears to be a target for Cdk5 [30]. Furthermore, HSPA2 expression was correlated with DNA damage (as measured by TUNEL) and prolactin-induced protein [29]. Notwithstanding certain criticisms of this study [31], the implications are interesting. It is possible that many infertile males have a "common" cause. Such would be the case if, for example, the proteasome is deregulated. Not only would this lead to fundamental physiological outcomes, but a seemingly consistent pattern of change in the proteomic composition of spermatozoa in the infertile population. The latest study looking at the semen profile of fertile and infertile men found semenogelin II precursor and clusterin isoform 1 were not present in the infertile men. However, given the limited number of biological replicates used ($n=1$ fertile, $n=3$ infertile), such protein differences would need to be validated in independent data sets [32].

It is beyond the scope of this article to include all of the research employing 2D proteomics addressing reproductive issues, however others have used a 2D-PAGE approach to look for primary binding proteins to the bull zona pellucida, [33], proteins involved in the regulation of sperm motility [34], and the protein composition of sperm chromatin [35].

Use of LC-MS/MS to Study Mammalian Spermatozoa

Compared to 2D technology, greater and, at times, complementary coverage of the sperm proteome was achieved when newer technologies, including 2D-liquid chromatography directly coupled to an ion-trap mass spectrometer, were employed [19]. The first published study of this kind occurred when pooled human sperm ejaculates were purified using Percoll gradients, then subjected to 1 % triton X-100 solubilization [19], SDS-PAGE, and LC-MS/MS analysis. Over 1,000 proteins were documented, which is an accomplishment now repeated for spermatozoa from the mouse [36], rat [2], bull [37], and fruit fly [38]. We have performed an analysis of the "common" proteins present within these species (common being found in at least two species) [31] and could show that no less than 18 different kinases were found in most, if not all of the proteomes.

One remarkable facet was the identification of different isoforms of Protein kinase A (PKA) present within sperm cells. PKA has been reported to play a role in many aspects of sperm function [39–45]. Several PKA knockout mice have been produced, with intriguing results. The enzyme itself is a tetramer, consisting of both regulatory and catalytic subunits. Targeted deletion of the sperm regulatory subunit IIα (rIIα) delocalized PKA in mouse spermatozoa, but did not affect motility or fertility [46, 47]. However, haplo-insufficiency of PKArIα gave rise to fertility defects in male mice and men [48], suggesting that the latter is important and can act in a redundant role if PKArIIα is missing [41]. Genetic approaches to abolish the

PKAcα gene (and thereby remove both the PKAcα1 and PKAcαII catalytic subunits) led to reduced sperm cell motility and consequent infertility [39]. To clarify individual roles, specific deletion of PKAcαII isoform produced spermatozoa that could not undergo either hyperactivation or the normal pattern of protein tyrosine phosphorylation seen during capacitation [49]. Despite these advances, proteomic studies suggest more work needs to be done on PKA isoforms in spermatozoa. For example, a non-redundant peptide hit (i.e., a peptide that only matches to one isoform) was found for the catalytic subunit of PKAβ in spermatozoa [50], suggesting that this isoform may also play a key role in sperm metabolism. Given the evident importance of kinases such as PKA in the regulation of sperm function, several reports have focused on describing the phosphorylation changes that occur during epididymal transit and capacitation.

Epididymal Transit

By exploiting the ability of titanium dioxide to bind negatively charged compounds, we have examined 1 % triton X-100 soluble sperm proteins that were enriched for their phosphopeptide content. In total, 77 peptide changes were found as spermatozoa traversed the rat epididymis [51]. Of these, eight peptides presented with an absolute change (i.e. the entire protein was lost), which included some abundant proteins like testis lipid binding proteins, heat shock protein 90-α ornithine decarboxylase antizyme 3 (OAZ3), and retinol dehydrogenase. Many of these changes were ratified through orthogonal approaches, including Western blot analysis. From this analysis, it appears that polyamine regulation undergoes substantial changes during epididymal transit since we found that total loss of OAZ3 during epididymal maturation coincided with the observation that caudal epididymal sperm cells possess no OAZ3 activity [52]. OAZ3 is an inhibitor of ornithine decarboxylase (ODC); however, the precise role of ODC and, by extension, polyamines in sperm maturation is not clear. Why is this inhibitor no longer needed in the caudal epididymal cells? Clearly our understanding of polyamines is still in its infancy, since only recently was it reported that OAZ3 may also be regulated (inhibited) by another enzyme termed Antizyme Inhibitor 2 [53]. Interestingly, this enzyme has restricted tissue expression, being present only in the testis and the brain [54]. Furthermore, the highest expression of antizyme inhibitor 2 (which also functions to inhibit ODC) was found in haploid germ cells, the same as OAZ3. In light of the aforementioned data, it would be interesting to look at polyamine regulation in infertile males.

Capacitation

Capacitation begins upon ejaculation when spermatozoa enter the female reproductive tract. This transition results in an immediate influx of calcium and bicarbonate, which then stimulates soluble adenylyl cyclase (sAC) activity, leading to a rise in intracellular cAMP. This initial increase in cAMP appears to initiate forward progressive motility [55, 56] and allows the spermatozoa to ascend the female reproductive tract to the site of fertilization in the ampullae of the Fallopian tubes. During their ascent of the female tract, spermatozoa experience a second rise in cAMP levels, which, via PKA, generates a global increase in tyrosine phosphorylation [57]. In support of this general scheme, deletion of the sperm-specific PKACαII generates an infertility phenotype associated with clear disruption of the tyrosine phosphorylation cascade responsible for promoting sperm capacitation [49]. PKA, being a serine/threonine kinase, cannot, of its own accord, play a direct role in the stimulation of tyrosine phosphorylation. This pathway must therefore involve an intermediate kinase(s) that, once activated by PKA, orchestrates the complex array of tyrosine phosphorylations associated with the induction of sperm capacitation [58]. Interestingly, one such candidate is pp60c-src (c-Src), the activity of which is stimulated by PKA [59]. Downstream targets known to become tyrosine phosphorylated in the spermatozoa of various species include A-kinase anchoring proteins (AKAP) 3 and 4, axoneme-associated protein, calcium binding protein 56 [60], heat shock protein 90 [61], endoplasmin and heat shock protein 60 [62] sp32 [63], and glycerol-3-phosphate dehydrogenase. Nevertheless, it appears that the majority of tyrosine phosphorylated proteins have yet to be clearly identified.

Attempts to achieve this objective have focused on either phosphorylated proteins isolated using immobilized metal ion affinity chromatography [64] or, specifically, tyrosine phosphorylated proteins, excised from 2D gels [65]. In the case of the former, 55 unique in vivo phosphorylation sites were identified, corresponding to 42 different phosphopeptides. Many of the identified proteins have roles in capacitation, including AKAP4 and hexokinase. One interesting finding was the phosphorylation of dynein axonemal intermediate chain 1 [64]. Capacitated cells are often defined by their ability to undergo a change in their flagella beat frequency, in a process known as hyperactivation [66, 67]. However, the molecular mechanisms underpinning hyperactivation are yet to be established. Protein phosphorylation is clearly central to this process since, as previously mentioned, the PKAαII knockout mice cannot exhibit either tyrosine phosphorylation or hyperactivation [49]. It is tempting to speculate therefore that the dynein intermediate chain may be involved, at least in part, in the hyperactivation process.

Our own studies using titanium dioxide (as opposed to IMAC [(Immobilized Metal Ion Affinity Chromatography]) to isolate phosphopeptides have contributed to the literature on the role of protein phosphorylation in the regulation of sperm function. In one study [68] we found 15 differentially phosphorylated proteins during capacitation and, in the process, confirmed the same phosphorylated dynein intermediate chain serine residue that was found in the Platt et al. [64] study. In addition, we saw changes never previously reported, including phosphorylation of the sperm-egg fusion protein Izumo1 [69]. The *Izumo1* knockout mouse is infertile due to a failure of the spermatozoa to fuse with the egg [69]. Interestingly, although many of the pups die at birth, a small number of mice that lack testis-specific kinase 6 (*TSSK6)* do survive to reproductive age. The spermatozoa from these mice fail to re-localize Izumo1 to its site of action in the equatorial segment during the acrosome reaction and are therefore infertile [70]. These results raise the possibility that this kinase is involved in orchestrating the phosphorylation of Izumo1 during capacitation that control its subcellular relocation during acrosomal exocytosis [70]. Although still in their infancy, it is evident that proteomic studies are making significant contributions to our understanding of many fundamental aspects of sperm biology in addition to sperm-oocyte fusion. Recent examples of such studies include proteomic analyses of sperm–zona recognition and sperm capacitation [71–74].

Conclusions

Advances in mass spectrometry are revolutionizing biological sciences. It is our belief that over the next decade a systems-biology 'omics' revolution will come to dominate our thinking. As a result of this revolution we shall be able to provide detailed insights into the composition and structure of specified cells and biological fluids in different physiological and pathological states. This information will be invaluable in its own right as a source of biomarkers for diagnostic purposes and will, in addition, facilitate our understanding of some of the biochemical pathways associated with normal and abnormal cell function. In the microcosm of andrology, the application of 'omics' technologies will not only facilitate our understanding of how sperm biology is regulated, but also help us to resolve the defects that underpin male infertility and provide insights into possible approaches to male contraception. Never before have we had such sophistication at the call of researchers determined to resolve the molecular mechanisms regulating sperm function.

References

1. Pascal LE, True LD, Campbell DS, Deutsch EW, Risk M, Coleman IM, et al. Correlation of mRNA and protein levels: cell type-specific gene expression of cluster designation antigens in the prostate. BMC Genomics. 2008;9:246.

2. Baker MA, Hetherington L, Reeves G, Muller J, Aitken RJ. The rat sperm proteome characterized via IPG strip prefractionation and LC-MS/MS identification. Proteomics. 2008;8:2312–21.
3. Baker MA, Witherdin R, Hetherington L, Cunningham-Smith K, Aitken RJ. Identification of Post-translational modifications that occur during sperm maturation using Difference in 2D-Gel electrophoresis. Proteomics. 2005;5:1003–12.
4. Bitton DA, Smith DL, Connolly Y, Scutt PJ, Miller CJ. An integrated mass-spectrometry pipeline identifies novel protein coding-regions in the human genome. PLoS One. 2010;5:e8949.
5. Stapels MD, Barofsky DF. Complementary use of MALDI and ESI for the HPLC-MS/MS analysis of DNA-binding proteins. Anal Chem. 2004; 76:5423–30.
6. Stapels MD, Cho JC, Giovannoni SJ, Barofsky DF. Proteomic analysis of novel marine bacteria using MALDI and ESI mass spectrometry. J Biomol Tech. 2004;15:191–8.
7. Julka S, Regnier F. Quantification in proteomics through stable isotope coding: a review. J Proteome Res. 2004;3:350–63.
8. Chulavatnatol M, Panyim S, Wititsuwannakul D. Comparison of phosphorylated proteins in intact rat spermatozoa from caput and cauda epididymidis. Biol Reprod. 1982;26:197–207.
9. Tash JS, Kakar SS, Means AR. Flagellar motility requires the cAMP-dependent phosphorylation of a heat-stable NP-40-soluble 56 kd protein, axokinin. Cell. 1984;38:551–9.
10. Yano-Toyoshima Y. Two heavy chains of 21S dynein from sea urchin sperm flagella. J Biochem. 1985;98: 767–79.
11. Maekawa M, O'Brien DA, Allen RL, Eddy EM. Heat-shock cognate protein (hsc71) and related proteins in mouse spermatogenic cells. Biol Reprod. 1989;40: 843–52.
12. Verdier Y, Chaffaux S, Boue F. Identification of post-vasectomy sperm auto-antigens in fox (Vulpes vulpes) by two-dimensional gel electrophoresis and Western blotting. J Reprod Immunol. 2002;54:65–80.
13. Martinez-Heredia J, Estanyol JM, Ballesca JL, Oliva R. Proteomic identification of human sperm proteins. Proteomics. 2006;6:4356–69.
14. Oliva R, de Mateo S, Estanyol JM. Sperm cell proteomics. Proteomics. 2009;9:1004–17.
15. Cao W, Gerton GL, Moss SB. Proteomic profiling of accessory structures from the mouse sperm flagellum. Mol Cell Proteomics. 2006;5:801–10.
16. Miki K, Qu W, Goulding EH, Willis WD, Bunch DO, Strader LF, et al. Glyceraldehyde 3-phosphate dehydrogenase-S, a sperm-specific glycolytic enzyme, is required for sperm motility and male fertility. Proc Natl Acad Sci USA. 2004;101:16501–6.
17. de Mateo S, Castillo J, Estanyol JM, Ballesca JL, Oliva R. Proteomic characterization of the human sperm nucleus. Proteomics. 2011;11:2714–26.
18. Baker MA, Hetherington L, Reeves GM, Aitken RJ. The mouse sperm proteome characterized via IPG strip prefractionation and LC-MS/MS identification. Proteomics. 2008;8:1720–30.
19. Baker MA, Reeves G, Hetherington L, Muller J, Baur I, Aitken RJ. Identification of gene products present in Triton X-100 soluble and insoluble fractions of human spermatozoa lysates using LC-MS/MS analysis. Proteomics Clin Appl. 2007;1:524–32.
20. Baker MA. The 'omics revolution and our understanding of sperm cell biology. Asian J Androl. 2011;13:6–10.
21. Voglmayr JK, White IG. Effects of rete testis and epididymal fluid on the metabolism and motility of testicular and post-testicular spermatozoa of the ram. Biol Reprod. 1979;20:288–93.
22. Evans RW, Setchell BP. The effect of rete testis fluid on the metabolism of testicular spermatozoa. J Reprod Fertil. 1978;52:15–20.
23. Voglmayr JK, Murdoch RN, White IG. Metabolism of ram testicular spermatozoa in the presence of testosterone and related steroids. Acta Endocrinol (Copenh). 1970;65:565–76.
24. O'Shea T, Voglmayr JK. Metabolism of glucose, lactate, and acetate by testicular and ejaculated spermatozoa of the ram. Biol Reprod. 1970;2:326–32.
25. Voglmayr JK, Scott TW, Setchell BP, Waites GM. Metabolism of testicular spermatozoa and characteristics of testicular fluid collected from conscious rams. J Reprod Fertil. 1967;14:87–99.
26. Ijiri TW, Merdiushev T, Cao W, Gerton GL. Identification and validation of mouse sperm proteins correlated with epididymal maturation. Proteomics. 2011;11:4047–62.
27. Yuan H, Liu A, Zhang L, Zhou H, Wang Y, Zhang H, et al. Proteomic profiling of regionalized proteins in rat epididymis indicates consistency between specialized distribution and protein functions. J Proteome Res. 2006;5:299–307.
28. Cao W, Aghajanian HK, Haig-Ladewig LA, Gerton GL. Sorbitol can fuel mouse sperm motility and protein tyrosine phosphorylation via sorbitol dehydrogenase. Biol Reprod. 2009;80:124–33.
29. de Mateo S, Martinez-Heredia J, Estanyol JM, Dominguez-Fandos D, Vidal-Taboada JM, Ballesca JL, et al. Marked correlations in protein expression identified by proteomic analysis of human spermatozoa. Proteomics. 2007;7:4264–77.
30. Rosales JL, Lee BC, Modarressi M, Sarker KP, Lee KY, Jeong YG, et al. Outer dense fibers serve as a functional target for Cdk5.p35 in the developing sperm tail. J Biol Chem. 2004;279:1224–32.
31. Baker MA, Aitken RJ. Proteomic insights into spermatozoa: critiques, comments and concerns. Expert Rev Proteomics. 2009;6:691–705.
32. Thacker S, Yadav SP, Sharma RK, Kashou A, Willard B, Zhang D, et al. Evaluation of sperm proteins in infertile men: a proteomic approach. Fertil Steril. 2011;95:2745–8.

33. van Gestel RA, Brewis IA, Ashton PR, Brouwers JF, Gadella BM. Multiple proteins present in purified porcine sperm apical plasma membranes interact with the zona pellucida of the oocyte. Mol Hum Reprod. 2007;13:445–54.
34. Thepparat T, Katawatin S, Vongpralub T, Duangjinda M, Thammasirirak S, Utha A. Separation of bovine spermatozoa proteins using 2D-PAGE revealed the relationship between tektin-4 expression patterns and spermatozoa motility. Theriogenology. 2012;77(9): 1816–21.
35. Oliva R. Protamines and male infertility. Hum Reprod Update. 2006;12:417–35.
36. Baker MA, Reeves G, Hetherington L, Aitken RJ. The mouse sperm proteome characterised via IPG strip prefractionation and LC-MS/MS identification. Proteomics. 2008;8:1720–30.
37. Peddinti D, Nanduri B, Kaya A, Feugang JM, Burgess SC, Memili E. Comprehensive proteomic analysis of bovine spermatozoa of varying fertility rates and identification of biomarkers associated with fertility. BMC Syst Biol. 2008;2:19.
38. Dorus S, Busby SA, Gerike U, Shabanowitz J, Hunt DF, Karr TL. Genomic and functional evolution of the Drosophila melanogaster sperm proteome. Nat Genet. 2006;38:1440–5.
39. Skalhegg BS, Huang Y, Su T, Idzerda RL, McKnight GS, Burton KA. Mutation of the Calpha subunit of PKA leads to growth retardation and sperm dysfunction. Mol Endocrinol. 2002;16:630–9.
40. Schmitt JM, Stork PJ. PKA phosphorylation of Src mediates cAMP's inhibition of cell growth via Rap1. Mol Cell. 2002;9:85–94.
41. Amieux PS, McKnight GS. The essential role of RI alpha in the maintenance of regulated PKA activity. Ann N Y Acad Sci. 2002;968:75–95.
42. Baker MA, Aitken RJ. Identification of pp 60c-src as a key PKA-stimulated tyrosine kinase involved in the capacitation and hyperactivation of murine spermatozoa. J Cell Sci. 2006;119:3182–92.
43. Harrison RA. Rapid PKA-catalysed phosphorylation of boar sperm proteins induced by the capacitating agent bicarbonate. Mol Reprod Dev. 2004;67: 337–52.
44. Carr DW, Fujita A, Stentz CL, Liberty GA, Olson GE, Narumiya S. Identification of sperm-specific proteins that interact with A-kinase anchoring proteins in a manner similar to the type II regulatory subunit of PKA. J Biol Chem. 2001;276:17332–8.
45. Baker MA, Hetherington L, Curry B, Aitken RJ. Phosphorylation and consequent stimulation of the tyrosine kinase c-Abl by PKA in mouse spermatozoa; its implications during capacitation. Dev Biol. 2009;333:57–66.
46. Burton KA, Treash-Osio B, Muller CH, Dunphy EL, McKnight GS. Deletion of type IIalpha regulatory subunit delocalizes protein kinase A in mouse sperm without affecting motility or fertilization. J Biol Chem. 1999;274:24131–6.
47. Burton KA, McKnight GS. PKA, germ cells, and fertility. Physiology (Bethesda). 2007;22:40–6.
48. Burton KA, McDermott DA, Wilkes D, Poulsen MN, Nolan MA, Goldstein M, et al. Haploinsufficiency at the protein kinase A RI alpha gene locus leads to fertility defects in male mice and men. Mol Endocrinol. 2006;20:2504–13.
49. Nolan MA, Babcock DF, Wennemuth G, Brown W, Burton KA, McKnight GS. Sperm-specific protein kinase A catalytic subunit C{alpha}2 orchestrates cAMP signaling for male fertility. Proc Natl Acad Sci USA. 2004;101:13483–8.
50. Baker MA, Hetherington L, Reeves G, Müller J, Aitken RJ. The rat sperm proteome characterised via IPG strip pre-fractionation and LC-MS/MS identification. Proteomics. 2008;8:2312–21.
51. Baker MA, Smith ND, Hetherington L, Pelzing M, Condina MR, Aitken RJ. Use of titanium dioxide to find phosphopeptide and total protein changes during epididymal sperm maturation. J Proteome Res. 2010;10:1004–7.
52. Qian ZU, Tsai YH, Steinberger A, Lu M, Greenfield AR, Haddox MK. Localization of ornithine decarboxylase in rat testicular cells and epididymal spermatozoa. Biol Reprod. 1985;33:1189–95.
53. Lopez-Contreras AJ, Lopez-Garcia C, Jimenez-Cervantes C, Cremades A, Penafiel R. Mouse ornithine decarboxylase-like gene encodes an antizyme inhibitor devoid of ornithine and arginine decarboxylating activity. J Biol Chem. 2006;281:30896–906.
54. Tosaka Y, Tanaka H, Yano Y, Masai K, Nozaki M, Yomogida K, et al. Identification and characterization of testis specific ornithine decarboxylase antizyme (OAZ-t) gene: expression in haploid germ cells and polyamine-induced frameshifting. Genes Cells. 2000;5:265–76.
55. Esposito G, Jaiswal BS, Xie F, Krajnc-Franken MA, Robben TJ, Strik AM, et al. Mice deficient for soluble adenylyl cyclase are infertile because of a severe sperm-motility defect. Proc Natl Acad Sci USA. 2004;101:2993–8.
56. Xie F, Garcia MA, Carlson AE, Schuh SM, Babcock DF, Jaiswal BS, et al. Soluble adenylyl cyclase (sAC) is indispensable for sperm function and fertilization. Dev Biol. 2006;296:353–62.
57. Visconti PE, Bailey JL, Moore GD, Pan D, Olds-Clarke P, Kopf GS. Capacitation of mouse spermatozoa. I. Correlation between the capacitation state and protein tyrosine phosphorylation. Development. 1995;121:1129–37.
58. Arcelay E, Salicioni AM, Wertheimer E, Visconti PE. Identification of proteins undergoing tyrosine phosphorylation during mouse sperm capacitation. Int J Dev Biol. 2008;52:463–72.
59. Baker MA, Hetherington L, Aitken RJ. Identification of pp 60c-src as a key PKA-stimulated tyrosine kinase involved in the capacitation and hyperactivation of murine spermatozoa. J Cell Sci. 2006;119:3182–92.
60. Ficarro S, Chertihin O, Westbrook VA, White F, Jayes F, Kalab P, et al. Phosphoproteome analysis of capacitated human sperm. Evidence of tyrosine phosphorylation of a kinase-anchoring protein 3 and

valosin-containing protein/p97 during capacitation. J Biol Chem. 2003;278:11579–89.
61. Ecroyd H, Jones RC, Aitken RJ. Tyrosine phosphorylation of HSP-90 during mammalian sperm capacitation. Biol Reprod. 2003;69:1801–7.
62. Asquith KL, Baleato RM, McLaughlin EA, Nixon B, Aitken RJ. Tyrosine phosphorylation activates surface chaperones facilitating sperm-zona recognition. J Cell Sci. 2004;117:3645–57.
63. Dube C, Leclerc P, Baba T, Reyes-Moreno C, Bailey JL. The proacrosin binding protein, sp32, is tyrosine phosphorylated during capacitation of pig sperm. J Androl. 2005;26:519–28.
64. Platt MD, Salicioni AM, Hunt DF, Visconti PE. Use of differential isotopic labeling and mass spectrometry to analyze capacitation-associated changes in the phosphorylation status of mouse sperm proteins. J Proteome Res. 2009;8:1431–40.
65. Kota V, Dhople VM, Shivaji S. Tyrosine phosphoproteome of hamster spermatozoa: role of glycerol-3-phosphate dehydrogenase 2 in sperm capacitation. Proteomics. 2009;9:1809–26.
66. Baker MA, Lewis B, Hetherington L, Aitken RJ. Development of the signalling pathways associated with sperm capacitation during epididymal maturation. Mol Reprod Dev. 2003;64:446–57.
67. Yanagimachi R. Mammalina fertilization. In: Knobil E, Neil JD, editors. The physiology of reproduction. 2nd ed. New York: Raven Press, Ltd.; 1994. p. 189–317.
68. Baker MA, Smith ND, Hetherington L, Taubman K, Graham ME, Robinson PJ, et al. Label-free quantitation of phosphopeptide changes during rat sperm capacitation. J Proteome Res. 2010;9:718–29.
69. Inoue N, Ikawa M, Isotani A, Okabe M. The immunoglobulin superfamily protein Izumo is required for sperm to fuse with eggs. Nature. 2005;434:234–8.
70. Sosnik J, Miranda PV, Spiridonov NA, Yoon SY, Fissore RA, Johnson GR, et al. Tssk6 is required for Izumo relocalization and gamete fusion in the mouse. J Cell Sci. 2009;122:2741–9.
71. Baker MA, Reeves G, Hetherington L, Aitken RJ. Analysis of proteomic changes associated with sperm capacitation through the combined use of IPG-strip pre-fractionation followed by RP chromatography LC-MS/MS analysis. Proteomics. 2009;10:482–95.
72. Dun MD, Smith ND, Baker MA, Lin M, Aitken RJ, Nixon B. The chaperonin containing TCP1 complex (CCT/TRiC) is involved in mediating sperm-oocyte interaction. J Biol Chem. 2011;286:36875–87.
73. Krapf D, Arcelay E, Wertheimer EV, Sanjay A, Pilder SH, Salicioni AM, et al. Inhibition of Ser/Thr phosphatases induces capacitation-associated signaling in the presence of Src kinase inhibitors. J Biol Chem. 2010;285:7977–85.
74. Visconti PE, Florman HM. Mechanisms of sperm-egg interactions: between sugars and broken bonds. Sci Signal. 2010;3:pe35.

19 Proteomic Analysis of Embryo Viability

Mandy G. Katz-Jaffe and Susanna McReynolds

The selection of the most competent embryo(s) for transfer is a crucial component of assisted reproductive technologies (ART). Currently, detailed morphological assessment is used to predict the embryos with the highest implantation potential [1, 2]. Though this method is relatively successful in improving pregnancy rates and reducing multiple gestations, morphology has limitations, with more than 70 % of in vitro fertilization (IVF) embryos failing to implant. This failure is likely due to both our inability to select the most competent embryo(s) present as well as the absence of developmentally competent embryos in an IVF cohort. Hence, the field of human ART would benefit from more accurate and quantitative methods of embryo viability determination. The ability to select the most viable embryo in a cohort could allow for routine single embryo transfer, while maintaining or improving pregnancy rates [3].

The recent developments in omics technologies (genomics, transcriptomics, proteomics, and metabolomics), including improvements in platform sensitivity, has enabled us to investigate new approaches other then morphology to improve embryo viability selection. Assessment of the embryonic proteome can provide a snapshot of cellular physiology and function. In addition, analysis of the embryonic secretome (proteins that are produced and secreted by the developing embryo) would represent a noninvasive approach to embryo assessment [4]. Defining and characterizing the embryonic secretome will also expand our knowledge of early embryogenesis and advance our understanding of the embryonic role during implantation.

M.G. Katz-Jaffe (✉) • S. McReynolds
National Foundation for Fertility Research,
Lone Tree, CO, USA
e-mail: mkatz-jaffe@fertilityresearch.org

Proteomic Analysis of Embryo Viability in ART

The human proteome is complex and dynamic, with over one million proteins constantly changing through both internal and external interactions and stimuli. The proteome represents all the proteins translated from a cell's gene expression products that are responsible for cellular function. Studies investigating gene expression do not always predict protein presence or abundance due to mechanisms that degrade mRNA transcripts prior to translation. Consequently, in order to fully understand cellular function and comprehend biological processes an investigation of the proteome is vital. Knowledge of the human embryonic proteome is very limited even despite recent advances in proteomic technologies. The main hurdles include limited template, low protein concentration, deficient platform sensitivity, and limited protein database information. Of particular interest to researchers trying to identify proteins involved in specific disease states is the secretome, defined as those proteins produced by cells and secreted at any given time [5, 6].

D.K. Gardner et al. (eds.), *Human Gametes and Preimplantation Embryos: Assessment and Diagnosis*,
DOI 10.1007/978-1-4614-6651-2_19, © Springer Science+Business Media New York 2013

In ART, the secretome includes those proteins that are produced by embryos and secreted into the surrounding culture medium. Proteomic assessment of secreted embryonic proteins would represent a noninvasive method of embryo selection. Identifying noninvasive biomarkers that reflect developmental competence and embryo viability may improve ART outcome [7]. To date, this has proven to be a challenging task, but holds promise with recent developments of increased sensitivity for both targeted and proteomic profiling approaches.

Targeted Single Protein and Molecular Analysis

Early studies of the human embryonic secretome involved targeted analysis of individual proteins or molecules. The soluble factor, 1-o-alkyl-2-acetyl-sn-glycero-3-phosphocholine (PAF), was one of the first molecules to be identified in the human embryonic secretome [8]. PAF is produced and secreted by mammalian embryos during preimplantation development and has been shown to act as a survival factor in an autocrine fashion. The release of PAF also influences a range of maternal physiology alterations including platelet activation and maternal immune function [8].

While studying the interaction between the embryo and endometrial epithelial cells (EEC), Leptin, a 16 kDa small pleotrophic peptide was observed in blastocyst-conditioned medium [9]. Competent human blastocysts were shown to secrete higher leptin concentrations into the surrounding medium than arrested embryos. Leptin has been hypothesized to initiate and establish a molecular dialogue with leptin receptors in the maternal endometrium during the window of implantation [10]. Another reciprocal embryo–endometrial interaction that could transform the local uterine environment, impacting both embryo development and the implantation process, is HOXA10. HOXA10 is expressed by epithelial endometrial cells and its regulation is modulated by an unknown soluble molecule secreted by human blastocysts [11].

Human leukocyte antigen G (HLA-G) has been hypothesized to play a role at the maternal embryonic interface during implantation. HLA-G is produced by human oocytes and embryos at both the mRNA and protein level and has also been detected in embryo spent culture media [12–14]. The presence of soluble HLA-G (sHLA-G) in embryo spent culture media has been reported in several publications to be associated with successful pregnancy outcome. It has been suggested that in conjunction with current morphological embryo assessment, sHLA-G represents a noninvasive marker for prediction of embryo quality and implantation success [15]. These results however have not been absolute with pregnancies established from sHLA-G negative embryos and studies revealing undetectable levels of sHLA-G in embryo spent culture media [15–17].

In a multicenter study, a wide range of sHLA-G concentrations were observed in embryo spent culture media across different ART clinics. Indeed, a significant association between sHLA-G-positive embryo spent culture media and successful implantation was only established in one of the three clinics involved in the study [18]. Another recent study was unable to detect any association between sHLA-G expression and implantation rates, but concluded that miscarriage rates were significantly lower when embryos were selected based on a graduated embryo morphology score and sHLA-G levels vs. the morphology score alone [19]. However, no correlation was observed between the concentration of sHLA-G in embryo spent culture media and either embryo morphology [20], or chromosome aneuploidy by FISH for up to 11 chromosomes (8, 9, 13, 15, 16, 17, 18, 21, 22, X, and Y) [21].

There are numerous factors that could influence the presence of sHLA-G in embryo spent culture media including the culture system itself, the extent of cumulus removal, single vs. group embryo culture, media composition, microdrop volume, and the day of media collection [15, 16]. Another explanation for the lack of reproducibility and association observed to date could be the lack of sensitivity of the current sandwich ELISA assays used for most sHLA-G analysis. It would appear that a more sensitive (picogram level) and reproducible quantitative method for analysis is required in order to determine the significance of sHLA-G in relation to embryo development and implantation outcome [16].

Protein Profiling of the Embryonic Secretome

The targeted secretome studies described above have been focused on only a single protein or molecule; however, it would be reasonable to assume that more than one factor would be required to predict developmental competence and/or implantation potential considering the multifactorial nature of embryonic development. With the recent advances in proteomic technologies including increased sensitivity, it has become possible for more extended investigations of the proteins and molecules produced and secreted by the human embryos.

Mass Spectrometry (MS) has rapidly become an important technology in proteomics research. Searching for reliable and reproducible changes in protein expression have revealed underlying molecular mechanisms of physiological processes and disease states [22]. MS incorporates an ion source for production of a charged species in the gas phase, coupled to an analyzer, which can separate ions by their mass-to-charge (*m/z*) ratio. A variety of ionization methods exist including electrospray ionization (ESI), matrix-attenuated laser desorption/ionization (MALDI) and surface-enhanced laser desorption/ionization (SELDI). Common analyzers include time-of-flight (TOF) and ion trap analyzers, which can occur in tandem for peptide sequencing. Strict quality control is a crucial prerequisite for reliable and reproducible proteomic data including, running samples in replicates, routinely performing internal and external calibrations and including suitable control samples with every run [23]. Additionally, tight protocols need to be followed for sample collection, storage and handling, due to the dynamic and sensitive nature of the human proteome.

SELDI-TOF MS, with specific surface affinity protein chips, was developed for fast, cost-effective, high-throughput application of small sample volumes (μL range) and enabled sensitivity to be in the picomole to femtomole range, crucial for use in oncoproteomics when there is limited biological material [24]. Using SELDI, Katz-Jaffe et al. [25] were the first to successfully analyze the protein profile of individual human embryos. The authors observed distinctive protein secretome signatures every 24 h during preimplantation development, from the time of fertilization to the blastocyst stage. Maternal proteins were observed during the first 24 h of development and unique embryonic proteins were observed in the human embryonic secretome after the activation of the embryonic genome post day 3. A clear association was observed between protein expression profiles and morphology, with degenerating embryos exhibiting significant up-regulation of several potential biomarkers that might be involved in apoptotic and growth-inhibiting pathways.

In addition, an 8.5 kDa protein was observed to be increased in expression in the secretome of developing blastocysts when compared to the secretome of degenerating embryos, potentially indicating an association between this protein and developmental competence. Protein identification using tandem MS and peptide sequencing indicated that the best candidate for this 8.5 kDa protein was ubiquitin, a component of the ubiquitin-dependent proteosome system that is involved in a number of physiological processes including proliferation and apoptosis. Recently, secreted ubiquitin has been shown to be up-regulated in body fluids in certain disease states and this accumulation provides evidence for an increased protein turnover [26, 27]. Ubiquitin has also been implicated to play a crucial role during mammalian implantation by controlling the activities and turnover of key signaling molecules [28].

Protein microarrays have also been investigated in the characterization of the embryonic secretome. In a retrospective study by Dominguez et al. in 2008, protein microarrays that contained 120 targets were used to compare pooled conditioned media from implanted versus non-implanted blastocyst following single embryo transfer [29]. An increased expression of the soluble TNF receptor 1 and IL-10, and the decreased expression of MSP-alpha, SCF, CXCL13, TRAILR3, and MIP-1beta were observed in the embryo-conditioned media compared to control media [29]. Upon comparison of conditioned media of implanted blastocysts compared to non-implanted blastocysts, no proteins were significantly increased and two proteins were significantly decreased, CXCL13 and GM-CSF. The authors hypothesized that the decrease in CXCL13 and GM-CSF indicated consumption of these proteins by the human blastocyst. Indeed, GM-CSF has been shown to promote embryo development and implantation when present in both human and murine blastocyst culture media [30].

A follow-up study by the same group comparing protein secretome profiles between the EEC co-culture system and sequential microdrop culture media also revealed differential protein secretome profiles [31]. Several molecules were increased in the EEC co-culture profile including Interleukin-6 (IL-6), PLGF, and BCL (CXCL13), while other proteins were decreased such as FGF-4, IL-12p40, VEGF, and uPAR. IL-6 displayed the highest protein concentration in the EEC co-culture system, and upon assessment of the sequential culture media secretome using an IL-6 ELISA assay, viable blastocysts displayed an increased uptake of IL-6 compared to blastocysts that failed to result in a pregnancy, thereby suggesting a potential role for IL-6 in blastocyst development and implantation [31].

Two-dimensional (2D) gel electrophoresis and tandem MS have also been utilized to identify proteins in spent culture media from human preimplantation embryos. Using 2D-gel electrophoreses in combination with ELISA analysis of spent culture media, Apolipoprotein A1 (ApoA1) was identified in the embryonic secretome with increased levels associated with blastocysts of higher morphological grade [32]. The presence of ApoA1 mRNA was also confirmed to be expressed in blastocysts but not early cleavage stage embryos suggesting that ApoA1 is a part of the embryonic transcriptome and secretome [32]. However, in relation to IVF outcome, no association was observed with ApoA1 levels in the embryonic secretome.

Chromosome aneuploidies, defined as the gain or loss of an entire chromosome, is responsible for up to 70 % of spontaneous miscarriage in human reproduction. Current methods used to screen for chromosome aneuploidy in embryos involve biopsy procedures which are invasive and could compromise subsequent development. A noninvasive method for aneuploidy screening would be a significant addition to embryo selection methods. Using SELDI-TOF MS, protein profiles of embryo spent culture media from individual blastocysts relative to their chromosomal constitution were investigated [4]. Discrimination between euploid (correct number of chromosomes) and aneuploid chromosomal constitutions was observed in the secretome of individual blastocysts [4]. A novel set of nine differentially expressed biomarkers classified a euploid blastocyst from an aneuploid blastocyst with statistical significance and reproducibility.

Further investigation of the blastocyst protein secretome in relation to chromosome aneuploidy was performed using an LC-MS/MS platform. The protein profile of a euploid blastocyst secretome was again notably different from the protein profile of the aneuploidy blastocyst secretome. Nine novel candidate biomarkers characteristically classified chromosome aneuploidy in a cohort of transferable-quality blastocysts. Lipocalin-1 was identified as the first potential biomarker for noninvasive aneuploidy screening [33]. The increased expression of Lipocalin-1 was confirmed using an ELISA assay that examined both pooled and individual embryo spent culture media. Lipocalin-1 has a large variety of ligands and is overproduced under conditions of stress, infection, and inflammation. The increased secretion of Lipocalin-1 from an aneuploid blastocyst could represent an overall compromised state of the embryo itself that reflects the aneuploid chromosome complement.

Ongoing research by this group is focused on further validation of identified biomarkers to reliably discriminate between euploid and aneuploid blastocysts including a blinded prospective study (Fig. 1). The ability to noninvasively assay for embryonic developmental competence that includes euploidy would represent a powerful selection tool in ART.

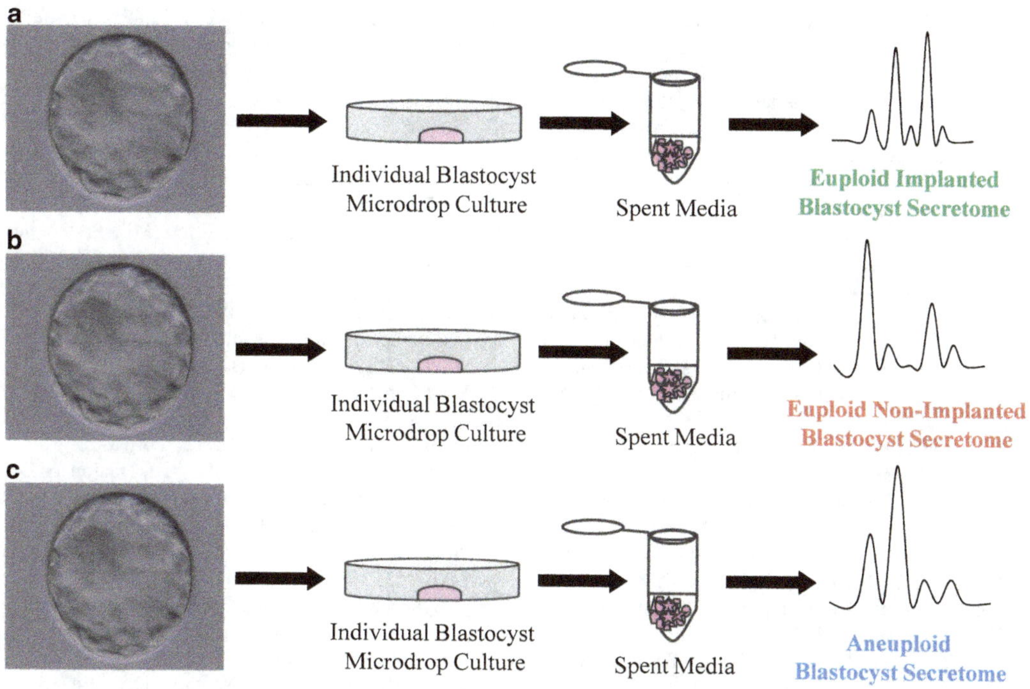

Fig. 19.1 Ongoing research is focused on validation of identified biomarkers to reliably discriminate between euploid implanted (**a**), euploid non-implanted (**b**), and aneuploid blastocyst (**c**) secretome

Summary

Proteomic analysis is a promising technology for the development of noninvasive methods for embryo selection in the field of ART. Taking into account the complexity and diversity of the human embryo, the challenge ahead still includes the reliable and reproducible identification of proteins associated with embryo viability and IVF success. However once identified, immunodetection using ELISA or radioimmunoassay will allow for sensitivity, high throughput, and cost-effectiveness for application in an IVF clinical setting. To date, no omics platform, including proteomics, has proven to be of true clinical predictive value or been examined in prospective randomized control trials to be better than current morphology-based selection methods. However, the combination of a quantitative noninvasive assay alongside morphology assessment could represent the greatest improvement in embryo selection techniques and could lead to routine single embryo transfers with healthy singleton deliveries.

References

1. Ebner T, Moser M, Sommergruber M, Tews G. Selection based on morphological assessment of oocytes and embryos at different stages of preimplantation development: a review. Hum Reprod Update. 2003;9(3):251–62.
2. Racowsky C, Ohno-Machado L, Kim J, Biggers JD. Is there an advantage in scoring early embryos on more than one day? Hum Reprod. 2009;24(9):2104–13.
3. Seli E, Vergouw CG, Morita H, et al. Noninvasive metabolomic profiling as an adjunct to morphology for noninvasive embryo assessment in women undergoing single embryo transfer. Fertil Steril. 2010; 94(2):535–42.
4. Katz-Jaffe MG, McReynolds S, Gardner DK, Schoolcraft WB. The role of proteomics in defining the human embryonic secretome. Mol Hum Reprod. 2009;15(5):271–7.
5. Hu S, Loo JA, Wong DT. Human body fluid proteome analysis. Proteomics. 2006;6(23):6326–53.
6. Kulasingam V, Diamandis EP. Proteomics analysis of conditioned media from three breast cancer cell lines: a mine for biomarkers and therapeutic targets. Mol Cell Proteomics. 2007;6(11):1997–2011.
7. Katz-Jaffe MG, Gardner DK. Embryology in the era of proteomics. Theriogenology. 2007;68 Suppl 1: S125–30.

8. O'Neill C. The role of paf in embryo physiology. Hum Reprod Update. 2005;11(3):215–28.
9. Gonzalez RR, Caballero-Campo P, Jasper M, et al. Leptin and leptin receptor are expressed in the human endometrium and endometrial leptin secretion is regulated by the human blastocyst. J Clin Endocrinol Metab. 2000;85(12):4883–8.
10. Cervero A, Horcajadas JA, Dominguez F, Pellicer A, Simon C. Leptin system in embryo development and implantation: a protein in search of a function. Reprod Biomed Online. 2005;10(2):217–23.
11. Sakkas D, Lu C, Zulfikaroglu E, Neuber E, Taylor HS. A soluble molecule secreted by human blastocysts modulates regulation of HOXA10 expression in an epithelial endometrial cell line. Fertil Steril. 2003; 80(5):1169–74.
12. Jurisicova A, Casper RF, MacLusky NJ, Librach CL. Embryonic human leukocyte antigen-G expression: possible implications for human preimplantation development. Fertil Steril. 1996;65(5):997–1002.
13. Jurisicova A, Casper RF, MacLusky NJ, Mills GB, Librach CL. HLA-G expression during preimplantation human embryo development. Proc Natl Acad Sci USA. 1996;93(1):161–5.
14. Yao YQ, Barlow DH, Sargent IL. Differential expression of alternatively spliced transcripts of HLA-G in human preimplantation embryos and inner cell masses. J Immunol. 2005;175(12):8379–85.
15. Warner CM, Lampton PW, Newmark JA, Cohen J. Symposium: innovative techniques in human embryo viability assessment. Soluble human leukocyte antigen-G and pregnancy success. Reprod Biomed Online. 2008;17(4):470–85.
16. Vercammen M, Verloes A, Haentjens P, Van de Velde H. Can soluble human leucocyte antigen-G predict successful pregnancy in assisted reproductive technology? Curr Opin Obstet Gynecol. 2009;21(3):285–90.
17. Vercammen MJ, Verloes A, Van de Velde H, Haentjens P. Accuracy of soluble human leukocyte antigen-G for predicting pregnancy among women undergoing infertility treatment: meta-analysis. Hum Reprod Update. 2008;14(3):209–18.
18. Tabiasco J, Perrier d'Hauterive S, Thonon F, et al. Soluble HLA-G in IVF/ICSI embryo culture supernatants does not always predict implantation success: a multicentre study. Reprod Biomed Online. 2009; 18(3):374–81.
19. Kotze DJ, Hansen P, Keskintepe L, Snowden E, Sher G, Kruger T. Embryo selection criteria based on morphology VERSUS the expression of a biochemical marker (sHLA-G) and a graduated embryo score: prediction of pregnancy outcome. J Assist Reprod Genet. 2010;27(6):309–16.
20. Noci I, Fuzzi B, Rizzo R, et al. Embryonic soluble HLA-G as a marker of developmental potential in embryos. Hum Reprod. 2005;20(1):138–46.
21. Coulam CB, Roussev RG, Lerner S, Zlatopolsky Z, Ilkevitch Y, Tur-Kaspa I. How to predict implantation? No correlation between embryonic aneuploidy and soluble human leukocyte antigen G-concentrations. Fertil Steril. 2009;91(6):2408–13.
22. Dominguez DC, Lopes R, Torres ML. Proteomics: clinical applications. Clin Lab Sci. Fall 2007;20(4): 245–8.
23. Hu J, Coombes KR, Morris JS, Baggerly KA. The importance of experimental design in proteomic mass spectrometry experiments: some cautionary tales. Brief Funct Genomic Proteomic. 2005;3(4):322–31.
24. Cho WC. Contribution of oncoproteomics to cancer biomarker discovery. Mol Cancer. 2007;6:25.
25. Katz-Jaffe MG, Schoolcraft WB, Gardner DK. Analysis of protein expression (secretome) by human and mouse preimplantation embryos. Fertil Steril. 2006;86(3):678–85.
26. Delbosc S, Haloui M, Louedec L, et al. Proteomic analysis permits the identification of new biomarkers of arterial wall remodeling in hypertension. Mol Med. 2008;14(7–8):383–94.
27. Sandoval JA, Hoelz DJ, Woodruff HA, et al. Novel peptides secreted from human neuroblastoma: useful clinical tools? J Pediatr Surg. 2006;41(1):245–51.
28. Wang HM, Zhang X, Qian D, et al. Effect of ubiquitin-proteasome pathway on mouse blastocyst implantation and expression of matrix metalloproteinases-2 and -9. Biol Reprod. 2004;70(2):481–7.
29. Dominguez F, Gadea B, Esteban FJ, Horcajadas JA, Pellicer A, Simon C. Comparative protein-profile analysis of implanted versus non-implanted human blastocysts. Hum Reprod. 2008;23(9):1993–2000.
30. Robertson SA. GM-CSF regulation of embryo development and pregnancy. Cytokine Growth Factor Rev. 2007;18(3–4):287–98.
31. Dominguez F, Gadea B, Mercader A, Esteban FJ, Pellicer A, Simon C. Embryologic outcome and secretome profile of implanted blastocysts obtained after coculture in human endometrial epithelial cells versus the sequential system. Fertil Steril. 2010;93(3):774–82.e771.
32. Mains LM, Christenson L, Yang B, Sparks AE, Mathur S, Van Voorhis BJ. Identification of apolipoprotein A1 in the human embryonic secretome. Fertil Steril. 2011;96(2):422–7.e422.
33. McReynolds S, Vanderlinden L, Stevens J, Hansen K, Schoolcraft WB, Katz-Jaffe MG. Lipocalin-1: a potential marker for noninvasive aneuploidy screening. Fertil Steril. 2011;95(8):2631–3.

Metabolism of the Viable Human Embryo

20

David K. Gardner

Regulation of energy production is fundamental to the survival and propagation of any cell type. What makes the preimplantation mammalian embryo so fascinating to study is the fact that the embryo undergoes major changes in its physiology and gene expression profiles during development. As the fertilised oocyte develops and differentiates into the blastocyst, embryonic genes are successively turned on (with the concomitant destruction of maternally derived mRNAs). Subsequently there is a growing energy demand as mitoses and biosynthesis increase post-embryonic-genome activation and as the blastocoel subsequently forms (through the activity of Na/K ATPase in the trophectoderm). Concomitantly, there are major changes in the regulation and relative activities of energy generating pathways. Of clinical interest is the fact that should an embryo at any stage of development have substantially altered energy production, i.e. if the flux of a specific nutrient through a metabolic pathway alters to a significant degree, even for a brief period, then this is associated with significantly impaired development in culture and reduction of viability post-transfer. Clearly it is in our interest to understand how the preimplantation embryo regulates its energy production, and to develop culture systems that best support an 'optimal' metabolism. Furthermore, it is evident that analysis of embryo metabolism is an appropriate means of assessing embryonic health and predicting subsequent viability. The task ahead is to determine the optimal range of metabolic functions that reflect viability at successive stages of embryo development.

D.K. Gardner (✉)
Department of Zoology, University of Melbourne, Melbourne, VIC 3010, Australia
e-mail: david.gardner@unimelb.edu.au

Changes in Metabolism with Development

The fertilised oocyte exhibits low utilisation of oxygen [1] and has a limited capacity to utilise glucose as an energy source [2]. In fact, glycolytic activity is restricted in the fertilised oocyte and early embryo by the allosteric regulation of phosphofructokinase (PFK) due to a high ATP:ADP ratio [3]. High ratio of these nucleotides is a consequence of the low energy demands at these stages, reflecting the dormant status of the oocyte from which it was derived. Consequently, in the absence of amino acids, the early embryo generates its energy from low levels of oxidation of pyruvate (fertilised oocyte) and lactate (from the 2-cell stage onwards), derived directly from oviduct fluid (and the cumulus cells in the case of the oocyte [4–6]) (Fig. 1). However, the early embryo can also utilise the malate-aspartate shuttle, and in the presence of specific amino acids, e.g. aspartate, the embryo can utilise lactate as an energy source through the conversion of lactate to pyruvate [7]. In the immediate post-fertilisation period of mouse zygotes, there is an absolute requirement

D.K. Gardner et al. (eds.), *Human Gametes and Preimplantation Embryos: Assessment and Diagnosis*, DOI 10.1007/978-1-4614-6651-2_20,

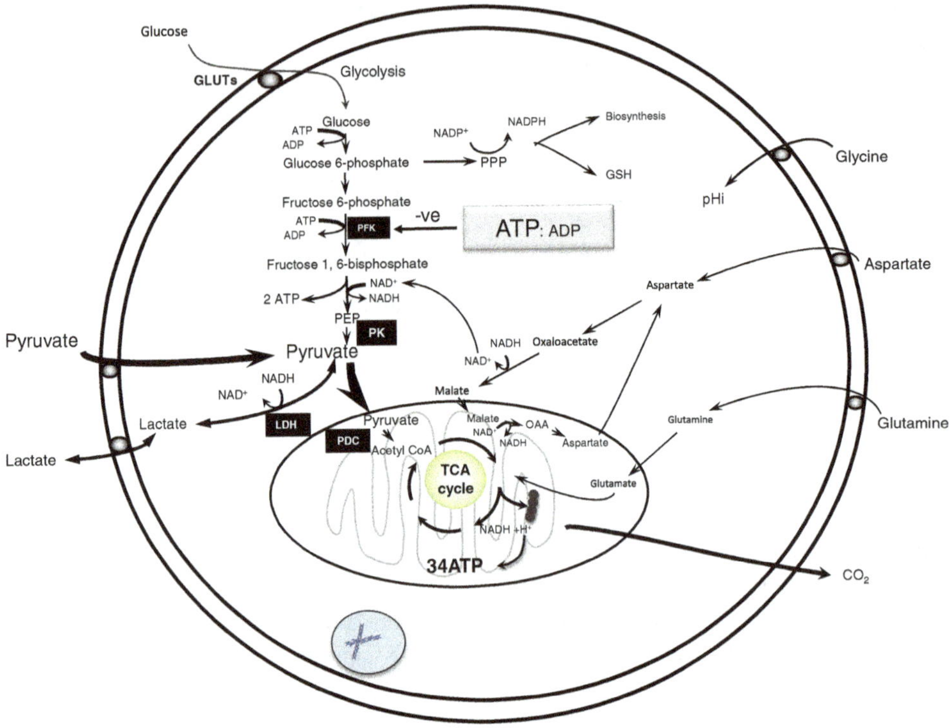

Fig. 20.1 Metabolism of the pronucleate oocyte and cleavage stage embryo. Prior to compaction the embryo has a metabolism based around low levels of oxidation of pyruvate, lactate and specific amino acids. The ovulated oocyte is surrounded by and is directly connected to cumulus cells, which actively produce pyruvate and lactate from glucose [4, 6]. This creates a high concentration of pyruvate and lactate and a low concentration of glucose around the fertilised oocyte. Upon dispersal of the cumulus cells, the human zygote and cleavage stage embryo still find themselves in a relatively high concentration of pyruvate (0.32 mM) and lactate (10.5 mM), and low levels of glucose (0.5 mM) [6]. Significantly, the relative abundance of nutrients affects the metabolism of the embryo. For example, the ratio of pyruvate:lactate in the surrounding environment directly affects the ratio of NADH:NAD$^+$ in the embryo, which in turn controls the redox state of the cells and hence the flux of nutrients through specific energy generating pathways [85]. Lactate dehydrogenase comprises ~5 % of the total protein of the mouse oocyte [86]. The oocyte, pronucleate oocyte and all stages of development to the blastocyst exhibit LDH isoform I [87], which then changes to predominantly isoform V at the late blastocyst stage upon outgrowth [88]. Isoform I favours the formation of pyruvate, and is typically found in heart tissue. Isoform V favours lactate formation, and is typically found in muscle tissues. This switch in isoforms is consistent with the changes in patterns of energy metabolism as the embryo develops, but cannot explain the significant production of lactate by the blastocyst (see Fig. 2). The early embryo is characterised by a high ATP:ADP level [3], which in turn allosterically inhibits PFK, thereby limiting the flux of glucose through the glycolytic pathway. Amino acids fill several niches in embryo physiology, such as the use of glycine as buffer of intracellular pH (pHi). Several amino acids are also utilised as energy sources by the early embryo such as glutamine and aspartate. Aspartate can be utilised through the malate-aspartate shuttle [7], the significance of which during embryo development we are only beginning to understand. The thickness of the lines represents the relative flux of metabolites through the pathway. *PFK* phosphofructokinase; *PK* pyruvate kinase; *LDH* lactate dehydrogenase; *PDC* pyruvate dehydrogenase complex; *PPP* pentose phosphate pathway; *OAA* oxaloacetate; *pHi* intracellular pH

for oxidative metabolism of pyruvate to support the completion of the second meiotic division and subsequent development [8].

With an increase in cell divisions and biosynthesis following the activation of the embryonic genome, the formation of a transporting epithelium when the morula is formed, and subsequent creation of the blastocyst, the need for cellular energy increases dramatically. Consequently there is a decline in the ATP:ADP ratio (and a dramatic increase in AMP levels) as ATP is readily consumed, thereby alleviating inhibition on PFK and facilitating the flux of glucose through glycolysis. However, the overall regulation of carbon flux through glycolysis is also regulated at a number of sites (Fig. 2).

Interestingly, although the blastocyst exhibits a much higher oxygen consumption than the cleavage stage embryo [9–11], the late stage embryo does not oxidise all of the glucose consumed, but rather converts approximately 50 % (somewhat species-dependent) of glucose carbon to lactate, this even in the presence of adequate oxygen for complete oxidation of the glucose. This latter metabolic phenomenon is referred to as 'aerobic glycolysis' (not to be confused with anaerobic glycolysis found in tissues such as muscle when oxygen is limited). Aerobic glycolysis is a trait found in cancers and rapidly dividing cells, a phenomenon also known as the Warburg effect [12, 13] (Fig. 2).

What Is the Role of Aerobic Glycolysis/ Warburg Effect in the Blastocyst?

In the blastocyst of primates and rodents, high levels of aerobic glycolysis, have been interpreted as the embryos adaptation to its imminent invasion of the endometrium, which remains avascular for a period of up to 12 h, and will therefore be relatively anoxic [14, 15]. During the initial stages of blastocysts invasion, glycolysis will plausibly be the predominant means of generating energy. However, this may not be the sole explanation for the high levels of glycolysis observed in blastocysts of domestic animals, as they do not 'implant' for a further week. An alternative explanation for the rather idiosyncratic metabolism of the blastocyst was proposed by Gardner in 1998 [16]. A high level of aerobic glycolysis is a common characteristic of proliferating cells and tumours, with which the mammalian blastocyst shares several traits [17–19]. As well as being used to generate energy for increased mitoses and blastocoel expansion, high levels of glucose utilisation will be required for the synthesis of triacylglycerols and phospholipids and as a precursor for complex sugars of mucopolysaccharides and glycoproteins. Glucose metabolised by the pentose phosphate pathway (PPP) will generate ribose moieties required for nucleic acid synthesis and the NADPH and carbon skeletons required for the biosynthesis of lipids and other complex molecules [18, 20]. NADPH is also required for pathways of one carbon metabolism, which are vital for the methylation of various intracellular substrates, including DNA. It is now well appreciated that embryos undergo dramatic changes in the epigenetic modifications of their genomes including DNA methylation during preimplantation development [21]. NADPH is also required for the reduction of intracellular glutathione, an important antioxidant for the embryo [22]. Interestingly, although the absolute amount of glucose metabolised through the PPP increases with development [23], the percentage of the total glucose consumed which is metabolised through this pathway appears to be lowest at the blastocyst stage [24]. This again raises the question as to why such high levels of aerobic glycolysis are required? It is plausible that high levels of aerobic glycolysis, such as that observed in the mammalian blastocyst, will ensure that there is sufficient substrate and cytosolic ATP available for biosynthetic pathways, such as the synthesis of nucleic acids, proteins and new membranes, at the required times during cellular proliferation [25, 26]. This in turn suggests that there are times within the cell cycle when the PPP is more active than others (Fig. 2). Analysis of embryo energy metabolism with respect to cell cycle has not been thoroughly analysed, but it is speculated that at specific times during the cell cycle there will be increased energy demands, particularly during cytokinesis.

A further explanation for the high levels of aerobic glycolysis by the blastocyst could lie in the activity of mitochondrial shuttles in the oxidation of hydrogen equivalents formed through glycolysis. The malate-aspartate is one such shuttle that allows cytosolic NADH to be exchanged for NAD^+ that is derived from the mitochondrion. Once within the mitochondrion, the NADH can be more efficiently converted to ATP through oxidative phosphorylation. Interestingly, the malate-aspartate (NADH) shuttle of different tumours can contribute between 20 and 80 % of

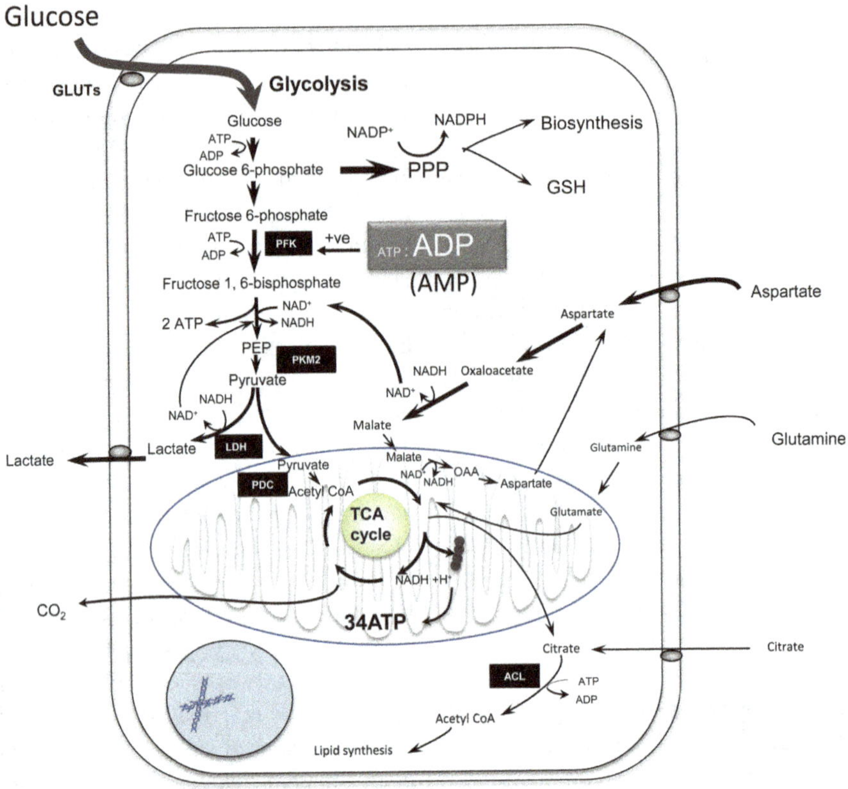

Fig. 20.2 Metabolism of the blastocyst. After compaction the embryo exhibits greatly increased oxygen consumption [1, 9, 10] and an increased capacity to use glucose as an energy source. The increase in oxygen consumption plausibly reflects the considerable energy required for the formation and maintenance of the blastocoel, while the increase in glucose utilisation reflects an increased demand for biosynthetic precursors [16]. Consequently, there is a reduction in the ATP:ADP ratio [3], and a concomitant increase in AMP, which will have a positive allosteric effect on PFK, thereby facilitating a higher flux of glucose through glycolysis. Rather than oxidise the glucose consumed, the blastocyst exhibits high levels of aerobic glycolysis [5]. Although this may appear energetically unfavourable, it does ensure that the biosynthetic arm of the pentose phosphate pathway has maximum substrate availability at all times. Activity of the pentose pathway will ensure that reducing equivalents are available for biosynthesis and ensure production of glutathione (reduced), a key intracellular antioxidant. In order for high levels of glycolysis to proceed the blastomeres need to regenerate cytosolic NAD^+. This can be achieved through the generation of lactate from pyruvate. A second means of generating cytosolic NAD^+ is through the activity of the malate-aspartate shuttle. Although it is evident that blastocysts do use aerobic glycolysis, it is proposed that the significant increase in oxygen utilisation at this stage of development could be largely attributed to the activity of the malate-aspartate shuttle and the resulting demand for oxygen to convert intramitochondrial NADH to ATP. Indeed many tumours that exhibit aerobic glycolysis also have high levels of the malate-aspartate shuttle [28]. Furthermore, inhibition of this shuttle has dire consequences for subsequent fetal development [21, 89]. A further key regulatory enzyme in glycolysis is pyruvate kinase (PK). In proliferating cells and in cancer cells, a specific isoform is present, PKM2 [90, 91]. This particular isoform of PK has been shown to promote aerobic glycolysis and anabolic metabolism [92], and recently has been identified in the mammalian blastocyst [93]. Further work is warranted on establishing the regulation of PKM2 in the embryo, with specific reference to its control by exogenous factors and signalling pathways involved. The pyruvate dehydrogenase complex catalyses the irreversible conversion or pyruvate to acetyl Co-A, and consequently functionally linking glycolysis to the activity of the oxidative TCA cycle. The activity of this enzyme complex is tightly regulated through three main mechanisms; (1) phosphorylation/dephosphorylation, (2) the redox state (NAD^+:NADH, ATP:ADP and the acetylCoA:CoA ratios) and (3) transcriptional regulation. However, relatively little is known about the regulation of this complex in mammalian embryos during the preimplantation period. Citrate, formed from either mitochondrial metabolism, or provided in the culture medium, could serve as a precursor in lipid synthesis, required for membrane generation associated with proliferation. As the embryo develops, it

the total respiratory rate [27, 28]. As the mammalian blastocyst has a high respiratory quotient [1] combined with high levels of lactate production [5], it is plausible that glycolysis is used to derive ATP oxidatively through the malate-aspartate shuttle. In support of this it has recently been demonstrated that in the mouse preimplantation embryo malate-aspartate shuttle activity is essential for the regulation of metabolism during the preimplantation period [7]. Furthermore, if the activity of the shuttle is inhibited in the blastocyst, then subsequent implantation and fetal development are significantly reduced [29]. Such data further highlight the significance of maintenance of embryonic metabolism to subsequent viability and normality.

Comparison of Metabolic Activities of Embryos Developed In Vitro Compared to In Vivo

One advantage of working with an animal model, such as the mouse, is the ability to access and analyse embryos developed in vivo, thereby being able to determine how similar, or otherwise, embryos are when maintained in vitro. If a mouse blastocyst is collected from the uterus and its metabolism quantitated immediately, it is observed that just less than 50 % of glucose consumed will be released into the surrounding medium as lactate [5]. It has been established that when developed in simple culture conditions (i.e. a culture medium lacking amino acids and vitamins, and with only glucose, pyruvate and lactate as energy sources, which is typical of the early human embryo culture media such as HTF [30]), resultant blastocysts exhibit a significant increase in lactate production [5, 31] and a concomitant reduction in carbohydrate oxidation [32], which has been documented to be associated with a significant loss of viability [33]. Lane and Gardner [34] demonstrated that placing a mouse blastocyst that had developed in vivo and collected directly from the uterus, into a simple culture medium induced aberrant metabolism within just 3 h of incubation. They went on to show that collecting mouse blastocysts in the presence of amino acids and vitamins greatly reduced this metabolic trauma. Furthermore, when in vivo developed blastocysts were incubated for just 6 h in a simple medium prior to transfer, they exhibited a significant reduction in implantation rate and subsequent fetal development. In contrast, blastocysts incubated in the presence of amino acids and vitamins for the 6 h period were not significantly compromised post-transfer.

Key points arising from the aforementioned study are: that culture-induced metabolic stress, i.e. incubation in a medium lacking amino acids and vitamins, resulted in a *rapid* loss of metabolic regulation, and that secondly, this metabolic perturbation not only reduced implantation but also impacted fetal development, culminating in lighter foetuses. So an incubation of just a few hours in a stressful environment can induce metabolic changes that have downstream effects leading to compromised fetal development. Hence, several studies have used this model to develop culture conditions which ensure that embryos

Fig. 20.2 (continued) exhibits a growing number of receptors for specific growth factors [94]. Given that growth factor signalling can reorganise metabolic fluxes independently of traditional allosteric means, it will be important to determine how exogenous factors affect key metabolic processes within the embryo. Analysis of blastocyst metabolism is a measurement of the relative activity of two cell types, the trophectoderm and inner cell mass (ICM). In the mouse blastocyst it has been determined that whereas the trophectoderm converts around half of the glucose consumed to lactate, the ICM is almost exclusively glycolytic [95]. It is not know what the relative activities of the two cell types are in the human blastocyst, but given that human embryonic stem cells are dependent upon a high glycolytic activity [96], it would be prudent to assume that the human ICM also exhibits low levels of glucose oxidation. Although the number of trophectoderm cells far outnumbers those of the ICM, it remains important to consider these cell-specific differences when analysing metabolic data. The thickness of the lines represents the relative flux of metabolites through the pathway. *PFK* phosphofructokinase; *PK* pyruvate kinase; *LDH* lactate dehydrogenase; *PDC* pyruvate dehydrogenase complex; *ACL* acetyl-citrate lyase; *OAA* oxaloacetate; *PPP* pentose phosphate pathway; *OAA* oxaloacetate; *GSH* reduced glutathione. From 97 with permission

in vitro exhibit a metabolic profile similar to those embryos developed in vivo [35]. These data firmly establish that quantifying embryo metabolism is an appropriate physiological parameter to relate to subsequent viability after transfer. Furthermore, the above study was performed on in vivo developed blastocysts, and it has been shown that embryos post-compaction are far more resilient to environmental stress than the cleavage stage embryo. Consequently, exposing cleavage stage embryos to stress, i.e. prior to compaction, may have even greater downstream effects [36, 37].

Relationship Between Carbohydrate Metabolism and Embryo Viability

As discussed, substantial perturbations in the relative activity of pathways involved in intermediary metabolism culminate in compromised embryo development in culture and a reduction of viability post-transfer. Data from such studies have been invaluable in the development of modern culture systems that support normal metabolic function in the developing embryo, thereby promoting the development of viable human embryos [38]. A relationship between carbohydrate utilisation by embryos and resultant viability has been established both in animal models [33, 39, 40] and the human [41, 42] (reviewed in detail in Chap. 23). Post-compaction glucose consumption is positively correlated with subsequent viability. Furthermore, should the metabolism of glucose by the blastocyst differ from that expected, i.e. excessive glycolytic activity, then it has been established that viability is significantly compromised in the mouse model. These data support the hypothesis that it is not only the rate at which a nutrient is consumed that reflects developmental potential but also the metabolic fate of the nutrient measured. Of further interest is the observation that female embryos are metabolically more active than males [41, 43]. This finding is consistent with the observed differences in gene expression profiles [44, 45], and subsequent proteome [46], between male and female embryos.

Beyond the Carbohydrate Triad: Analysis of Amino Acid Utilisation

Alternative energy sources for cells, other than those present in typical embryo culture media (i.e. glucose, pyruvate and lactate) include free fatty acids (FFA) and amino acids. Although FFA may have a role in the development embryos of certain species (typically those with a high endogenous lipid content, such as the cow and pig), and their uptake by human embryos has been quantitated [47], further work is required to understand how FFA impact the metabolism of the embryo. Consequently they will not be discussed further here. However, it would be prudent to watch developments in this area, especially with regard to the role of FFA metabolism in oocyte maturation [48]. The beneficial effects of amino acids on embryos in culture have been demonstrated for several years. Amino acids are abundant in oviduct and uterine fluids [49, 50] and are important regulators of embryonic function. As well as their documented effects as biosynthetic precursors [51], buffers of intracellular pH in the embryo [52], antioxidants [53] and in signalling and differentiation [54–56], amino acids also serve as energy sources [23]. Furthermore, our understanding of how embryo energy metabolism is regulated has changed recently with the determination that the malate-aspartate shuttle is involved in the control of carbohydrate metabolism [7]. A paradigm held for over 40 years was that the fertilised oocyte had an absolute requirement for pyruvate [2]. However, recent analysis of embryo physiology has revealed that lactate and aspartate can substitute for pyruvate at the 1-cell stage, the two nutrients presumably generating sufficient energy through the malate-aspartate shuttle to support development.

The relationship between amino acid utilisation and embryo development and viability has been analysed by Leese and colleagues [57–59], and reviewed in detail by Houghton (Chap. 24). Using HPLC to quantitate amino acids in embryo culture medium, it was observed that a different pattern of amino acid utilisation existed between embryos that went on to form a blastocyst compared to those embryos that failed to develop in vitro. It was observed that leucine was taken up from the culture medium more by embryos which went on to develop [57]. The profiles of the amino acids alanine, arginine, asparagine, glutamine and methionine utilisation also correlated with blastocyst formation, although no relationship between amino acid utilisation and blastocyst quality or viability was established. Subsequently, Brison et al. [58] reported that changes in concentration of amino acids in the spent medium of human zygotes cultured for 24 h to the 2-cell stage in an embryo culture medium containing a mixture of amino acids, using HPLC. It was found that asparagine, glycine and leucine were all significantly associated with clinical pregnancy and live birth. Furthermore, and consistent with the data on glucose consumption, there appears to be gender differences with regard to amino acid utilisation [59, 60], consistent with differences in the proteomes of male and female embryos [43].

An important point to note is that all of the studies analysing the utilisation of amino acids by human embryos have been performed in the presence of 20 % oxygen, the significance of which is just now being realised and is discussed below.

Impact of the Culture Environment on Embryonic Metabolism

The relative concentrations of nutrients present in culture media directly affects embryo metabolism [61]. However, other factors of the culture system such as medium pH [62] and the concentration of oxygen used in the incubator can impact metabolic function. Historically, atmospheric oxygen (~20 %) has been in tissue culture, and human IVF laboratories subsequently adopted this level of oxygen for embryo culture. However, the physiological concentration of oxygen within the female reproductive tract has been reported to be below 10 % [63–65]. Consistent with such data, embryo development in all mammals studied to date is significantly improved by culture in an oxygen concentration of 5–7 %, compared to 20 % [66–69], with a high oxygen concentration having its most detrimental effects at the cleavage stages [70]. Similar data sets are now being documented for the human embryo [71–74].

A significant body of work has been amassed on the effects of oxygen concentration on mammalian embryo development. It transpires that atmospheric oxygen has a significant negative impact on blastocyst gene expression [36, 75], the embryonic proteome [76] and more recently it has been established that oxygen concentration has a significant impact on embryo metabolism, impacting the utilisation of both carbohydrates and amino acids [77] (Fig. 3). Of interest the effects of oxygen on metabolism were stage-specific. During the cleavage stages, 20 % oxygen was associated with an overall increase in amino acid turn over and pyruvate uptake by embryos. In contrast, post-compaction 20 % oxygen was associated with a decrease in amino acid turnover and glucose uptake. Given that it has been established that glucose uptake by the embryo post-compaction is positively correlated with viability, such findings are consistent with reports of lower pregnancy rates following culture in 20 % oxygen, i.e. the decrease in glucose utilisation in the presence of 20 % oxygen is related to the reduction in viability. Given the documented harm atmospheric oxygen imparts on the developing embryo and its physiology, its continued use in human IVF can no longer be condoned.

What Are the Accepted Patterns of Metabolic Activity? Quietness Revisited

A novel hypothesis proposed by Leese [78] suggested that those embryos with a less active, or a ‘quiet’ metabolism are those that go on to give rise to pregnancies. Data to support this hypothesis have been obtained from different species and reviewed recently [79]. In essence it was proposed that embryos with a low metabolic activity reflected a less stressed physiology, and consequently those embryos classified as viable would be those that had low nutrient uptake and turn

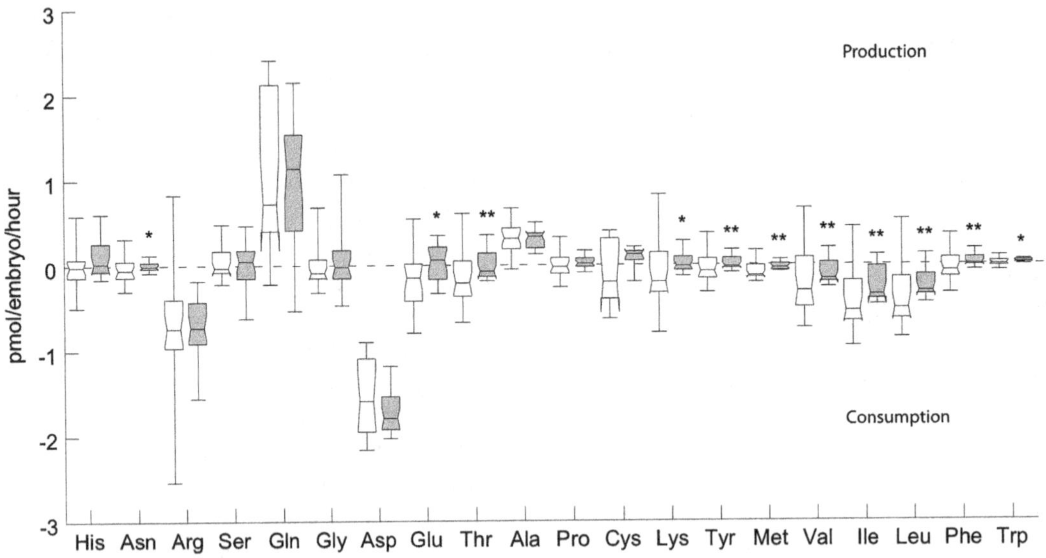

Fig. 20.3 Effect of oxygen concentration on amino acid utilisation by mouse post-compaction embryos from day 4 to 5. Five per cent oxygen, *open box* and 20 % oxygen, *grey box* (25 replicates per treatment, groups of 3, $n = 75$ embryos). The line across the box is the median uptake or release. There were significant differences in the utilisation of asparagine, glutamate, tryptophan and lysine ($P < 0.05$), with greater significance for utilisation of threonine, tyrosine, methionine, valine, isoleucine, leucine and phenylalanine ($P < 0.01$), between the two oxygen concentrations. Consumption for each of these amino acids was greater at 5 % oxygen than atmospheric oxygen, and overall amino acid utilisation was higher at 5 % compared to 20 % ($P < 0.05$). Notches represent the confidence interval of the median, and the depth of the box represents the interquartile range (50 % of the data), whiskers represent the 5 and 95 % quartiles. *Asterisks* indicate significant differences from embryos cultured in 5 % oxygen (*$P < 0.05$, **$P < 0.01$) (From 77 with permission)

over [79]. However, a growing number of recent studies have generated data that do not provide support for this hypothesis [33, 41, 80, 81], rather they indicate that viability is associated with increased metabolic activity. So how can this apparent paradox be resolved? An analysis of the studies upon which the 'quiet hypothesis' was built reveals that a common factor among them is the use of 20 % oxygen, either for embryo culture and analysis, or during the actual analysis of metabolism. Given the documented negative impact of 20 % oxygen on embryonic gene expression, proteome and metabolism described above, the significance of the 'quiet hypothesis' for embryos cultured under physiological oxygen conditions must be carefully reviewed and studies performed to determine what is the optimal nutrient utilisation profile under physiological conditions.

We know that when mammalian embryos are stressed, especially by 20 % oxygen, their metabolic profile changes significantly [77]. Data to date [79] indicate that those embryos cultured in 20 % oxygen which are able to develop do have a lower turnover of nutrients. One explanation for this finding may be related to the inability of unhealthy or developmentally compromised embryos to tolerate oxidative stress. Suboptimal embryos may have lower endowments of antioxidants or less robust systems for responding to oxidising agents and consequently may have to resort to other energetically consuming mechanisms to preserve their redox status. In this context, the quiet embryo hypothesis would pertain more to the embryo's ability to respond to oxidative stress than to its innate metabolic characteristics under physiologic conditions. Studies evaluating the metabolism of the same embryos in both low and high oxygen conditions could test this hypothesis. Thus far, little attention has been devoted to the development and application of stress tests, i.e., exposing embryos to safe, well-controlled stresses and monitoring their responses, to evaluate embryonic health and developmental potential. There are certainly many clinical situations in which stress tests are used to diagnose disease or disease susceptibility such as exercise stress tests for cardiac disease and glucose tolerance tests for gestational diabetes. The challenge for the development of an embryonic stress test is to ensure that the stressor does not cause lasting harm. As mentioned previously, exposure to high oxygen tension is not an acceptable stressor based on our understanding of the short- and long-term effects of this exposure.

It is evident that when a 5 % oxygen concentration is used during culture, the metabolism of embryos on day 4 and 5 at the morula and blastocyst stages, is significantly higher in those embryos that give rise to pregnancies, compared to those embryos that fail to develop post-transfer. Such data, therefore, do not support the 'quiet hypothesis' for embryos beyond the 8-cell stage. In contrast, the data obtained for day 4 and 5 human embryos and their subsequent pregnancy outcome, were collected under low oxygen conditions. These data that reveal those embryos with the *more active* metabolism give rise to pregnancies. Interestingly, recent data on oxygen consumption by cleavage stage human embryos indicates that at the cleavage stage viability is associated with an increased oxygen consumption rate, reflecting an increase in respiration rate [81]. At present, we do not know if there is a value that is too high to be consistent with viability, although it is most plausible. There will likely be upper and lower values of metabolic normality, outside which embryo will show a decline in viability. Given that there is an overall increase in most metabolic activities as the preimplantation embryo proceeds through development, it would seem more likely for compromised embryos to have lower rather than higher metabolic activities relative to their healthy cohorts. Furthermore, as glucose uptake [41, 43] and amino acid utilisation [59] are related to the sex of embryo, such data need to be factored in to further hypotheses on embryo metabolism and optimal rates of metabolic activity for embryo selection.

Conclusions

Some 30 years after Renard et al. showed a relationship between glucose uptake by day 10 cow blastocysts and subsequent pregnancy outcome [39], data sets relating the patterns of nutrient utilisation by the human embryo with pregnancy outcome, are growing [41, 58, 59]. Further analysis of human embryo physiology will assist in establishing the metabolic algorithms for embryo selection. Growing data indicate that stage-specific and sex-specific differences in metabolism exist during the preimplantation period. Understanding the nature of these differences, the impact of culture conditions (such as medium composition and the concentration of oxygen used) has important implications for embryo selection. As development proceeds, there is an increase in asynchrony amongst embryos of a cohort and this will be manifest as an increased variation in nutrient utilisation (Fig. 4). Consequently it is predicted that differences in

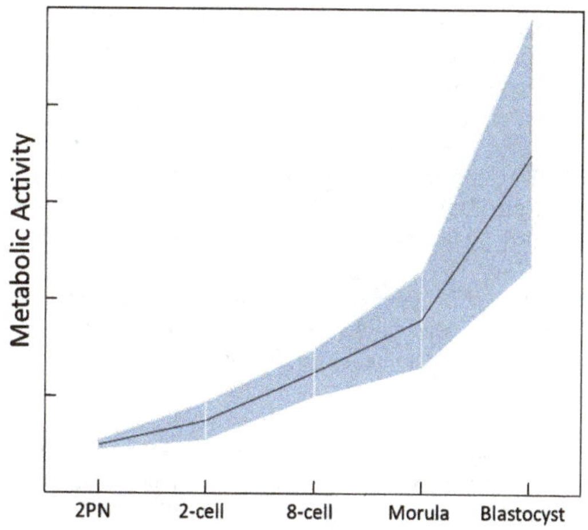

Fig. 20.4 Distribution of metabolic activity with respect to preimplantation embryo development. As development proceeds, asynchrony between embryos and metabolic activity increase. Consequently, it may be easier to identify a viable embryo within a cohort later in development

embryo metabolism will be more readily detected with increasing developmental stage.

It is also evident that changes in metabolic activity not only affect subsequent implantation potential, but have downstream effects through to fetal development and beyond. Given that perturbations in metabolic activity are linked to epigenetic regulation of cell function [82], assessment of a viable metabolism should facilitate the creation of conditions that support the genetic stability and epigenetic integrity of the embryo.

Whereas the technologies for such work currently resides in a handful of laboratories around the world, the rapid developments in laboratory-on-a-chip technologies may well ensure that the assays required will be able to be housed in microfluidic devices and subsequently such analyses will be readily available to the general IVF community [83, 84].

Acknowledgments The author is indebted to Dr Mark Johnson for his comments on the manuscript.

References

1. Trimarchi JR, Liu L, Porterfield DM, Smith PJ, Keefe DL. Oxidative phosphorylation-dependent and -independent oxygen consumption by individual preimplantation mouse embryos. Biol Reprod. 2000;62: 1866–74.
2. Biggers JD, Whittingham DG, Donahue RP. The pattern of energy metabolism in the mouse oocyte and zygote. Proc Natl Acad Sci USA. 1967;58:560–7.
3. Leese HJ, Biggers JD, Mroz EA, Lechene C. Nucleotides in a single mammalian ovum or preimplantation embryo. Anal Biochem. 1984;140:443–8.
4. Leese HJ, Barton AM. Production of pyruvate by isolated mouse cumulus cells. J Exp Zool. 1985;234: 231–6.
5. Gardner DK, Leese HJ. Concentrations of nutrients in mouse oviduct fluid and their effects on embryo development and metabolism in vitro. J Reprod Fertil. 1990;88:361–8.
6. Gardner DK, Lane M, Calderon I, Leeton J. Environment of the preimplantation human embryo in vivo: metabolite analysis of oviduct and uterine fluids and metabolism of cumulus cells. Fertil Steril. 1996;65:349–53.
7. Lane M, Gardner DK. Mitochondrial malate-aspartate shuttle regulates mouse embryo nutrient consumption. J Biol Chem. 2005;280:18361–7.
8. Johnson MT, Freeman EA, Gardner DK, Hunt PA. Oxidative metabolism of pyruvate is required for meiotic maturation of murine oocytes in vivo. Biol Reprod. 2007;77:2–8.
9. Mills RM, Brinster RL. Oxygen consumption of preimplantation mouse embryos. Exp Cell Res. 1967;47: 337–44.
10. Thompson JG, Partridge RJ, Houghton FD, Cox CI, Leese HJ. Oxygen uptake and carbohydrate metabolism by in vitro derived bovine embryos. J Reprod Fertil. 1996;106:299–306.
11. Houghton FD, Sheth B, Moran B, Leese HJ, Fleming TP. Expression and activity of hexokinase in the early mouse embryo. Mol Hum Reprod. 1996;2:793–8.
12. Vander Heiden MG, Cantley LC, Thompson CB. Understanding the Warburg effect: the metabolic requirements of cell proliferation. Science. 2009;324: 1029–33.
13. Warburg O. On the origin of cancer cells. Science. 1956;123:309–14.
14. Rogers PAW, Murphy CR, Gannon BJ. Absence of capillaries in the endometrium surrounding the implanting rat blastocyst. Micron. 1982;13:373–4.
15. Rogers PA, Murphy CR, Rogers AW, Gannon BJ. Capillary patency and permeability in the endometrium surrounding the implanting rat blastocyst. Int J Microcirc Clin Exp. 1983;2:241–9.
16. Gardner DK. Embryo Development and culture techniques. In: Clark J, editor. Animal breeding: technology for the 21st century. London: Harwood Academic; 1998. p. 13–46.
17. Hume DA, Weidemann MJ. Role and regulation of glucose metabolism in proliferating cells. J Natl Cancer Inst. 1979;62:3–8.
18. Morgan MJ, Faik P. Carbohydrate metabolism in cultured animal cells. Biosci Rep. 1981;1:669–86.
19. Mandel LJ. Energy metabolism of cellular activation, growth, and transformation. Curr Top Membr Transp. 1986;27:261–91.
20. Reitzer LJ, Wice BM, Kennell D. The pentose cycle. Control and essential function in HeLa cell nucleic acid synthesis. J Biol Chem. 1980;255:5616–26.
21. Shi L, Wu J. Epigenetic regulation in mammalian preimplantation embryo development. Reprod Biol Endocrinol. 2009;7:59.
22. Rieger D. Relationships between energy metabolism and development of early mammalian embryos. Theriogenology. 1992;37:75–93.
23. Rieger D, Loskutoff NM, Betteridge KJ. Developmentally related changes in the uptake and metabolism of glucose, glutamine and pyruvate by cattle embryos produced in vitro. Reprod Fertil Dev. 1992;4:547–57.
24. Rieger D, Guay P. Measurement of the metabolism of energy substrates in individual bovine blastocysts. J Reprod Fertil. 1988;83:585–91.
25. Newsholme EA, Crabtree B, Ardawi MS. The role of high rates of glycolysis and glutamine utilization in rapidly dividing cells. Biosci Rep. 1985;5:393–400.
26. Newsholme EA. Application of metabolic-control logic to the requirements for cell division. Biochem Soc Trans. 1990;18:78–80.

27. Greenhouse WV, Lehninger AL. Occurrence of the malate-aspartate shuttle in various tumor types. Cancer Res. 1976;36:1392–6.
28. Greenhouse WV, Lehninger AL. Magnitude of malate-aspartate reduced nicotinamide adenine dinucleotide shuttle activity in intact respiring tumor cells. Cancer Res. 1977;37:4173–81.
29. Mitchell M, Cashman KS, Gardner DK, Thompson JG, Lane M. Disruption of mitochondrial malate-aspartate shuttle activity in mouse blastocysts impairs viability and fetal growth. Biol Reprod. 2009;80: 295–301.
30. Quinn P, Kerin JF, Warnes GM. Improved pregnancy rate in human in vitro fertilization with the use of a medium based on the composition of human tubal fluid. Fertil Steril. 1985;44:493–8.
31. Gardner DK, Sakkas D. Mouse embryo cleavage, metabolism and viability: role of medium composition. Hum Reprod. 1993;8:288–95.
32. Menke TM, McLaren A. Mouse blastocysts grown in vivo and in vitro: carbon dioxide production and trophoblast outgrowth. J Reprod Fertil. 1970;23: 117–27.
33. Lane M, Gardner DK. Selection of viable mouse blastocysts prior to transfer using a metabolic criterion. Hum Reprod. 1996;11:1975–8.
34. Lane M, Gardner DK. Amino acids and vitamins prevent culture-induced metabolic perturbations and associated loss of viability of mouse blastocysts. Hum Reprod. 1998;13:991–7.
35. Gardner D, Lane M. Towards a single embryo transfer. Reprod Biomed Online. 2003;6:470–81.
36. Gardner DK, Lane M. Ex vivo early embryo development and effects on gene expression and imprinting. Reprod Fertil Dev. 2005;17:361.
37. Lane M, Gardner DK. Understanding cellular disruptions during early embryo development that perturb viability and fetal development. Reprod Fertil Dev. 2005;17:371–8.
38. Gardner DK, Lane M. Culture and selection of viable blastocysts: a feasible proposition for human IVF? Hum Reprod Update. 1997;3:367–82.
39. Renard JP, Menezo Y, Heyman Y. Alternative tests to assess viability of bovine embryos. Theriogenology. 1982;17:106.
40. Gardner DK, Leese HJ. Assessment of embryo viability prior to transfer by the noninvasive measurement of glucose uptake. J Exp Zool. 1987;242:103–5.
41. Gardner DK, Wale PL, Collins R, Lane M. Glucose consumption of single post-compaction human embryos is predictive of embryo sex and live birth outcome. Hum Reprod. 2011;26:1981–6.
42. Conaghan J, Hardy K, Handyside AH, Winston RM, Leese HJ. Selection criteria for human embryo transfer: a comparison of pyruvate uptake and morphology. J Assist Reprod Genet. 1993;10:21–30.
43. Gardner DK, Larman MG, Thouas GA. Sex-related physiology of the preimplantation embryo. Mol Hum Reprod. 2010;16:539–47.
44. Kobayashi S, Isotani A, Mise N, Yamamoto M, Fujihara Y, Kaseda K, et al. Comparison of gene expression in male and female mouse blastocysts revealed imprinting of the X-linked gene, Rhox5/Pem, at preimplantation stages. Curr Biol. 2006;16: 166–72.
45. Bermejo-Alvarez P, Rizos D, Rath D, Lonergan P, Gutierrez-Adan A. Sex determines the expression level of one third of the actively expressed genes in bovine blastocysts. Proc Natl Acad Sci USA. 2010; 107:3394–9.
46. Epstein CJ, Smith S, Travis B, Tucker G. Both X chromosomes function before visible X-chromosome inactivation in female mouse embryos. Nature. 1978; 274:500–3.
47. Haggarty P, Wood M, Ferguson E, Hoad G, Srikantharajah A, Milne E, et al. Fatty acid metabolism in human preimplantation embryos. Hum Reprod. 2006;21:766–73.
48. Dunning KR, Cashman K, Russell DL, Thompson JG, Norman RJ, Robker RL. Beta-oxidation is essential for mouse oocyte developmental competence and early embryo development. Biol Reprod. 2010;83: 909–18.
49. Casslen BG. Free amino acids in human uterine fluid. Possible role of high taurine concentration. J Reprod Med. 1987;32:181–4.
50. Harris SE, Gopichandran N, Picton HM, Leese HJ, Orsi NM. Nutrient concentrations in murine follicular fluid and the female reproductive tract. Theriogenology. 2005;64:992–1006.
51. Crosby IM, Gandolfi F, Moor RM. Control of protein synthesis during early cleavage of sheep embryos. J Reprod Fertil. 1988;82:769–75.
52. Edwards LJ, Williams DA, Gardner DK. Intracellular pH of the mouse preimplantation embryo: amino acids act as buffers of intracellular pH. Hum Reprod. 1998;13:3441–8.
53. Liu Z, Foote RH. Development of bovine embryos in KSOM with added superoxide dismutase and taurine and with five and twenty percent O2. Biol Reprod. 1995;53:786–90.
54. Martin PM, Sutherland AE. Exogenous amino acids regulate trophectoderm differentiation in the mouse blastocyst through an mTOR-dependent pathway. Dev Biol. 2001;240:182–93.
55. Martin PM, Sutherland AE, Van Winkle LJ. Amino acid transport regulates blastocyst implantation. Biol Reprod. 2003;69:1101–8.
56. Lane M, Gardner DK. Differential regulation of mouse embryo development and viability by amino acids. J Reprod Fertil. 1997;109:153–64.
57. Houghton FD, Hawkhead JA, Humpherson PG, Hogg JE, Balen AH, Rutherford AJ, et al. Non-invasive amino acid turnover predicts human embryo developmental capacity. Hum Reprod. 2002;17:999–1005.
58. Brison DR, Houghton FD, Falconer D, Roberts SA, Hawkhead J, Humpherson PG, et al. Identification of viable embryos in IVF by non-invasive measurement

of amino acid turnover. Hum Reprod. 2004;19: 2319–24.
59. Picton HM, Elder K, Houghton FD, Hawkhead JA, Rutherford AJ, Hogg JE, et al. Association between amino acid turnover and chromosome aneuploidy during human preimplantation embryo development in vitro. Mol Hum Reprod. 2010;16:557–69.
60. Sturmey RG, Bermejo-Alvarez P, Gutierrez-Adan A, Rizos D, Leese HJ, Lonergan P. Amino acid metabolism of bovine blastocysts: a biomarker of sex and viability. Mol Reprod Dev. 2010;77:285–96.
61. Gardner DK. Changes in requirements and utilization of nutrients during mammalian preimplantation embryo development and their significance in embryo culture. Theriogenology. 1998;49:83–102.
62. Edwards LJ, Williams DA, Gardner DK. Intracellular pH of the preimplantation mouse embryo: effects of extracellular pH and weak acids. Mol Reprod Dev. 1998;50:434–42.
63. Mastroianni Jr L, Jones R. Oxygen tension within the rabbit fallopian tube. J Reprod Fertil. 1965;147: 99–102.
64. Ross RN, Graves CN. O_2 levels in female rabbit reproductive tract. J Anim Sci. 1974;39:994.
65. Fischer B, Bavister BD. Oxygen tension in the oviduct and uterus of rhesus monkeys, hamsters and rabbits. J Reprod Fertil. 1993;99:673–9.
66. Quinn P, Harlow GM. The effect of oxygen on the development of preimplantation mouse embryos in vitro. J Exp Zool. 1978;206:73–80.
67. Harlow GM, Quinn P. Foetal and placenta growth in the mouse after pre-implantation development in vitro under oxygen concentrations of 5 and 20%. Aust J Biol Sci. 1979;32:363–9.
68. Thompson JG, Simpson AC, Pugh PA, Donnelly PE, Tervit HR. Effect of oxygen concentration on in-vitro development of preimplantation sheep and cattle embryos. J Reprod Fertil. 1990;89:573–8.
69. Batt PA, Gardner DK, Cameron AW. Oxygen concentration and protein source affect the development of preimplantation goat embryos in vitro. Reprod Fertil Dev. 1991;3:601–7.
70. Wale PL, Gardner DK. Time-lapse analysis of mouse embryo development in oxygen gradients. Reprod Biomed Online. 2010;21:402–10.
71. Kovacic B, Vlaisavljevic V. Influence of atmospheric versus reduced oxygen concentration on development of human blastocysts in vitro: a prospective study on sibling oocytes. Reprod Biomed Online. 2008;17:229–36.
72. Kovacic B, Sajko MC, Vlaisavljevic V. A prospective, randomized trial on the effect of atmospheric versus reduced oxygen concentration on the outcome of intracytoplasmic sperm injection cycles. Fertil Steril. 2010;94:511–9.
73. Waldenstrom U, Engstrom AB, Hellberg D, Nilsson S. Low-oxygen compared with high-oxygen atmosphere in blastocyst culture, a prospective randomized study. Fertil Steril. 2009;91:2461–5.
74. Meintjes M, Chantilis SJ, Douglas JD, Rodriguez AJ, Guerami AR, Bookout DM, et al. A controlled randomized trial evaluating the effect of lowered incubator oxygen tension on live births in a predominantly blastocyst transfer program. Hum Reprod. 2009;24:300–7.
75. Rinaudo PF, Giritharan G, Talbi S, Dobson AT, Schultz RM. Effects of oxygen tension on gene expression in preimplantation mouse embryos. Fertil Steril. 2006; 86(4 Suppl):1252–65.
76. Katz-Jaffe MG, Linck DW, Schoolcraft WB, Gardner DK. A proteomic analysis of mammalian preimplantation embryonic development. Reproduction. 2005; 130:899–905.
77. Wale PL, Gardner DK. Oxygen regulates amino acid turnover and carbohydrate uptake during the preimplantation period of mouse embryo development. Biol Reprod. 2012;87:24, 1–8.
78. Leese HJ. Quiet please, do not disturb: a hypothesis of embryo metabolism and viability. Bioessays. 2002; 24:845–9.
79. Leese HJ, Baumann CG, Brison DR, McEvoy TG, Sturmey RG. Metabolism of the viable mammalian embryo: quietness revisited. Mol Hum Reprod. 2008; 14:667–72.
80. Ingerslev HJ, Hindkjaer J, Kirkegaard K. Effect of oxygen concentration on human embryo development evaluated by time-lapse monitoring. Hum Reprod. 2012;27:ii22–4.
81. Meseguer M, Tejera A, Herrero J, de los Santos M, Viloria T, Remohi J, et al. Oxygen consumption increases during cytokinesis in implanting human embryos; a time-lapse and microsensor combined analysis. Hum Reprod. 2012;27:ii22–4.
82. Donohoe DR, Bultman SJ. Metaboloepigenetics: interrelationships between energy metabolism and epigenetic control of gene expression. J Cell Physiol. 2012;227:3169–77.
83. Urbanski JP, Johnson MT, Craig DD, Potter DL, Gardner DK, Thorsen T. Noninvasive metabolic profiling using microfluidics for analysis of single preimplantation embryos. Anal Chem. 2008;80:6500–7.
84. Heo YS, Cabrera LM, Bormann CL, Smith GD, Takayama S. Real time culture and analysis of embryo metabolism using a microfluidic device with deformation based actuation. Lab Chip. 2012;12: 2240–6.
85. Lane M, Gardner DK. Lactate regulates pyruvate uptake and metabolism in the preimplantation mouse embryo. Biol Reprod. 2000;62:16–22.
86. Brinster RL. Lactate dehydrogenase activity in the preimplanted mouse embryo. Biochim Biophys Acta. 1965;110:439–41.
87. Auerbach S, Brinster RL. Lactate dehydrogenase isozymes in the early mouse embryo. Exp Cell Res. 1967;46:89–92.
88. Gibbons J, Hewitt E, Gardner DK. Effects of oxygen tension on the establishment and lactate dehydrogenase activity of murine embryonic stem cells. Cloning Stem Cells. 2006;8:117–22.
89. Wakefield SL, Lane M, Mitchell M. Impaired mitochondrial function in the preimplantation embryo perturbs fetal and placental development in the mouse. Biol Reprod. 2011;84:572–80.

90. Mazurek S. Pyruvate kinase type M2: a key regulator of the metabolic budget system in tumor cells. Int J Biochem Cell Biol. 2011;43:969–80.
91. Vander Heiden MG, Lunt SY, Dayton TL, Fiske BP, Israelsen WJ, Mattaini KR, et al. Metabolic pathway alterations that support cell proliferation. Cold Spring Harb Symp Quant Biol. 2011;76: 325–34.
92. Christofk HR, Vander Heiden MG, Harris MH, Ramanathan A, Gerszten RE, Wei R, et al. The M2 splice isoform of pyruvate kinase is important for cancer metabolism and tumour growth. Nature. 2008;452: 230–3.
93. Redel BK, Brown AN, Spate LD, Whitworth KM, Green JA, Prather RS. Glycolysis in preimplantation development is partially controlled by the Warburg effect. Mol Reprod Dev. 2012;79:262–71.
94. Hardy K, Spanos S. Growth factor expression and function in the human and mouse preimplantation embryo. J Endocrinol. 2002;172:221–36.
95. Hewitson LC, Leese HJ. Energy metabolism of the trophectoderm and inner cell mass of the mouse blastocyst. J Exp Zool. 1993;267:337–43.
96. Abu Dawud R, Schreiber K, Schomburg D, Adjaye J. Human embryonic stem cells and embryonal carcinoma cells have overlapping and distinct metabolic signatures. PLoS One. 2012;7:e39896.
97. Gardner DK, Wale PL. Analysis of metabolism to select viable human embryos for transfer. Fertil Steril. 2013;99:1062–72.

21 Analysis of Respiration as an Indicator of Oocyte and Embryo Developmental Potential

David L. Keefe

Women experience age-related decline in reproductive function even while other physiological systems continue to function at near peak capacity [1]. Fecundity declines beginning about 15 years before menopause and the last conception typically occurs about 10 years before menopause, even though thousands of primary oocytes remain within the ovary. Reproductive aging in women decreases the chances of conception, increases miscarriage and aneuploidy rates, and increases variability in fecundity among woman of the same chronological age. Fertility treatments that depend on the woman's own oocytes provide decreasing efficacy with reproductive aging, and donation of oocytes from younger to older women completely abrogates the effects of aging on reproduction, demonstrating the central role of the oocyte in reproductive aging.

Accurate prediction of oocyte quality, i.e., the capacity to produce a viable, normal offspring, is one of the most urgent priorities in infertility research today. Maternal age provides the best available predictor of oocyte quality, but as women age, the variability of oocyte quality among women of the same age increases, so measures of biological aging are needed. The localization of biological aging to a single cell, the oocyte, provides a unique opportunity to test hypotheses derived from model organisms about the cellular origins of aging. Moreover, the widespread use of ART by women of various ages provides a unique opportunity to apply newly available methods of noninvasive analysis of single cells to a pressing clinical problem.

D.L. Keefe (✉)
Department of Obstetrics and Gynecology, New York University School of Medicine, NYU Langone Medical Center, 550 First Avenue, NBVN91A, New York, NY 10016, USA
e-mail: david.keefe@nyumc.org

Mitochondria, Free Radicals, and the Pathophysiology of Aging

A number of pathobiological processes have been reported to underlie cellular aging and one of the most compelling involves disruption of respiration via mitochondrial dysfunction and associated free radical production [1, 2]. Mitochondria contain their own chromosomes and are transmitted exclusively through the female germ line. Indeed, oocytes are highly enriched in mitochondria compared to other cells in the body. Mitochondrial function has been linked to aging in many long lived, post-mitotic cell types. The mitochondrial genome is highly susceptible to free radicals and genotoxic damage. Mitochondria DNA (mtDNA) lacks nucleosomes and the DNA damage repair pathways that protect against oxidative stress over the course of an organism's life span [1]. MtDNA is localized within the organelle that primarily produces free radicals, which in turn promotes DNA mutations, exacerbates free radical production, and generates more mtDNA damage, creating a vicious cycle culminating in cell senescence and death.

D.K. Gardner et al. (eds.), *Human Gametes and Preimplantation Embryos: Assessment and Diagnosis*, DOI 10.1007/978-1-4614-6651-2_21, © Springer Science+Business Media New York 2013

Accumulation of mtDNA damage during the prolonged prophase I arrest of the oocytes provides a compelling explanation for age-related changes in the oocyte. Indeed, mtDNA mutations in oocytes and follicular cells increase with age [2, 5]. Advancing age reduces the capacity mitochondria to produce ATP [3] and the quality of preimplantation embryos is related to the ATP content [4]. The mtDNA in eggs of older women express the most common age-related deletion, a 5 kb deletion flanked by direct repeats [5]. In an attempt to model mitochondrial dysfunction in human embryos, chemically induced mitochondrial dysfunction [6] resulted in decreased ATP production, increased reactive oxygen, and gross chromosome misalignment on the meiotic spindle, culminating in cell death. Other studies have described a relationship between oocyte function and mtDNA content. Oocytes with lower total mtDNA content demonstrate poor development [7], and women with lower mtDNA copy number have lower ovarian reserve [8]. Depletion of mitochondria organelle numbers through selective knockout of essential genes in mice, such as *Tfam*, fail to affect ovarian reserve though they dramatically affect the ability to produce competent pregnancies [9].

The bottleneck theory of mtDNA inheritance suggests that primordial follicles contain a limited number of copies of mtDNA that expand to populate a new organism. As the germ cell passes from oogonia to oocyte, mtDNA copy number increases from 200 to hundreds of thousands [10]. Theoretically, limiting inheritance initially to a few copies with later expansion would allow oogenesis to select for high-quality mtDNA [11]. The consequence of selection for normal mitochondria would be deselection of abnormal mitochondria, cell death of germ cells, and infertility in the mother if no viable germ cells remain. While mtDNA pathology as a cause of reproductive aging is an attractive theory, a recent study suggests that selection of mitochondria in primordial follicles occurs randomly [12], allowing equal opportunity for transmission of mutant and normal mtDNA to subsequent generations. Moreover, women who harbor germ line mtDNA mutations and deliver offspring with severe mtDNA diseases appear to have normal fertility, arguing for a complex role of mtDNA in age-related oocyte dysfunction [13–15].

Oxygen Consumption by Oocytes and Preimplantation Embryos

Mitochondrial DNA can be damaged by oxidative stress, a wide variety of mtDNA rearrangements appear in oocytes from infertile women [16, 17] and the heteroplasmy of oocyte mtDNA challenges limits the ability of molecular genetic approaches to predict mitochondrial function noninvasively in individual oocytes and embryos. Measurements of oxygen consumption from oocytes and embryos, on the other hand, could provide a more direct and noninvasive assay of mitochondrial function.

The first oxygen measurements were taken from groups of mammalian oocytes and embryos over 70 years ago [18, 19]. A Cartesian diver technique showed groups of blastocysts consumed more oxygen than groups of cleavage-stage embryos. Changing the concentration of metabolic substrates in culture medium altered the amount of oxygen consumed by embryos [18–23]. Later studies employed microspectrophotometry to analyze spectral shifts in extracellular oxyhemoglobin resulting from oxygen consumption by embryos [24–26]. Stationary solid-state oxygen electrodes also have been employed to measure oxygen consumption from groups of embryos as well as from individual embryos. Overstrom et al. [27] and Magnusson et al. [24] independently employed spectrophotometry to show that embryos with higher rates of oxygen consumption developed to blastocysts at higher rates than those with lower oxygen consumption. Benos and Balaban [28] employed oxygen electrodes to demonstrate that 50–70 % of the oxygen consumed by blastocysts derived from oxidative phosphorylation (OXPHOS) to generate ATP for the plasma membrane Na/K-ATPase, and Manes and Lai [29] demonstrated that a significant part of the total oxygen consumed by embryos was not utilized by mitochondrial OXPHOS, but rather by

OXPHOS-independent oxygenases. Houghton et al. [30] used an ultrafluorescence technique to measure oxygen consumption in individual embryos and to study the association between metabolites secreted into culture media and consumption of oxygen by preimplantation embryos.

We applied a novel self-referencing oxygen sensor to assess oxygen consumption by individual oocytes and embryos. The self-referencing oxygen electrode [31, 32] provides noninvasive measurements of oxygen flux across the membranes of individual cells by measuring differences in the concentration of oxygen dissolved in the culture media at two locations, close and far from the cell, then uses Fick's Law to calculate flux. The self-referencing principle underlying this technology provides exquisite sensitivity and specificity. By moving the oxygen sensor between two positions, about 10 μm apart, the sensor serves as its own control, thus minimizing drift and other sources of electrophysiologic noise, which otherwise become problematic when dealing with the low signal-to-noise ratio of single cells. One excursion of the senor's oscillation measures oxygen concentration near the cell while the other excursion of the sensor's oscillation measures oxygen concentration at a position about 10 μm from the cell. Knowing the diffusion constant of oxygen in water, Fick's Law can be solved to calculate flux of oxygen into the embryo. This technique has been used to measure oxygen consumption from a variety of cell types [33], including oocytes and preimplantation embryos [34].

Our system used a Zeiss Axiovert 100 TV inverted microscope (Carl Zeiss, Inc., Thornwood, NY) equipped with a modified stage plate and computer-controlled micromanipulators (BioCurrents Research Center, MBL, Woods Hole, MA) [31–34]. The microscope rested on a Kinetic Systems Vibraplane vibration-resistant table (Boston, MA) enclosed in a stainless steel, insulated chamber. The temperature of the chamber and its contents, including the microscope and manipulators, was maintained at a constant 37 °C by a thermostat-controlled heater, purchased from an automobile supply store. We conducted physiological measurements in 4 mL of HEPES-buffered KSOM (HKSOM) containing reduced $NaHCO_3$ (4 mM) and elevated HEPES (14 mM) with no oil overlay and at atmospheric gas pressures. Recordings were obtained from embryos in plastic Petri dishes with a coverglass bottom (MatTek Corp., Ashland, MA) that enabled stabilization of the embryos on the dish, but also were easy to manipulate the embryo after completion of the study. Typically, we studied a set of four to six embryos in each dish, and obtained at least three independent recordings from each embryo over several minutes. We observed that mouse embryos exposed to these conditions developed to blastocysts and live pups at rates similar to control embryos not exposed to measurements of oxygen consumption. In the absence of intentional perturbations, the oxygen gradients around embryos measured by the self-referencing oxygen electrode remained stable throughout experimental measurement periods lasting over 1 h.

Oxygen-sensitive electrodes with a tip diameter of 2–4 μm were purchased from Diamond General Corp. (Ann Arbor, MI) [33, 34]. A silver/silver chloride reference electrode completed the electrical circuit in solution via a 3 mol L^{-1} KCl/3 % agar bridge. All electrodes were calibrated both in saturated oxygen (high range) and saturated nitrogen solutions (low range). During recordings, the electrode was oscillated in a square wave parallel to the electrode axis over a distance of 10 μm with a frequency of 0.3 Hz. Initially, the near position of this oscillation was 1.5–2.5 μm from the zona pellucida or plasma membrane in cases where the zona pellucida was removed by brief pronase (0.5 % in HKSOM) digestion. Mathematical modeling of the gradients around embryos, however, suggested that more reliable signals could be obtained at a distance of 6 μm away from embryos. Accordingly, all subsequent recordings were obtained at this distance. The hardware and software controlling electrode movements, signal amplification, and data acquisition were designed and constructed by the BioCurrents Research Center at the Marine Biological Laboratory, Woods Hole, MA (www.mbl.edu/BioCurrents [case sensitive]) [31–34]. The lower limit of detection, with a signal-to-noise ratio of 3, was approximately a 0.01 μM difference in oxygen concentration between the two excursion points, and the oxygen signals were greater than ten times this lower detection limit. We also captured digital images of embryos using a Cohu analog video camera (Cambridge Research Instruments, Cambridge, MA) and a personal computer running Metamorph Software (Universal Imaging Corp., West Chester, PA).

The self-referencing oxygen electrode measures oxygen consumption noninvasively, so it can be used in conjunction with other single-cell techniques, such as polarized light and Nomarski differential interference light microscopy, polymerase chain reaction (PCR) of mtDNA deletions [17], metabolite-uptake/lactate-secretion assays [35–37], mitochondria redistribution dynamics [38], preimplantation genetic diagnosis [39, 40], in vivo protein dynamic studies using green-fluorescent protein (GFP) [41], and fluorescence resonance energy transfer (FRET) [42]. The ability of self-referencing oxygen electrode technique to measure subtle changes in oxygen consumption from individual embryos also makes it more sensitive to detect changes that otherwise might be hidden in the variation endogenous to groups of asynchronous embryos and may eventually provide a diagnostic tool for assessing the level of mitochondria dysfunction and developmental potential of individual embryos.

We used this method to investigate the effects of a number of experimental interventions on oxygen consumption by oocytes and preimplantation mouse embryos. We treated oocytes and preimplantation mouse embryos with mitochondrial toxins, various metabolic substrates in the culture media, and cell death-inducing agents known to collapse the mitochondrial membrane potential [35]. mtDNA rearrangements had not yet been reported in wild-type or genetically engineered mouse oocytes, so we could not test our original hypothesis, that mtDNA mutations could be detected noninvasively by preimplantation mouse embryos using oxygen consumption. Instead we employed pharmacological agents to perturb OXPHOS in mouse embryos. This allowed us to study the contributions of mitochondrial OXPHOS-dependent and OXPHOS-independent processes to total oxygen consumption of individual oocytes and preimplantation mouse embryos.

To study the effects of perturbing mitochondrial function on oxygen flux, we added concentrated solutions of the experimental compounds calculated to yield the final desired concentrations: 1 μM FCCP, 1 μM antimycin A, 1 mM sodium cyanide, 0.01 % solvent. To disrupt mitochondria and induce cell death, we pretreated embryos with diamide for 3 h [43]. To investigate the influence of metabolic substrates such as pyruvate on oxygen consumption, we studied embryos incubated overnight in pyruvate-free KSOM and compared them to controls cultured overnight in pyruvate-containing KSOM.

Embryos came from female B6C3F1 mice (6 weeks old) superovulated by standard methods using PMSG and hCG, and mated individually. Zygotes (~30/animal) enclosed in cumulus masses were released from the ampullae into HKSOM supplemented with 0.03 % hyaluronidase. Cumulus cells were gently removed from one-cell embryos by pipetting. Cumulus-free one-cell embryos were washed in HKSOM three times and then in pre-equilibrated modified KSOM three times. Modified KSOM used for in vitro culture was supplemented with nonessential amino acids (1 mL of 100× stock/100 mL medium) and 2.5 mM HEPES. Embryos were pooled, randomly distributed, and cultured in 50-μL droplets (7–16 embryos/drop) under mineral oil at 37 °C in a humidified atmosphere of 7 % CO_2 in air. These methods provided a high yield of development to blastocysts (>90 %) and after transfer they developed to term at the same rate whether exposed to oxygen measurements or not.

Oxygen Flux from Individual Preimplantation Mouse Embryos

The concentration of dissolved oxygen in the medium surrounding individual mouse embryos could be measured reliably and remained stable during experimental recordings, which lasted up to 1 h. The concentration of dissolved oxygen in the culture medium near the one-cell embryos was reduced by 0.33 ± 0.07 μM relative to that of the rest of the culture media (0.21 mM), such that a gradient of depleted dissolved oxygen surrounded each embryo (Fig. 1a). The concentration of oxygen in the medium was less depleted at increasing distances from embryos, but a gradient in the concentration of dissolved oxygen concentration could be measured at distances of over 10 μm away from the embryo (Fig. 2).

The oxygen gradient changed across preimplantation embryo development. The oxygen gradient around two-cell embryos (−0.43 ± 0.10 μM, $n = 22$) compared to media surrounding one-cell embryos (−0.33 ± 0.07 μM, $n = 8$) (Fig. 1b).

The variable cell size of blastomeres across preimplantation development provides a potential confounder in these experiments. The radius of blastomeres in two-cell embryos (26.9 ± 0.6 μm; $n = 22$) is less than the radius of one-cell embryos (37.3 ± 0.7 μm; $n = 16$). The position of the oxygen sensor relative to the geometric center of the specimen, therefore, differs among embryos at different developmental stages. To adjust for these geometric differences at different stages of preimplantation embryo development, we derived a mathematical function to control for these geometric differences (Fig. 2b). The only assumption intrinsic to this function was that oxygen consumption would be relatively homogeneous around each embryo. Actual measurements from different locations around embryos confirmed this assumption.

We obtained a series of 120 measurements at various distances (>6 μm) from nine blastocysts, and a standard curve was generated with the function:

$$f = 0.015 + 0.461 \times e^{(-0.028 \times x)} \quad (1)$$

where x is the distance from the electrode tip to the geometric center of the cell as determined from images of embryos taken at an equatorial focal plane (Fig. 2b). Scaling to a common radius of 40 μm occurred by (2).

$$\text{scaled } \Delta[O_2] = (\text{measured } \Delta[O_2] / [0.015 + 0.461 \times e^{(-0.028 \times x)}]) \times [0.015 + 0.461 \times e^{(-0.028 \times 40)}] \quad (2)$$

We validated this set of equations in more than a dozen subsequent experiments on over 80 embryos at various developmental stages, with and without removal of zona pellucidae, and in each case the data fit this function. We found that one-, two-, and four-cell embryos exhibited similar levels of oxygen gradients, about 0.3 μM. Oxygen gradients around blastocysts, in contrast, were about two times greater than those surrounding cleavage-stage embryos, 0.6 ± 0.1 μM (Fig. 1b).

To calculate oxygen consumption by each individual embryos, Fick's law was used to calculate flux = oxygen diffusion coefficient × ($\Delta[O_2]$/probe excursion) [31–34]. Oxygen consumption by individual cleavage-stage embryos was 7.7 pmol O_2 cm^{-2} h^{-1} (or 0.1 nL embryo^{-1} h^{-1}) and by individual blastocysts was 15.8 pmol O_2 cm^{-2} h^{-1} (or 0.3 nL embryo^{-1} h^{-1}).

Oxygen gradients among embryos showed normal distribution with a median (±95 % confidence intervals) of 0.31 ± 0.03 μM and range of 0.27–0.41 μM (Fig. 3). Ninety percent of two-cell embryos reached the blastocyst stage of development. We did not observe a correlation between oxygen consumption and the probability of reaching blastocyst, but almost all the mouse embryos reached blastocyst, so the experimental paradigm was not optimal for answering this question.

Contribution of OXPHOS to Oxygen Consumption

Oxygen consumption could result from OXPHOS and/or oxygen consumption by OXPHOS-independent oxygenases within embryos. To determine the relative contributions of OXPHOS

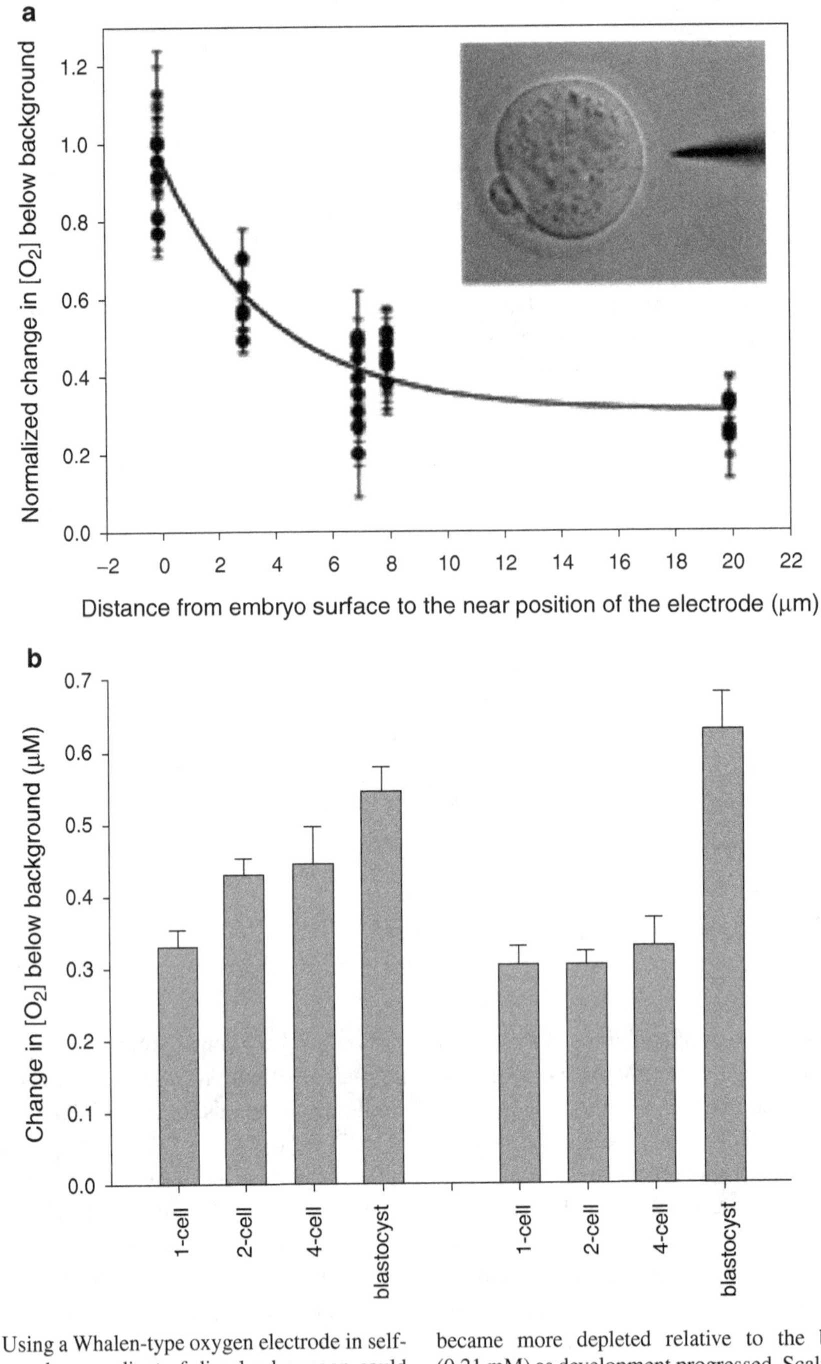

Fig. 21.1 Using a Whalen-type oxygen electrode in self-referencing mode, a gradient of dissolved oxygen could be measured around individual embryos. (**a**) The gradient of depleted oxygen extended tens of microns into the medium away from one-cell embryos ($n=7$). The closest probe position (0) was 0.25–0.75 µm away from the zona pellucida surface. Each point is the mean ± standard deviation of >25 samples taken during a 3–5-min period of self-referencing with the electrode position nearest to the embryo plotted. (*Inset*) Image of a mouse one-cell embryo and juxtaposed oxygen electrode. (**b**) Different developmental stages depleted the surrounding medium of oxygen to different extents ($n=7$–22 for each group). The concentration of oxygen in the medium nearest embryos became more depleted relative to the bulk medium (0.21 mM) as development progressed. Scaling of the data to account for variations in embryo size (see text) demonstrated that the medium surrounding blastocysts was twice as depleted of oxygen as that surrounding cleavage-stage embryos, suggesting at least a twofold increase in oxygen consumption by blastocysts. Data are presented as the change in dissolved oxygen concentration near embryos relative to that of the bulk medium (background = 0.21 mM) (From Trimarchi JR, Liu L, Porterfield DM, Smith PJ, Keefe DL. Oxidative phosphorylation-dependent and -independent oxygen consumption by individual preimplantation mouse embryos. Biol Reprod. 2000 Jun;62(6):1866–74, with permission)

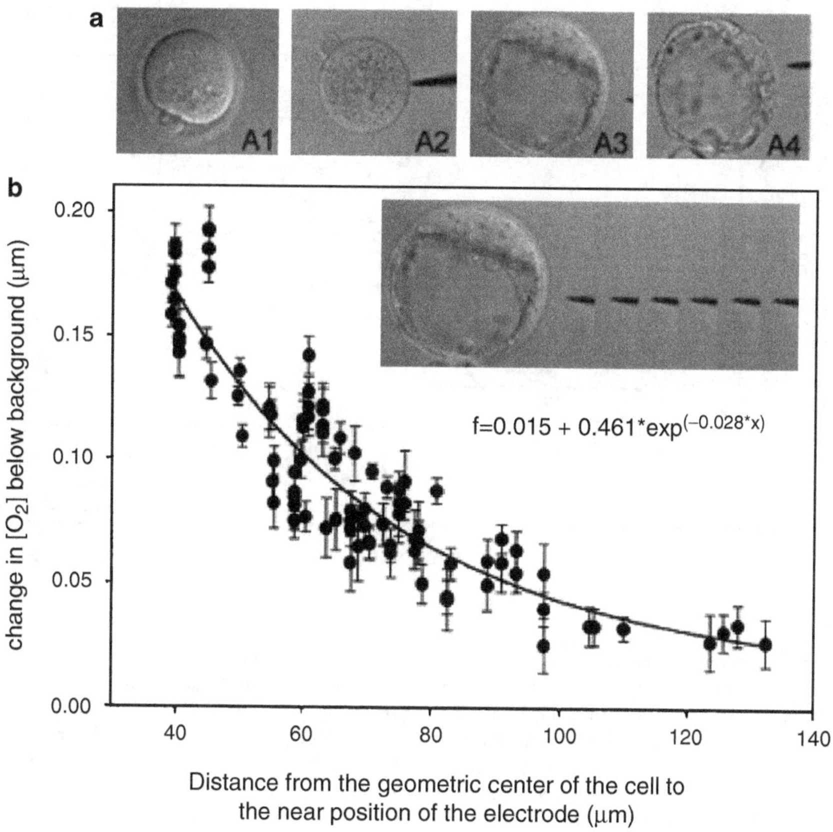

Fig. 21.2 Quantification of oxygen consumption by embryos that varied in size required a mathematical scaling function. (**a**) Embryos of different developmental stages exhibit significantly different radii. (A1) One-cell embryo, zona pellucida intact. (A2) One-cell embryo, zona pellucida remove. (A3) Blastocysts, zona pellucida intact. (A4) Blastocysts, zona pellucida removed. Removal of the zona did not alter the embryo morphology or the surrounding oxygen gradients. Dark point in A2–A4 was the oxygen-selective electrode. (**b**) A mathematical function was determined that allowed oxygen gradients surrounding embryos of different sizes to be adjusted geometrically and quantitatively compared. A series of 120 measurements were obtained at various distances (>6 μM) from nine blastocysts that ranged in radii from 32 to 62 μm, and a standard curve was fitted with the equation noted. Data presented as the change in dissolved oxygen concentration near embryos relative to that of the bulk medium (background = 0.2102 mM). Each point is the mean ± standard deviation of >25 samples taken during a 3–5-min period of self-referencing with the electrode position nearest to the embryo plotted as the distance from geometric center of the embryo. (*Inset*) Oxygen electrode at various distances from a blastocyst

and non-OXPHOS oxygen consumption, we measured oxygen consumption before and after exposure to various pharmacological agents known to perturb OXPHOS. FCCP increases oxygen consumption by uncoupling the proton gradient from OXPHOS and sodium cyanide and antimycin A reduce mitochondrial oxygen consumption by blocking OXPHOS electron flow [43]. We found that FCCP (1 μM) increased oxygen consumption (Fig. 4a, b) by 89.2 ± 31.2 % compared to pre-FCCP treatment. The effect of FCCP on oxygen consumption in blastocysts was more modest compared to its effect on cleavage stage embryos, showing a 49.5 ± 25.9 % increase in oxygen consumption compared to pre-FCCP treatment.

Cyanide (1 mM) and antimycin A (1 μM) decreased oxygen consumption by embryos (Fig. 4a, b), with 77 % of oxygen consumption by cleavage-stage embryos cyanide/antimycin A resistant. Oxygen consumption by cleavage stage embryos was 60–70 % less sensitive to

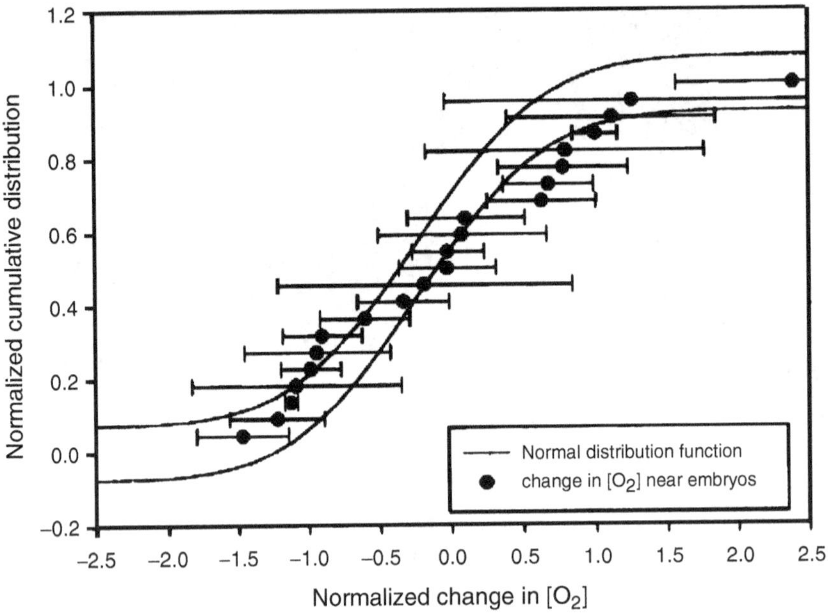

Fig. 21.3 Oxygen-gradient measurements from a population of 22 two-cell embryos exhibited a normal distribution as evident by an overlap between the standard error bars for the normalized change in oxygen concentration surrounding each embryo and the 95 % confidence intervals of a normal distribution function (*gray lines*) in a Kolmogorov-Smirnov plot. There appeared to be no obvious correlation between the magnitude of the oxygen gradient around an embryo and its developmental competence (see text) (From Trimarchi JR, Liu L, Porterfield DM, Smith PJ, Keefe DL. Oxidative phosphorylation-dependent and -independent oxygen consumption by individual preimplantation mouse embryos. Biol Reprod. 2000 Jun;62(6):1866–74, with permission)

cyanide and antimycin A compared to blastocysts, suggesting higher rates of OXPHOS-related oxygen consumption in blastocysts (Fig. 4b). Interestingly, the level of OXPHOS-independent oxygen consumption remained relatively constant across preimplantation embryo development, while mitochondrial OXPHOS-dependent oxygen consumption doubled from the cleavage- to blastocyst stages of development (Fig. 4c).

Pyruvate Concentration in the Culture Media Modulates Oxygen Consumption by the Embryo

Culturing embryos overnight from the late one-cell to the two-cell stage in pyruvate-free KSOM (pyruvate-free embryos) reduced oxygen consumption compared to control embryos cultured overnight in pyruvate-containing media (0.2 mM) (Fig. 5). This difference in the degree of oxygen consumption was partially masked by the smaller size of pyruvate-free embryos, which allowed positioning of the electrode closer to the center of pyruvate-free embryos, thereby artifactually increasing the signal (Fig. 5a). After controlling for embryo size, oxygen consumption around embryos cultured in pyruvate-free media was 26 % less than those cultured in media containing pyruvate.

Diamide Oxidation Modulates Oxygen Consumption

Diamide, a glutathione oxidizing agent, induces cell death in mammalian embryos [35]. Exposure to diamide (50 μM) for 3 h significantly reduced oxygen consumption. After controlling for size differences among embryos, diamide treatment of one-cell embryos decreased oxygen consumption by 32 % (0.12 ± 0.02 μM vs. 0.18 ± 0.01 μM, $P<0.005$).

In summary, the self-referencing oxygen electrode technique can measure oxygen consumption by individual oocytes and preimplantation

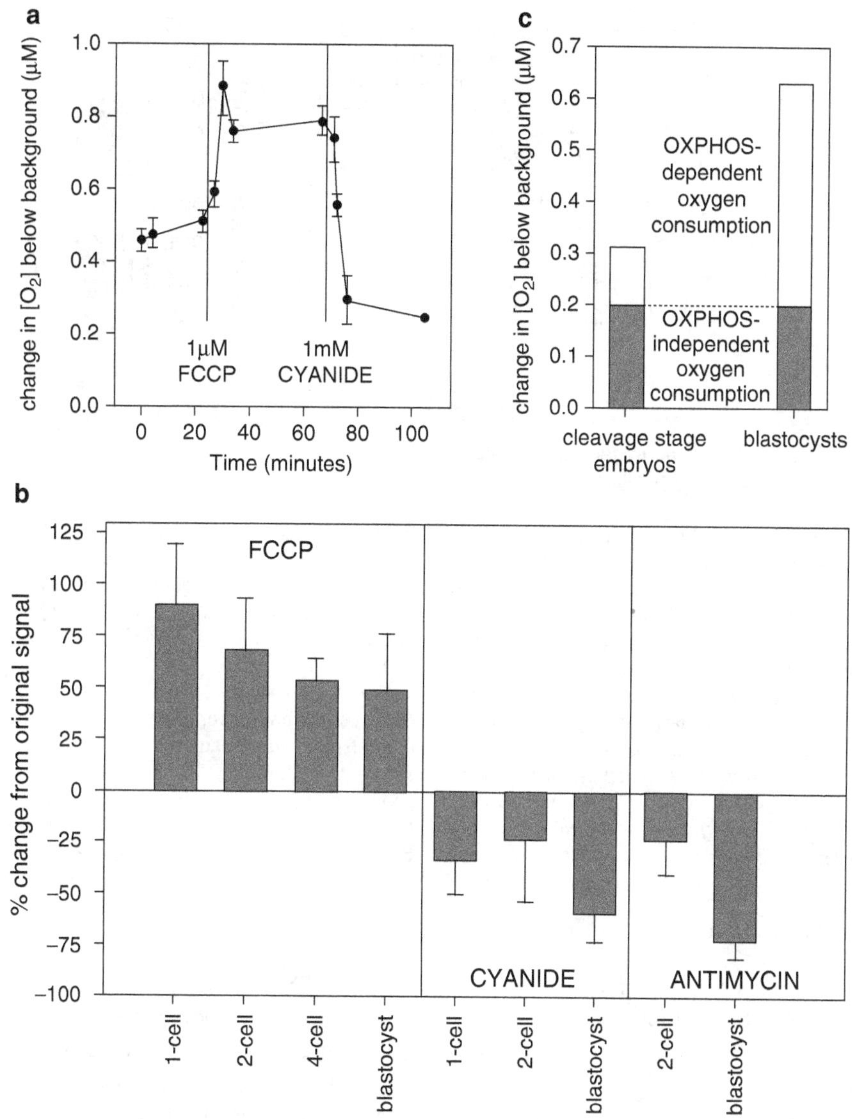

Fig. 21.4 Mitochondrial toxins modulated the oxygen consumed by embryos. (**a**) The FCCP (1 μM) rapidly increased and cyanide (1 mM) quickly decreased the oxygen consumed by an individual blastocyst as evident by alterations in the dissolved oxygen concentration in the surrounding medium relative to that of the bulk medium. Each point is the mean ± standard deviation of >25 samples taken during a 3–5-min period of self-referencing and plotted at the median sample time. (**b**) The FCCP (1 μM) increased oxygen consumption by cleavage-stage embryos and blastocysts. Cyanide (1 mM) and antimycin A (1 μM) greatly decreased oxygen consumption by blastocysts but only modestly decreased oxygen consumption by cleavage-stage embryos (single factor ANOVA, cyanide, $P<0.03$; antimycin A, P 0.01). Mean ± standard deviation; $n=22$ FCCP-treated embryos with more than 4 embryos in each group, $n=15$ cyanide-treated embryos with more than 4 embryos in each group $n=16$ antimycin A-treated embryos with more than 6 embryos in each group. (**c**) Calculations of the contribution of OXPHOS-dependent and OXPHOS-independent oxygen consumption, based upon FCCP, cyanide, and antimycin A data. The majority of oxygen consumed by cleavage-stage embryos was not utilized by OXPHOS (OXPHOS-independent oxygen consumption), whereas the majority of oxygen consumed by blastocysts was utilized by OXPHOS (OXPHOS-dependent oxygen consumption). The OXPHOS-independent oxygen consumption remains relatively constant throughout development, while OXPHOS in blastocysts consumed six times more oxygen than did OXPHOS of cleavage-stage embryos. Data are presented as the change in the dissolved oxygen concentration near embryos relative to that of the bulk medium (background = 0.21 mM) (From Trimarchi JR, Liu L, Porterfield DM, Smith PJ, Keefe DL. Oxidative phosphorylation-dependent and -independent oxygen consumption by individual preimplantation mouse embryos. Biol Reprod. 2000 Jun;62(6):1866–74, with permission)

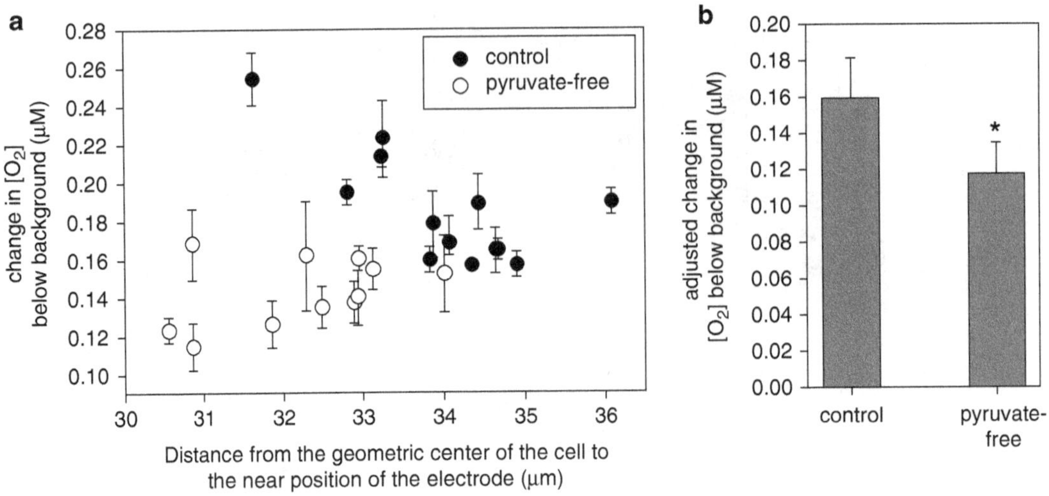

Fig. 21.5 Late one-cell embryos cultured overnight in pyruvate-free medium, cleaved to two cells but consumed less oxygen than did control embryos cultured in medium containing 0.2 mM pyruvate. Data are presented as the change in dissolved oxygen concentration near embryos relative to that of the bulk medium (background = 0.21 mM). (**a**) Unscaled data illustrating the relationship between, treatment, embryo size, and change in oxygen concentration of the medium near embryos. Each point is the mean ± standard deviation of >25 samples taken during a 3–5-min period of self-referencing with the electrode position nearest to the embryo plotted as the distance from the embryo center. Measurements were taken 6 μm away from the surface of embryos from which the zona had been removed ($n = 11$ pyruvate-free embryos, 13 control embryos). Pyruvate-free embryos were smaller and consumed less oxygen than did control embryos. (**b**) Scaling of data from A using the mathematical function described in the text demonstrated that control embryos depleted the surrounding medium of 26 % more oxygen than did embryos cultured overnight in pyruvate-free medium (mean ± standard deviation; $P << 0.005$) (From Trimarchi JR, Liu L, Porterfield DM, Smith PJ, Keefe DL. Oxidative phosphorylation-dependent and -independent oxygen consumption by individual preimplantation mouse embryos. Biol Reprod. 2000 Jun;62(6):1866–74, with permission)

embryos. This gradient can be measured even as far as 50 μm from the embryo surface. Embryos group cultured in microdrops, therefore, presumably could influence the concentration of oxygen for their neighboring embryos. This physiological interaction between embryos in culture may account, in part, for the enhanced development of embryos cultured in groups vs. individually [44, 45]. Blastocysts consume two to four times more oxygen than cleavage-stage embryos [20–23, 30, 46]. The proportion of total oxygen consumed by OXPHOS-dependent and OXPHOS-independent processes changes across preimplantation development [21, 23, 30, 46–48], with the bulk (70 %) of oxygen consumed by blastocysts fueling OXPHOS, as evidenced by its cyanide-sensitivity [21, 28]. This finding is consistent with changes in the morphology of mitochondria reported in blastocysts. Benos and Balaban [28] estimated that 50–70 % of oxygen consumed by blastocysts was used by mitochondria to generate ATP for the Na/K-ATPase. Only 20–30 % of oxygen consumed by cleavage-stage embryos is OXPHOS-dependent, suggesting that OXPHOS-independent oxygenases contribute significantly to their oxygen consumption. OXPHOS-independent oxygen consumption by blastocysts contributes to surface H_2O_2 production [49] and H_2O_2-producing oxygenases [29]. Because cleavage-stage embryos produce only limited amounts of H_2O_2 [38] the two mixed, multifunctional oxidase systems functioning in cleavage-stage embryos [50, 51] could contribute to the OXPHOS-independent oxygen consumption at this developmental stage. The OXPHOS-dependent/OXPHOS-independent ratio of 30 %/70 % in cleavage-stage embryos and 70 %/30 % in blastocysts is consistent with prior investigations using different methods to measure oxygen consumption [47, 48] and with studies of oxygen consumption by somatic cells [52, 53]. Our observations of OXPHOS-independent oxygen consumption during early development and OXPHOS-dependent oxygen consumption in the blastocyst are consistent with morphological changes of mitochondria across preimplantation embryo development. Mitochondria in oocytes and early embryos have reduced cristae and blastocytes have swollen cristae [54–59]. The number of mitochondria and copies of mtDNA [56–61], and the concentration of OXPHOS enzymes also increase in blastocysts [62, 63]. Total ATP content and ATP/ADP+ P ratio decrease in blastocysts, which would be expected to stimulate OXPHOS [47, 64, 65]. Metabolic substrate preferences also change across development [30, 36, 37, 46–48, 66, 67]. At the two-cell stage, when mitochondria are condensed, and total ATP content, as well as the ATP/ADP ratio high, pyruvate provides the preferred energy substrate, lactate secretion is low, total oxygen consumption is low, and OXPHOS-independent mechanisms account for the majority of oxygen consumption. By blastocyst stage mitochondria exhibit extensive cristae, high concentrations of OXPHOS enzymes, and low total ATP content and ATP/ADP ratio. These stimulate aerobic glycolysis and OXPHOS-dependent mechanisms that increase lactate secretion and oxygen consumption.

Oxygen Consumption to Predict Embryo Outcome

Magnusson et al. [24] suggested that human blastocysts consuming more oxygen developed to blastocysts at higher rates than those consuming less oxygen. Overstrom et al. [27] confirmed this result in bovine blastocysts. Studying healthy mouse embryos cultured in the robust culture media KSOM, we could not find a significant association between oxygen consumption and embryo development, but nearly all the embryos developed to blastocyst. Consistent with the findings of Magnusson et al. and Overstrom et al., we demonstrated that healthy control one-cell embryos and blastocysts consumed more oxygen than those undergoing cell death. Since the early phases of cell death are associated with changes in mitochondria [35, 68, 69], and changes in oxygen consumption were detectable only 3 h after treatment with an agent (diamide) known to induce death of embryos [35], these results suggest that changes in oxygen consumption might be indicative of disruptions in mitochondria and a decline in developmental competence.

Various modifications of the self-referencing oxygen sensor have demonstrated the ability to predict embryo fate in preclinical and clinical settings. A modification of the self-referencing probe concept, which measures the oxygen gradients of embryos placed inside glass capillaries rather than in bulk media, found that the respiration rates of individual bovine embryos provided information that was complementary to embryo morphology [70]. Later studies on bovine embryos established that the method did not appear to disrupt embryo viability, that in vitro produced bovine embryos had higher respiration rates than in vivo produced bovine embryos [71], and that the sex of the embryo did not influence its respiration [72]. Oxygen consumption by embryos appears to be affected by ovarian stimulation regimens. A self-referencing oxygen sensor demonstrated decreased oxygen consumption in vitrified blastocysts after warming compared to control blastocysts [73, 74]. In summary, while much work remains, the self-referencing oxygen sensor holds promise to provide a noninvasive physiologic assay of embryo viability [75].

References

1. Wilding M, Di Matteo L, Dale B. The maternal age effect: a hypothesis based on oxidative phosphorylation. Zygote. 2005;13(4):317–23.
2. Seifer DB, DeJesus V, Hubbard K. Mitochondrial deletions in luteinized granulosa cells as a function of age in women undergoing in vitro fertilization. Fertil Steril. 2002;78(5):1046–8.
3. Shigenaga MK, Hagen TM, Ames BN. Oxidative damage and mitochondrial decay in aging. Proc Natl Acad Sci USA. 1994;91(23):10771–8.

4. Van Blerkom J, Davis PW, Lee J. ATP content of human oocytes and developmental potential and outcome after in-vitro fertilization and embryo transfer. Hum Reprod. 1995;10(2):415–24.
5. Keefe DL et al. Mitochondrial deoxyribonucleic acid deletions in oocytes and reproductive aging in women. Fertil Steril. 1995;64(3):577–83.
6. Thouas GA et al. Mitochondrial dysfunction in mouse oocytes results in preimplantation embryo arrest in vitro. Biol Reprod. 2004;71(6):1936–42.
7. Reynier P et al. Mitochondrial DNA content affects the fertilizability of human oocytes. Mol Hum Reprod. 2001;7(5):425–9.
8. May-Panloup P et al. Low oocyte mitochondrial DNA content in ovarian insufficiency. Hum Reprod. 2005;20(3):593–7.
9. Wai T et al. The role of mitochondrial DNA copy number in mammalian fertility. Biol Reprod. 2010; 83(1):52–62.
10. Wai T, Teoli D, Shoubridge EA. The mitochondrial DNA genetic bottleneck results from replication of a subpopulation of genomes. Nat Genet. 2008;40(12): 1484–8.
11. Bentov Y et al. The contribution of mitochondrial function to reproductive aging. J Assist Reprod Genet. 2011;28(9):773–83.
12. Inoue K et al. Generation of mice with mitochondrial dysfunction by introducing mouse mtDNA carrying a deletion into zygotes. Nat Genet. 2000;26(2):176–81.
13. Pikó L, Matsumoto L. Number of mitochondria and some properties of mitochondrial DNA in the mouse egg. Dev Biol. 1976;49:1–10.
14. Jansen RP, de Boer K. The bottleneck: mitochondrial imperatives in oogenesis and ovarian follicular fate. Mol Cell Endocrinol. 1998;145:81–8.
15. Taanman JW. The mitochondrial genome: structure, transcription, translation and replication. Biochim Biophys Acta. 1999;1410:103–23.
16. Keefe DL, Niven-Fairchild T, Powell S, Buradagunta S. mtDNA deletion in oocytes and reproductive aging in women. Fertil Steril. 1995;64:577–83.
17. Barritt JA, Brenner CA, Cohen J, Matt DW. Mitochondrial DNA rearrangements in human oocytes and embryos. Mol Hum Reprod. 1999;5:927–33.
18. Dragiou I, Benetato G, Opreanu R. Recherches sur la respiration des ovocytes des mammiféres. C R Soc Biol. 1937;126:1044–6.
19. Boell EJ, Needham J. Morphogenesis and metabolism: studies with the Cartesian diver apparatus I, II, III, IV. Proc R Soc Lond (B). 1939;127:322–87.
20. Boell EJ, Nicholas JS. Respiratory metabolism of mammalian eggs and embryos. Anat Rec. 1939; 75(Suppl):66.
21. Fridhandler I, Hafez ESE, Pincus G. Developmental changes in the respiratory activity of rabbit ova. Exp Cell Res. 1957;13:132–9.
22. Boell EJ, Nicholas JS. Respiratory metabolism of the mammalian egg. J Exp Zool. 1948;109:267–81.
23. Mills RM, Brinster RL. Oxygen consumption of preimplantation mouse embryos. Exp Cell Res. 1967;47: 337–44.
24. Magnusson C, Hillensjö T, Hamberger L, Nillson L. Oxygen consumption by human oocytes and blastocysts grown in vitro. Hum Reprod. 1986;1:183–4.
25. Magnusson C, Hillensjö T, Tsafriri A, Hultborn R, Ahrén K. Oxygen consumption of maturing rat ovaries. Biol Reprod. 1977;17:9–15.
26. Nilsson BO, Magnusson C, Widéhn S, Hillensjö T. Correlation between blastocysts oxygen consumption and trophoblast cytochrome oxidase reaction and initiation of implantation of delayed mouse blastocysts. J Embryol Exp Morphol. 1982;71:75–82.
27. Overstrom EW, Duby RT, Dobrinsky J, Roche JF, Boland MP. Viability and oxidative metabolism of the bovine blastocyst. Theriogenology. 1992;37:269.
28. Benos DJ, Balaban RS. Energy requirements of the developing mammalian blastocyst for active ion transport. Biol Reprod. 1980;23:941–7.
29. Manes C, Lai NC. Nonmitochondrial oxygen utilization by rabbit blastocysts and surface production of superoxide radicals. J Reprod Fertil. 1995;104:69–75.
30. Houghton FD, Thompson JG, Kennedy CJ, Leese HJ. Oxygen consumption and energy metabolism of the early mouse embryo. Mol Reprod Dev. 1996;44: 476–85.
31. Smith PJS. The non-invasive probes—tools for measuring transmembrane ion flux. Nature. 1995;378: 645–6.
32. Smith PJS, Hammar K, Porterfield DM, Sanger RH, Trimarchi JR. A self-referencing, non-invasive, ion-selective electrode for single cell detection of trans-plasma membrane calcium flux. Microsc Res Tech. 1999;46:398–417.
33. Land SC, Porterfield DM, Sanger RH, Smith PJS. The self-referencing oxygen-selective microelectrode: detection of transmembrane oxygen flux from single cells. J Exp Biol. 1999;202:211–8.
34. Porterfield DM, Trimarchi JR, Keefe DL, Smith PJS. Characterization of oxygen and calcium fluxes from early mouse embryos and oocytes. Biol Bull. 1998;195:208–9.
35. Liu L, Trimarchi JR, Keefe DL. Thiol oxidation-induced embryonic cell death in mice is prevented by the antioxidant dithiothreitol. Biol Reprod. 1999;61: 1162–9.
36. Lane M, Gardner DK. Selection of viable mouse blastocysts prior to transfer using metabolic criterion. Hum Reprod. 1996;11:1975–96.
37. Gott AL, Hardy K, Winston RM, Leese HJ. Non-invasive measurement of pyruvate and glucose uptake and lactate production by single human preimplantation embryos. Hum Reprod. 1990;5:104–8.
38. Wokosin DL, White JG, Bavister BD, Squirrell JM. Long-term two-photon fluorescence imaging of mammalian embryos without compromising viability. Nat Biotechnol. 1999;17:763–7.
39. Ray PF, Ao A, Taylor DM, Winston RM, Handyside AH. Assessment of the reliability of single blastomere analysis for preimplantation diagnosis of the delta F508 deletion causing cystic fibrosis in clinical practice. Prenat Diagn. 1998;18:1402–12.

40. Muggleton-Harris AL, Glazier AM, Pickering S, Wall M. Genetic diagnosis using polymerase chain reaction and fluorescent in-situ hybridization analysis of biopsied cells from both the cleavage and blastocyst stages of individual cultured human preimplantation embryos. Hum Reprod. 1995;10:183–92.
41. Emmanouilidou E, Teschemacher AG, Pouli AE, Nicholls LI, Seward EP, Rutter GA. Imaging Ca(2+) concentration changes at the secretory vesicle surface with a recombinant targeted cameleon. Curr Biol. 1999;9:915–8.
42. Pollok BA, Heim R. Using GFP in FRET-based applications. Trends Cell Biol. 1999;9:57–60.
43. Stryer L. Biochemistry. New York: WH Freeman and Company; 1988.
44. Moessner J, Dodson WC. The quality of human embryo growth is improved when embryos are cultured in groups rather than separately. Fertil Steril. 1995;64:1034–5.
45. Gardner DK, Lane MW, Lane M. Development of the inner cell mass in mouse blastocysts is stimulated by reducing the embryo:incubation volume ratio. Hum Reprod. 1997;12:182–3.
46. Fridhandler L. Pathways of glucose metabolism in fertilized rabbit ova at various pre-implantation stages. Exp Cell Res. 1961;22:303–16.
47. Biggers JD, Borland RM. Physiological aspects of growth and development of the preimplantation embryo. Annu Rev Physiol. 1976;38:95–119.
48. Leese HJ. Metabolic control during preimplantation mammalian development. Hum Reprod Update. 1995;1:63–72.
49. Manes C. Cyanide-resistant reduction of nitroblue tetrazolium and hydrogen peroxide production by the rabbit blastocyst. Mol Reprod Dev. 1992;31:114–21.
50. Balling R, Haaf H, Maydl R, Metzler M, Beier HM. Oxidative and conjugative metabolism of diethylstilbestrol by rabbit preimplantation embryos. Dev Biol. 1985;109:370–4.
51. Filler R, Lew KJ. Developmental onset of mixed function oxidase activity in preimplantation embryos. Proc Natl Acad Sci USA. 1981;78:6991–5.
52. Curnutte JT, Babior BM. Chronic granulomatous disease. Adv Hum Genet. 1987;16:229–97.
53. Kumar S, Acharya SK. 2,6-Dichloro-phenol indophenol prevents switch-over of electrons between the cyanide-sensitive and -insensitive pathway of the mitochondrial electron transport chain in the presence of inhibitors. Anal Biochem. 1999;268:89–93.
54. Mackler B, Grace R, Haynes B, Bargman GJ, Shepard TH. Studies of mitochondrial energy systems during embryogenesis in the rat. Arch Biochem Biophys. 1973;158:885–8.
55. Shepard TH, Muffley LA, Smith LT. Ultrastructural study of mitochondria and their cristae on embryonic rats and primates (*N. nemistrina*). Anat Rec. 1998;252:383–92.
56. Hillman N, Tasca R. Ultrastructural autoradiographic studies of mouse cleavage stages. Am J Anat. 1969;126:151–74.
57. Stern S, Biggers J, Anderson E. Mitochondria and early development of the mouse. J Exp Zool. 1971;176:179–92.
58. Calarco PG, Brow EH. An ultrastructural and cytological study of preimplantation development of the mouse. J Exp Zool. 1969;171:253–83.
59. Chech S, Sedlácková M. Ultrastructure and morphometric analysis of preimplantation mouse embryos. Cell Tissue Res. 1983;230:661–70.
60. Pikó L. Synthesis of macromolecules in early mouse embryos cultured in vitro: RNA, DNA, and polysaccharide component. Dev Biol. 1970;21:257–79.
61. Pikó L, Chase DG. Role of the mitochondrial genome during early development in mice. Effects of ethidium bromide and chloramphenicol. J Cell Biol. 1973;58:357–78.
62. Taylor KD, Pikó L. Mitochondrial biogenesis in early mouse embryos: expression of the mRNAs for subunits IV, Vb, and VIIc of cytochrome C oxidase and subunit 9 (PI) of H+-ATP synthase. Mol Reprod Dev. 1995;40:29–35.
63. Pikó L, Taylor KD. Amounts of mitochondrial DNA and abundance of some mitochondrial gene transcripts in early mouse embryos. Dev Biol. 1976;123:364–74.
64. Ginsberg L, Hillman N. Shifts in ATP synthesis during preimplantation stages of mouse embryos. J Reprod Fertil. 1975;43:83–90.
65. Ginsberg L, Hillman N. ATP metabolism in cleavage-staged mouse embryos. J Embryol Exp Morphol. 1973;30:267–82.
66. Brinster RL. Carbon dioxide production from glucose by the preimplantation mouse embryo. Exp Cell Res. 1967;47:271–7.
67. Gardner DK, Lane M. Culture of viable human blastocysts in defined sequential serum-free media. Hum Reprod. 1998;13(Suppl):148–59.
68. Crompton M. The mitochondria permeability transition pore and its role in cell death. Biochem J. 1999;341:233–49.
69. Gross A, McDonnell JM, Korsmeyer SJ. BCL-2 family members and the mitochondria in apoptosis. Genes Dev. 1999;13:1899–911.
70. Lopes AS, Larsen LH, Ramsing N, Løvendahl P, Räty M, Peippo J, et al. Respiration rates of individual bovine in vitro-produced embryos measured with a novel, non-invasive and highly sensitive microsensor system. Reproduction. 2005;130(5):669–79.
71. Lopes AS, Madsen SE, Ramsing NB, Løvendahl P, Greve T, Callesen H. Investigation of respiration of individual bovine embryos produced in vivo and in vitro and correlation with viability following transfer. Hum Reprod. 2007;22(2):558–66.
72. Agung B, Otoi T, Abe H, Hoshi H, Murakami M, Karja NW, et al. Relationship between oxygen consumption and sex of bovine in vitro fertilized embryos. Reprod Domest Anim. 2005;40(1):51–6.

73. Tejera A, Herrero J, de Los Santos MJ, Garrido N, Ramsing N, Meseguer M. Oxygen consumption is a quality marker for human oocyte competence conditioned by ovarian stimulation regimens. Fertil Steril. 2001;96(3):618–623.e.2.
74. Yamanaka M, Hashimoto S, Amo A, Ito-Sasaki T, Abe H, Morimoto Y. Developmental assessment of human vitrified-warmed blastocysts based on oxygen consumption. Hum Reprod. 2011;26(12):3366–71.
75. Trimarchi JR, Liu L, Porterfield DM, Smith PJ, Keefe DL. Oxidative phosphorylation-dependent and -independent oxygen consumption by individual preimplantation mouse embryos. Biol Reprod. 2000; 62(6):1866–74.

22 Mitochondrial Activity as a Biomarker of Gamete and Embryo Health

Jonathan Van Blerkom

The use of descriptors such as *health*, *potential*, and *viability* when applied to human oocytes and preimplantation stage embryos is intended to provide the observer of their performance in vitro some meaningful indication as to developmental competence. As a descriptor for development, competence implies an ability to predict with some measure of certainty both fertilizability and the ability of the fertilized oocyte to progress normally through the preimplantation stages. For the embryo, competence is typically used to gauge the likelihood of implantation and possibly, the likelihood of subsequent gestation to birth. Because certain elements of embryo competence are already largely determined in oocyte (e.g., occurrence of aneuploidy), there are few overt biological or physiological characteristics that can realistically distinguish between the "health" of an oocyte and the competence of the resulting embryo. However, meiotically mature human oocytes (metaphase II, MII) routinely obtained for in vitro fertilization (IVF) after controlled ovarian hyperstimulation and ovulation induction do exhibit certain cytoplasmic characteristics detectable by light microscopy that have been correlated with developmental competence [1–3]. Indeed, for the oocyte considerable efforts have been devoted to characterizing oocyte morphology with respect to competence [4], and for the embryo, both static and morphokinetic (time-lapse) imaging of performance will likely produce standard set of time- and stage-related morphological markers of competence [5] associated with a specific pattern of gene expression [6].

The characterization of morphological cues to create a uniform scheme for competence evaluation has two purposes: (1) to standardize assessments between observers and IVF programs by the use of a common "language" and (2) to provide biologically based criteria for selection where the number of oocytes that can be inseminated or embryos transferred is limited by local convention or is mandated by law. One of the positive features of a morphokinetic/performance-based paradigm is that characteristics and features can be added, removed, or modified as outcome findings demonstrate predictive strengths or limitations for each. The weakness inherent in this type of competence evaluation is that it is empirical by nature, and in the absence of quantitative biometric algorithms, even a common language can be largely subjective. Although there have been some attempts to introduce objective parameters, such as determinations of blastomere and nuclear volumes and shapes, similar biometrics designed to measure cytoplasmic loss to cytoplasts that were spontaneously extruded (fragments) have not entered routine use in the IVF laboratory. This is evidenced by subjective estimates of cytoplasmic loss listed in percentile form as for example, <10 %, <40 %, or >50 %, when performance findings from embryo culture are described in the literature or reported to

J. Van Blerkom (✉)
Department of Molecular, Cellular and Developmental Biology, University of Colorado, Boulder, CO 80309, USA
e-mail: jonathan.vanblerkom@colorado.edu

D.K. Gardner et al. (eds.), *Human Gametes and Preimplantation Embryos: Assessment and Diagnosis*, DOI 10.1007/978-1-4614-6651-2_22,

national IVF registries. Where empirical schemes truly fail, regardless of the criteria or characteristics used, is their inability to suggest which oocyte or embryo to select when they are all literally morphologically equivalent. It is common in clinical IVF that after insemination of such oocytes, or transfer of two embryos between days 2 and 5 with equivalent stage-appropriate appearance and performance characteristics, no implantation is indicted by a rise in circulating levels of human chorionic gonadotropin (hCG), or if a positive hCG occurs, the pregnancy is a singleton. While there is a relatively moderate-to-high probability, depending upon maternal age and fertility history, that some MII oocytes will be aneuploid at insemination, chromosomal defects cannot account for similar failures when embryos with positive morphological and performance characteristics (the so-called high grade) are shown to be euploid by preimplantation genetic diagnosis. Likewise, while poor or inadequate "uterine receptivity" is a known factor that can compromise postimplantation embryogenesis owing to specific molecular and cellular defects in endometrial structure and function [7], a normal singleton birth would seem to preclude this as a factor in the developmental failure of the other embryo.

Introduction of Objective Criteria for Competence Selection in Clinical IVF

The questionable reliability of subjective assessments and the need for higher levels of confidence for selection have been the primary driving forces behind alternative methods to assess oocyte and embryo developmental "health." For such assessment schemes to be widely applicable in routine clinical IVF practice, the following conditions would seem self-evident, regardless of methodology: (1) noninvasive, in the sense that it poses no risk of an iatrogenic contribution to failure; (2) objective, with respect to the provision quantitative values that have a biological basis; (3) largely operator-independent, but able to be used to assist to the operator with a final selection if weighted towards objective criteria; (4) ease of adoption and use in the IVF laboratory, i.e., highly specialized analytical methods, equipment and expertise are kept to a minimum, if possible. The final and most important criterion of all is that of outcome. Whatever "alternative" to a strictly empirically based method of selection is used, the percent of normal births/treatment cycle must be clearly demonstrated to be significantly superior to successful outcomes obtained with the same experienced IVF laboratory personnel who were involved in selection by morphological criteria alone. Under this circumstance, the fourth caveat noted above is unnecessary, and if outcome results are found to be consistently higher that previously under the same conditions of oocyte retrieval, fertilization, and embryo culture, the added expense for selection that is objectively based should be considered justifiable.

In clinical practice, biochemical analysis of culture medium in which early embryogenesis is occurring is truly noninvasive and can be completely operator-independent. A simultaneous morphokinetic sequence of performance during in vitro culture imaged by time-lapse could be of benefit if used to distinguish between embryos in which objective/analytical criteria for selection were essentially identical. Selection of oocytes for insemination presents a different set of requirements. First, there is value for morphology, if only to eliminate immature oocytes and those with cytoplasmic defects known to compromise competence [1–3]. However, these oocytes must be denuded of all surrounding somatic cells, which can be an iatrogenic factor in fertilization failure by conventional IVF, thus requiring invasive insemination by ICSI. Second, whatever oocyte biochemical parameters are being measured, if they are to reflect oocyte competence directly, the somatic cumulus and coronal cells will still have to be removed. At present, most research efforts that have focused on the identification of potential competence biomarkers by noninvasive means have analyzed the medium in which human oocytes and preimplantation stage embryos were cultured. The biological basis of this approach is a relatively simple one, namely, that the presence of an oocyte or embryo will effect changes in medium composition and their quantitation may reflect normal cellular activities that can be correlated with outcome and therefore, competence markers detectable at the earliest stages of development. In practice, analytical methods considered useful in competence assessments are designed to measure different aspects of cellular metabolism that may be detected by rates of depletion or uptake of medium constituents, the presence of molecules secreted into culture medium, and the synthesis or turnover of bioactive molecules, which would include secreted small polypeptides and proteins.

Mitochondria as Biomarker of Developmental Health

Recently, the notion that mitochondria could be a significant factor in the developmental competence of human oocytes and embryos has received considerable interest, especially with respect to their fundamental role in supporting cellular bioenergetics [8–12]. Indeed, the notion that a bioenergetic deficiency in the human oocyte could be a primary cause of compromised developmental competence has led to parallel avenues of investigation including the following: (1) analysis of oxygen consumption as an indicator of mitochondrial activity [13, 14]; (2) measurements of pyruvate and glucose uptake [15, 16]; (3) determinations of what is a net cytoplasmic ATP content for the mature oocyte that is consistent with competence [17–19]; (4) detection of putative molecular signatures of metabolites in culture medium by Raman spectroscopy or proton nuclear magnetic resonance that may indicate levels of mitochondrial metabolism [20–22]; (5) the possibility that competence may be restored to normalcy by "therapeutic" mitochondrial donation [23]; and (6) that dietary supplementation, including the use of certain polyunsaturated fatty acids, may benefit "mitochondrial health" by enhancing their functions, including bioenergetic performance [24, 25]. Each of these investigational paths is based on the single premise that mitochondrial health and ATP production are directly related, and directly determine oocyte and preimplantation embryo competence; this implies the existence of threshold bioenergetic levels that determine whether or not an oocyte undergoes normal preovulatory maturation, is fertilization competent, and can develop through the preimplantation stages with sufficient ATP to support energy-requiring processes during cleavage, cavitation, blastocyst formation, expansion, and hatching. The intent of this review is to examine what is known about mitochondrial function during early mammalian development, whether the assumption that mitochondria are a proximal cause of early developmental failure is credible, and whether it is possible to reliably assess mitochondrial activity noninvasively as metric of competence.

All mitochondria in the mammal are maternally inherited from a relative handful present in the primordial germ cell [26]. Mitochondrial replication occurs during the growth phase and reaches a terminal complement size when the oocyte is fully grown (germinal vesicle stage) and usually competent to reinitiate meiosis, which had been arrested at prophase I (from the fetal stages). The origin of an expanded maternal complement from such a small number of progenitors is the basis of metabolic (OXPHS) diseases if a pathogenic mutation in mitochondrial DNA (mtDNA) that affects certain functions, such as ATP production, is differentially expressed (mutant load) between oocytes [27, 28], resulting in varying degrees of phenotypic expression (severity of clinical symptoms) in affected individuals. The usual familiarity clinical and basic researchers have with mitochondria is in the context of their being termed the "powerhouse of a cell" that supplies the energy required to drive biological processes. Less familiar to most are their roles in calcium and redox signaling [29–32], signal transduction [33], apoptosis and cell cycle regulation [34], β-oxidation [35], steroidogenesis [36] and more recently, possible roles in tumor suppression [37].

The archetypical photographic image of mitochondria is commonly one of an electron micrograph taken from a differentiated cell showing fully developed, highly elongated organelles with numerous well-defined cristae traversing a matrix of low electron density. This is the impression most have of this organelle, because it is the usual representation of their fine structure presented in biology textbooks. Some of the micrographs still used for illustrative purposes are from the original fine structural studies of Sjostrand [38] and Palade [39, 40] in the early 1950s! In the same respect, the notion that mitochondrial structure and function are indicators of the health or age of somatic cells, and that changes in structure parallel cellular pathogenesis, has been a central element in studies of cellular aging, cancer, degenerative neuromuscular and metabolic diseases for decades [41–46].

Given the fundamental contribution of mitochondria to normal cell function and the known pathophysiological consequences of mitochondrial dysfunction, a similar role in the establishment of developmental competence for the human oocyte and preimplantation stage embryo is not too surprising. When it is also considered that mitochondrial replication (fission) does not begin until well after implantation [47], the presence of a numerically suboptimal complement, or a dysfunctional subpopulation, could have a significant impact on competence if stage-specific energy supply and demand are not in balance. In part, this explains the current emphasis on mitochondria as a principle determinant of human oocyte and embryo competence, and interest in whether noninvasive methods exist or could be developed to assess mitochondrial "health" at the oocyte or early preimplantation stages for purposes of selection. In order to address these possibilities, important differences between mitochondria in differentiated cells and those common to mammalian oocytes and early embryos, including the human, need to be considered.

The State of Mitochondrial Development in Mature Oocytes and Early Embryos

The classic view of a mitochondrion noted above bears little resemblance to their fine structure in the mature human oocyte and newly fertilized egg [48]. Similar to their counterparts in other mammals (e.g., mouse, rabbit [49, 50]), mitochondria in MII human oocytes are small (~1 μm in diameter [26]), spherical to slightly oblong, contain a large, electron dense matrix with no well-defined internal membranous architecture that normally defines the interior compartment. Indeed, the relatively few detectable cristae are truncated and located near the outer mitochondrial membrane, rarely penetrating the dense matrix to any significant degree. Because of this organization, mitochondria at these stages are referred to "undeveloped," but that does not mean they are metabolically inactive [51, 52] or that signs of dysfunction evident at the fine structural level in fully developed organelles are not evident in oocyte mitochondria. One of the first detailed studies relating the structure and biochemistry of mitochondria in oocytes of women of advanced reproductive age was undertaken by Muller-Hocker et al. [53], who reported increased mitochondrial volume (swelling) and changes in fine structure indicative of reduced respiratory function were common features associated with advanced age. Despite the varied mitochondrial functions and activities noted above to have essential roles in normal cell function, their role in ATP production is generally considered the primary factor responsible for early developmental failure in the human. In this context, a cytoplasmic bioenergetic deficit has been suggested as the cause of certain cytoplasmic defects, chromosomal aneuploidies, and failed fertilization for the human oocyte, and for the preimplantation embryo, chromosomal mosaicism and developmental arrest [17, 18, 54–60]. If a reduced capacity to generate ATP is related to mitochondrial swelling and other structural defects, a bioenergetic deficit may indeed be a causative factor in the age-related decline in fertility and fecundity that occurs with advancing maternal age [53].

The ATP requirements of the oocyte and newly fertilized egg are supplied by mitochondria that while structurally undeveloped are nevertheless metabolically active, as demonstrated by the kinetics of cytoplasmic ATP turnover under conditions that inhibit electron transport or oxidative phosphorylation [61]. To meet demands for the oocyte or early embryo as a whole, an intrinsically low ATP output for each mitochondrion is likely compensated for by the size of the mitochondrial complement, the progenitor population for the next generation, prior to their postimplantation replication. It is here where mitochondrial activity, cytoplasmic bioenergetics, and developmental competence converge to become an active area of investigation with respect to human oocyte and embryo developmental ability. The most obvious and practical question for clinical IVF is: if mitochondrial "health" could be assessed non-invasively, would it serve as a reliable biomarker of competence for oocyte and embryo selection?

What Is the Normal Mitochondrial Complement of a Mature Human Oocyte: Mitochondrial Mass vs. MtDNA Copy Number?

The numerical size of the mitochondrial complement in a MII human oocyte and whether certain threshold levels exist that can be clearly associated with competence and fundamental cell biological and fundamental cell biological issues remain to be resolved. For example, could a bioenergetic deficit be associated with a suboptimal population that resulted from a defect in mitochondrial replication during the growth phase of oogenesis? Most studies that have asked these questions have assumed that each oocyte mitochondrion contains a single genomic copy and that mtDNA copy and organelle numbers (mitochondrial mass) are largely equivalent; some early reports related low mtDNA copy numbers to the normality of preovulatory maturation in vivo, fertilizability and early development in vitro [57, 62]. Yet other studies using similar PCR methodologies showed mtDNA contents for mature (MII) oocytes differing by several orders of magnitude, from the low thousands to high hundreds of thousands to over one million copies [18, 52, 59, 63–67]. If based on size alone, the sea urchin oocyte and human MII oocyte are both about 100 μm in diameter, and early morphometric analyses indicated a mitochondrial complement in the sea urchin of about 150,000 organelles [68]. It would seem unlikely that fully grow human oocytes have mitochondrial numbers close to one million organelles, and studies designed to estimate this number, report a complement size that is at least an order of magnitude lower [69], suggesting that mitochondrial mass and mtDNA copy number are not synonymous. Indeed, threshold values reported to be associated with normal competence are difficult to reconcile with each other as what one study may describe as an mtDNA threshold for competence can be significantly different from another that with the same methodology, has reached a similar conclusion but at a much higher mtDNA value [18, 59]. It would appear that the notion of one mtDNA copy/organelle may need to be revisited, and that additional determinations of threshold organelle numbers for competence in the human oocyte and early embryo are warranted. It may well be that a mtDNA copy number around 100K is a reasonable consensus figure for competence, as suggested by some [69], but whether this translates to a mitochondrial population at MII of 20,000 or 100,000 organelles remains to be determined [70].

The relationship between mtDNA copy number and ATP generation in structurally undeveloped oocyte mitochondria is presumably similar to the one identified for differentiated cells, where respiratory rates and mtDNA copy number are associated [52, 71]. However, this association may be more complicated in the oocyte than in the somatic cell. In several species, a significant burst of mtDNA synthesis occurs during preovulatory meiotic maturation, i.e., in the fully grown oocyte immediately preceding ovulation [72]. However, these authors reported that during the early cleavage stages, most of these new copies were degraded and mtDNA content returned to near previous levels. A transient increase in mtDNA in the oocyte may allow higher levels of ATP generation to support of energy-intensive activities during the terminal stages of oogenesis, fertilization, and early cleavage. Why nearly 80 % of the mtDNA copies are apparently degraded prior to morulation and cavitation, which are presumably high-energy demanding processes, is unclear [72]. Perhaps the beginning of a structural transformation from an undeveloped to more developed form is associated with a progressive upregulation of respiratory capacity and ATP output/organelle such that demand and supply are in balance [12, 50]. Whether this is a realistic explanation for stage-specific mtDNA kinetics, or whether a similar transient expansion of mtDNA occurs in the maturing human oocyte, is unknown. However, if the health of an oocyte or nascent embryos is to be assessed on mitochondrial properties and activities (e.g., levels of β-oxidation, superoxide generation), these are the types of basic cell biological questions that will need to be answered and defined with respect to "normal" stage-specific mtDNA and organelle numbers and ATP supply and demand. In this regard, we are currently investigating different analytical methods for their ability to accurately measure and correlate mitochondrial mass and mitochondrial activity in mature human oocytes and preimplantation embryos [73].

Mitochondria and Free Calcium Homeostasis

The regulatory relationship between mitochondrial activity and ambient free calcium levels is another aspect of mitochondrial bioenergetics found in differentiated cells that also applies to the oocyte and early embryo, despite their structurally undeveloped forms [12, 74]. Recently, Van Blerkom [52, 75] reported that unusually high net cytoplasmic ATP contents occurred in some MII human oocytes and could be correlated with defects in the regulation of intracellular free calcium. The elevated ATP content did not appear to result from a mitochondrial mass (organelle complement) that was higher than normal, but rather from levels of intracellular free calcium measured after calcium ionophore activation that were significantly higher than normally recorded for the first calcium-transient maxima detected either after fertilization, or in normal ionophore-activated human oocytes [74]. Also atypical was the finding that high intracellular free calcium levels persisted for significantly longer than usual after activation or fertilization. The origin of this atypical bioenergetic state was suggested to result from a defect in the organization of the smooth surfaced endoplasmic reticulum (sER) from which free calcium was released en mass from highly condensed, rather than dispersed cisternae. In somatic cells, the release of calcium from sER elements in proximity to mitochondria regulates levels of ATP production [76] and by means of both calcium-induced calcium-release (CIRC [77]) and the mitochondrial CIRC signaling pathways (mCIRC [52, 78]); mitochondrial ATP generation can be up-or down-regulated. Dumollard et al. [79] showed that mitochondrial activity in mouse oocytes was regulated by free calcium released from sER elements in proximity to these organelles. For the human, small clusters of mitochondria surrounded by cisternae of the sER has been suggested to be a normal feature of the subplasmalemmal cytoplasm in the mature oocyte [51]. These authors suggested that ATP production by subplasmalemmal mitochondria may be upregulated by proximity to sER clusters and that an elevated bioenergetic capacity may be needed to support various oolemmal functions (e.g., transport, signaling, endo- and exocytosis). By means of regulating mitochondrial activity through modulation of free calcium levels, ATP supply and demand can be balanced focally and without changing mitochondrial activity in the entire cytoplasm, or where a higher bioenergetic state was not needed. In the absence of focal regulation, a global increase in mitochondrial activity could be associated with unwanted increases in superoxide generation [79], which if beyond the endogenous capacity of the oocyte to detoxify this oxygen-free radical, has the potential to induce damaging effects on cell structure and function.

Assessing mitochondrial "health" as a measure of oocyte or embryo competence by direct quantification of ATP or mtDNA content is obviously not a viable method as cell lysis is required. Quantification of superoxide levels may provide an indication of mitochondrial activity that could be related to mitochondrial health, as described below. However, lysis of oocytes or embryos for the first two mitochondrial parameters noted above could be clinically helpful if used retrospectively, i.e., as part of a diagnostic scheme to examine possible etiologies of total fertilization or preimplantation developmental failure in a cohort. In the same respect, failure analysis using direct assessments of mitochondrial mass by quantitative fluorescent analysis with mitochondria-specific probes could show whether developmentally significant differences existed between oocytes, assuming that a standard curve of relative fluorescent intensity (RFI) and mitochondrial mass could be generated [73]. For selective purposes for fertilization or embryo transfer, use of most currently available mitochondria-specific fluorescent probes is problematic. While a particular probe or stain may not be cytotoxic or cause defects in cell function when associated with mitochondria, this can change when the fluorophore is excited by ultraviolet illumination, and depending upon probe, concentration, duration of illumination, and the relative intensity of fluorescence, mitochondrial damage and disruption can have lethal developmental effects that are essentially immediate (Van Blerkom, unpublished) or manifest during the pre- or early postimplantation implantation stages [80].

Another factor to be considered in assessment schemes that contemplate the use of mitochondria as a biomarker of oocyte and embryo developmental health, is that they can be disproportionately inherited (segregated) during the first and subsequent cleavage divisions of the human embryo [81]. The resulting cells have different ATP contents and RFI reported by mitochondria-specific probes. One potentially clinically useful aspect of this finding is that it may be possible to relate mitochondrial mass with a bioenergetic state for each blastomere during early cleavage, as noted above. The differences observed in ATP content and RFI for embryos in which blastomeres were examined individually were related to the intact embryo with regard to normal or abnormal performance characteristics during cleavage to the 12-cell stage. Where mitochondrial segregation between blastomeres was relatively uniform at the 2- and 4-cell stages, development to the 12-cell stage was normal with respect to stage and time-appropriate cell divisions. In instances where disproportionate segregation occurred, blastomeres with a significantly lower RFI than their siblings either arrested cell division, divided more slowly or in the extreme; where RFI and ATP content values (measured in similar cells) were quite low, blastomeres underwent abrupt lysis. What these studies showed was that total ATP measured for a cleavage stage embryo can be misleading as far as relating mitochondrial health to competence is concerned. Total ATP levels for embryos showing disproportionate inheritance were within normal ranges for cleavage stage embryos, which could indicate healthy organelles; how they are numerically distributed among blastomeres, however, can have variable developmental consequences that differentially affect the developmental "health" of each cell within the embryo [81]. The results also suggest threshold levels exist for ATP and mitochondrial mass that can be related to the competence of individual blastomeres. However, ATP analysis required cell lysis so any estimates of bioenergetic status based on mitochondrial RFI would require the derivation of standard curve of blastomere-specific RFI for each potential probe (e.g., rhodamine 123, MitoTracker family), a standard staining time and concentration, followed by blastomere lysis for ATP quantification by chemiluminescent methods [17].

In this experimental context, relative mitochondrial fluorescence determined in the living state can be related to quantitative measurements of ATP content after lysis. In unpublished studies by this author, the mitochondrial mass for individual blastomeres in 2- and 4-cell human embryos could be estimated based on the cell-specific intensities of mitochondrial fluorescence measured with different fluorescent probes [73] and correlated with bioenergetic state by quantitative ATP measurements in the corresponding lysed blastomeres [17]. However, as is often the case in translating experimental findings into clinically applicable and acceptable methods, the process of quantifying mitochondrial RFI in oocytes or early embryos intended for IVF or transfer can have adverse downstream consequences likely related to subtle damage to mitochondrial membranes during the duration of fluorophore excitation required to obtain meaningful quantitative values by scanning laser confocal microscopy. In these instances, cleavage continued for 1 or 2 divisions and then ceased. Fine structural analysis showed delayed alterations in mitochondrial fine structure, such as vacuolation within the matrix and distended or fragmented cristae, which are also characteristics of mitochondria in differentiated cells undergoing pathological changes related to disease or acute exposure to toxic agents.

The advantage of direct microscopic observation and quantitation of mitochondrial fluorescence is the ability to image individual cells as well as the entire embryo. Thus, subtle differences between oocytes and embryos or within embryos (i.e., blastomeres) with respect to mitochondrial mass should translate to estimates of bioenergetic status and competence. However, imaging by traditional fluorescent microscopy (e.g., epifluorescence or scanning laser confocal) with current probes is associated with a risk of iatrogenic damage that could compromise subsequent cell function and embryo competence, as noted above. Additional studies in which different reporters are tested for their ability to accurately quantify mitochondrial RFI, or advantage is taken of nonlethal mitochondrial autofluorescence [82], or live cell measurements of cytosolic metabolites that reflect mitochondrial activity [83], offer novel possibilities to correlate mitochondrial health and bioenergetic status for use as biomarkers of competence for selection in clinical IVF. As discussed below, colorimetric measurements of enzymatic reactions or bioactivities that are ATP-driven may provide an indirect indication of cytoplasmic bioenergetics and may be useful for assessing relative mitochondrial activity levels. However, it is worthwhile mentioning that all current methods that attempt to relate mitochondrial function in human oocytes or early embryos with competence, whether by rates or levels of oxygen uptake, metabolite depletion, or by biochemical alterations detectable in culture medium (the so-called molecular signatures detected by Raman spectroscopy), are ultimately associating competence with some metabolic activity that has a mitochondrial component. However, it should be emphasized that these assessments are made for intact embryos, and that blastomere-specific differences related to mitochondrial activity or bioenergetic status would go undetected. It may well be that spontaneously occurring differences in mitochondrial content that arise between blastomeres during cleavage are not only commonplace in clinical IVF, but ultimately have a greater influence on developmental competence than apparent differences in mtDNA copy number between oocytes. It is in this context that future efforts related to mitochondrial health by quantifying stage-specific activity levels or functions may be better directed for competence assessments.

Spatial Compartmentalization of Mitochondrial Activity in Oocytes and Preimplantation Stage Embryos: Potential Biomarkers of Competence

Van Blerkom and Davis [84] introduced the notion that mitochondria in the mature oocyte and nascent embryo may functionally compartmentalized whereby activity in the subplasmalemmal cytoplasm was different from levels in more interior regions. These authors suggested that mitochondria in proximity to the oocyte surface may have a higher inner mitochondrial membrane potential ($\Delta\Psi m$) than those more distant and as a result, higher levels of ATP generation [52]. Further studies [85] indicated that high potential in the subplasmalemmal domain likely occurs at the terminal stages of preovulatory maturation, while for the newly fertilized egg and early embryo, high potential in this region is constitutive. It is not until the blastocyst stage, and for the trophectoderm specifically, that intracellular distinctions between high and low potential mitochondria no longer exist; virtually all trophectodermal mitochondria are high potential whereas $\Delta\Psi m$, reflective of mitochondrial bioenergetic activity in the inner cell mass is lower [86], which is consistent with quantitative measurements of ATP generation in the inner cell mass showing lower levels of ATP production than in trophectoderm [87].

In the context of location-dependent mitochondrial activity as a possible determinant of human oocyte and competence, potentiometric probes can provide useful spatial and metabolic information that may enable competent oocytes and embryos to be distinguished from those that are more likely to be developmentally compromised. For example, normal appearing human MII oocytes found to be unpenetrated after conventional IVF often showed scant or undetectable high potential mitochondria in the subplasmalemmal cytoplasm [51, 88]. Wilding et al. [89] observed abnormal distributions of high ΔΨm in cytoplasmic mitochondrial aggregates and correlated these atypical formations with high frequencies of chromosomal aneuploidies and catastrophic mosaicisms in human IVF. In this study, the presence of distinct clusters of high potential mitochondria were observed in the cytoplasm, whereas others, using the same potentiometric fluorescence probe (JC1), found high potential forms localized to the subplasmalemmal cytoplasm [23, 51, 74, 90]. In this regard, Aw [91] showed that mitochondrial clustering could upregulate ΔΨm within the cluster by virtue of a reduced ambient pHi resulting from ATP hydrolysis, which increases the magnitude of the chemi-osmotic gradient across the inner mitochondria membrane that establishes ΔΨm. Whether subtle differences in reactive oxygen species (ROS) generation or redox state could have local influence on signal transduction pathways that are ROS- or redox-dependent [52, 92], or on ROS-induced mitochondrial ROS release pathways [93] remain to be investigated as possible determinants of developmental competence that have a mitochondrial association.

In our studies, we have found that current mitochondria-specific potentiometric probes such as JC1, which can report relative activity levels, are highly useful in assessing mitochondrial "health" after the fact; that is, in oocytes that failed to mature, fertilize, or develop normally after penetration [51, 88]. However, for proactive use in selection, they would have to be shown to be nontoxic and developmentally benign in stained oocytes and embryos with or without excitation. It is unlikely that current methods and probes used to report different aspects of mitochondrial physiology, activity (e.g., ΔΨm), or mass, would be clinically acceptable for selection prior to fertilization or transfer, but they could be a useful diagnostic in determining whether mitochondria had a role in failed IVF cycles, as noted above. However, continued studies are warranted, because the "right" probe could offer a direct indication of mitochondrial "health" if the findings can be quantitated and correlated with other omic parameters, such as oxygen or substrate utilization, molecular signatures in culture medium, embryo performance in vitro, and outcome after transfer. The right probe of course needs to be one where its detection does not have adverse or lethal downstream effects on embryogenesis, as has been shown to occur with the fluorescent probes currently used to study mitochondria during early mammalian development. In this regard, the following section presents other approaches to assess mitochondrial health that have come from the animal industry or from new research findings relevant to mitochondrial physiology.

Novel Biomarkers of Mitochondrial Function and Cellular Bioenergetic Status: Potential Applications in Clinical IVF

Superoxide Flashes

More speculative in terms of possible methods to assess mitochondrial function and activity is the recent detection of the so-called superoxide flashes that result from the spontaneous openings of the mitochondrial transition pore complex that induces superoxide generation by the electron transport chain [93–96]. Superoxide is a ROS generated by the "leakiness" of the electron transport chain that under normal cytoplasmic conditions plays an important role in cellular functions, including ROS-dependent signaling (see above). Cellular toxicity can result when superoxide generation is abnormally high (e.g., oxidative stress) and endogenous ROS scavenger pathways (e.g., glutathione) are insufficient to return levels to a homeostatic state. The detection of superoxide flashes and their relationship to mitochondrial physiology, bioenergetic and calcium homeostasis, ROS signaling and redox state is a comparatively new area of mitochondrial research that has already contributed new insights into understanding normal cell function and the pathophysiology of disease [97, 98]. Different analytical methods have been developed to detect superoxide flashes (i.e., the superoxide ion) including fluorescence microscopy, chemiluminescence, and electron spin resonance with stable spin probes [99, 100]. However, quantitation can be problematic and especially challenging with fluorescent methods that use an endogenous superoxide biosensor, such as a circularly permuted yellow fluorescent protein (cpYFP; 101), whose presence in the mitochondrial matrix currently requires genetically targeting transfection. Nevertheless, optimism expressed in recent studies for this aspect of mitochondrial physiology has centered on its potential to assess the state of mitochondrial activity under different environmental and physiological conditions that can be related to normal or abnormal cellular states. Whether technology of this type has applications in clinical IVF for the assessment of mitochondrial health is difficult to predict at the present time. Clearly, gene transfection that results in the translation of a protein-based superoxide biosensor is not a reasonable use of this technology for clinical purposes. However, continued studies will likely see the development of cell permeable superoxide biosensors that can be introduced in vitro and targeted to mitochondria [101]. Under ideal circumstances, flash quantitation using chemiluminescent detection could be applied to oocytes and early embryos for assessments of mitochondrial health and related to developmental viability, but only if (1) no downstream toxicity is evident, (2) superoxide production in the structurally undeveloped mitochondria of the human oocytes and pre-expansion stage embryo occurs with sufficient sensitivity for purposes of competence selection, and (3) the biosensor can be incorporated into the oocyte or blastomere without genetic manipulations. Measuring superoxide flashes for clinical purposes in infertility treatment is an intriguing possibility, especially if it can be shown to assess mitochondrial function and activity as presently indicated for cultured somatic cells, and analytical means appropriate for the IVF laboratory can be developed [102]. This technology may also identify important differences between oocytes and early embryos in their endogenous ability to react to oxidative stress that may occur during in vitro culture and, therefore, provide an additional parameter to assess developmental health or competence.

Oxygen Uptake and Mitochondrial Health

The possibility of measuring subtle physiological processes that may be directly related to mitochondrial health for purposes of selection, such as superoxide flashes, is necessarily speculative because this field of research is still developing and it is unclear whether methods used in experimental research can readily translate to the clinical IVF laboratory. However, other methods suggested to indirectly report mitochondrial activity in oocytes and preimplantation stage embryos, such as quantitation of rates and levels of oxygen uptake from culture medium, have been used to assess oocyte and embryo competence in different species, including the human [13, 103–106]. Whether uptake findings can be related to outcome and, therefore, serve as the primary criterion for noninvasive oocyte or embryo selection is still unclear in human IVF [107]; reliable stage-specific threshold levels of oxygen consumption below which developmental competence can be clearly and reproducibly shown to be compromised, based on fertilizability, embryo performance in vitro, and outcome after transfer, have yet to be determined or established definitively. It should also be recalled that for the oocyte, uptake measurements of oxygen or other metabolites and small molecules require compete denudation of the somatic cumulus and coronal cell compartment, which could compromise conventional IVF and thus require the added costs of ICSI. For oxygen uptake kinetics in particular, there are several unknowns related to use in human IVF that need to be resolved: (1) what percent of dissolved oxygen extracted by the oocyte or embryo from culture medium is used for oxidative metabolism? In other species, a significant proportion does not go to oxidative respiration [13]; (2) to what extent do uptake and utilization kinetics differ between morphologically equivalent MII oocytes and preimplantation stage embryos? (3) can stage-specific threshold levels be established that with respect to outcome, have high predictive power for competence selection? and (4) to what extent are these putative threshold levels consistent with a specific mitochondrial mass, mtDNA copy number, bioenergetic state, or spatial localization of high $\Delta\Psi m$ forms? The value of this approach to assessments of mitochondrial health will only be demonstrated by consistent outcome findings where oocyte and embryo selection is standardized in well-designed and controlled clinical studies.

Brilliant Cresyl Blue Staining

Current methods proposed for competence assessment that may be related to mitochondrial health or metabolic activity described above involve the use of relatively complex analytical equipment that can detect and quantitate at high sensitivity, changes in molecular signatures, metabolomic and biochemical profiles, and oxygen uptake from culture medium. The use of these physiological parameters is largely intended to provide objective information that is independent of, or an assist to, subjective assessments (oocyte or embryo morphology or certain in vitro performance characteristics), with sufficient predictive power with regard to outcome as to become the primary means of competence selection. However, there are other methods that have been used in the animal industry to assess competence that may have clinical applications and are considerably simpler in concept and laboratory application than those described above. It is often forgotten, or possibly unrecognized by those whose only experience with IVF is in the clinical arena, that virtually all important protocols, culture media, and knowledge about the molecular and cellular biology of oogenesis, fertilization, and preimplantation embryogenesis derive from experimental models (e.g., mouse) and commercially important species (e.g., bovine).

Brilliant Cresyl Blue staining (BCB) is one of the most widely used methods for oocyte selection for commercial embryo production that use oocytes derived from slaughterhouse ovaries for in vitro maturation and IVF in a variety of important species including the bovine [108], ovine [109], porcine [56, 110], caprine [111], and others [112]. BCB is a noninvasive method that measures glucose-6-phosphate dehydrogenase activity [108–113]. At high activity levels, such as in growing oocytes, BCB is reduced to a colorless compound, where as in fully grown oocytes, in which enzyme activity is lower, BCB retains it color. The developmental competence of BCB^+ and BCB^- oocytes has been demonstrated by outcome after IVM and IVF, or IVF alone with embryos transfers from MII oocytes selected on the basis of coloration (BCB^+) or its absence (BCB^-). In the bovine and ovine systems, superior rates of in vitro development to the blastocyst stage were observed in oocytes classified as BCB^+ and in most studies, differences in blastocyst formation between embryos from BCB negative and positive oocytes have been marked higher, often threefold higher [111–113]. In animal studies, including the mouse [114] intact cumulus-oocyte complexes are stained with BCB, and after denudation, cytoplasmic coloration for the oocyte determined empirically under a dissecting microscope with BCB^- oocytes distinguished from their BCB^+ counterparts simply by the absence of any detectable coloration. Since BCB is nontoxic, oocyte selection with BCB in the bovine system has been used for cloning by somatic cell nuclear transfer or IVF in commercial embryo production enterprises with BCB^+ oocytes detected while immature and after IVM to MII, shown to have superior competence when compared to BCB^- oocytes in the same cohort when maturation was initiated [113]. The collective results from animal studies support the use of BCB staining as a noninvasive method for developmental competence assessment in oocyte selection.

Studies of levels of oxidative phosphorylation and gene expression in BCB$^+$ and BCB$^-$ bovine oocytes showed marked differences that would be expected to be of developmental significance during preimplantation embryogenesis (e.g., upregulation of genes involved in cell cycle regulation), and significant differences in apparent levels of mitochondrial metabolic activity reported by ATP content analysis and the mitochondria-specific fluorescent probes [115]. Torner et al. [115] reported that apparent levels of mitochondrial activity were higher in BCB$^-$ oocytes with corresponding high G6PDH activity when compared to BCB$^+$ oocytes, and suggested this difference could reflect increased respiratory activity required to supply ATP at higher levels to complete preovulatory maturation that, in the BCB$^-$ oocyte, may be delayed or slower. This notion is supported by their detection of upregulated levels of expression for genes involved in ATP synthesis and electron transport in the BCB$^-$ state. An association between oocyte developmental competence and mitochondria was also suggested by the recent studies of Silva et al. [116] and Catala et al. [117] in the bovine and ovine systems, respectively. Silva et al. found that the central distribution of mitochondria in MII bovine oocytes that is consistent with normal nuclear and cytoplasmic maturation and higher rates of blastocyst formation on day 7 was associated with a BCB$^+$ status in the fully grown oocyte at the outset of maturation in vitro. Catala et al. found immature BCB$^+$ sheep oocytes were the most competent to develop to the blastocyst stage after in vitro maturation and fertilization, and showed significantly higher levels of mitochondrial activity at the completion of oocyte maturation (i.e., MII) than their BCB$^-$ counterparts. In these studies, MitroTracker Orange CMTMRos, a probe that reports relative mitochondrial oxidative activity based on RFI was used.

A common theme to come from BCB staining studies is that selection of fully grown oocytes for IVM/IVF in animal models consistently results in rates of development to the blastocyst stage that are several-fold higher when oocytes are BCB positive, thus indicating that a low level of G6PDH activity at the time of insemination is associated with developmental competence after fertilization. Although G6PDH is a cytosolic enzyme in the pentose phosphate pathway that generates NADPH, the association of BCB staining with mitochondrial activity described above (e.g., higher ATP concentrations in BCB$^+$ oocytes) suggests that this method could also be an indirect indicator of mitochondrial health related to mitochondria bioenergetic capacity [118]. Any clinical application of BCB staining would appear to be most relevant for in vitro maturation, where selection based on coloration at the GV stage could indicate both maturation and postfertilization competence, and if studies from animal models apply to the human, potentially useful information about the size and normality of follicles from which the oocytes were derived. Preliminary studies in this author's laboratory on BCB staining of human oocytes from the GV-to-MII stages have shown mixed results in terms of coloration that could be useful for selection. To date, 11 of 27 fully grown GV stage oocytes showed BCB positive cytoplasmic staining ranging from barely detectable to clearly blue after a standard 90 min exposure to BCB at a concentrations of 35 μM (time and concentration similar to those used for other species [108–114]). After BCB classification by light microscopy (e.g., BCB$^-$: BCB$^+$, BCB^{++}, BCB^{+++}), oocytes were washed and returned normal medium. Preliminary findings showed no correlation between BCB positive or negative staining, or the relative intensity of staining, and the ability of the corresponding oocyte to mature to MII. Similar findings were obtained with oocytes whose maturational status was classified as pre-MII owing to the absence to an germinal vesicle or first polar body. In these instances ($n=35$), and for similar oocytes that matured to MII in vitro ($n=80$), the range of ATP levels [17] was similar in immature and mature BCB$^-$ and BCB$^+$ oocytes. However, the patterns of BCB staining in both immature and mature oocytes may be relevant for competence selection even if the bioenergetic status is largely similar. At MII, 23 of the 80 in vitro matured MII oocytes examined show well-defined foci of relatively dense BCB staining against a cytoplasm that was largely, if not entirely BCB⁻. Staining with rhodamine 123, a mitochondria-specific fluorescent dye, showed corresponding higher levels of fluorescence in these BCB⁺ foci, indicating a BCB pattern that seems to report abnormal mitochondrial aggregations that could have negative developmental consequences. In a similar preliminary study of in vivo matured oocytes, BCB staining intensities of denuded unfertilized ($n=30$) and dispermic oocytes (3 PN, $n=9$) showed no significant differences, although a blue coloration was initially detectable and in 12 unfertilized oocytes, dark cytoplasmic foci of BCB staining were evident.

These initial findings warrant further study with respect to whether BCB can identify a subset of human oocytes derived from hyperstimulated cycles that should not be subjected to insemination either by ICSI or conventional means. Whether differences in BCB coloration are associated with spindle organization and function at MII that could compromise subsequent embryonic development, despite a similar bioenergetic status between oocytes (i.e., ATP content), is currently under investigation. However, it is worth mentioning that the utility of BCB staining for competence selection of immature oocytes reported for other species involves oocytes that were retrieved directly from unstimulated ovaries and transported from slaughterhouse to laboratory. These GV stage oocytes mostly reside in intact cumulus-oocyte complexes and are stained in situ, allowed to mature under conditions optimized for each species, and then inseminated in vitro. In this context, BCB staining appears to be a very positive element in increasing the efficiency of low cost embryo production, which is the goal of this enterprise for commercially important species. For the human, IVM may be the most useful application of BCB selection methodology as it is currently applied in animals. In normal IVF cycles, immature oocytes are aspirated from expanded antral follicles after ovarian hyperstimulation and ovulation induction. The fact that they have not initiated or completed nuclear maturation in vivo, but will often do so spontaneously in vitro after cumulus/coronal cell denudation (required to confirm normal fertilization, i.e., two pronuclei), indicates a possible intrafollicular signaling defect associated with LH/hCG induction of the resumption of arrested meiosis (i.e., nuclear maturation). Whether the cytoplasmic component of preovulatory maturation is equally perturbed is unknown. However, it will be relevant in assessing the utility of BCB in clinical IVF to determine whether atypical BCB⁺ regions in an otherwise clear cytoplasm, which appear to involve foci of mitochondrial aggregations, is an indirect biomarker of aberrant cytoplasmic maturation. If confirmed, staining of type may be a simpler approach to competence selection.

It is evident that additional studies are required to assess whether BCB has a place in clinical IVF and whether its putative use for oocyte selection could be extended into the preimplantation period. Although some studies have tried to associate BCB staining with mitochondrial function or activity, more specific correlations with normal and abnormal spatial distributions of mitochondria, and differences in organelle number (i.e., mitochondrial mass) and bioenergetic activity are needed. Resolution of these issues will go a long way in assessing the value of BCB staining in human oocyte competence assessment. What may ultimately be more useful is the principle behind BCB staining as applied in the animal industry. The stain and method of staining per se are nontoxic and current evidence indicates that it poses no apparent developmental hazard. In this regard, BCB is an indirect indicator of stage-specific "health" as related to subsequent developmental competence, and while mitochondria are known to contribute directly to competence, the extent to which BCB coloration reflects this contribution is unknown. For clinical IVF, it may be useful to examine the extensive list of other vital stains that can be readily detected by light microscopy for those whose coloration may be responsive to known mitochondria-specific activities (e.g., superoxide/ROS production) or influences on cytoplasmic physiology (e.g., intracellular pH/redox potential). Preliminary studies in animal systems would have to demonstrate safety, sensitivity, specificity, and efficacy. While this approach could be viewed as somewhat "retro" by revisiting an earlier period of light microscopy histology of living cells, it may well be that stains exist or can be modified for this purpose. Alternatively, sufficient interest in assessment by this means could lead to the design stains that detect important mitochondrial properties and functions that by virtue of cytoplasmic coloration, report oocyte- or embryo-specific differences of developmental significance.

Summary and Needed Research

The notion that noninvasive metabolic or bioenergetic measurements of human oocytes and preimplantation embryos can indicate the status of mitochondrial health as related to function, and that the state of mitochondrial function is a biomarker of developmental competence, is an appealing one from a clinical perspective in IVF. In practice however, what mitochondrial activities may be the most relevant competence markers, and whether they can be assessed directly without inducing developmental toxicity, are essential issues that need to be addressed and answered by experimentation. In the same respect, while it is largely assumed that mitochondria have a central role in multiple aspects of cell function in the oocyte and early embryo, and that their normal activity at these stages is a direct determinant of developmental health, certain fundamental aspects of their biology in the mature human oocyte remain to be defined. These aspects need to be understood more completely if mitochondria are to be considered and studied as a biomarker of competence for the human oocyte and early embryo. For example, values for mitochondrial mass and mtDNA copy number that can be universally considered normal for the MII human oocyte need to be established, and noninvasive methods that can estimate these values in living oocytes developed. While not easy tasks, the clinical IVF field is a robust one with many talented individuals up to the challenge.

At present, the detection and quantitation of changes in molecular composition or molecular signatures in culture medium due to addition or depletion by an oocyte or preimplantation stage embryo are "omic"-based approaches to competence assessment that may have a significant mitochondrial component. Oxygen depletion/uptake is a current method suggested to be an indicator of competence and mitochondrial activity, but its use for selection in clinical IVF needs to be clearly validated. Each technology required to make omic or uptake determinations from samples of culture medium is complex and often costly. However, the decisions based on assessments of this type are crucial in clinical IVF because it is upon these findings that an oocyte(s) may be inseminated, or not, or embryo(s) transferred, cryopreserved, or "deselected" for either. Recently, the notion that compromised mitochondrial health may underlie fertilization and early developmental failure has led to the consideration of mitochondrial rescue by transferring organelles with normal function isolated from a patient's somatic cells (autologous transfer: e.g., cumulus cells) at the time of insemination (ICSI). Autologous transfers would address the issue of heteroplasmy associated with cytoplasmic transfers from donor oocytes, and mitochondrial transfers of this type have been shown to increase net cytoplasmic ATP concentrations [119]. With the exception of known pathogenic mutations in mtDNA however, there must be compelling and unambiguous evidence that compromised embryonic development has a definable mitochondrial etiology.

In summary, it is largely assumed that defects in mitochondrial function are proximate cause of failure in clinical IVF, and most likely, conceptions occurring in natural cycles as well. In this author's opinion, this assumption is generally correct. However, evidence in support of a very significant or primary role in developmental incompetence for the mature human oocyte and preimplantation embryo is often contradictory; for example, what is a normal mtDNA copy number or net cytoplasmic ATP content (i.e., threshold levels for competence)? To what extent are mitochondrial superoxide/ROS, calcium signaling, and their regulation of redox state critical activities in the oocyte and early embryo that if perturbed, can be developmentally lethal? Why do certain mature human oocytes exhibit a subplasmalemmal cytoplasm that is deficient in high

$\Delta\Psi m$ forms and why is this associated with penetration or fertilization failures? These studies can provide the type of basic information needed for a clear physiological understanding of "mitochondrial function" and its association with the health of the human oocyte and early embryo. How such an understanding will fit into current omic paradigms of competence selection in clinical IVF remains to be determined. However, given the necessity for competence selection in clinical IVF and the prominent role mitochondria have in the establishment and maintenance of developmental competence, it seems likely that methods currently considered novel or used in the animal industry will be investigated for human application. While novel methods that can detect and quantify newly discovered mitochondrial activities such as superoxide flashes may be currently impractical for human IVF, as this area of research progresses, new methods of detection will likely emerge which will have clinical applications. Likewise, vital (nontoxic) stains whose colorimetric properties reflect changes in cytoplasmic physiology influenced or regulated by mitochondria warrant investigation, and would be ideal if they can report differences in metabolic activity or state in general, and between individual blastomeres in particular, that can be detected by light microscopic methods common to IVF programs. Although there is reason for optimism that methods to assess mitochondrial activity and function (i.e., health) in living oocytes and embryos will be developed, the major issue, as always, will be whether translation from research to clinical IVF laboratory is warranted on evidence-based outcomes. There is reason for optimism that new findings and methods will likely support this diagnostic approach in clinical IVF in the near future.

References

1. Van Blerkom J, Henry G. Oocyte dysmorphism and aneuploidy in meiotically mature human oocytes after controlled ovarian stimulation. Hum Reprod. 1992;7:379–90.
2. Meriano J, Alexis J, Visram-Zaver J, et al. Tracking of oocyte dysmorphisms for ICSI patients may prove relevant to outcome in subsequent patient cycles. Hum Reprod. 2001;16:2118–23.
3. de Cássia S Figueira S, de Almeida Ferreira Braga DP, Semiao-Francisco L, Madaschi C, Iaconeli A, Borges E. Metaphase II human oocyte morphology: contributing factors and effects on fertilization potential and embryo developmental ability in ICSI cycles. Fertil Steril. 2010;94:1115–7.
4. Balaban B et al. Alpha scientists in reproductive medicine and ESHRE special interest group of embryology. The Istanbul consensus workshop on embryo assessment: proceedings of an expert meeting. Hum Reprod. 2011;26:1270–83.
5. Lemmen J, Agerholm I, Ziebe S. Kinetic markers of human embryo quality using time-lapse recordings of IVF/ICSI-fertilized oocytes. Reprod Biomed Online. 2008;17:385–91.
6. Wong C, Loewke K, Bossert N, Behr B, De Jong C, Baer T, et al. Non-invasive imaging of human embryos before embryonic genomic activation predicts development to the blastocyst stage. Nat Biotechnol. 2010;28:1115–21.
7. Singh M, Chaudhry P, Asselin E. Bridging endometrial receptivity and implantation: network of hormones, cytokines and growth factors. J Endocrinol. 2011;210:5–14.
8. Huttemann M, Lee I, Sanavati L, Yu H, Doan J. Regulation of mitochondrial oxidative phosphorylation through cell signaling. Biochim Biophys Acta. 2007;1773:1701–20.
9. Brown G. Control of respiration and ATP synthesis in mammalian mitochondria and cells. Biochem J. 1992;284:1–13.
10. Van Blerkom J. The role of mitochondria in human oogenesis and preimplantation embryogenesis: engines of metabolism, ionic regulation and developmental competence. Reproduction. 2004;128:269–80.
11. Wilding M, Coppola G, Dale B, Di Matteo L. Mitochondria and human preimplantation embryo development. Reproduction. 2009;137:619–24.
12. Dumollard R, Duchen M, Carroll J. The role of mitochondrial function in the oocyte and embryo. Curr Top Dev Biol. 2007;77:21–49.
13. Trimarchi J, Liu L, Porterfield D, Smith P, Keefe D. Oxidative phosphorylation-dependent and-independent oxygen consumption by individual preimplantation mouse embryos. Biol Reprod. 2000;62:1866–74.
14. Yamanaka M, Hashimoto S, Arno A, Ito-Sasaki T, Abe H, Morimoto Y. Developmental assessment of human vitrified-warmed blastocysts based on oxygen consumption. Hum Reprod. 2011;26:3366–71.
15. Hardy K, Hooper M, Handyside A, Rutherford A, Winston R, Leese H. Non-invasive measurements of glucose and pyruvate uptake by individual human oocytes and preimplantation embryos. Hum Reprod. 1989;4:188–91.
16. Gardner D, Wale P, Collins R, Lane M. Glucose consumption of single post-compaction human embryos is predictive of embryo sex and live birth outcome. Hum Reprod. 2011;26:1981–6.

17. Van Blerkom J, Davis P, Lee J. ATP content of human oocytes and developmental potential and outcome after in-vitro fertilization and embryo transfer. Hum Reprod. 1995;10:415–24.
18. Zeng H, Ren Z, Yueng S, Shu Y, Xu Y, Zhuang G, et al. Low mitochondrial DNA and ATP contents contribute to the absence of birefringent spindle imaged with PolScope in in-vitro matured human oocytes. Hum Reprod. 2007;22:1681–6.
19. Manipalviratn S, Tong Z, Stegmann B, Widra E, Carter J, DeCherney A. Effect of vitrification and thawing on human oocyte ATP concentration. Fertil Steril. 2011;95:1839–41.
20. Seli E, Sakkas D, Scott R, Kwok S, Rosendahl S, Burns D. Noninvasive metabolomic profiling of embryo culture media using Raman and near-infrared spectroscopy correlates with reproductive potential of embryos in women undergoing in vitro fertilization. Fertil Steril. 2007;88:1350–7.
21. Seli E, Botros L, Sakkas D, Burns D. Noninvasive metabolomic profiling of embryo culture medium using proton nuclear magnetic resonance correlates with reproductive potential of embryos in women undergoing in vitro fertilization. Fertil Steril. 2008;90:2183–9.
22. Hardarson T, Ahlstrom A, Rogberg L, Botros L, Hillensjo T, Westlander G, et al. Non-invasive metabolomic profiling of Day 2 and Day 5 embryo culture medium: a prospective randomized trial. Hum Reprod. 2012;27:89–96.
23. Mahler H, Cohen J. Ooplasmic transfer: animal models assist human studies. Reprod Biomed Online. 2002;5:26–35.
24. Wakefield S, Lane M, Schultz S, Hebart M, Thompson J, Mitchell M. Maternal supply of omega-3 polyunsaturated fatty acids alter mechanisms involved in oocyte and early embryo development in the mouse. Am J Physiol Endocrinol Metab. 2008;294:E425–34.
25. Bentov Y, Esfandiari N, Burnstein E, Casper R. The use of mitochondrial nutrients to improve the outcome of fertility treatment in older patients. Fertil Steril. 2010;93:272–5.
26. Motta P, Nottola S, Makabe S, Makabe S, Heyn R. Mitochondrial morphology in human fetal and adult female germ cells. Hum Reprod. 2000;15 Suppl 2:128–47.
27. Shoffner J, Wallace D. Oxidative phosphorylation diseases and mitochondrial DNA mutations: diagnosis and treatment. Ann Rev Nutr. 1994;14:535–68.
28. Jacobs L, de Wer G, Geraedts J, de Coo I, Smeets H. The transmission of OXPHOS disease and methods to prevent this. Hum Reprod. 2006;12:11–136.
29. Collins Y, Chouchani T, James A, Menger K, Cocheme H, Murphy M. Mitochondrial redox signalling at a glance. J Cell Sci. 2012;125:801–6.
30. Eichenlaub-Ritter U, Wieczorek M, Seidel T. Age related changes in mitochondrial function and new approaches to study redox regulation in mammalian oocytes in response to age or maturation conditions. Mitochondrion. 2011;11:783–96.
31. Cao X, Chen Y. Mitochondria and calcium signaling in embryonic development. Semin Cell Dev Biol. 2009;20:337–45.
32. Van Blerkom J. The mitochondria in early development. Semin Cell Dev Biol. 2009;20:191–200.
33. Klymkowsky M. Mitochondrial activity, embryogenesis, and the dialogue between the big and little brains of the cell. Mitochondrion. 2011;11:814–9.
34. McBride H, Neuspiel M, Wasiak S. Mitochondria: more than just a powerhouse. Curr Biol. 2006;16: R551–60.
35. Eaton S, Bartlett K, Pourfarzm M. Mammalian mitochondrial beta-oxidation. Biochem J. 1996;320: 345–57.
36. Miller W. Role of mitochondria in steroidogenesis. Endocrinol Dev. 2011;20:1–19.
37. Cuezva J, Ortega A, Willers I, Sanchez-Cenizo L, Aldea M, Sanchez-Arago M. The tumor suppressor function of mitochondria: translation into the clinics. Biochim Biophys Acta. 2009;1792:1145–58.
38. Sjostrand F. Electron microscopy of mitochondria and cytoplasmic double membranes. Nature. 1953;202:1075–8.
39. Palade G. The fine structure of mitochondria. Anat Rec. 1952;114:427–52.
40. Palade G. An electron microscope study of mitochondrial structure. J Histochem Cytochem. 1953;1: 188–211.
41. Fisher ER, Danowski TS. Mitochondrial myopathy. Am J Clin Pathol. 1969;51:619–30.
42. Seo A, Joseph A-M, Dutta D, Hwang J, Aris J, Leeuwenburgh C. New insights into the role of mitochondria in aging: mitochondrial dynamics and more. J Cell Sci. 2010;123:2533–42.
43. Warburg O. On the origin of cancer cells. Science. 1956;123:309–14.
44. Carew J, Huang P. Mitochondrial defects in cancer. Mol Cancer. 2002;1:9–18.
45. DiMauro S, Schon E. Mitochondrial respiratory-chain diseases. N Engl J Med. 2003;248:2656–68.
46. Stadhouders A, Sengers R. Morphological observations in skeletal muscle from patients with mitochondrial myopathy. J Inherit Metab Dis. 1987;10 Suppl 1:62–80.
47. Larsson N, Wang J, Wilhemsson H, Oldfors A, Rustin P, Lewandoski M, et al. Mitochondria transcription factor A is necessary for mtDNA maintenance and embryogenesis in mice. Nat Genet. 1998;18:231–6.
48. Zamboni L, Mishell D, Bell J, Baca M. Fine structure of the human ovum in the pronuclear stage. J Cell Biol. 1966;30:579–600.
49. Calarco P, Brown E. An ultrastructural and cytological study of preimplantation development of the mouse. J Exp Zool. 1969;171:253–83.
50. Van Blerkom J, Manes C, Daniel J. Development of preimplantation rabbit embryos in vivo and in vitro: I. An ultrastructural comparison. Dev Biol. 1973;35:262–82.
51. Van Blerkom J, Davis P, Mawhig V, Alexander S. Domains of high and low polarized mitochondria in

mouse and human oocytes and early embryos. Hum Reprod. 2002;17:393–406.
52. Van Blerkom J. Mitochondrial function in the human oocyte and embryo and their role in developmental competence. Mitochondrion. 2011;11:797–813.
53. Muller-Hocker J, Shafer S, Weis S, Munscher C, Strowitzki T. Morphological, cytochemical and molecular genetic analysis of mitochondria in isolated human oocytes and reproductive age. Mol Hum Reprod. 1996;2:951–8.
54. Wakefield S, Lane M, Mitchell M. Impaired mitochondrial function in the preimplantation embryo perturbs fetal and placental development in the mouse. Biol Reprod. 2011;84:572–80.
55. Schon E, Kim S, Ferreora J, Magalhaes P, Grace M, Warburton D, et al. Chromosomal non-disjunction in human oocytes: is there a mitochondrial connection? Hum Reprod. 2000;15 Suppl 2:160–72.
56. Shahinaz H, El-Shourbagy S, Spikings E, Freitas M, St John J. Mitochondria directly influence fertilisation outcome in the pig. Reproduction. 2006;131:233–45.
57. Reynier P, May-Panloup P, Chretien M, Morgan C, et al. Mitochondrial DNA content effects the fertilizability of human oocytes. Mol Hum Reprod. 2001;7:425–9.
58. Almedia-Santos T, El Shourbagy S, St John C. Mitochondrial content reflects oocyte variability and fertilization outcome. Fertil Steril. 2006;85:584–91.
59. Santos T, El-Shourbagy S, St John J. Mitochondrial content reflects oocyte variability and fertilization outcome. Fertil Steril. 2006;85:584–92.
60. Au H, Yeh T, Kao S, Tzeng C, Hsieh R. Abnormal mitochondrial structure in human unfertilized oocytes and arrested embryos. Ann N Y Acad Sci USA. 2005;1042:177–85.
61. Van Blerkom J, Davis P. Mitochondrial signaling and fertilization. Mol Hum Reprod. 2007;13:759–70.
62. Lin D, Huang C-C, Wu H-M, Cheng T-C, Chen C-I, Lee M-S. Comparison of mitochondrial DNA contents in human embryos with good or poor morphology at the 8-cell stage. Fertil Steril. 2004;81:73–9.
63. Barrit J, Kokot M, Cohen J, Steuerwald N, Brenner C. Quantification of human ooplasmic mitochondria. Reprod Biomed Online. 2002;4:243–7.
64. Steuerwald N, Barrit J, Alder R, Mahler H, Schimmel T, Cohen J, et al. Quantification of mtDNA in single oocytes, polar bodies and subcellular components by real-time rapid fluorescence monitored. Zygote. 2000;9:209–15.
65. May-Panloup P, Chretien M-F, Jacques C, Vasseur C, Malthiery Y, Reynier P. Low oocyte mitochondrial DNA content and oocyte insufficiency. Hum Reprod. 2005;20:593–7.
66. May-Panloup P, Chretien M-F, Malthiery Y, Reynier P. Mitochondrial DNA in the oocyte and the developing embryo. Curr Top Dev Biol. 2007;77:51–83.
67. Van Blerkom J. The enigma of fragmentation in early human embryos: possible causes and clinical relevance. In: Van Blerkom J, Gregory L, editors. Essential IVF: basic research and clinical applications. Boston: Kluwer; 2004. p. 377–421.
68. Afzelius B. Electron microscopy of sea urchin eggs. Uppsala: Almqvist and Wiksell; 1957. p. 1–20.
69. Shoubridge E, Wai T. Mitochondrial DNA and the mammalian oocyte. Curr Top Dev Biol. 2007;77:87–111.
70. Van Blerkom J. Mitochondria as regulatory forces in oocytes, preimplantation embryos and stem cells. Reprod Biomed Online. 2008;16:553–69.
71. Tatuch Y, Robinson B. The mitochondrial DNA mutation at 8993 associated with NARP slows rate of ATP synthesis in isolated lymphoblast mitochondria. Biochem Biophys Res Commun. 1993;192:124–8.
72. Spikings E, Alderson J, St John J. Regulated mitochondrial DNA replication during oocyte maturation is essential for successful porcine embryonic development. Reproduction. 2007;76:327–35.
73. Agnello M, Morici G, Rinaldi M. A method for measuring mitochondrial mass and activity. Cytotechnology. 2008;56:145–9.
74. Van Blerkom J, Davis P, Alexander S. Inner mitochondrial membrane potential cytoplasmic ATP content and free calcium levels in metaphase II mouse oocytes. Hum Reprod. 2003;18:2429–40.
75. Van Blerkom J. The role of mitochondria in the establishment of developmental competence in early human development. In: Nagy Z, Varghese A, Agarwal A, editors. Practical manual of in vitro fertilization. New York: Springer;2012.
76. Jouaville L, Pinton P, Bastianutto C, Rutter G, Rizzuto R. Regulation of mitochondrial ATP synthesis by calcium: evidence for long-term metabolic priming. Proc Natl Acad Sci USA. 1999;96:13807–12.
77. Whitaker M. Calcium at fertilization and in early development. Physiol Rev. 2005;86:25–88.
78. Ichas F, Jouaville L, Sidash S, Mazat J-P, Holmuhamedov E. Mitochondrial calcium spiking: a transduction mechanism based on calcium-induced permeability transition in cell calcium signalling. FEBS Lett. 1994;348:211–5.
79. Dumollard R, Hammar K, Porterfield M, Smith P, Cibert C, Rouviere C, et al. Mitochondrial respiration and Ca^{2+} waves are linked during fertilization and meiosis completion. Development. 2003;130:83–692.
80. Thouas G, Trounson A, Wolvestag E, Jones G. Mitochondrial dysfunction in mouse oocytes results in preimplantation embryo arrest in vitro. Biol Reprod. 2004;16:1936–42.
81. Van Blerkom J, Davis P, Alexander S. Differential mitochondrial inheritance between blastomeres in cleavage stage human embryos: determination at the pronuclear stage and relationship to microtubular organization, ATP content and developmental competence. Hum Reprod. 2000;15:2621–33.
82. Squirrell JM, Schramm RD, Paprocki AM, Wokosin L, Bavister B. Imaging mitochondrial organization in living primate oocytes and embryos using multiphoton microscopy. Microsc Microanal. 2003;9:190–201.
83. Dumollard R, Carroll J, Duchen M, Campbell K, Swan K. Mitochondrial function and redox state in

mammalian embryos. Semin Cell Dev Biol. 2009; 20:346–53.
84. Van Blerkom J, Davis P. High-polarized ($\Delta\Psi m_{HIGH}$) mitochondria are spatially polarized in human oocytes and early embryos in stable subplasmalemmal domains: developmental significance and the concept of vanguard mitochondria. Reprod Biomed Online. 2006;13:246–54.
85. Van Blerkom J, Davis P, Thalhammer V. Regulation of mitochondrial polarity in mouse and human oocytes: the influence of cumulus derived nitric oxide. Mol Hum Reprod. 2008;14:431–44.
86. Van Blerkom J, Cox H, Davis P. Mitochondrial regulation of development during the preimplantation period: cell and location-specific $\Delta\Psi m$ in normal, diapausing and outgrowing mouse blastocysts. Reproduction. 2006;131:961–70.
87. Houghton F. Energy metabolism of the inner cell mass and trophectoderm of the mouse blastocyst. Differentiation. 2006;7:11–8.
88. Van Blerkom J. The role of the plasma membrane, subplasmalemmal and subcortical cytoplasm in early mammalian development. In: Coticchio G, De Santis L, Albertini D, editors. New York: Springer; 2012.
89. Wilding M, Dale B, Marino M, di Mattero L, Alviggi C, Pisaturo M, et al. Mitochondrial aggregation patterns and activity in human oocytes and preimplantation embryos. Hum Reprod. 2001;16:909–17.
90. Jones A, Van Blerkom J, Davis P, Toledo A. Cryopreservation of metaphase II human oocytes effects mitochondrial inner membrane potential: implications for developmental competence. Hum Reprod. 2004;19(8):1861–6.
91. Aw T-Y. Intracellular compartmentalization of organelles and gradients of low molecular weight species. Int Rev Cytol. 2000;192:223–53.
92. Zhang X, Li X-H, Ma X, Wang Z-H, Lu S, Guo Y-L. Redox induced apoptosis of human oocytes in resting follicles in vitro. J Soc Gynecol Investig. 2006;13:451–8.
93. Zorov D, Filburn C, Klotz L, Zweier J, Sollott S. Reactive oxygen species (ROS)-induced ROS release: a new phenomenon accompanying induction of the mitochondrial permeability transition in cardiac myocytes. J Exp Med. 2000;192:1000–4.
94. Wang W, Fang H, Groom L, Cheng A, Zhang W, Liu J, et al. Superoxide flashes in single mitochondria. Cell. 2008;134:279–90.
95. Wang X, Jian C, Zhang X, Huang Z, Xu J, Hou T, et al. Superoxide flashes: elemental events of mitochondrial ROS signaling in the heart. J Mol Cell Cardiol. 2012;52:940–8.
96. Pouvreau S. Superoxide flashes in mouse skeletal muscle are produced by discrete arrays of active mitochondria operating coherently. PLoS One. 2010;5(9):e13035.
97. Mantel C, Messina-Graham S, Broxmeyer H. Superoxide flashes, reactive oxygen species, and the mitochondrial permeability transition pore: potential implications for hematopoietic stem cell function. Curr Opin Hematol. 2011;18:208–13.
98. Wei L, Salahura G, Boncompagni S, Kasischke K, Protasi F, Sheu S-S, et al. Mitochondrial superoxide flashes: metabolic markers of skeletal muscle activity and disease. FASEB J. 2011;25:3068–78.
99. Robinson K, Janes M, Beckman J. The selective detection of mitochondrial superoxide by live cell imaging. Nat Protoc. 2008;3:941–7.
100. Warwar N, Mor A, Fluhr R, Pandian R, Kuppusamy P, Blank A. Detection and imaging of superoxide in roots by an electron spin resonance spin-probe method. Biophys J. 2011;101:1529–38.
101. Ma Q, Fang H, Shang W, Liu L, Xu Z, Ye T, et al. Superoxide flashes: early mitochondrial signals for oxidative stress-induced apoptosis. J Biol Chem. 2011;286:27573–81.
102. Li K, Zhang W, Fang H, Xie W, Liu J, Zheng M, et al. Superoxide flashes reveal novel properties of mitochondrial reactive oxygen species excitability in cardiomyocytes. Biophys J. 2012;102:1011–21.
103. Magnusson C, Hillensjo T, Hamberger L, Nilsson L. Oxygen consumption by human oocytes and blastocysts grown in vitro. Hum Reprod. 1986;1:183–4.
104. Houghton F, Thompson J, Kennedy C, Leese H. Oxygen consumption and energy metabolism of the early mouse embryo. Mol Reprod Dev. 1996;44: 476–85.
105. Lopes A, Larsen L, Ramsing N, Lovendahl P, Raty M, Peippo J, et al. Respiration rates of individual bovine in vitro-produced embryos measured with a novel, non-invasive and highly sensitive microsensor system. Reproduction. 2005;130:669–79.
106. Tejera A, Herrero J, de los Santos M, Garrido N, Ramasing N, Meseguer M. Oxygen consumption is a quality marker for human oocyte competence conditioned by ovarian stimulation regimens. Fertil Steril. 2011;96:618–23.
107. Scott L, Berntsen J, Davies D, Gundersen J, Hill J, Ramsing N. Human oocyte respiration-rate measurement—a potential to improve oocyte and embryo selection? Reprod Biomed Online. 2008;17:461–9.
108. Alm H, Toner H, Lohrke B, Viergutz T, Ghoneim I, Kanitz W. Bovine blastocyst developmental rate in vitro is influences by selection of oocytes by brilliant cresyl blue staining before IVM as an indicator for glucose-6-phosphate dehydrogenase activity. Theriogenology. 2005;63:2194–205.
109. Catala M, Izquierdo D, Rodriguez-Prado M, Hammami S, Paramio M. Effect of oocyte quality on blastocyst development after in vitro fertilization (IVF) and intracytoplasmic sperm injection (ICSI) in a sheep model. Fertil Steril. 2012;97:1004–8.
110. Wongsrikeao P, Otoi T, Yamasaki H, Agung B, Taniguchi M, Naoi H, et al. Effects of single and double exposure to brilliant cresyl blue on the selection of porcine oocytes for in vitro production of embryos. Theriogenology. 2006;15:366–72.
111. Rodriguez-Gonzalez E, Lopez-Bejar M, Velilla E, Paramio M. Selection of prepubertal goat oocytes

using the brilliant cresyl blue test. Theriogenology. 2002;57:1379–409.

112. Manjuntha B, Gupta P, Devaraj M, Ravindra J, Nandi S. Selection of developmentally competent buffalo oocytes by brilliant cresyl blue staining before IVM. Theriogenology. 2007;68:1299–304.

113. Bhojwani S, Alm H, Toner H, Kanitz W, Poehland R. Selection of developmentally competent oocytes through brilliant cresyl blue stain enhances blastocyst development rate after bovine nuclear transfer. Theriogenology. 2007;67:341–5.

114. Wu Y-G, Lin Y, Zhou P, Lan G-C, Han D, Miao D-Q, et al. Selection of oocytes for in vitro maturation by brilliant cresyl blue staining: a study using the mouse model. Cell Res. 2007;17:722–31.

115. Torner H, Ghanem N, Ambros C, Holker M, Toomek W, Phatsara C, et al. Molecular and subcellular characterization of oocytes screened for their developmental competence based on glucose-6-phosphate dehydrogenase activity. Reproduction. 2008;135: 197–212.

116. Silva D, Rodroguez P, Galuppo A, Arruda N, Rodrigues J. Selection of bovine oocytes by brilliant cresyl blue staining: effect on meiosis progression, organelle distribution and embryo development. Zygote. 2011;19:1–6.

117. Catala M, Izquierdo D, Uzbekova S, Morato R, Roura M, Romageura R, et al. Brilliant cresyl blue staining selects largest oocytes with highest mitochondrial activity, maturation-promoting factor activity and embryo developmental competence in prepubertal sheep. Reproduction. 2011;142:517–27.

118. Lopes A, Wrenzycki C, Ramsing N, Hermann D, Niemann H, Lovendahl P, et al. Respiration rates correlated with mRNA expression of G6PD and GLUT1 genes in individual bovine oocytes in in vitro-produced blastocysts. Theriogenology. 2007;68:223–36.

119. Van Blerkom J, Sinclair J, Davis P. Mitochondrial transfer between oocytes: potential applications of mitochondrial donation and the issue of heteroplasmy. Hum Reprod. 1998;12:2857–68.

23 Carbohydrate Analysis and Embryo Viability

Michelle Lane and David K. Gardner

A key component in a successful single embryo transfer program within an IVF unit is a robust method for identification of the relative viability of embryos. The capacity to rank a patient's embryos with respect to their viability in a quantitative, accurate, and repeatable manner is an important aspect of moving towards single embryo transfers for the majority of patients. Ideally viability markers for human embryos should be noninvasive and provide quantitative measures that are repeatable and are able to transverse different patient populations such as different aetiologies, stimulation regimes, and other health and lifestyle factors of the sub-fertile couple. In order to be incorporated into a fresh embryo transfer program they also need to have rapid turnaround times and need ultimately to provide additional information over the associative morphology assessments that are used today. Quantification of carbohydrate utilization by embryos and its relationship to subsequent fetal development post transfer has been well established in animal models. Analysis of carbohydrate metabolism by human embryos, particularly post-compaction, provides a most promising candidate as a noninvasive marker of embryo viability.

M. Lane (✉)
Repromed, 180 Fullarton Road, Dulwich, SA 5165, Australia
e-mail: MLane@repromed.com.au

D.K. Gardner
Department of Zoology, University of Melbourne, Melbourne, VIC, Australia
e-mail: david.gardner@unimelb.edu.au

Preimplantation Embryo Development: Pre-compaction vs. Post-compaction

In order to understand the importance of embryo metabolism and how it might reflect embryo development and viability it is important to understand the dynamic nature of preimplantation development. The preimplantation mammalian embryo represents a highly dynamic period of development where it develops following fertilization from a single pluripotent cell to the complex structure of the blastocyst containing around 80–100 cells having undergone the first differentiation event. During early stages of preimplantation development, a series of highly coordinated developmental events occur, in the human in a period of 4–5 days, involving the completion of the sperm-derived calcium waves that initiate activation [1, 2] and continue with zygotic gene expression [3], reductive cleavage divisions every 12–15 h, and initial activation of the embryonic genome [4]. During development up to the 8-cell stage, cells are loosely connected and the embryo resembles closely a unicellular organism with quite primitive mechanisms for the regulation of cellular homeostasis [5–8]. The early embryo also appears to lack robust systems for protection against reactive oxygen species (ROS) and has been shown to be particularly sensitive to oxidative stress in culture [9–11].

At the 8-cell stage, compaction begins where the blastomeres polarize, begin to flatten against

D.K. Gardner et al. (eds.), *Human Gametes and Preimplantation Embryos: Assessment and Diagnosis*, DOI 10.1007/978-1-4614-6651-2_23, © Springer Science+Business Media New York 2013

one another increasing cell to cell contacts, forming gap, and tight junctions to produce the morula. Many metabolic and physiological changes occur around the time of compaction, including an increase in transcription resulting in more robust homeostatic regulatory pathways such as antioxidant defense mechanisms, which are lacking at the early stage of development [12]. The creation of the blastocoelic cavity, via Na^+/K^+ ATPase [13], and the first differentiation of blastomeres into the inner cell mass (ICM) and the trophectoderm (TE) results in the blastocyst.

Preimplantation Embryo Metabolism

Concomitantly with the distinct changes in physiology that occur during development from the zygote to the blastocyst stage are dynamic changes in the metabolism of the embryo. At the zygote stage, the embryo is initially quiescent with a low metabolic and biosynthetic activity. At these early stages the embryo predominantly uses the carboxylic acids pyruvate and lactate as its preferred energy substrates [14–16]. Therefore, at these early stages of development the embryo is completely reliant on mitochondrial-based metabolism for ATP generation. However, the embryo does take up low levels of glucose [14, 15], which are likely metabolized by the pentose-phosphate pathway for the maintenance of reducing power in the cell particularly in the production of reduced glutathione for protection against oxidative stress. Furthermore, there is a recent understanding that the metabolism of glucose by the hexosamine biosynthesis pathway in the early embryo may be important in establishing O-linked glycosylation that is important for later stage development [17, 18]. Therefore, it may be that this metabolism of glucose, although at a low level during the early stages of preimplantation development, is essential for setting the subsequent metabolic program.

With the onset of the embryonic genome and as the embryo undergoes compaction there is a switch in nutrient preference to a glucose-based metabolism and by the blastocyst stage, glucose has become the preferred nutrient [14, 15], although uptake of carboxylic acids still occurs. However, unlike most somatic cells that metabolize virtually all of the glucose taken up via the TCA cycle, glucose taken up by the blastocyst is metabolized by both the TCA cycle as well as around half of all of the glucose being converted to lactate by aerobic glycolysis [19, 20]. This unusual conversion of glucose to lactate in the presence of significant levels of oxygen is thought to result from the high biosynthetic demand or as a result of an inability to maintain redox control in the cell and has been shown to occur in other rapidly dividing cells such as tumor cells. Interestingly, there appears to be a significant difference in the metabolism of the inner cell mass cells of the blastocyst compared to the cells of the surrounding trophectoderm. Inner cell mass cells have been shown to be completely reliant on glycolysis for their energy and do not appear to have any functional oxidative metabolism while trophectoderm cells metabolize the majority of glucose through oxidative-based metabolism [21, 22].

Relationship of Carbohydrate Metabolism to Embryo Viability: Animal Models

The impact of poor culture conditions on embryo metabolism was demonstrated as early as 1970 by Menke and McLaren, who determined that when 8-cell mouse embryos were cultured in a simple medium the resultant blastocysts exhibited compromised carbon dioxide production compared to in vivo-developed control embryos [23]. As such, these observations indicated that the oxidative capacity of the blastocyst was impaired by culture. Ten years later, the first study that directly measured carbohydrate metabolism of individual embryos and related this to transfer outcome was published. Renard et al. demonstrated that increased levels of glucose metabolism by day 10 cow blastocysts were related to the ability of the blastocyst to subsequently implant and produce a viable pregnancy, providing the first evidence that glucose metabolism in the blastocyst could be used as a viability marker [24]. This work was further extended by

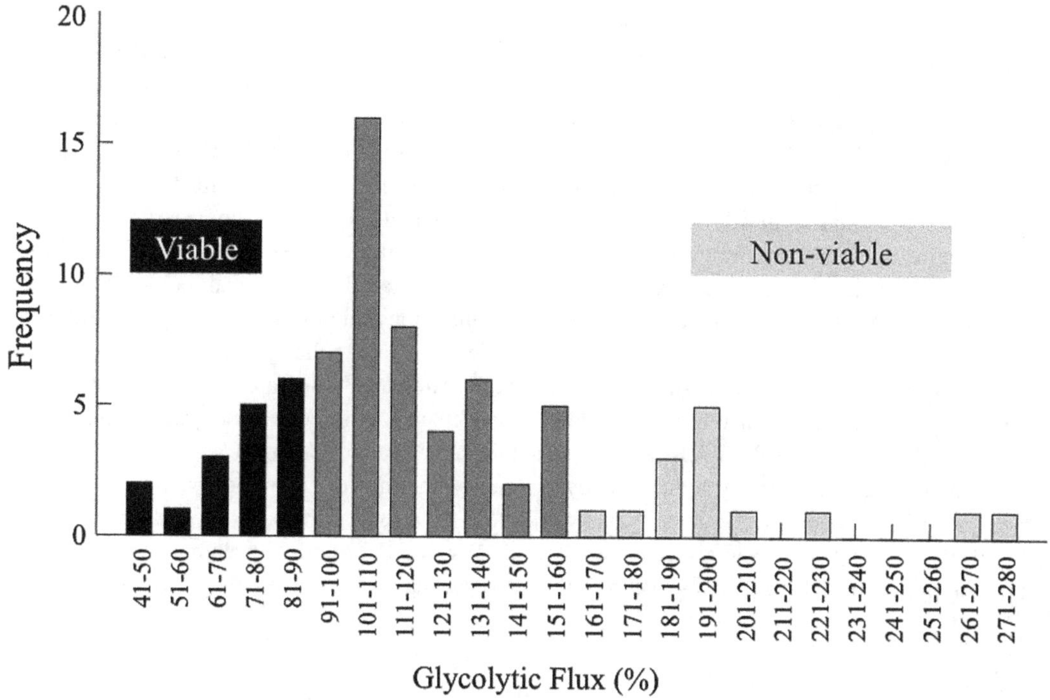

Fig. 23.1 Fetal development of mouse blastocysts selected for transfer using glycolytic activity as a biochemical marker. "Viable" blastocysts were classified as those with a glycolytic rate close to in vivo-developed blastocysts (<88 %), while "Non-viable" blastocysts had a glycolytic rate in the highest 15 % of the distribution (<160 %). On each day of the experiment, a selection of blastocysts were transferred at random, along with those selected as either viable or nonviable (adapted from Lane M, Gardner DK. Selection of viable mouse blastocysts prior to transfer using a metabolic criterion. Hum Reprod. 1996;11:1975–8, with permission)

Gardner and Leese in 1987 who were able to demonstrate in a retrospective study that the glucose uptake of morphologically similar mouse blastocysts was correlated with its viability after transfer, with viable blastocysts taking up increased rates of glucose [25]. Interestingly, they also determined that glucose uptake was elevated in female embryos compared to male embryos, a finding that was later confirmed in further studies where the sex of the embryo could be established using a GFP tag [26].

In 1996, Lane and Gardner determined that the viability of morphologically similar mouse blastocysts (of the same diameter) could be predicted based on the levels of glucose metabolism in a prospective study [27]. In this seminal paper it was revealed that the discriminatory and predictive nature of the glucose metabolism between viable and nonviable mouse embryos was improved when additional measures that provide information regarding the fate of the glucose taken up by the embryo were also included in the analysis [27]. Glycolytic activity, calculated as the amount of glucose that was taken up by the embryo and converted to lactate, was highly variable with a large range in values between blastocysts, despite them being of a similar morphology (Fig. 1). Demonstrating that metabolic activity was adding additional information over morphology alone which is an important feature for any measure that is to be used in a clinical program.

Relationship of Carbohydrate Metabolism to Embryo Viability: Human Embryos

The early human embryo prior to compaction has a pyruvate-based metabolism and is relatively quiescent [28]. Although there have been some attempts at the assessment of pyruvate uptake as a maker of human embryo metabolism, these studies demonstrated that there was no correlation between cleavage stage metabolism and pyruvate uptake [29, 30]. This is plausbily a result of the low metabolic activity of the cleavage stage embryo and the smaller metabolic differences between embryos during the first couple of cell cycles [31]. Furthermore, observations in animal models would indicate that the fate of the metabolite is as important as the uptake itself.

In contrast, post-compaction stage human embryo has a significantly increased metabolic rate and similar to the animal models, the uptake of glucose increases significantly at the blastocyst stage [14, 15]. Studies on the metabolism of donated human embryos determined that the uptake of pyruvate and glucose by the morula were higher in embryos that developed to the blastocyst stage. Further, on day 5, blastocysts of higher morphological grades had highest rates of glucose uptake, demonstrating that glucose was the most important carbohydrate for the human blastocysts [16]. Similar to animal studies, it was confirmed that there was considerable range in glucose uptakes between human blastocysts that had a similar morphological grade even from within a population of blastocysts from the same patient, indicating that glucose consumption may be discriminatory compared to morphology alone. Of 13 blastocysts of the same grade, and all from the same patient, there was over 100 pmol/embryo/h range of glucose consumption.

In a recent retrospective study in patients undergoing IVF/ICSI with a single embryo transfer, we have determined that there is a highly

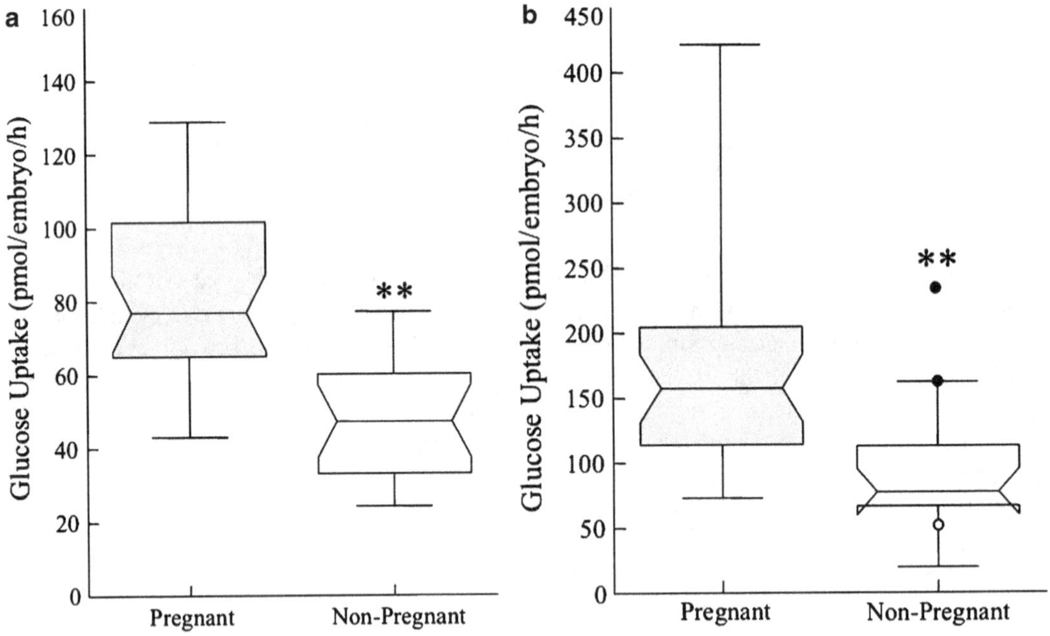

Fig. 23.2 (**a**) Glucose uptake on day 4 of embryonic development and pregnancy outcome (positive fetal heart beat). Notches represent the interquartile range (50 % of the data), whiskers represent the 5 and 95 % quartiles. The line across the box is the median glucose consumption. ** significantly different from pregnant ($P<0.01$). (**b**) Glucose uptake on day 5 of embryonic development and pregnancy outcome (positive fetal heart beat). Notches represent the confidence interval of the median, and the depth of the box represents interquartile range (50 % of the data), whiskers represent the 5 and 95 % quartiles. The line across the box is the median glucose consumption. *Closed circles* represent two blastocysts that gave rise to a positive fetal sac, but no subsequent fetal heart. The *open circle* represents a blastocyst that resulted in a positive hCG but not fetal sac. ** significantly different from pregnant ($P<0.01$) (from Gardner DK, Wale PL, Collins R, Lane M. Glucose consumption of single post-compaction human embryos is predictive of embryo sex and live birth outcome. Hum Reprod. 2011;26:1981–6, with permission)

significant association between the uptake of glucose from both day 3 to day 4 (compaction and morula formation) and also from day 4 to day 5 (blastocyst development) and both pregnancy and live birth rates [32]. Embryos that resulted in a successful pregnancy had a higher mean glucose uptake compared to embryos that failed in implant (Fig. 2). In this study, it was also reported that glucose uptake by the embryos was independent of the morphological grade of the embryo, indicating that metabolic activity could serve as a valuable independent maker of developmental potential. Intriguingly, this study also demonstrated sex-related difference in glucose uptake consistent with animal studies, reflecting the fact that male and female embryos have difference proteomes [25, 26, 33] (Fig. 3).

It must be noted that in all of the studies to date, there is notable overlap between populations of embryos that produced a pregnancy and those that did not. In animal studies it is clear that an increased level of differentiation between viable and nonviable embryos results from assessments not only of glucose uptake but of metabolic fate [27].

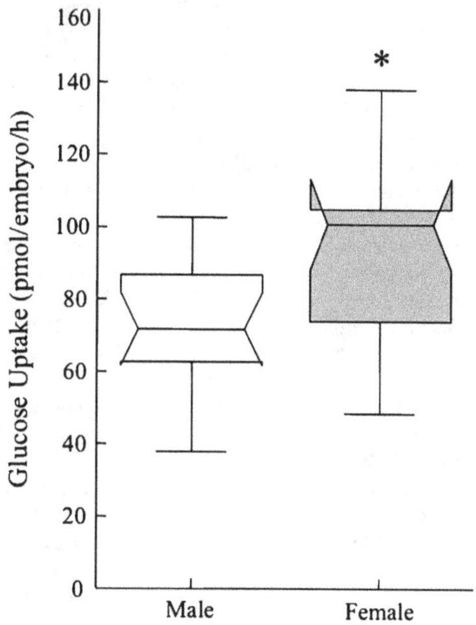

Fig. 23.3 Glucose uptake by male and female embryos on day 4 of development. Notches represent the interquartile range (50 % of the data), whiskers represent the 5 and 95 % quartiles. The line across the box is the median glucose consumption. * significantly different from male embryos ($P<0.05$) (from Gardner DK, Wale PL, Collins R, Lane M. Glucose consumption of single post-compaction human embryos is predictive of embryo sex and live birth outcome. Hum Reprod. 2011;26:1981–6, with permission)

Although glucose metabolism is a promising candidate marker in predicting subsequent viability, a clear limitation of the current technology is the need to markers to be proven in randomized controlled trials.

Current Challenges for Adoption of Assessment of Metabolic Activity as a Viability Marker

Technical

Introduction of metabolic assessment criteria into a busy IVF laboratory does present some challenges and changes to protocols to ensure that results are repeatable. Aspects such as consistent volume of the culture drops are critical both at the set up of the dishes and also when the embryo is added to the drop. Contamination of media from a previous step by incomplete washing of the embryo can also render results meaningless. Therefore, in our experience the introduction of a metabolic measure requires an update of protocols and increase in QA and monitoring of procedures associates with embryo culture. This aspect of assessment is often understated and may be a limitation for the widespread application of this technology.

Environmental

Metabolism of a cell is an essential aspect to cell health. When faced with a hostile environment most cells can make metabolic adaptations in order to survive and maintain function. The mammalian embryo is no different. Whilst it has been established that the human embryo has a degree of plasticity this does come at a cost to viability. The controlled usage of substrates (correct fate of substrate) at the appropriate stage of development is essential for optimal viability [34–36]. We have determined in animal embryos that exposure to conditions such as high oxygen [37] or amino acid-free media [20] can result in a loss of control of metabolism that make interpretation of data difficult and change reference ranges between laboratories. In the case of removal of amino acids, glucose uptake has actually shown to increase in stressed blastocysts to compensate for change in substrate fate away from a mitochondrial (efficient production of ATP) to a cytoplasmic (aerobic glycolysis and 18-fold reduced ATP production)-based metabolism. Therefore, it is likely that metabolism markers will need to be interpreted carefully between laboratories that employ different conditions, such as oxygen levels, as direct comparison between uptake studies alone may be misleading. Further, it is likely that measures that can effectively demonstrate the most efficient carbohydrate metabolism of an embryo are likely to be the most robust measures.

Conclusion

The capacity to be able to rank embryos in a quantitative fashion in the laboratory is highly sort after with many different approaches being tried, both refining morphological assessments that have been used for many years as well as the development and adoption of new technologies either genomic, transcriptomic, proteomic, or metabolic approaches. Carbohydrate metabolism of the embryo, particularly the later stage embryo, is an attractive option as it is noninvasive, provides measures post-embryonic genome activation, thereby including aspects of maternal and paternal genomes, and can easily be performed in the timeframe required for a fresh transfer. Animal studies highlight carbohydrate metabolism as an important feature in viability, and recent human studies have shown similar promise. The advent of platforms such as lab-on a-chip technologies should enable integration of technology in laboratories and facilitate large multicenter randomized controlled trials [38, 39].

References

1. Dumollard R, Duchen M, Sardet C. Calcium signals and mitochondria at fertilisation. Semin Cell Dev Biol. 2006;17:314–23.
2. Jones KT. Mammalian egg activation: from Ca2+ spiking to cell cycle progression. Reproduction. 2005;130:813–23.
3. Schultz RM. The molecular foundations of the maternal to zygotic transition in the preimplantation embryo. Hum Reprod Update. 2002;8:323–31.
4. Braude P, Bolton V, Moore S. Human gene expression first occurs between the four- and eight-cell stages of preimplantation development. Nature. 1988;332:459–61.
5. Lane M, Gardner DK. Blastomere homeostasis. In: Gardner DK, Lane M, editors. Art and the human blastocyst. Boston: Serono Symposia; 2001. p. 69–90.
6. Lane M, Baltz JM, Bavister BD. Regulation of intracellular pH in hamster preimplantation embryos by the sodium hydrogen (Na+/H+) antiporter. Biol Reprod. 1998;59:1483–90.
7. Lane M, Baltz JM, Bavister BD. Bicarbonate/chloride exchange regulates intracellular pH of embryos but not oocytes of the hamster. Biol Reprod. 1999;61: 452–7.
8. Phillips KP, Baltz JM. Intracellular pH regulation by HCO3-/Cl- exchange is activated during early mouse zygote development. Dev Biol. 1999;208:392–405.
9. Nasr-Esfahani MH, Winston NJ, Johnson MH. Effects of glucose, glutamine, ethylenediaminetetraacetic acid and oxygen tension on the concentration of reactive oxygen species and on development of the mouse preimplantation embryo in vitro. J Reprod Fertil. 1992;96:219–31.
10. Nasr-Esfahani MM, Johnson MH. The origin of reactive oxygen species in mouse embryos cultured in vitro. Development. 1991;113:551–60.
11. Wale PL, Gardner DK. Time-lapse analysis of mouse embryo development in oxygen gradients. Reprod Biomed Online. 2010;21:402–10.
12. Lane M, Gardner DK. Regulation of ionic homeostasis by mammalian embryos. Semin Reprod Med. 2000;18:195–204.
13. Watson AJ, Kidder GM. Immunofluorescence assessment of the timing of appearance and cellular distribution of Na/K-ATPase during mouse embryogenesis. Dev Biol. 1988;126:80–90.
14. Gott AL, Hardy K, Winston RM, Leese HJ. Non-invasive measurement of pyruvate and glucose uptake and lactate production by single human preimplantation embryos. Hum Reprod. 1990;5:104–8.
15. Hardy K, Hooper MA, Handyside AH, Rutherford AJ, Winston RM, Leese HJ. Non-invasive measurement of glucose and pyruvate uptake by individual human oocytes and preimplantation embryos. Hum Reprod. 1989;4:188–91.

16. Gardner DK, Lane M, Stevens J, Schoolcraft WB. Noninvasive assessment of human embryo nutrient consumption as a measure of developmental potential. Fertil Steril. 2001;76:1175–80.
17. Jansen S, Cashman K, Thompson JG, Pantaleon M, Kaye PL. Glucose deprivation, oxidative stress and peroxisome proliferator-activated receptor-alpha (PPARA) cause peroxisome proliferation in preimplantation mouse embryos. Reproduction. 2009;138:493–505.
18. Pantaleon M, Scott J, Kaye PL. Nutrient sensing by the early mouse embryo: hexosamine biosynthesis and glucose signaling during preimplantation development. Biol Reprod. 2008;78:595–600.
19. Gardner DK, Leese HJ. Concentrations of nutrients in mouse oviduct fluid and their effects on embryo development and metabolism in vitro. J Reprod Fertil. 1990;88:361–8.
20. Lane M, Gardner DK. Amino acids and vitamins prevent culture-induced metabolic perturbations and associated loss of viability of mouse blastocysts. Hum Reprod. 1998;13:991–7.
21. Hewitson LC, Leese HJ. Energy metabolism of the trophectoderm and inner cell mass of the mouse blastocyst. J Exp Zool. 1993;267:337–43.
22. Hewitson LC, Martin KL, Leese HJ. Effects of metabolic inhibitors on mouse preimplantation embryo development and the energy metabolism of isolated inner cell masses. Mol Reprod Dev. 1996;43:323–30.
23. Menke TM, McLaren A. Mouse blastocysts grown in vivo and in vitro: carbon dioxide production and trophoblast outgrowth. J Reprod Fertil. 1970;23:117–27.
24. Renard JP, Philippon A, Menezo Y. In-vitro uptake of glucose by bovine blastocysts. J Reprod Fertil. 1980;58:161–4.
25. Gardner DK, Leese HJ. Assessment of embryo viability prior to transfer by the noninvasive measurement of glucose uptake. J Exp Zool. 1987;242:103–5.
26. Gardner DK, Larman MG, Thouas GA. Sex-related physiology of the preimplantation embryo. Mol Hum Reprod. 2010;16:539–47.
27. Lane M, Gardner DK. Selection of viable mouse blastocysts prior to transfer using a metabolic criterion. Hum Reprod. 1996;11:1975–8.
28. Leese HJ. Metabolism of the preimplantation embryo: 40 years on. Reproduction. 2012;143:417–27.
29. Conaghan J, Hardy K, Handyside AH, Winston RM, Leese HJ. Selection criteria for human embryo transfer: a comparison of pyruvate uptake and morphology. J Assist Reprod Genet. 1993;10:21–30.
30. Turner K, Martin KL, Woodward BJ, Lenton EA, Leese HJ. Comparison of pyruvate uptake by embryos derived from conception and non-conception natural cycles. Hum Reprod. 1994;9:2362–6.
31. Gardner DK. Analysis of embryo metabolism and the metabolome to identify the most viable embryo within a cohort. In: Gardner DK, Risk RMB, Falcone T, editors. Human assisted reproductive technology: future trends in laboratory ad clinical practice. Cambridge: Cambridge University Press; 2011. p. 301–12.
32. Gardner DK, Wale PL, Collins R, Lane M. Glucose consumption of single post-compaction human embryos is predictive of embryo sex and live birth outcome. Hum Reprod. 2011;26:1981–6.
33. Epstein CJ, Smith S, Travis B, Tucker G. Both X chromosomes function before visible X-chromosome inactivation in female mouse embryos. Nature. 1978;274:500–3.
34. Gardner DK, Pool TB, Lane M. Embryo nutrition and energy metabolism and its relationship to embryo growth, differentiation, and viability. Semin Reprod Med. 2000;18:205–18.
35. Lane M, Gardner DK. Understanding cellular disruptions during early embryo development that perturb viability and fetal development. Reprod Fertil Dev. 2005;17:371–8.
36. Leese HJ, Baumann CG, Brison DR, McEvoy TG, Sturmey RG. Metabolism of the viable mammalian embryo: quietness revisited. Mol Hum Reprod. 2008;14:667–72.
37. Wale PL, Gardner DK. Oxygen regulates amino acid turnover and carbohydrate uptake during the preimplantation period of mouse embryo development. Biol Reprod. 2012;87(1):24.
38. Urbanski JP, Johnson MT, Craig DD, Potter DL, Gardner DK, Thorsen T. Noninvasive metabolic profiling using microfluidics for analysis of single preimplantation embryos. Anal Chem. 2008;80:6500–7.
39. Heo YS, Cabrera LM, Bormann CL, Smith GD, Takayama S. Real time culture and analysis of embryo metabolism using a microfluidic device with deformation based actuation. Lab Chip. 2012;12:2240–6.

Identification of Viable Embryos by Noninvasive Measurement of Amino Acids in Culture Media

24

Francesca D. Houghton

Amino acids are an essential component of human preimplantation culture media and have several physiological roles. They form the building blocks of protein, chelate heavy metals, act as osmolytes, regulate intracellular pH, are precursors for nucleotides, polyamines, signalling molecules and may be metabolised for energy production. Thus, being intrinsic to so many cellular functions, it is not surprising that there has been a resurgence of interest in the role of amino acids in human preimplantation development over recent years. This review does not intend to give a historical account of the role of amino acids during embryo development, such information can be found elsewhere [1]. Suffice to say, the inclusion of amino acids in culture media has been shown to be beneficial for early embryo development in a number of species [2–8]. This chapter concentrates on data obtained in the human and specifically the emerging evidence which highlights the ability of amino acid utilisation to noninvasively predict the viability of individual preimplantation embryos.

In vivo, embryos will be exposed to a complete, physiological mixture of amino acids found in the Fallopian tube and uterus. However, in terms of human nutrition, amino acids are generally categorised into two groups: either essential or nonessential. Essential amino acids are those which cannot be formed de novo from other compounds in the body and thus must be obtained from the diet. In contrast, nonessential amino acids are not required in the diet as they can be synthesised in vivo. However in practice, this nomenclature is somewhat more complex as some nonessential amino acids become essential and are required in the diet under certain conditions and disease states and are termed conditionally essential (CE) [9, 10]. In terms of this review an understanding of which amino acids fall into each category is important since this method of segregation has been used to supplement the medium at different stages of embryo development (Table 1).

Effect of Amino Acids on Human Preimplantation Embryos

Initially studies investigated the effect of adding individual or small groups of amino acids to human preimplantation culture medium. One of the first amino acids to be added was glutamine which was found to improve development to the blastocyst stage [6]. However, following data obtained from mouse embryos it was found that human embryos cultured in the presence of nonessential amino acids up until the 8- to 16-cell stage (day 3 of development), followed by the inclusion of a complete mixture of amino acids for the remainder of preimplantation development was beneficial for blastocyst formation and

F.D. Houghton (✉)
Centre for Human Development, Stem Cells & Regeneration, Faculty of Medicine, University of Southampton, Tremona Road, Southampton, SO16 6YD, UK
e-mail: F.D.Houghton@soton.ac.uk

D.K. Gardner et al. (eds.), *Human Gametes and Preimplantation Embryos: Assessment and Diagnosis*, DOI 10.1007/978-1-4614-6651-2_24, © Springer Science+Business Media New York 2013

Table 24.1 Amino acid classification

Essential	Histidine, isoleucine, leucine, lysine, methionine, phenylalanine, threonine, tryptophan, valine
Nonessential	Alanine, arginine (CE), asparagine, aspartic acid, cysteine (CE), glutamic acid, glutamine (CE), glycine (CE), proline (CE), serine (CE), tyrosine (CE)

improved viability post-transfer [11–13]. These landmark studies highlighted the beneficial effects of amino acids for embryo development and revolutionised human IVF with the advent of sequential culture media.

Ability of Amino Acid Profiling to Noninvasively Predict Future Blastocyst Formation

One of the most recently discovered and intriguing roles of amino acids is the ability of their utilisation to predict future embryo development [14–16]. Interestingly, these experiments were performed in a defined medium composed of Earle's balanced salt solution containing 0.5 % human serum albumin, 1 mM glucose, 0.47 mM pyruvate and 5 mM lactate, together with a complete mixture of amino acids at near physiological levels found in the Fallopian tube [17]. Human embryos derived from fresh cycles of IVF were cultured individually for 24 h periods in sequential 4 μL drops of medium from day 2 post-fertilisation, and development to the blastocyst stage was monitored [14]. The concentration of 18 amino acids in the spent drops was analysed retrospectively using reverse phase HPLC and compared to that observed in embryo-free drops which were cultured alongside the embryos. This allowed the amino acid appearance into, and depletion from the medium by the embryo to be determined. The results obtained were somewhat surprising as there was a significant difference in the utilisation of asparagine, glutamine, arginine, alanine and methionine by embryos from day 2 to day 3 which developed to the blastocyst stage compared to those which arrested prior to blastocyst formation. Counter intuitively, total amino acid depletion by those individual embryos which developed to the blastocyst stage was significantly lower than those which arrested [14]. Similarly, total amino acid depletion from the compacting 8-cell to morula stage was also significantly lower in those embryos which developed to the blastocyst stage compared to those which arrested before blastocyst formation.

When amino acid turnover (sum of the amino acids that appeared into, and disappeared from the medium) was investigated similar results were observed; embryos cultured from day 2 to day 3, as well as from the compacting 8-cell to morula stage that developed to the blastocyst stage displayed an amino acid turnover which was significantly less than their arresting counterparts [14]. These results were fascinating, particularly since there was no morphological difference in embryo grade between the groups. Thus, by using morphological criteria alone it would not be possible to predict which embryo would progress to the blastocyst stage suggesting that the difference in amino acid profile does not simply reflect embryo quality.

Another interesting finding from this study was the observation of which specific amino acids were depleted from the medium at each stage of development. As might be expected there was an increase in the number of amino acids depleted as development progressed. Leucine was the only amino acid depleted from day 2 to 3, compared to leucine, arginine and serine from the compacting 8-cell to morula stage and finally leucine, arginine, serine, methionine and valine over the morula to blastocyst transition [14]. This not only indicates the importance of these particular amino acids to preimplantation development but also highlights a potential concern with commercially available human embryo culture medium. Currently, many companies do not disclose the precise composition of the media used to culture preimplantation embryos and hence it is difficult to assess what impact this may have on metabolism and future development. This is particularly important in light of recent evidence showing that there is an associaton between the medium used for human embryo culture and subsequent birthweight [18, 19]. The majority of sequential media only contain nonessential amino acids until day 3 of development before including both essential and nonessential amino acids for culture to the blastocyst stage. This is surprising since:

- The premise was based largely on data obtained from the mouse.
- In vivo, an embryo would never be exposed to only a subset of amino acids, but rather a complete mixture of amino acids.
- If a near to physiological concentration of amino acids is used to culture an embryo from day 2 to day 3, the only amino acid which is depleted from the medium is leucine, an essential amino acid.

Thus, by artificially limiting the amino acids present in the medium, the nutrition of developing embryos is being restricted. In this era of transparency, it is surprising that information on something as critical as human preimplantation embryo culture media composition is not made freely available. This lack of information makes it very difficult for clinics to make fully informed choices on which are the best media to use in Assisted Reproductive Technologies.

Ability of Amino Acid Profiling to Predict Subsequent Development of Frozen-Thawed Embryos to the Blastocyst Stage

The ability of amino acid profiling to predict the development of fresh embryos to the blastocyst stage was a significant breakthrough in the attempt to devise a noninvasive technique of embryo health. However, many good quality supernumerary embryos from fresh cycles of IVF are routinely cryopreserved for use in subsequent treatment cycles and thus, it was necessary to validate whether amino acid profiling could also predict embryo survival post-thaw. This was important since one of the predominant risks to future embryo survival following cryopreservation is the formation of ice crystals during either the freezing or thawing processes [20] which may result in blastomere lysis due to cell membrane damage [21]. Although embryos are notoriously malleable and can adapt to both environmental stresses e.g. variations in culture medium, as well as physical insults such as removal of blastomeres for preimplantation genetic diagnosis, the potential damage that freeze-thawing may have on the integrity of blastomere membranes is also likely to affect cellular homeostasis including metabolism and thus may explain the reduced success rates obtained in frozen cycles.

The amino acid profile of embryos thawed on day 2 and cultured for 24 h was similar to that observed for fresh embryos. Specifically, there was a significant difference in the utilisation of glutamate, glutamine, glycine, arginine, alanine and lysine between frozen-thawed embryos which developed to the blastocyst stage and those which arrested prior to blastocyst formation [16]. This corresponded to developmentally competent embryos displaying significantly lower overall rates of amino acid appearance, depletion and turnover compared to those which arrested before the blastocyst stage. When this data was interrogated further and only the utilisation of glutamine, glycine and alanine was considered, the sum of these amino acids was significantly higher in those embryos which arrested prior to the blastocyst stage compared to those which formed a blastocyst (Fig. 1). What was intriguing was by investigating the use of these 3 amino acids from day 2 to day 3, it was possible to predict with 87 % accuracy which spare, frozen-thawed embryo would develop to the blastocyst stage [16]. Interestingly, as with the results obtained for fresh embryos, there was no difference in embryo grade between these two groups suggesting that amino acid profiling may be a better mechanism to assess embryo development rather than assessing morphology.

This conclusion was further substantiated when the amino acid utilisation of only the best quality, grade I embryos were investigated. There was a significant difference in the utilisation of glutamate, glutamine, glycine, arginine, tryptophan and lysine between grade I embryos which arrested and those which developed to the

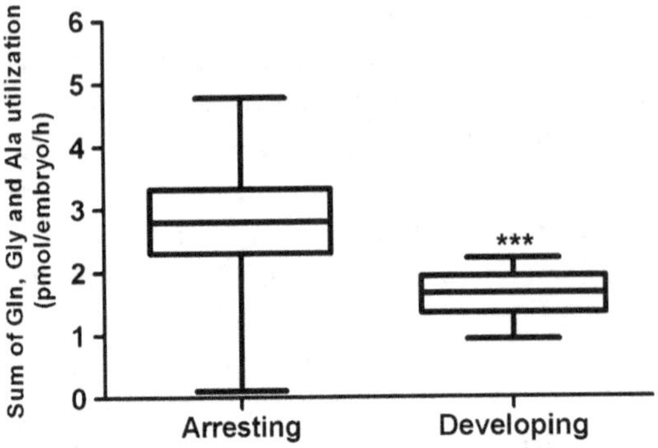

Fig. 24.1 Box and whisker plot of the sum of glutamine, glycine and alanine for individual frozen-thawed human embryos from day 2 to day 3 of development which either arrested prior to blastocyst formation (arresting), or subsequently developed to the blastocyst stage (developing). ***$P<0.001$ (adapted from Stokes PJ, Hawkhead JA, Fawthrop RK, Picton HM, Sharma V, Leese HJ, Houghton FD. Metabolism of human embryos following cryopreservation: implications for the safety and selection of embryos for transfer in clinical IVF. Hum. Reprod. 2007;22:829–835, with permission)

blastocyst stage [16]. These results suggest that developmentally competent embryos (both fresh and frozen-thawed) have a lower amino acid turnover than their arresting counterparts. These findings were fascinating since:

1. They highlight a noninvasive metabolic assay to predict future developmental competency.
2. Amino acid profiling was able to predict development before embryonic genome activation at the 8-cell stage suggesting that egg quality is likely to be of critical importance.
3. They suggest that morphological scoring systems do not adequately reflect viability especially in embryos of the highest apparent quality.

Ability of Amino Acid Profiling to Predict Embryo Development After Transfer

These data were exciting and offered the prospect that as well as being able to predict development to the blastocyst stage, amino acid profiling of early preimplantation embryos might also be able to distinguish which embryos are capable of generating a pregnancy and live birth following transfer. To test this proposition, a trial was initiated in a clinical IVF programme. In contrast to the previous studies, amino acid utilisation was measured from day 1 to day 2 post-fertilisation. Briefly, oocytes were fertilised using intracytoplasmic sperm injection (ICSI) and incubated individually in 4 μL drops of medium containing a close to physiological concentration of amino acids for 24 h. Two (or exceptionally one or three) resultant embryos were selected for transfer back into the uterus using standard, morphological criteria which also took into account the blastomere cell number. The concentration of amino acids in the spent medium was retrospectively measured and subsequently analysed to determine whether amino acid utilisation for each embryo was correlated with implantation, pregnancy and subsequent live birth [15]. Overall in this study, 113 embryos were transferred into 52 patients with a clinical pregnancy being achieved in 18 of the cycles which comprised 4 sets of twins and 14 singleton births. All data was included in the analysis. Obviously, it was not possible to determine which embryo it was that implanted when two or more were transferred and only a singleton pregnancy was generated but this experimental design was deliberately chosen to be inclusive and representative of clinical IVF, rather than simply include cycles where a 100 % implantation rate was achieved from either a one or two embryo transfer. Moreover, this fact was taken into consideration in the statistical analysis.

Analysis of the spent medium found that the utilisation of asparagine, glycine and leucine by single embryos from day 1 to day 2 of development were significantly correlated with pregnancy and live birth [15]. Moreover, this effect was independent of other indicators currently used to assess pregnancy outcome such as basal FSH levels, maternal age, embryo morphology and cell number. This amino acid correlation was intriguing particularly since the majority of cycles contained data from 2 embryos even though only a singleton pregnancy resulted. Thus, these data would be expected to be even more highly predictive of a live birth in cycles where all the embryos transferred successfully implanted.

This study represented one of the first noninvasive, quantitative, metabolic assays capable of predicting the future viability of preimplantation embryos in clinical IVF and has the potential to revolutionise how embryos are selected for transfer. However, it is first necessary to perform a prospective, randomised study to determine the power of amino acid profiling by transferring single embryos based either on their amino acid profile alone, or in combination with morphological grade. A further major benefit of amino acid profiling is that embryos are only required to be cultured in an artificial environment in vitro for 24 h, allowing transfer on either day 2 or day 3 of development. In contrast, traditional methods of embryo selection based on blastocyst formation rely on embryos being cultured in vitro for 5–6 days. Although blastocyst formation has been used successfully to predict future viability [22], such extended culture has recently been associated with the induction of epigenetic alterations at least in mice [23, 24]. Thus, amino acid profiling has great potential as a method to prospectively select viable embryos for transfer during early preimplantation development in clinical IVF and also negates the requirement for prolonged, potentially damaging in vitro culture.

Ability of Amino Acid Profiling to Predict the Genetic Health of Embryos

The mechanisms which underlie the ability of amino acid profiling to predict future embryo development remain unknown but recent data suggests an association with genetic health [25]. Human preimplantation embryos containing blastomeres which were 100 % euploid for chromosomes 13, 18, 21, X and Y were found to utilise significantly different levels of asparagine, glycine and valine compared to those containing no normal cells from day 2 to 3 of development. Similarly, from day 3 to 4 of development there was a significant difference in the turnover of leucine, lysine and serine between embryos which were uniformly normal (no abnormal blastomeres) or 100 % abnormal [25]. Thus, as well as being capable of predicting future embryo development, amino acid profiling is also able to differentiate between human preimplantation embryos which are completely chromosomally normal, or wholly abnormal. Unfortunately, amino acid turnover was not able to differentiate between mosaic embryos containing a mixture of normal and abnormal blastomeres.

The use of fluorescence in situ hydridisation (FISH) incorporating X and Y probes provided the ability to determine for the first time whether there was an association between embryo sex and amino acid profiling. As expected there was no difference in the amino acid profile of male and female embryos measured from day 1 to day 2 of development, presumably since the embryonic genome activation has yet to occur. However from day 2 to day 3 male embryos depleted significantly more leucine and tryptophan than female embryos [25]. These data were intriguing and suggest for the first time that human male and female embryos metabolise amino acids differently. Moreover, this technique offers the exciting potential to noninvasively select the gender of embryos at risk of inheriting X-linked genetic disorders.

Correlation of Amino Acid Turnover with Blastocyst Integrity

Integral to the formation of a functional blastocyst is the appropriate assembly of trophectoderm junctional complexes (Reviewed in [26–28]). Total amino acid turnover of compacting and cavitating embryos were both found to be correlated with the assembly of junctional proteins; ZO-1α^{+} and occludin. Embryos which displayed a greater total amino acid turnover were found to have an improved assembly of both ZO-1α^{+} and occludin [29]. Initially, this may appear to contradict previous data but it is worth noting that the current study was performed on a cohort of developing embryos and amino acid turnover was measured much later in development, during compaction and cavitation. Thus the high level of amino acid turnover which correlates with appropriate membrane assembly may simply reflect an increase in protein synthesis during blastocyst formation [30, 31]. These data are exciting and were the first to show an association between metabolism and trophectoderm integrity.

Ability of Amino Acid Profiling to Predict DNA Damage in Embryos

It is still not known why arresting embryos are more metabolically active but the amount of DNA damage may provide a clue. Recently, a positive correlation was observed between the amino acid turnover of human embryos from day 2 to day 3 of development and the percentage of DNA damage in that same resultant blastocyst [32]. Thus, embryos which were more metabolically active in terms of amino acid turnover from day 2 to day 3 also had a significantly increased amount of DNA damage at the blastocyst stage. In contrast, embryos with a low amino acid turnover formed blastocysts with little DNA damage. A further interesting finding of this study was that no correlation was found between embryo grade and mean DNA damage [32]. This highlights once again that embryo morphology is not a good predictor of embryo health in clinical IVF data which is supported by metabolic assays using amino acid profiling [15] and metabolomic assessment [33] which were both able to predict embryo viability independently of embryo grade.

Several lines of evidence now suggest that the noninvasive monitoring of amino acid profiling is beneficial for selecting future embryo health [14–16, 25, 29, 32]. Although the mechanisms which regulate these effects have yet to be determined, they are all consistent with the quiet embryo hypothesis [34] which proposes that metabolically quiet embryos are more viable than their active counterparts. There are several reasons why an embryo may be developmentally compromised and these can be broadly categorised into either intrinsic or extrinsic effects. Intrinsic factors are likely to be due to a maternal stress, poor oocyte quality, chromosomal abnormalities etc. Whereas extrinsic effects relate largely to the culture-induced stressors such as the type of medium used, amount of time the embryos are handled, environmental temperature control etc. Compromised embryos appear to have lost some of the control mechanisms which regulate "normal" nutrient utilisation and results in embryos having a greater requirement for exogenous nutrients in an attempt to overcome damage and facilitate development [35].

Summary

This chapter has highlighted many important roles of amino acids for human preimplantation embryos. Amino acids are not only beneficial to embryo development but their utilisation by the embryo is also predictive of future viability, genetic health, DNA damage and trophectoderm integrity. These findings were remarkable and highlight how integral amino acids are to the physiology of the embryo. Thus, it is important that much consideration is given to the media used in clinical IVF. This will require suppliers to provide details of media formulations so that informed choices can be made. The use of amino acid profiling in a clinical setting offers the exciting prospect to nonsubjectively select the most developmentally competent embryo for transfer with the greatest chance of producing a live birth.

Acknowledgment I thank Prof. Tom Fleming for his helpful comments on this chapter.

References

1. Sturmey RG, Brison DR, Leese HJ. Assessing embryo viability by measurement of amino acid turnover. Reprod Biomed Online. 2008;17:486–96.
2. Gardner DK, Lane M. Amino acids and ammonium regulate mouse embryo development in culture. Biol Reprod. 1993;48:377–85.
3. Ho Y, Wigglesworth K, Eppig JJ, Schultz RM. Preimplantation development of mouse embryos in KSOM: augmentation by amino acids and analysis of gene expression. Mol Reprod Dev. 1995;14:232–8.
4. Liu Z, Foote RH. Effects of amino acids on the development of in vitro matured/in vitro fertilization bovine embryos in simple protein-free medium. Hum Reprod. 1995;10:2985–91.
5. Steeves TE, Gardner DK. Temporal and differential effects of amino acids on bovine embryo development in culture. Biol Reprod. 1999;61:731–40.

6. Devreker F, Winston RM, Hardy K. Glutamine improves human preimplantation development *in vitro*. Fertil Steril. 1998;69:293–9.
7. Devreker F, Hardy K, Van den Bergh M, Vannin AS, Emiliani S, Englert Y. Amino acids promote human blastocyst development in vitro. Hum Reprod. 2001;16:749–56.
8. Beebe LF, Vassiliev I, McIlfatrick S, Nottle MB. Adding essential amino acids at a low concentration improves the development of in vitro fertilized porcine embryos. J Reprod Dev. 2009;55:373–7.
9. Reeds PJ. Dispensable and indispensable amino acids for humans. J Nutr. 2000;130:1835S–40S.
10. Fűrst P, Stehle P. What are the essential elements for the determination of amino acid requirements in humans? J Nutr. 2004;134 Suppl 6:1558S–65S.
11. Gardner DK, Lane M. Culture of viable human blastocysts in defined sequential serum-free media. Hum Reprod. 1998;13 Suppl 3:148–59.
12. Gardner DK, Vella P, Lane M, Wagley L, Schlenker T, Schoolcraft WB. Culture and transfer of human blastocysts increases implantation rates and reduces the need for multiple embryo transfers. Fertil Steril. 1998;69:84–8.
13. Jones GM, Trounson AO, Gardner DK, Kausche A, Lolatgis N, Wood C. Evolution of a culture protocol for successful blastocyst development and pregnancy. Hum Reprod. 1998;13:169–77.
14. Houghton FD, Hawkhead JA, Hupherson PG, Hogg JE, Balen AH, Rutherford AJ, et al. Non-invasive amino acid turnover predicts human embryo developmental capacity. Hum Reprod. 2002;17:999–1005.
15. Brison DR, Houghton FD, Falconer D, Roberts SA, Hawkhead J, Humpherson PG, et al. Identification of viable human embryos in IVF by non-invasive measurement of amino acid turnover. Hum Reprod. 2004;19:2319–24.
16. Stokes PJ, Hawkhead JA, Fawthrop RK, Picton HM, Sharma V, Leese HJ, et al. Metabolism of human embryos following cryopreservation: implications for the safety and selection of embryos for transfer in clinical IVF. Hum Reprod. 2007;22:829–35.
17. Tay JI, Rutherford AJ, Killick SR, Maguiness SD, Partridge RJ, Leese HJ. Human tubal fluid: production, nutrient composition and response to adrenergic agents. Hum Reprod. 1997;12:2451–6.
18. Dumoulin JC, Land JA, Van Montfoort AP, Nelissen EC, Coonen E, Derhaag JG, et al. Effect of in vitro culture of human embryos on birthweight of newborns. Hum Reprod. 2010;25:605–12.
19. Nelissen EC, Van Montfoort AP, Coonen E, Derhaag JG, Geraedts JP, Smits LJ, et al. Further evidence that culture media affect perinatal outcome: findings after transfer of fresh and cryopreserved embryos. Hum Reprod. 2012;27(7):1966–76.
20. Liebermann J, Nawroth F, Isachenko V, Isachenko E, Rahimi G, Tucker MJ. Potential importance if vitrification in reproductive medicine. Biol Reprod. 2002;67:1671–80.
21. Pal L, Kovacs G, Witt B, Jindal S, Santoro N, Barad D. Post thaw blastomere survival is predictive of the success of frozen-thawed embryo transfer cycles. Fertil Steril. 2004;82:821–6.
22. Gardner DK, Lane M, Stevens J, Schlenker T, Schoolcraft WB. Blastocyst score affects implantation and pregnancy outcome: towards a single blastocyst transfer. Fertil Steril. 2000;73:1155–8.
23. Fernandez-Gonzalez R, Ramirez MA, Pericuesta E, Calle A, Gutuerrez-Adan A. Histone modifications at the blastocyst Axin1(Fu) locus mark the heritability of in vitro culture-induced epigenetic alterations in mice. Biol Reprod. 2010;83:720–7.
24. Market-Velker BA, Fernandes AD, Mann MR. Side-by-side comparison of five commercial media systems in a mouse model: suboptimal in vitro culture interferes with imprint maintenance. Biol Reprod. 2010; 83:938–50.
25. Picton HM, Elder K, Houghton FD, Hawkhead JA, Rutherford AJ, Hogg JE, et al. Association between amino acid turnover and chromosome aneuploidy during human preimplantation embryo development in vitro. Mol Hum Reprod. 2010;16:557–69.
26. Fleming TP, Sheth B, Fesenko I. Cell adhesion in the preimplantation mammalian embryo and its role in trophectoderm differentiation and blastocyst morphogenesis. Front Biosci. 2001;6:D1000–7.
27. Hardy K, Warner A, Winston RM, Becker DL. Expression of intercellular junctions during preimplantation development of the human embryo. Mol Hum Reprod. 1996;8:621–32.
28. Ghassemifar MR, Eckert JJ, Houghton FD, Picton HM, Leese HJ, Fleming TP. Gene expression regulating epithelial intercellular junction biogenesis during human blastocyst development in vitro. Mol Hum Reprod. 2003;9:245–52.
29. Eckert JJ, Houghton FD, Hawkhead JA, Balen AH, Leese HJ, Picton HM, et al. Human embryos developing in vitro are susceptible to impaired epithelial junction biogenesis correlating with abnormal metabolic activity. Hum Reprod. 2007;22:2214–24.
30. Sellens MH, Stein S, Sherman MI. Protein and free amino acid content in preimplantation mouse embryos and in blastocysts under various culture conditions. J Reprod Fertil. 1981;61:307–15.
31. Lamb VK, Leese HJ. Uptake of a mixture of amino acids by mouse blastocysts. J Reprod Fertil. 1994;102: 169–75.
32. Sturmey RG, Hawkhead JA, Barker EA, Leese JH. DNA damage and metabolic activity in the preimplantation embryo. Hum Reprod. 2009;24:81–91.
33. Vergouw CG, Botros LL, Roos P, Lens JW, Schats R, Hompes PG, et al. Metabolomic profiling by near-infrared spectroscopy as a tool to assess embryo viability: a novel, non-invasive method for embryo selection. Hum Reprod. 2008;23:1499–504.
34. Leese HJ. Quiet please, do not disturb: a hypothesis of embryo metabolism and viability. Bioessays. 2002;24:845–9.
35. Baumann CG, Morris DG, Sreenan JM, Leese HJ. The quiet embryo hypothesis: molecular characteristics favouring viability. Mol Reprod Dev. 2007;74: 1345–53.

Metabolomic Profiling of Embryos Using Spectroscopy

25

Denny Sakkas and Emre Seli

The hypothesis that there is a relationship between the metabolic activity of an embryo and its reproductive potential has been upheld in numerous studies over the past 30 years. In 1980, Renard et al. [1] reported that day 10 cattle blastocysts that demonstrated an elevated glucose uptake developed better, both in culture and in vivo, compared to blastocysts with a lower glucose uptake. In 1987, Gardner and Leese [2] measured glucose uptake by individual day 4 mouse blastocysts prior to transfer to recipient females. They found that embryos that went to term had a significantly higher glucose uptake in culture than those embryos that failed to develop after transfer. Consequently, Lane and Gardner [3] showed that the glycolytic rate of morphologically similar mouse blastocysts could be used to select embryos for transfer prospectively. In their study, mouse blastocysts that were identified as viable using metabolic criteria prior to transfer, had a fetal development rate of 80 %. In contrast, embryos that exhibited an abnormal metabolic profile compared to in vivo developed controls, developed at a rate of only 6 %. These data provide strong evidence that metabolic function is linked to embryo viability and is independent of the information provided by morphology.

Currently, there are three main approaches that are utilized by researchers to obtain metabolic information about embryos: (1) analysis of carbohydrate utilization, (2) analysis of amino acid uptake and secretion, and (3) analysis of the embryonic metabolome. The first two approaches provide more specific information about candidate metabolites or the activity of specific metabolic pathways (discussed in Chaps. 23 and 24).

The third option provides a systematic analysis of the inventory of metabolites that represent the functional phenotype at the cellular level. Depending upon the technology employed to analyse the metabolome (reviewed in [4]), one does not necessarily obtain identification of specific metabolites, but an algorithm is created that relates to cell function. In this chapter, we will briefly review the basic aspects of metabolomic assessment and summarize the attempts at clinical application for embryo assessment in IVF.

Metabolomics Technology

The metabolome refers to the complete inventory of small molecule (<1 kDa), non-proteinaceous compounds including metabolic intermediates (amino acids, lipids, nucleotides), ATP, hormones, and secondary metabolites that are present within a biological sample (reviewed in [4]).

D. Sakkas (✉)
Boston IVF, 130 Second Avenue,
Waltham, MA 02451, USA
e-mail: dsakkas@bostonivf.com

E. Seli
Department of Obstetrics, Gynecology and Reproductive Sciences, Yale School of Medicine,
310 Cedar Street LSOG 304D, New Haven, CT 06520-8063, USA
e-mail: emre.seli@yale.edu

D.K. Gardner et al. (eds.), *Human Gametes and Preimplantation Embryos: Assessment and Diagnosis*, DOI 10.1007/978-1-4614-6651-2_25, © Springer Science+Business Media New York 2013

These compounds are the products of cellular metabolism and display a diverse array of physical and chemical properties, and a wide concentration range.

Interestingly, the number of metabolites is typically lower than the number of genes and proteins in a cell or organism, allowing metabolomic analysis to be achieved relatively faster compared to genomic or transcriptomic analyses (reviewed in [4]). Indeed, it is estimated that there are approximately 25,000 genes in the human genome, encoding for approximately 100,000–200,000 transcripts (through alternative splicing), whereas there may be as few as 2,500–3,000 small molecule metabolites that make up the human metabolome. Due to high intensity of labor and cost associated with transcriptomic and proteomic approaches, analysis of the metabolome is being increasingly used to understand the "global picture" of systems biology.

Metabolomics is the systematic study of the dynamic inventory of metabolites, as small molecular biomarkers representing the functional phenotype in a biological system. To investigate complex metabolic profiles within a biological milieu, nonselective, but specific analytical technologies must be utilized. Many spectroscopic/spectrometric and chromatographic techniques are available, and provide automated, high throughput methodologies that generate profiles of target biological fluids (reviewed in [4]).

To describe the analysis of biological fluids by spectroscopic technologies, the term "biospectroscopy" is commonly used; the scientific platform that incorporates biospectroscopy and metabolomic profiling is referred to as "biospectroscopy-based metabolomics." Common techniques applied in biospectroscopy-based metabolomics studies include nuclear magnetic resonance (NMR) spectroscopy, mass spectrometry (MS), which can be coupled with separation methods like gas chromatography (GC-MS), liquid chromatography (LC-MS) or high performance liquid chromatography (HPLC-MS), and capillary electrophoresis (CE-MS). Optical spectroscopies, such as near infrared (NIR), Fourier transform infrared (FT-IR), and Raman spectroscopies provide potentially complementary profiles of the various components within biological fluids due to the different physical mechanisms involved in each technique. Ultimately, using various forms of spectral and analytical approaches, metabolomics attempts to determine metabolites associated with physiologic and pathologic states [5].

Application of Metabolomics to the Study of Embryo Viability

Initial Studies

In 2007, Seli et al. [6] analyzed 69 day 3 spent embryo culture media samples from 30 patients with known outcome (0 or 100 % sustained implantation) using Raman and/or NIR spectroscopy. The mean spectrum of embryos that resulted in a pregnancy and live birth was compared to that of embryos that failed to implant. Spectral regions most predictive of pregnancy outcome were identified. Then, an algorithm based on these spectral regions was established and used to generate a viability score for each embryo (Fig. 1). With both Raman and NIR, the mean viability score of embryos that implanted and resulted in a live birth were significantly higher compared to those that failed to implant [6].

The algorithm established in the initial study [6] was then tested in a blinded trial using Raman spectroscopy to analyze day 3 and day 5 spent culture media collected at a different center, where embryos were cultured in a different type and volume of culture medium [7]. In this study, the viability scores of day 3 and day 5 embryos that resulted in a live birth were significantly higher compared to the viability scores of embryos that failed to implant [7].

Larger analyses of single embryo transfer cycles were also undertaken whereby NIR spectral analysis of frozen day 2 or 3 embryo culture media samples was performed blinded to outcome [8]. Individual metabolic profiles were established from as small as 7 μL of the samples with each measurement taking less than 1 min. Statistical analysis performed on the metabolic profiles established a viability score (as generated

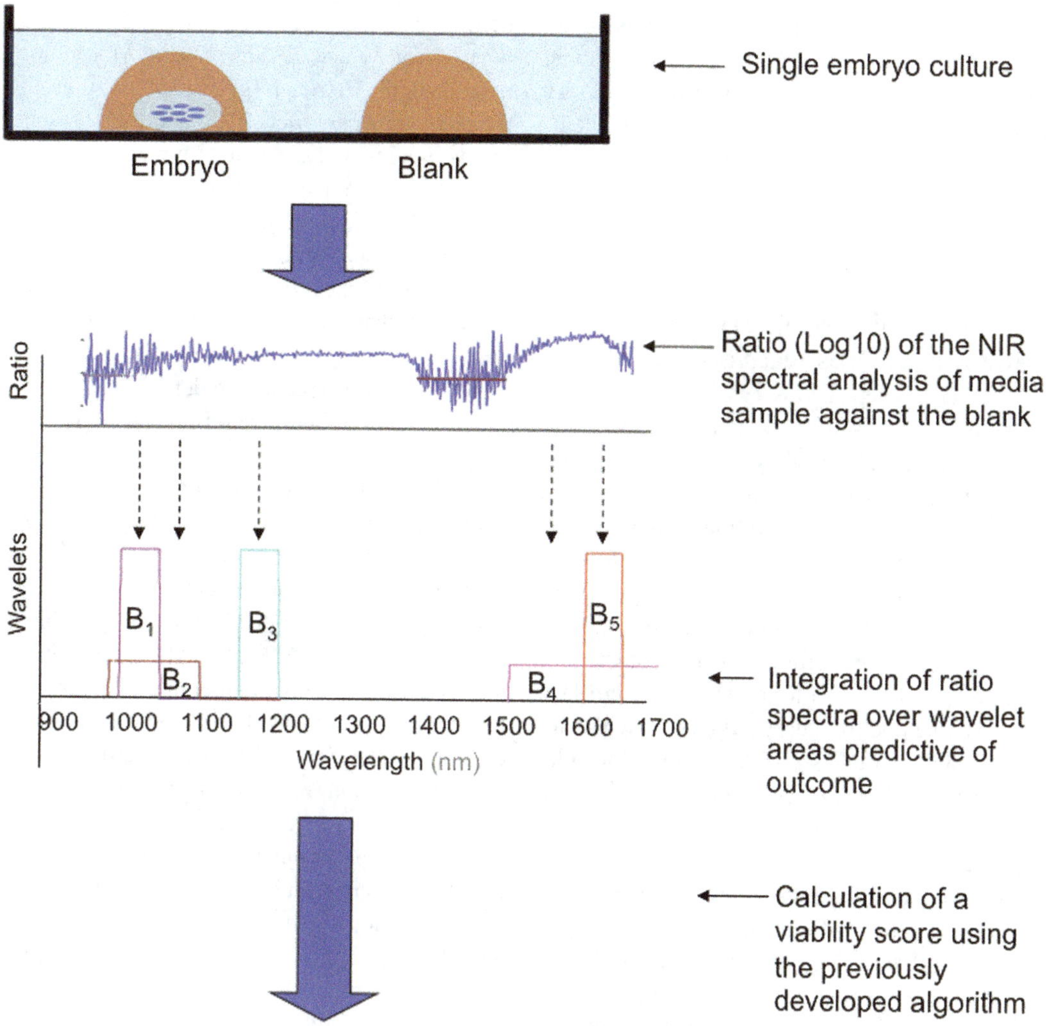

$$\text{Viability Score: } 0.35 + 0.081B_5 - 0.061B_4 - 0.023B_3 - 0.0015B_2 + 0.0026B_1$$

Fig. 25.1 Development of a viability score using NIR spectroscopic metabolomics. Culture media arising from a single embryo and a control blank media are measured to generate a spectral profile. The blank media is subtracted from the embryo media and then a previously developed predictive algorithm interrogates specific wavelet regions known to be associated with pregnancy outcome. The final Viability Score is then used to discern which embryo to transfer from a patient's own embryo cohort

above) that was significantly different ($P<0.001$) between the pregnant and nonpregnant patients. For these studies, a cut off value for predicting pregnancy was determined to be at >0.3. When this cut off was used to examine embryos of excellent and good morphology that underwent single embryo transfer a significant difference was found in the establishment of pregnancy [9]. Indeed, when human embryos of similar morphology were examined using the same NIR spectral profile, their viability scores varied remarkably in relation to morphology indicating that the metabolome of embryos that looked similar differed significantly. This observation was in agreement with the study of Katz-Jaffe et al. [10, 11] who revealed that the proteome of individual human blastocysts of the same grade differed between embryos, again indicating that embryo morphology is not completely linked to its physiology. Subsequent studies, using the SET model [9, 12, 13], demonstrated that increasing viability scores are associated with an increasing likelihood of embryo implantation, providing a semi-quantitative parameter that can be used as an adjunct to morphology.

Commercialization Efforts and Randomized Prospective Trials

Although a series of preliminary studies suggested a potential benefit with this technology, these studies were largely retrospective, and were performed in a single research laboratory as distinct from a real clinical setting. Therefore, to ascertain the potential of this technology, it was further developed by a private company, for clinical use. A series of prototypes and commercial instruments were then tested as an on-site, fast, and easy method for embryo assessment. The in-house clinical studies conducted by Molecular Biometrics Inc. using a NIR (ViaMetrics™) system reported inconsistent findings. The largest of these studies were performed as randomized clinical trials (RCTs) in centers performing SET and using prototype instruments. In these studies, women in the control arm underwent SET with embryos selected using standard morphological embryo assessment protocols. In the treatment arm, a combination of metabolomic profiling and morphologic assessment was used; by first identifying embryos with a good morphology suitable for transfer or cryopreservation, and then selecting the embryo to be transferred based on the metabolomic Viability Score™ generated by the NIR instrument.

In one of theses studies performed in Gothenburg [14], both day 2 and day 5 SETs were performed. Although not statistically significant, the results indicated a potential benefit of embryo selection through addition of NIR on day 2 transfer. Of 83 and 87 SETs in the Morphology alone and ViaMetrics [NIR]/morphology groups the pregnancy rates were 26.5 % and 31 %, respectively. In the same study no benefit for selection of day 5 SET was observed, whereby of 80 and 77 SETs in the Morphology alone and ViaMetrics [NIR]/morphology groups the pregnancy rates were 45 % and 39 %, respectively. Interestingly, when comparing the two groups significant differences were observed in this study in respect to the overall morphology of the day 2 embryos and blastocysts selected in the morphology alone group. The data also highlights the belief that selecting a single good quality blastocyst on day 5 remains as one of the best selection criteria available to date [15].

In another randomized trial performed by Vergouw et al. in Amsterdam, women undergoing SET on day 3 were similarly studied [16]. Authors found no difference in live birth rates between the groups (live birth rate was 29.5 % in the Viametrics [NIR]/morphology group [N= 146 patients] compared to the 31.3 % in Morphology alone group [N=163 patients]). Interestingly, there was a significantly higher rate of fragmented embryos and lower number of top quality day 3 embryos in the Viametrics-assisted group, which did not seem to impact pregnancy outcome [16].

Conversely, two concurrent RCTs were conducted using the commercial platform where 2 or 3 embryos were selected for transfer on the basis of Morphology alone or ViaMetrics [NIR]/Morphology; both showed improvements in the Viametrics-assisted selection group. In one of these, Sfontouris et al. [17] performed a study in which for every two patients where embryos were selected based on morphology, one patient had a transfer based on ViaMetrics [NIR]-assisted embryo selection (randomly allocated with a 2:1 ratio). They reported implantation rates (IR) with fetal cardiac activity that were significantly (P=0.04) improved in the Viametrics [NIR]/morphology group [N=39 patients, IR=33/102 (32.4 %)] compared to the Morphology alone group [N=86 patients, 55/257 (21.4 %)] [17].

One of the underlying problems encountered in the NIR system was that the different instruments were variable in performance, which in turn masked the low intensity of the signal generated from the embryo within the culture media. This meant that any algorithm created on one group of instruments suffered when translated on other instruments as their noise thresholds and behavior may have differed significantly. The commercial version of the NIR instrument was unfortunately withdrawn due to the wide variability in performance between clinics and inconsistent results in clinical trials. The technology will hopefully be improved and be tested again in the near future. This is not dissimilar to the situation faced by aneuploidy screening of embryos, whereby chromosomal screening of preimplantation embryos has always thought to be a strong theory, however, using FISH proved to be inadequate [18], while it now appears that modern comprehensive screening techniques are providing more consistent results [19].

Summary and Conclusions

The main aim when establishing a noninvasive technology is to provide an accurate and meaningful clinical tool and to limit the time taken to assess the samples, making it possible to perform the analysis just prior to embryo transfer. So far, while NIR spectroscopy met some of these criteria, it appears to have failed to consistently predict viability when selecting a single embryo for transfer.

Meanwhile, the promise of assessing culture media using a noninvasive platform remains. Studies describing markers in embryo culture media that are indicative of viability have been evident since 1980 (reviewed in [20]) hence the hypothesis that a factor or factors related to embryo viability exists in media appears hard to ignore. The pitfall is that relatively small amounts of these factors exist and, in addition, trying to discern differences in these factors between embryos that are viable or nonviable adds a further level of difficulty. Finally, not the hypothesis but how quickly a particular technology will allow us to perform this difficult assessment and whether the same technology can do this consistently and accurately is possibly the main barrier to clinical use of noninvasive embryo assessment tests.

References

1. Renard JP, Philippon A, Menezo Y. In-vitro uptake of glucose by bovine blastocysts. J Reprod Fertil. 1980; 58:161–4.
2. Gardner DK, Leese HJ. Assessment of embryo viability prior to transfer by the noninvasive measurement of glucose uptake. J Exp Zool. 1987;242:103–5.
3. Lane M, Gardner DK. Selection of viable mouse blastocysts prior to transfer using a metabolic criterion. Hum Reprod. 1996;11:1975–8.
4. Botros L, Sakkas D, Seli E. Metabolomics and its application for non-invasive embryo assessment in IVF. Mol Hum Reprod. 2008;14:679–90.
5. Ellis DI, Goodacre R. Metabolic fingerprinting in disease diagnosis: biomedical applications of infrared and Raman spectroscopy. Analyst. 2006;131:875–85.
6. Seli E, Sakkas D, Scott R, Kwok JS, Rosendahl S, Burns DH. Non-Invasive metabolomic profiling of human embryo culture media using Raman and near infrared spectroscopy correlates with reproductive potential of embryos in women undergoing in vitro fertilization. Fertil Steril. 2007;88:1350–7.
7. Scott RT, Seli E, Miller K, Sakkas D, Scott K, Burns DH. Non-Invasive metabolomic profiling of human embryo culture media using Raman spectroscopy predicts embryonic reproductive potential: a prospective blinded pilot study. Fertil Steril. 2008;90:77–83.
8. Vergouw CG, Botros LL, Roos P, Lens JW, Schats R, Hompes PGA, et al. Metabolomic profiling by near-infrared spectroscopy as a tool to assess embryo viability: a novel, non-invasive method for embryo selection. Hum Reprod. 2008;23:1499–504.
9. Seli E, Vergouw CG, Kato O, Botros L, Roos P, Morita H, et al. Noninvasive metabolomic profiling as an adjunct to morphology for noninvasive embryo assessment in women undergoing single embryo transfer. Fertil Steril. 2010;94:535–42.
10. Katz-Jaffe MG, Gardner DK, Schoolcraft WB. Proteomic analysis of individual human embryos to identify novel biomarkers of development and viability. Fertil Steril. 2006;85:101–7.
11. Katz-Jaffe MG, Schoolcraft WB, Gardner DK. Analysis of protein expression (secretome) by human and mouse preimplantation embryos. Fertil Steril. 2006;86:678–85.
12. Ahlstrom A, Wikland M, Rogberg L, Barnett JS, Tucker M, Hardarson T. Cross-validation and predictive value of near-infrared spectroscopy algorithms for day-5 blastocyst transfer. Reprod Biomed Online. 2011.
13. Seli E, Bruce C, Botros L, Henson M, Roos P, Judge K, et al. Receiver operating characteristic (ROC) analysis of day 5 morphology grading and metabolomic viability scores on predicting implantation outcome. J Assist Reprod Genet. 2011;28:137–44.
14. Hardarson T, Ahlstrom A, Rogberg L, Botros L, Hillensjo T, Westlander G, et al. Non-invasive metabolomic profiling of day 2 and 5 embryo culture

medium: a prospective randomized trial. Hum Reprod. 2012;27:89–96.
15. Blake DA, Farquhar CM, Johnson N, Proctor M. Cleavage stage versus blastocyst stage embryo transfer in assisted reproduction. Cochrane Database Syst Rev. 2007;4:CD002118.
16. Vergouw CG, Kieslinger DC, Kostelijk EH, Botros LL, Schats R, Hompes PG, et al. Day 3 embryo selection by metabolomic profiling of culture medium with near infrared spectroscopy as an adjunct to morphology: a randomized controlled trial. Hum Reprod. 2012;27(8):2304–11.
17. Sfontouris IA, Lainas GT, Sakkas D, Zorzovilis IZ, Petsas GK, Lainas TG. Embryo selection using non-invasive metabolomic analysis indicates improvement in implantation rates with fetal cardiac activity. Hum Reprod. 2011;26 Suppl 1:i86.
18. Mastenbroek S, Twisk M, van Echten-Arends J, Sikkema-Raddatz B, Korevaar JC, Verhoeve HR, et al. In vitro fertilization with preimplantation genetic screening. N Engl J Med. 2007;357:9–17.
19. Wells D, Alfarawati S, Fragoui E. Use of comprehensive chromosomal screening for embryo assessment: microarrays and CGH. Mol Hum Reprod. 2008;12: 703–10.
20. Sakkas D, Gardner DK. Noninvasive methods to assess embryo quality. Curr Opin Obstet Gynecol. 2005;17:283–8.

26 Microfluidic Devices for the Analysis of Gamete and Embryo Physiology

George A. Thouas, David L. Potter, and David K. Gardner

Assisted reproductive technologies (ARTs) are dedicated to the production of healthy preimplantation embryos using laboratory-based interventions, toward enabling infertile couples to conceive and deliver a healthy child. While tools such as light microscopy are fundamental to the analysis of gamete and embryo morphology and development, technologies for analysis of biochemistry and molecular biology are becoming more commonplace, including "OMICs"-based diagnostics for embryo selection. Any diagnostic tool employed in clinical ART must provide reliable and accurate quantitative data, with a minimum of variability, while remaining easily implemented into clinical IVF practice.

Many of the complex metrologies discussed in this chapter may not yet be readily or directly available to most clinical IVF units, although previous chapters have provided pertinent examples of how quantitative analysis can be used to measure different biological parameters. The main hindrance to translation is currently the cost associated with implementation of more complex technologies, extensive training requirements and space limitations. There is also a time lag between proof-of-concept and application development, which is longer for technologies not originally designed to work within the physical constraints of ART, or at the scale of gametes or embryos. For example, a standard high-field nuclear magnetic resonance (NMR) analysis requires volumes which are more readily suited to blood or urine analysis than culture media from a single embryo. The obvious solution for any application is to develop or utilize a "gateway" technology that adapts existing diagnostic technologies to the specific requirements of ART, rather than the reverse.

To this end, microfluidics has grown considerably from its physical science and engineering origins, into a biotechnology foundry. Microfluidic systems function at the upper end of the scale of cellular systems, such as some of the molecular diagnostics outlined so far. Devices built on microfluidic principles can enable detailed manipulation and study of single cells and subcellular systems in their native states and scales, at comparable fluid volumes, and with precise control of physical and environmental variables. These capabilities match well with the specific scales of gametes and embryos, and their specific physical and biochemical constraints.

This chapter, therefore, focuses on the potential suitability and efficacy of microfluidics for gamete and embryo analysis, as novel or alternative assay platforms. Metrologies and diagnostic parameters used routinely in ART are discussed, followed by an overview of current and potential applications in the context of microfluidic devices, with focus on those which can readily be adapted to ART procedures. The application of microfluidic devices to in vitro manipulation or culture of gametes and embryos will not be

G.A. Thouas (✉) • D.L. Potter • D.K. Gardner
Department of Zoology, The University of Melbourne, Melbourne, Victoria, Australia
e-mail: gthouas@unimelb.edu.au

D.K. Gardner et al. (eds.), *Human Gametes and Preimplantation Embryos: Assessment and Diagnosis*, DOI 10.1007/978-1-4614-6651-2_26, © Springer Science+Business Media New York 2013

discussed unless integral to the understanding of specific examples of analysis metrologies or systems.

An Introduction to Microfluidics

Cellular and biomolecular systems function on the micro- (10^{-6}) to pico- (10^{-12}) scale, whereas manipulation technologies function within the milli-scale (10^{-3}) and greater (macro-scale) (Fig. 1). Microscopy and micromanipulation can bridge this scaling disparity, to accommodate our inability to manipulate structures beyond visual acuity (approximately 100 μm, 10^{-4} m). Thus, light microscopy enables visual discrimination of a human oocyte (150 μm, 1.5×10^{-4} m) or spermatozoan (5 μm, 5×10^{-6} m) with reasonable detail. However, even light microscopy resolution (~500 nm, 5×10^{-7} m) does not allow sub-nano-scale discrimination of features in structures such as the haploid genome (3 pg in mass, 3×10^{-12} g).

These scaling considerations may seem trivial, but they are fundamental to understanding micro-scale manipulation and metrology. Directly at this interface lies microfluidics, the study of the nature of fluid dynamics in sub-millimetre mechanical systems. Microfluidic devices are essentially fluid handling systems incorporating structural flow features (e.g. branched or unbranched channels) that exploit the unique physical differences between macro- and micro-scale fluids. At this scale, flow is non-turbulent, and defined largely by the device geometry, with channel cross-section being the most critical parameter. True microfluidic systems utilize rectilinear fluid channels which are typically wider (>100 μm) with respect to height (>10 μm), and up to centimetres long [1]. It is surprising to consider that a channel of this profile accommodating 10 μL of culture medium would need to be 10 m long. In contrast, a channel of similar profile and only 10 mm long would only hold 10 nL (volume = cross section area × length). By comparison, a human expanded blastocyst is approximately 175–225 μm in diameter, equating to approximately 5 nL in volume. Thus, microfluidic device constraints marry quite well with the volume limitations of embryo analysis, particularly at the single embryo level.

Along with volume miniaturization, and of potentially greater value to quantitative analysis, is the high level of volume-to-volume accuracy offered by a microfluidic channel. Channel geometry itself physically constrains, and hence defines the fluid volume, which is a critical consideration for the reliability and repeatability of analyses relying on molarity functions (moles of analyte per litre).

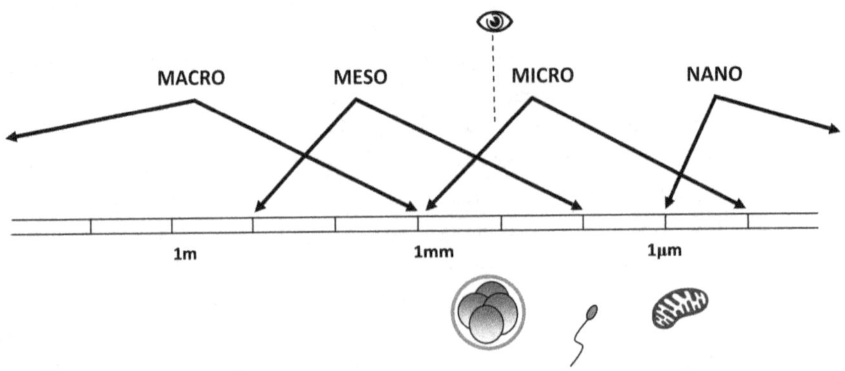

Fig. 26.1 Diagrammatic representation of conventional scale ranges relevant to biological systems. Microfluidic devices operate at the micro- to nano-scale, corresponding to the size of gamete and preimplantation embryos (eye symbol = limit of visual acuity)

This is preferable to conventional biological assays that require manual pipetting of microlitre volumes, with associated volumetric errors that occur randomly and cumulatively. Clearly, the highly accurate volume handling capabilities of microfluidic devices are advantageous for ART laboratories employing micron-scale or lower working volumes, for diagnostic assay of samples with very limited availability.

Aspects of Device Fabrication

In general, microfluidic devices are constructed in two-dimensional (2D or planar) functional layers of a solid material, through which variable height channels run independently, akin to the layout of printed electrical circuit boards. In some cases, multilayered three-dimensional (3D) devices have been fabricated, though are less common due the high level of manufacturing complexity involved [2]. In most cases, a pseudo-3D functionality is achieved through stacking of multiple planar layers, with intervening perpendicular conduits (vias) that allow communication between layers.

Microfluidic fabrication is defined by the material chosen for the structural layer, and relies on highly specialized and complex engineering methodology. In summary, a wide range of industrial scale methods are available, including photolithography, soft lithography, laser machining, micromilling, bead blasting, chemical etching, wax printing and hot embossing. These are essentially surface modification techniques capable of creating high resolution planar features, with micro-scale width and depth precision, and with high reproducibility. Devices for biological applications have been fabricated using a wide array of rigid and semi-rigid materials including borosilicate glass; light sensitive films (photoresists); polymers (e.g. poly(dimethyl)siloxane (PDMS), polycarbonate (PC), poly(methyl-methacrylate) (PMMA) and teflons); waxes; shrink-wrap films and even paper-based materials. The choice of material is normally dictated by the end use, or availability of the fabrication facility. To date, most microfluidic devices for biotechnology applications have been made from glass [3] or polymer, typically PDMS [4].

Glass devices are normally made by chemical etching or micromachining, which is costly and time consuming, but glass is well suited to bioassay systems owing to attributes such as minimal sample-surface interactions, resistance to organic solvents, lack of gas permeability and low optical background. Glass is also amenable to biochemical surface conjugation with proteins or linkers. Like glass, PDMS is silicon-based and optically clear, but is more rubber-like, with devices typically made using the microelectronics industry methods of photolithography and soft lithography (Fig. 2). Liquid polymer is typically poured over a rigid mould (master) produced as the inverse of the channel layout. The polymer is then cured by baking, and mounted on glass or other planar surfaces.

This process is considerably cheaper than for glass, but is equally time consuming, with most expenditure attributed to master design and production. Once completed, the same master can be reused to make multiple single-use or minimally reused device copies. Typical drawbacks of PDMS for biological device applications include its reactivity to organic solvents, heat sensitivity and porosity. This latter property can promote reactions with aqueous samples contained within the device, such as small molecule absorption into the bulk material [5] or release of trace amounts of PDMS monomers and oligomers [6] which may confound mass spectrometry studies, for example.

Operational Aspects of Microfluidic Devices

The functional unit of a microfluidic device is a single open-ended channel with smooth (non-turbulent or "laminar") fluid flow regulated by a defined head pressure, analogous to fluid moving in a vertical capillary under gravity. Laminar flow itself is based on the physical manner by which infinitely thin, adjacent "laminae" of fluid slide past each other in the direction of the pressure gradient, while remaining an intact "stack" (fluid bulk)

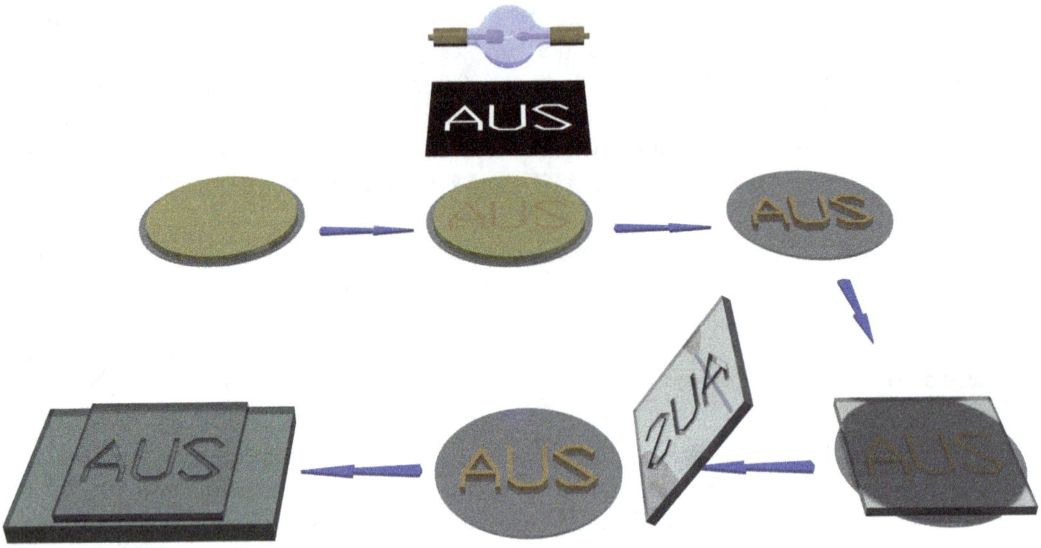

Fig. 26.2 Schematic of the process of soft lithography for fabricating microchannel features in microfluidic devices. A silicon wafer disc is first coated with a layer of photoresist (*upper left*). A template, the optical mask, containing the desired pattern is then overlaid, and the wafer is irradiated with ultraviolet light (*upper middle*), which cross-links only the area exposed by the pattern. The unexposed photoresist is removed using a solvent developer, leaving an intact 3D negative of the pattern, which is then hard-baked, creating a permanent moulding master (*upper right*). PDMS is poured over the master and cured (*bottom right*). The PDMS is peeled off the mould (*bottom middle*) and bonded onto a prepared glass substrate to create the finished device (*bottom left*). The master can then be reused to make multiple copies of the device as desired

similar to a deck of cards. As channel complexity and on-board integration increase to become more "chip-like" (e.g. incorporating sensors, electronics, tube feeds, control layers, etc.), so does coordination of the degree, timing and location of pressure controls in the fluid management system. Channels can also contain multiple inputs and outputs, forming branch-points that meet specific flow regimes for mixing, reaction or movement to a detection region (Fig. 3). Direct positive or negative fluid pressures can be generated mechanically via syringe pumps, internal or external peristaltic pumps, or indirectly by centripetal, gravitational or electromagnetic forces. Alternatively, chemically active methods at the device-fluid interface can be used, including surface tension (capillary action), electrowetting, electroosmosis or hydrophobic/hydrophilic interactions. In most cases, the pressure generating system is external to the microfluidic device.

Devices can be generally classified according to whether their internal fluid flow is free flowing (passively controlled) or valved (actively controlled). The former is strictly dependent on device geometry, while the latter type is subject to imposed mechanical, electrical or chemical switching methods (actuation). At the user end, the fluid flow rate input to the device is the most important control parameter, with the precision of fabrication dictating channel geometry, and thereby the effectiveness of downstream flow. Despite this level of engineering precision, the addition of active control imparts a far greater degree of flexibility of use in microfluidic devices. As a result, a plethora of actuation methods have been developed [7], such as pneumatic channel compression (one of the most common) (Fig. 4). While active control greatly reduces the geometric tolerance requirements of device channels, the off-board control system consequently becomes exponentially more cumbersome.

When the control system and device complexity are suitably optimized for a given endpoint analysis, there is the potential for "high order functional parallelism", a term describing the potential to perform massively parallel

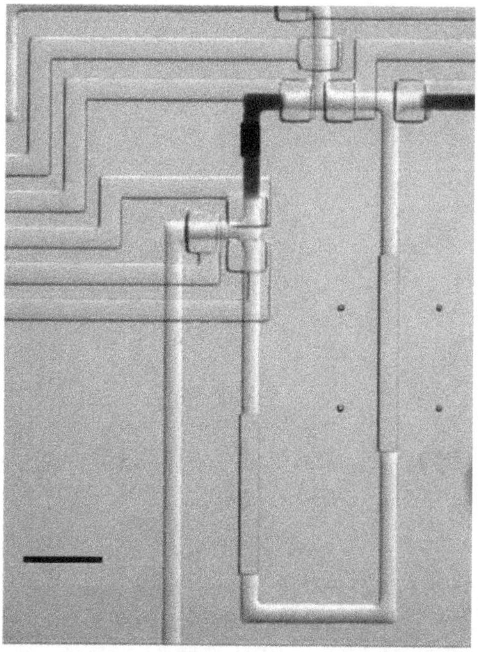

Fig. 26.3 Bright field micrograph of a PDMS microfluidic device used for metabolic analysis. Fluid flow channels are 100 μm wide by 50 μm in height; the volume of trapped blue dye is 2 nL. The channel section bounded by the four fiducial marker points represents the measurement region, where embryo culture media and metabolic reaction mix are coincubated and analyzed fluorometrically (measurement volume = 2.5 nL; scale bar = 500 μm [70])

assays in a single device footprint. Instead of repeated serial analysis, microfluidic devices can allow multiple analyses in parallel on a single sample, or defined fractions, greatly streamlining assay costs and analysis times, and maximizing available data. Combining metrologies (e.g. fluorometry and electrochemical detection) further increase data acquisition. Many existing sensor metrologies are unable to fit within the confines of microfluidic devices (e.g. NMR, mass spectroscopy (MS), photodetectors and lasers), with some metrologies having industrial scale space requirements. Hence most microfluidic analyses involve coupling of detection systems to the actual device, akin to microscopes coupled to a microscope slide. In one sense, the device can also be considered a kind of interface for these larger analysis and detection systems, rather than the analysis device itself, and overall system cost necessarily includes both.

Common Misconceptions About Microfluidics

Along with the popularization of microfluidics as a source of new biotechnologies has been the prevalence of a range of subtle but pervasive misconceptions. Microfluidic technology is considered a panacea, suitable for solving any scientific problem, most notably those of biological systems, which are inherently complex. In fact, microfluidic devices are simply tools, and essentially smaller scale versions of conventional tools designed for analysis of fluid-based systems of like scale. To this end, microfluidic devices are often considered overwhelmingly complex in operation. This perception is not helped by the abundance of bewildering jargon in scientific literature, which detracts from understanding the basic utility of a device for an end-use. The perceived complexity is more a product of the functional application, rather than the nature of the device itself. By analogy, a driver can operate a car precisely, unaware of the complexities of the systems involved in its operation, let alone knowing how to reconstruct one from spare parts. With some similarity, complex microfluidic systems can be appreciated as a group of unique subsystems working in unison (e.g. electrical timing and fuel delivery), or an array of like subsystems in parallel (e.g. cooling elements in a radiator), or both. The nature of laminar fluid flow in microfluidic devices is also a point of ambiguity and technical difficulty. At these scales, two adjacent fluid layers in a single channel cannot physically mix, except by very slow passive diffusion across their boundary. However, there are many attempts to circumvent this property in a majority of devices that adopt some form of mixing strategy, to emulate standard bench top tube-based bioassays. Furthermore, any level of fluid loading, mixing or on-board capture requires larger additional volumes to drive and direct movement beyond the claimed sample volumes of nano-, pico- or femtolitre scales. Thus one of the most pervasive

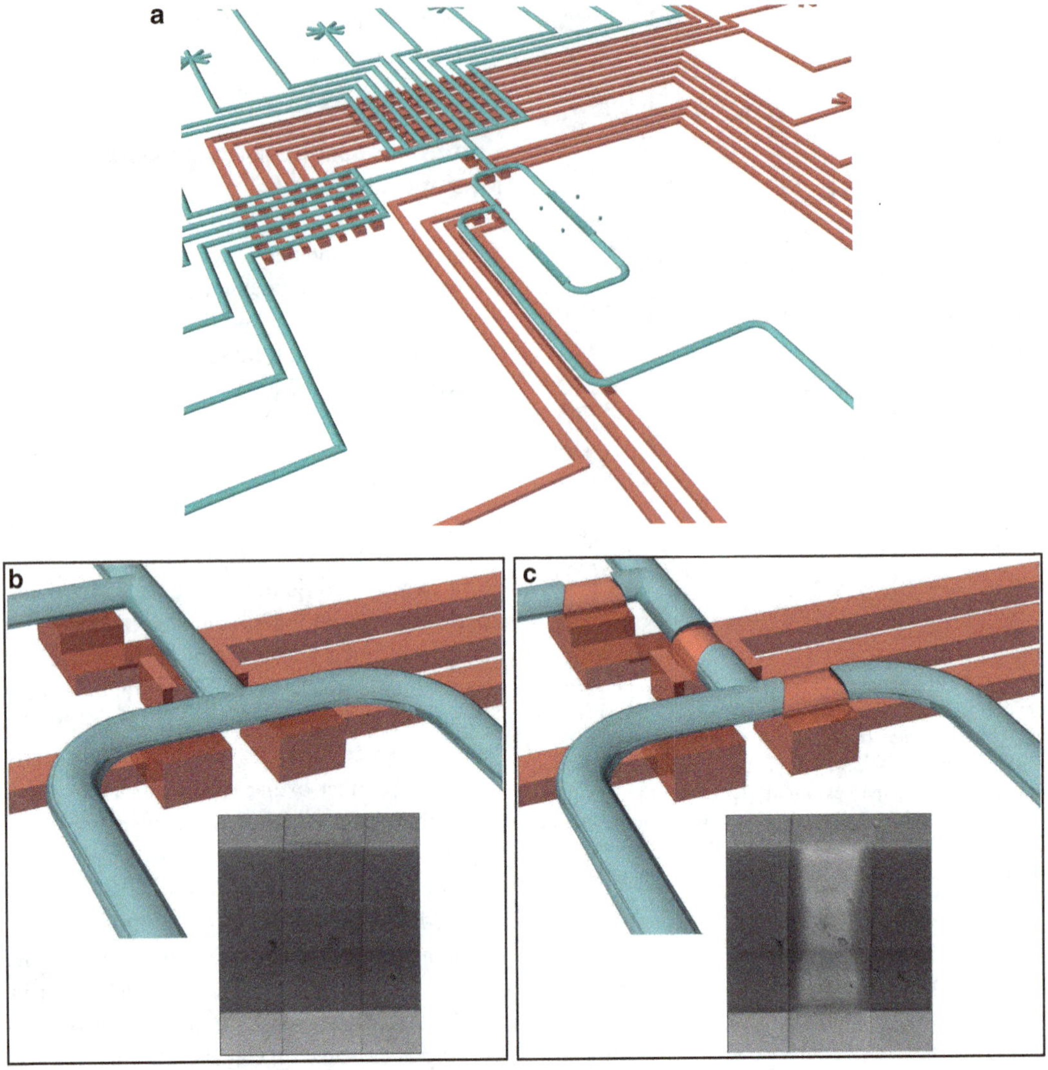

Fig. 26.4 Computer-generated rendering of the microfluidic device in Fig. 3, illustrating in 3D how the microchannel flow is controlled. The overall device format (**a**) shows individual fluid flow channels (*blue*) lying above a layer of control channels (*red*), which are driven pneumatically. Flow channels are a combination of rectilinear and rounded cross sections, with channel width uniformly around 100 μm. *Red boxes* represent valves that make contact with the blue flow channels from beneath, which appear in high density in the grid regions, representing the main control interface. A blow-up of a channel T-intersection (**b**, **c**) shows how each channel branch is positioned over three individual valves, the blind ending of a control line. When valves are open (**b**), no hydraulic pressure is in the line, and fluid can move freely in the flow channel (inset micrograph of a valve from a PDMS device, viewed from above). To close a valve, the hydraulic pressure in the control line is increased, pushing the channel floor upwards and preventing fluid flow in that region (inset photo with lighter region is where flow is blocked) (**c**)

misconceptions is that microfluidic devices are *micro*-fluidic. Taking into account total device working volume, which is usually continuous, except in the case of closed chambers or locked channels with defined volumes, they are more likely to be meso- or macro-fluidic. Some confusion can be resolved by the fact 1 mm^3 in capacity is equivalent to 1 μL of fluid, hence the discrepancies in describing geometry and fluid scale.

In general, these misconceptions are relevant to device design for a given diagnostic analysis, rather than to the end user. The following sections discuss similar microfluidic device aspects, but more specific to the methodology and analytical metrology in question.

Microfluidic Devices for Single Cell Morphology and Morphometric Analysis

As described in the introduction, imaging modalities are typically used as an off-board monitoring tool for microfluidic devices. However, integrated morphological assessment in a microfluidic device provides a unique opportunity for quantitation of a range of parameters. While the newer area of fusion between microfluidics and optical technology ("optofluidics") is still in its infancy, it may hold some promise for combining optics capabilities as built-in features of microfluidic chips, including magnification effects imparted by the chip material itself, or drawing from the physical actuation properties of light. One type of optofluidic chip is essentially lensless, employing a transparent PDMS microchannel flanked by a linear array of 2D light sensors in the base [8]. Actuated flow through the channel causes a contained object to roll across the channel base, projecting a transient shadow over each sensor at each point along its route. Computationally, images captured by the sensors at different orientations are then sequentially reconstructed to produce a high resolution 3D representation. This technique has been validated as an alternative to bright field microimaging of smaller multicellular organisms [9] and bacteria [10]. Combined with a tailored algorithm for quantitative image analysis, the device can also reveal internal cytoplasmic differences in real time, and has already proven suitable as an alternative to fluorescence-activated cell sorting (FACS) device [11]. Owing to its highly integrated operation, the device can be easily adapted for high-throughput quantitative imaging, provided an appropriate structural feature is targeted, which perhaps makes this type of device very useful for sorting of spermatozoa than single oocytes or embryos.

Beyond analysis of the visual morphology, microfluidic device chips have also proven extremely useful in accessing the biophysical nature of single cells. Parameters such as cell mass, size, density, volume and elasticity can be interrogated on passive microfluidic devices (e.g. using flow characteristics, variable width channels, in-flow geometric obstacles), or actively (e.g. using laser capture, electrostatics, acoustics, magnetic fields, etc.) or both [12]. One highly sensitive method of mass determination of single cells has been demonstrated using an ingenious microfluidic device, actuated electrically and coupled to a reflected laser and photosensor [13]. The device itself comprises a U-shaped, microfluidic channel suspended on a silicon cantilever, bonded to a sub-layer of electrodes and mounted inside a vacuum. The voltage driven across the cantilever causes it to resonate, and as a single cell traverses the channel, it causes a lag in the resonance monitored by the photosensor as a laser deflection. This provides incredibly accurate femtogram mass quantitation, suitable for even single bacteria and nanoparticles in suspension. Density can also be extrapolated based on the mass and volume (density = mass divided by volume), an approach taken using the same device to detect structurally abnormal erythrocytes in dilute blood samples from malarial patients [14]. While perhaps most suitable as a flow cytometry device, the method would be relatively non-invasive to cells. Another group constructed a similar device to discriminate between normal, abnormal and fertilized oocytes using a microfluidic channel subjected to a dielectrophoretic field in opposition to gravity, which could distinguish differences in buoyant density based on free-fall rate [15]. Although manually obtained visual morphology may still be more efficient for now, such as embryo size determination using a gradicule [16], these or other kinds of non-invasive mass determination microfluidic methods may prove useful in discriminating finer differences between oocytes in cohorts with similar morphology. This could relate to embryo developmental competence in terms of subsequent cell number, protein synthetic potential or inherent organelle complement.

Measurement of physical elasticity is another relatively overlooked method than can be performed very effectively in microfluidic devices, providing information that may relate to the type of morpho-dynamic observations described earlier. These methods are somewhat more invasive, whereby cells are subjected to graded physical deformation, and some methodologies have already shown tremendous potential for diagnosis of cancer cell phenotypes based on differences in cytoplasmic stiffness and membrane elasticity [17], possibly reflecting defects in cytoskeletal integrity or cell cycle status. While active device methods require cells to be immobilized for external forces to be applied, simpler flow-based passive techniques can also be employed. For example, flow of cells through constrictions in a channel can yield visually quantifiable data about compliance of the cells as they are being transiently compressed, with the exerted force quantifiable via micromechanical force transducers built into the flow channel [17]. This approach has been used effectively to demonstrate how a single erythrocyte can elicit a change in ATP production, measurable using fluorometry, following compression in a microfluidic channel constriction [18]. Thus, the "stiffness" of a single blastomere or oocyte could well be measured, which may relate to the complex interaction of cytoskeletal remodeling, membrane integrity or cytoplasmic viscocity, some of which are reportedly linked to developmental competence [19, 20]. Unfortunately, transient structural deformations may not necessarily be elastic, as illustrated by persistence of an injection furrow during ICSI; however, methods based on this type of physical quantitation may provide new insights into the nature of cell cycle length differences, cleavage dynamics or apoptotic phenotypes. The facts that preimplantation embryos in vivo remain in a dynamic fluid environment for several days, have a threshold of sensitivity to shear stress [21], and undergo a hydrostatic compression during blastocyst hatching may form the basis of a flow-based, minimally invasive, mechanical stress-response assay (Fig. 5) similar to the approach described by Kim and colleagues for deformation of bovine blastocysts [22].

Suitability of Microfluidics for Analysis of Oocyte and Embryo Morphology

Owing to their inherent compactness and optical transparency, microfluidic devices are easily adapted to bright field microscopy. While there are manual differences in loading protocols compared to dishes, microfluidic devices are advantageous as far as establishment of a robust and stable microenvironment for oocytes and embryos, and highly amenable to time-lapse imaging, which could be easily integrated with image capture and analysis technology. Incorporation of a method of cytostructural analysis, such as biophysical data, may also provide unique biological information relevant to the diagnostic assessment of developmental competence of oocytes and embryos, which may complement developmental kinetics. Further developments may entail on-board interrogation of an oocyte or growing embryo in a stand-alone device, possibly in an automated form, requiring only minimal manual intervention. This is a somewhat longer-term scenario, and in the meantime, it is envisaged that there will still remain a basic need for manual light microscopy as a proven tool in clinical IVF, combined with the sophisticated image discrimination skills of trained technicians.

Genomic Profiling Using Microfluidics

For convenience, the molecular approaches described can be categorized into: cell lysis or fractionation, DNA and RNA purification, amplification (e.g. for low-abundance templates of 3–6 pg genomic DNA per cell, ~30 pg total RNA per cell, ~10 cells in a blastocyst biopsy) and quantitative detection (e.g. fluorometric or spectrophotometric detection). Technological advances in all steps, most commercially available,

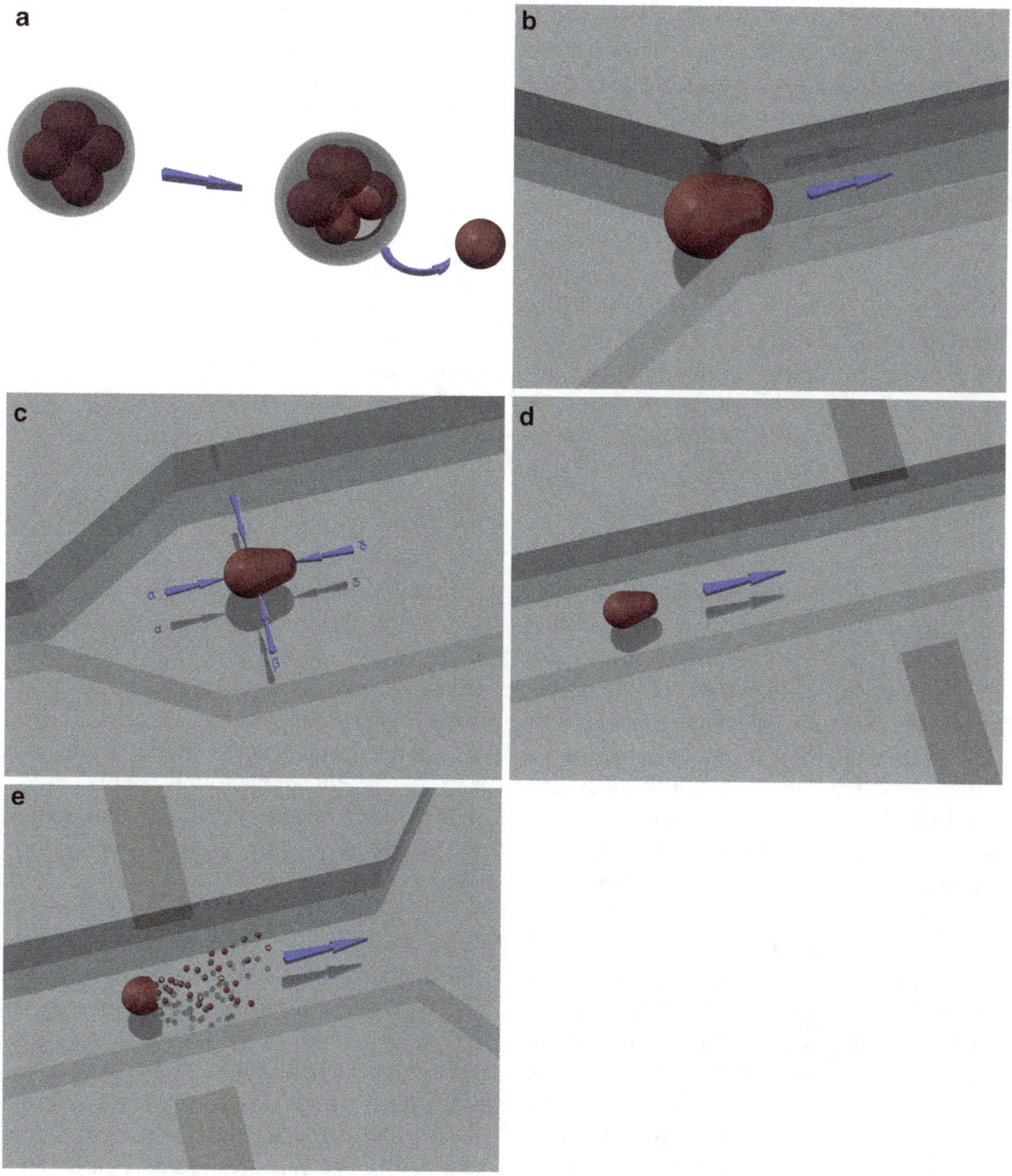

Fig. 26.5 Concept microfluidic device for biomechanical analysis of a preimplantation embryo. A blastomere is first biopsied from a cleavage stage embryo (**a**). The blastomere is then loaded into the microfluidic device and driven through a channel constriction (**b**). This causes morphological compression (**c**), from which some basic biomechanical properties can be calculated from curvatures of the rear (α), side (β) and front (δ) aspects of the plasma membrane. The same blastomere can then be moved to an actuation zone and lysed (**d**, **e**), with subcellular fragments divided by simple channel branching to other regions for parallel molecular analysis on-chip, or to other off-board platforms

have greatly decreased assay times without compromise in accuracy, a major consideration in the choice of a diagnostic assay for clinical genetic screening. Several hurdles to assay reliability, such as compensation for subtle genetic variations (e.g. mosaicism, copy number variation, random translocations) are still under continuous optimization.

Briefly, gamete or embryo fractionation is typically performed in-tube, using detergent and enzyme-based aqueous formulations with some thermal treatment and/or filtration, resulting in protein-free nanogram quantities of DNA or RNA in suspension. Further separation can also involve gel electrophoresis, allowing purification of specific mass ranges (10^3–10^6 Da) but requiring larger (microgram) amounts of starting material, with resolution down to tens or hundreds of nucleotides in length. Quantitation of extract yields prior to further analysis is typically fluorometric or spectrophotometric, based on nucleotide-specific probe binding or passive nucleotide absorbance relative to nucleotide amounts.

Once extracted, locus-specific amplification or whole genome amplification (WGA) is necessary, particularly from picogram quantities of DNA. Amplification most commonly involves variations of the PCR [23], a cyclic reaction in aqueous microlitre suspensions, that generates 10 to 20-fold increases in complementary DNA (cDNA) from short segments of gene-specific mRNA, between a pair of recognition sequences (primers). For whole genome approaches, oligonucleotide primers to randomly occurring repeat sequences (microsatellites) are targeted in specific chromosomes or across the genome. This forms the basis of degenerate oligonucleotide PCR (DOP) [24], which can be used to detect single nucleotide polymorphisms (SNPs), but may omit some regions due to incomplete coverage, resulting in allele drop-out (ADO). Expression levels can also be interrogated by analysis of gene-specific mRNA or total mRNA (transcriptome). For these applications, quantitative real-time PCR (q-PCR) has become the method of choice [25], whereby inactive fluorescent probes are incorporated into the PCR and monitored over a time-course fluorometrically, as they are activated with nascent cDNA copies. Fluorescence detection in this context is highly sensitive, allowing quantitation of very low amounts of transcript (1–10 cells worth). Further amplification can also be achieved by flanking or nesting adjacent primers, which effectively doubles the yield of cDNA. Similarly, combining multiple primer pairs (multiplexing) allows transcripts from several genes to be copied in one sample reaction, further enhancing data yield and assay.

Exponential improvement has been made in the characterization and quantitation of end products using this technique, which has greatly improved the accuracy and repeatability of analysis, with data comprehensiveness greatly aided by online gene databases and other bioinformatic software tools. This is exemplified by microarray technology, for which entire transcriptomes and genomes can be analysed in situ on two-dimensional planar "chips" containing nanogram quantities of deposited micro-spots of DNA or cDNA. Extracted cDNA from the oocyte or embryo is then applied, provided they have been suitably amplified to microgram quantities. Detection and quantitation is then performed by metrologies such as mass spectrometry (described later). Multiplex PCR technology has also converged with this approach, with the advent of PCR arrays, where multiple primer sets for specific gene families can be captured onto micro-well plate surfaces, and scanned using digital fluorescence imaging, as per qPCR. Both of these array approaches can be massively parallelized, in a similar way to microfluidic chip arrays, with microarrays perhaps the most similar in spatial scale, yet typically open devices.

An alternative high-throughput characterization with single nucleotide resolution is offered by DNA sequencing, which utilizes probes hybridized to each of the four bases (adenine, thymine, guanine and cytosine) [26]. Base detection in fractionated DNA extracts was previously performed using X-ray film exposure of radiolabelled probes bound to regions after electrophoresis. The use of fluorophores coupled to quantitative fluorescence imaging (e.g. charge-coupled devices, phosphor screens) then superseded this, or using smaller gel handling systems (e.g. microvolume capillary electrophoresis) [27] or suspensions (e.g. nano-scale particle suspensions). The latest automated sequencers are highly complex and rapid, using charge-detection based on semiconductor technology to monitor reaction rates at polymerase speeds (10–20 nucleotides per second) [28].

Microfluidic Alternatives to Genomic and Transcriptomic Analysis

Current analysis methods for quantitative genomics and transcriptomics in ART have followed quite obvious trends in micro-scaling, though mainly for static, openly accessible and scanned microdevices (e.g. DNA microarrays, microtitre plates for qPCR, PCR arrays) rather than dynamic microchannel devices. This is despite the fact that a large proportion of studies describing adaptation of a microfluidic device design to a biotechnology application have used molecular genetic endpoints for proof-of-concept, perhaps due to widespread accessibility of these techniques in experimental biosciences [29]. It may however be decades before such basic research and development are translated into practical diagnostic devices. Many adaptations therefore seek to replicate, or at least build on proven techniques, adopting the "gateway" approach.

For chromosomal analysis, there are several potentially relevant examples of microfluidic device equivalents for each of the genomic analyses outlined, which may have future benefits for ART. The first microfluidic device developed for FISH analysis of specific chromosomes was essentially a flow-through microchannel device suitable for simultaneous immobilization, hybridization and scanning of several hundred interphase cells at once, using two different flow formats and a static array [30, 31]. While only amenable to mass screening of hundreds of cells, the assay can be performed in hours, with tenfold less reagent than microscope slide assays. Other research groups have since demonstrated "FISH-on-a-chip" analysis of intact cells at metaphase [32], and most recently with interphase chromatin of a single cell nucleus in a single microchannel, taking advantage of the flow itself to linearly distend the chromatin [33], similar in principle to a COMET assay. This type of single cell application would be amenable to detect aneuploidy in combination with other structural anomalies not previously evident in an intact spread, and can be free-space coupled to standard microscopy apparatus.

Another microfluidic approach to chromosome-specific aneuploidy analysis, though again only suitable for analysis of DNA from large cell numbers is microfluidic digital PCR (μD-PCR). This commercial device uses a microarray containing 756 nL reaction wells per sample, with up to 12 samples per chip (9,072 samples in total) filled passively via evenly distributed feeder channels. Each well can support one reaction, with an incredible resolution down to one cDNA copy. Proof-of-concept of μD-PCR was first described for chromosome 21 screening of maternal and foetal blood DNA [34]. The same system is now being produced by Fluidigm Inc., also suitable as a qPCR device for transcriptomic analysis, in line with newer trends toward multiple capabilities offered by the same system. Similar microfluidic devices incorporate on-chip cell processing steps, based on reports dating back to the early 2000s [29], with recent single step examples of DNA [35] and RNA [36] fractionation; these can be run successfully on a multistep microfluidic device [37]. An ingenious microfluidic DNA sequencing chip uses electrowetting-on-dielectric (EWOD) to traffic, mix and separate sample drops containing nanobead conjugated DNA. The samples remain under oil which prevents evaporation. The electrowetting effect allows for precise control of fluid volume and mixing in an almost completely self-containined device. The DNA can be concentrated and further processed via the nanobead conjugates [38]. This system is now being commercialized by Advanced Liquid Logic Inc., as a microfluidic array pyrosequencer, a standard PCR device, a qPCR device and an SNP genotyper based on luminometry (excitation-free fluorometry), all within a similar footprint to a standard thermal cycler. A technical note has tested this system for multiplex qPCR analysis of human 8-cell embryos for up to 48 genes [39] using a commercial fluorescent probe system.

Concurrent studies have used a similar multiplex microfluidic array approach, claiming single blastomere resolution, using different microfluidic actuation principles. A landmark study from the Quake group has used the Fludigm Inc., system to analyse lineage-specific gene markers in single cells of mouse blastocysts [40]. A similar study demonstrated the use of a microwelled chip for standard PCR analysis of regulatory genes in single blastomeres, using a glass chip thermocycler

[41]; this device is less in-keeping with conventional microchannelled devices, although the same manufacturer now produces a single cell PCR channel-free device, using the microfluidic actuation method of acoustic mixing. The former study demonstrated the dynamics in coexpression of transcription factors from single cells disaggregated from morula to blastocyst stage embryos, showing differentiation into the three distinct populations, following multivariate analysis [40]. The investigators also used a preamplification step, which perhaps suggests further refinement would be required for application as a clinically relevant assay, even with sensitive luminescent probes [40]. This was very recently confirmed using the same system in a report demonstrating performance of a 24-plex qPCR reaction on single oocytes and blastocysts, with outputs that compare well statistically to pooled samples run in parallel [42]. It is therefore a matter of time before such systems become adopted clinically for single blastocyst biopsy and direct analysis, without the need for preamplification.

Suitability of Microfluidics for Genomic and Transcriptomic Analysis in ART

From a diagnostic viewpoint, perhaps the most likely platforms for both DNA and RNA analysis in ART based on microfluidics are μD-PCR devices, which are now hybrid DNA sequencers. It is probably not long before existing microarray manufacturers also venture down this path. These variants are already available in compact benchtop units, with high reproducibility and accuracy, lower cost per sample, better reaction efficiency (lower thermal masses and so faster thermal gradients), and with demonstrated proof-of-concept for oocyte and embryo analysis. There is also minimal requirement for preamplification steps, owing to improved signal-to-noise ratios and free-space coupling to highly sensitive detection systems (typically fluorescence or luminescence detection, depending on the chemistry of the probe system employed). Many of these advantages are aligned with the priorities for any clinical analysis as a diagnostic tool.

In relation to fluid handling, further advantages would be the elimination of fluid loss due to dispensing, or the need for excess fluid to drive samples into channels, should mixing be performed on-board, or using alternative forms of actuation. Fluid containment within a microfluidic channel format also ensures minimal contamination by foreign templates. Microfluidic operation systems represent the potential for integration with automation as well, providing opportunities for fractionation and other interventions, while eliminating manual handling steps. This also represents a significant purchasing and servicing cost for a complete system, although some cost may be recouped with increased sample density, increased assay variety, multiplexing or design modifications to allow for chip reuse for multiple patients per run.

Proteomic Profiling Using Microfluidics

Like genomic and transcriptomic analysis, proteomic analysis represents a destructive form of diagnostic testing, when whole or part of embryos or oocytes are assayed directly. Consequently, more attention has been paid to the non-invasive quantitation of secretory products released by embryos into the culture medium [43]. Analysis of specific proteins within cells requires protein extraction and precipitation steps, followed by fractionation (e.g. electrophoretic, chromatographic) and detection (spectroscopic, fluorometric). Similar technical limitations apply to the methodology and technology for extraction and analysis of proteins from the oocyte or embryo as for DNA and mRNA, except for differences in the overall amount of protein (>100 pg per cell, approximately three to four times the amount of total RNA), suggesting that amplification is less necessary, provided there is no significant loss during fractionation, and that detection methods are suitably sensitive. Of course, analysis of the protein component of all secreted molecules (secretome) bypasses these earlier preparatory steps completely, but remains an indirect biomarker of oocyte or embryo physiology.

Existing Proteomic Analysis in ART

Several groups have demonstrated proof-of-concept protein analysis of lysates from whole embryos or oocytes, largely in mammalian species, using traditional methods such as one- and two-dimensional (1D and 2D) gel electrophoresis [44–48]. These differ from electrophoresis techniques used for DNA and RNA separation, mainly due to the approximately tenfold higher molecular weight ranges of proteins (up to 100 kDa) compared to fractionated DNAs and RNAs (up to 10–15 kDa). Protein extracts electrophoresed vertically in one direction allows separation by size, whereas further separation across a gel at right angles using an increasing solvent pH gradient, allows the separation of proteins according to their molecular surface charge, revealing information about protein structure and relative abundances. These profiles form a type of fingerprint of gene translation products, which can be further processed for identification of specific proteins using conjugation of antibodies to specific protein sequences (e.g. Western analysis) or size quantitation of excised candidates by mass spectroscopy. Traditionally, the low sensitivity of protein purification has required extensive pooling of individual oocytes or embryos. Nowadays, methods such as difference in-gel electrophoresis (DIGE) have somewhat overcome this insensitivity, using fluorophore incorporation and quantitative digital imaging.

Another popular quantitative fluorescence-mediated approach applied to immobilized cells, whole cell lysates and secretory fractions is enzyme-linked immunosorbent assay (ELISA), which relies also on antibody-mediated recognition of specific amino acid sequences in proteins, followed by spectroscopic detection of a conjugated probe. Fluorometric ELISA has been used both to detect antigens on intact embryos [49] and secretory factors [50, 51]. For whole proteome analysis, cell lysates or spent media may also be applied to arrays of immobilized antibodies, similar to DNA microarrays, as shown previously for whole embryo detection based on mass spectroscopy [52].

Analysis of the protein composition of the secretome from the preimplantation embryo, and in some cases the oocyte [53], has typically been performed with more high resolution quantitation based on chromatographic separation coupled to mass spectroscopy [43]. Secretory proteins generally appear in lower molecular weight ranges, and in the case of embryos are lower in abundance than for more rapidly dividing cell types, a unique challenge to single embryo diagnostics. Contamination from high molecular weight albumins supplemented to culture medium is also a confounding factor, requiring a pre-separation step such as a molecular weight sieve or enzymatic digestions. Protein separation in aqueous liquids can be effectively performed using high performance liquid chromatography (HPLC), which employs linear solvent gradients to separate individual protein species from a mixture, based on subtle differences in their solubility and charge-to-molecular weight ratio. This fractionation technique is suitably sensitive for whole secretome analysis of single embryos, particularly for blastocysts that contain more protein synthetic cells. A wafer-based format, operating on similar protein adsorption principles, has enabled the embryo secretome to be interrogated with surface-enhanced laser-desorption/ionization mass spectroscopy (SELDI-TOF-MS) [54]. More recently, electron spray ionization mass spectroscopy (ESI-MS) has been used for the more sensitive detection of proteins in unfractionated culture media [55, 56]. The latter study also demonstrates a smaller scale variant called nano-scale ultra high performance liquid chromatography (nanoUPLC), which uses low-volume capillary electrophoresis, requiring less starting materials and greater yield for a wider range of protein types (e.g. hydrophobic, hydrophilic, acidic and basic), many of which are lost in standard electrophoresis and HPLC. That study still required pooling of cells and media [56], and laser-based mass spectroscopy also requires highly repetitive scanning of isolated protein fractions [52, 54]. Proteomics therefore can suffer from similar technical drawbacks to genomic analyses, in terms of a need for greater assay sensitivity, and therefore could greatly benefit from volume down-scaling.

Microfluidic Techniques Suitable for Proteomic Analysis for Oocytes and Embryos

Microfluidic devices are ideally suited to profiling of single blastocyst secretory proteins in culture media, and could easily accommodate cell lysates as well. To date, such applications have not been demonstrated exclusively for the analysis of preimplantation embryos, oocytes or accociated secretory products as an ART assay, although like genomic methods, many standard processing and analysis methods for proteins and the proteome have microfluidic equivalents. Microfluidic proof-of-concept devices have been demonstrated for on-board cell lysis and protein digestion [57], ELISA [58, 59], protein electrophoresis [60] and several examples of protein fractionation coupled to mass spectroscopy variants [61–63]. At present, these types of device concepts could offer very high efficiency and sensitivity, with some investigators claiming sub-femtomolar detection [64].

There are no commercially available microfluidic devices demonstrated for detecting oocyte or embryo biomarkers based on secretome differences. There is also still a lag to clinical translation of assays of specific protein candidates that have reported correlation to embryo implantation potential. Up- or down-regulation of secretion may however not necessarily correlate with normal expression, and many gene and protein functions are based on database sequence homology rather than precise functional characterizations. A more functional correlate may therefore be the metabolomic subset of the oocyte and embryo secretome, or at least combining known candidates in a multiplexed assay. Newer approaches in digital microfluidics, similar to the Advanced Liquid Logic Inc. device described earlier, are capable of multiple protein processing steps, and able to be coupled to mass spectrometry, for protein separation and identification for clinical assays [65]. Hence a proteomic adjunct to quantitative genomics in a microfluidic device, like the hybrid array types described earlier, may be the next "proteogenomic" development for embryo diagnostics.

Metabolomic Analysis Using Microfluidics

The metabolism of oocytes and preimplantation embryos (mainly) has proven to be one of the most critical functional parameters measured, regulating all aspects of development. All molecular processes (e.g. transcription, protein synthesis, organelle transport, cytokinesis, etc.) and homeostatic conditions have a requirement for continuous ATP supply. In turn, metabolic pathways are driven by complex molecular mechanisms, which are also heavily integrated into signal transduction pathways. While metabolism remains at a baseline level at all stages of oocyte maturation and embryo development, upregulation of activity coincides with increased energy demands, such as in association with programmed morphogenetic and differentiation steps, as determined for most mammalian species studied to date [66]. This is especially important to embryo production in vitro, where adverse culture conditions and nutrient deficits have proven, over several decades of culture system optimization, to have a direct effect on embryo developmental competence and viability [67]. Therefore, metabolic screening strategies derived from experimental methods have been recommended to be performed as routine assays for clinical IVF.

Existing Methodology Used for Metabolic Analysis of Embryos

Classical biochemical methods of metabolic analysis have proven to be highly useful in determining the metabolism of single in vitro produced embryos, being both quantitative and non-invasive, as far as indirect measurement of the culture medium composition. Broadly speaking, several techniques have been explored to quantitate specific pathway substrates (carbohydrates or amino acids, oxygen) and products (ammonium, carbon dioxide, lactate), although these will not be reviewed in depth here. A key method has been the analysis of a single aqueous metabolite (typically carbohydrate or amino acid) by enzymatic breakdown, coupled to production of a fluorescent co-factor, which is then quantitated using fluorescence microscopy. This method has recently been adapted to clinical IVF, via determination of glucose levels in culture media used to grow single human blastocysts [68]. This method is highly sensitive, relying on removal of nanolitre sized aliquots of culture medium using micromanipulation tools, and analyzing the contents in reaction nano-drops on a microscope slide by detection of fluorescence intensity. At this scale, rates of metabolic activity are typically expressed as picomoles per hour depending on the substrate and species.

This method is somewhat time-consuming and technically challenging, which has hampered its translation as a diagnostic tool to clinical IVF. Nevertheless, the concept of indirect analysis of single embryos based on altered medium nutrient levels remains one of the most well-matched functional assays to clinical IVF to date, ensuring that structural and developmental integrity of the embryo is maintained, and negating the need for any kind of biopsy procedure. More comprehensive analyses have been performed on spent media from clinical IVF embryos, to profile the entire pool of secreted metabolites (metabolome, approximately 3,000 known in the human, <3 kDa in size) or subsets such as all amino acids, using mature spectroscopic "footprinting" metrologies (e.g. (HPLC), Raman Spectroscopy, Fourier Transformed Infrared (FTIR) spectroscopy and near-infrared spectroscopy (NIR), NMR spectroscopy and mass spectroscopy (MS)) [69]. The metabolome itself is more closely aligned with the instantaneous developmental phenotype and physiological state of the embryo, than either the transcriptome or proteome, and therefore represents a defined, measureable outcome with predictive value for determination of implantation potential.

Microfluidic Approaches for Metabolic and Metabolomic Analysis

In terms of metrology type, micro-scale fluorometry is very well matched to microfluidic devices. Small volumes, which may ordinarily be a accessible to standard metrologies, provide increased analyte to volume molar ratio, with serial or parallel multi-analyte assays able to be scaled up on the same device. Also, microfluidic systems can be designed to process reactions on demand, and perform analysis at predetermined time-points following the reaction. Ordinarily, for microtitre plate-based fluorescence detection containing static volumes, multiple samples need to be reacted concurrently and scanned serially, resulting in sample analysis lag times. Upscaling volumes may not necessarily improve fluorescence analyses, even though signal intensity increases linearly with analyte level. Larger volumes can actually filter out some of the signal from within, when scanned through. In contrast, microfluidic devices may be scanned as a single image, with lower aspect ratio channels exhibiting virtually no optical filtration, autofluorescence or heterogeneous intensity effects due to free fluid surfaces (comparable to the parallel sides of a spectrophotometer cuvette). The culmination of this is increased signal-to-noise ratios, thereby enhancing the sensitivity of the measurement.

As is the case with protein secretome and morphometry analysis, there are currently no commercially available microfluidic devices appropriate for routine non-invasive assessment of embryo metabolism, based on any metrology. Using fluorometry, two important proof-of-concept studies have recently demonstrated that microfluidic devices can however be used as direct equivalents to current microscope-based methods used for embryo culture media analysis of carbohydrate level [70, 71]. The initial approach uses pneumatic actuation to merge and mix culture media volumes so they react in a nanolitre region, with feed channels able to deliver biological samples, three separate carbohydrate enzyme cocktails and five carbohydrate standards in the one device (Figs. 3 and 4a) [70]. The sensitivity of this microfluidic analysis was found to be an order of magnitude greater than standard microfluorescence analysis. A more recent approach is actually an adaptation of an electromechanically driven microfluidic culture device for embryos, modified for glucose analysis, although large feed-volumes and a macro-scale footprint suggest that the device is technically more "macrofluidic" [71].

Micro-scale spectroscopies may also be amenable to metabolic assay on a microfluidic device in specific cases, despite equipment complexity and size limitations. These methods are largely label- and preparation-free. Methods of chemical composition measurement based on absorbance of energy by molecular bond vibration (FTIR, NIR, Raman and NMR spectroscopy) have unique pros and cons for measurement of aqueous media in a microfluidic device. Infrared radiation is readily absorbed by device material, except for rarer materials such as ionic crystals or diamond. Water itself is also a prolific absorber of infrared wavelengths (1–14 μm); therefore, samples often require fixation and dehydration, which could chemically alter some metabolites. Infrared spectroscopy can also suffer from a decrease in the ability to resolve individual metabolites as the chemical complexity of the media increases, requiring extensive post-assay bioinformatics analysis of spectral peaks. Raman spectroscopy also interrogates molecular composition, though it utilizes inelastic scattering of light rather than absorbance like the other metrologies (except MS). Raman scattering signal strengths are extremely low (~10^7-fold loss of intensity), which requires very high energy light sources and long acquisition times. The method is however not wavelength-dependent like fluorometry, or water-dependent like infrared methods, and can allow measurement of specific ranges of metabolites using discrete wavelength sources (e.g. lasers). Device modifications such as metalized coatings and specific thickness ranges can also enhance and amplify the scattering signal. Like Raman spectroscopy, proton NMR spectroscopy is non-invasive, using radio waves to excite hydrogen protons in organic molecules, with the transient relaxation signal indicative of their molecular location. While requiring no external calibration, and suitable for measuring relative abundances and absolute levels of metabolites, there is major interference from water, the spatial resolution is low (there is no advantage to volume reduction, as entire chips are scanned within the device as one value), and large distances to the detector result in major loss of signal strength.

All of these spectroscopies have proven successful for their ability to obtain quantitative metabolomic profiles from used embryo culture media to predict implantation and pregnancy rates, and to correlate both using tailored bioinformatics [72]. Microfluidic devices have not yet been used to address these findings, perhaps because of continued requirements for downscaling of source and detector hardware to match the volume constraints of chips. Recent technological advancements may expedite this specific adaptation, such as via built-in detection components, such as remote coils for on-board NMR sensing [73] or micro-sized optics for enhanced infrared signals [74].

To this latter end, several interesting developments have been made in microfluidic device coupling to MS [74], which although requires extensive sample preparation, is perhaps the most prolific scientific tool for metabolite identification and structural analysis. MS is different than the other modalities discussed, as the metabolite mixture is essentially decomposed into submolecular fragments using a solvent, and sprayed over a distance, with deflection in electric fields determining the absolute composition (mass-to-charge ratio). This method is also capable of measurement of blastocoele metabolite levels after removal from human blastocysts [75], using a very similar approach to an earlier study using HPLC for amino acid detection [76]. Thus, MS offers a high level of sensitivity for native nanolitre fluid volumes relevant to embryo physiology, suggesting that non-invasive measurement of media on a chip may benefit from future improvements in device–detector interfaces, although the technique can be volume limited. Research is ongoing as to how chemical separation may be built into a device, such as via porous extraction bead injection into channels [77], or modification of device structure to match the requirements of detectors, such as converting channel outlets into spray nozzles for ESI/MS [78], or changing device materials to accommodate those used for matrix-assisted LDI/MS, as recently reviewed [79].

Suitability and Limitations of Microfluidics for Metabolic Analysis of Embryos

While microfluidic devices can enable quantitative analysis of single or multiple metabolite levels in embryo culture media, at the single embryo level, the technology is still in its infancy, despite a host of new proof-of-concept devices and device–detector combinations. The main hindrance for IVF laboratories is the cost associated with the detection metrologies that are coupled to microfluidic devices, as well as the need to tailor device design, fabrication, use and endpoint analysis to individual laboratory needs. Nevertheless, microfluidic devices have been demonstrated for fluorometric single metabolite detection, providing comparable (if not better) outcomes to conventional assays. Considering that metabolomic spectroscopy outcomes have also correlated with clinical implantation and pregnancy outcomes based on the same general sampling protocol in milli-scale volumes, with metabolite identification in some cases, a fully quantitative profile of known metabolites measured in a stage-specific manner is still highly conceivable. Such an approach would be even more informative if combined with some kind of continuous monitoring morphometric and culture device.

Concluding Thoughts

Microfluidic technology provides a unique means of interfacing known analytical methods for embryo developmental physiology and molecular phenotypes in real time. Proof of concept devices have been demonstrated for quantitation of all relevant biological parameters, with commercial translation more prevalent for genomic and proteomic detection, wherein microfluidic devices might form the next generation of PGS technologies. While PDMS devices are amenable to culture and microscopic visualization of growing embryos, there is still no easily implemented substitute for standard incubation techniques, although there is the very real prospect of integration of a microfluidic device for morphokinetic analysis, as an adjunct to time-lapse imaging. It may still be some time before the wealth of experimental concepts in microfluidic sciences are translated into a clinically relevant diagnostic tool for IVF, but these should provide a gateway to future devices with more automation and less user intervention, to systematize ART laboratories. An ideal device could be an active, continuous culture platform with integrated time-lapse imaging and metabolomic or secretomic endpoints, providing real-time physiological outputs as the embryo develops, as well as sampling for interface with more detailed molecular analyses.

References

1. Atencia J, Beebe DJ. Controlled microfluidic interfaces. Nature. 2005;437(7059):648–55.
2. DeMello AJ. Control and detection of chemical reactions in microfluidic systems. Nature. 2006;442(7101):394–402.
3. Szekely L, Guttman A. New advances in microchip fabrication for electrochromatography. Electrophoresis. 2005;26(24):4590–604.
4. Weibel DB, Diluzio WR, Whitesides GM. Microfabrication meets microbiology. Nat Rev Microbiol. 2007;5(3):209–18.
5. Wang JD et al. Quantitative analysis of molecular absorption into PDMS microfluidic channels. Ann Biomed Eng. 2012;40:1862–73.
6. Regehr KJ et al. Biological implications of polydimethylsiloxane-based microfluidic cell culture. Lab Chip. 2009;9(15):2132–9.
7. Lee CY et al. Microfluidic mixing: a review. Int J Mol Sci. 2011;12(5):3263–87.
8. Heng X et al. Optofluidic microscopy—a method for implementing a high resolution optical microscope on a chip. Lab Chip. 2006;6(10):1274–6.
9. Cui X et al. Lensless high-resolution on-chip optofluidic microscopes for Caenorhabditis elegans and cell imaging. Proc Natl Acad Sci USA. 2008;105(31):10670–5.
10. Lee LM, Cui X, Yang C. The application of on-chip optofluidic microscopy for imaging Giardia lamblia trophozoites and cysts. Biomed Microdevices. 2009; 11:951–8.
11. Cho SH et al. Human mammalian cell sorting using a highly integrated micro-fabricated fluorescence-activated cell sorter (microFACS). Lab Chip. 2010;10(12):1567–73.
12. Bao G, Suresh S. Cell and molecular mechanics of biological materials. Nat Mater. 2003;2(11):715–25.
13. Burg TP et al. Weighing of biomolecules, single cells and single nanoparticles in fluid. Nature. 2007; 446(7139):1066–9.

14. Grover WH et al. Measuring single-cell density. Proc Natl Acad Sci USA. 2011;108(27):10992–6.
15. Hwang H et al. Enhanced discrimination of normal oocytes using optically induced pulling-up dielectrophoretic force. Biomicrofluidics. 2009;3(1):14103.
16. Lane M et al. Assessment of metabolism of equine morulae and blastocysts. Mol Reprod Dev. 2001; 59(1):33–7.
17. Suresh S. Biomechanics and biophysics of cancer cells. Acta Biomater. 2007;3(4):413–38.
18. Wan J, Ristenpart WD, Stone HA. Dynamics of shear-induced ATP release from red blood cells. Proc Natl Acad Sci USA. 2008;105(43):16432–7.
19. Palermo GD et al. Oolemma characteristics in relation to survival and fertilization patterns of oocytes treated by intracytoplasmic sperm injection. Hum Reprod. 1996;11(1):172–6.
20. Ebner T et al. Developmental competence of oocytes showing increased cytoplasmic viscosity. Hum Reprod. 2003;18(6):1294–8.
21. Xie Y et al. Shear stress induces preimplantation embryo death that is delayed by the zona pellucida and associated with stress-activated protein kinase-mediated apoptosis. Biol Reprod. 2006;75(1):45–55.
22. Kim MS et al. A microfluidic in vitro cultivation system for mechanical stimulation of bovine embryos. Electrophoresis. 2009;30(18):3276–82.
23. Saiki RK et al. Enzymatic amplification of beta-globin genomic sequences and restriction site analysis for diagnosis of sickle cell anemia. Science. 1985; 230(4732):1350–4.
24. Telenius H et al. Degenerate oligonucleotide-primed PCR: general amplification of target DNA by a single degenerate primer. Genomics. 1992;13(3):718–25.
25. Steuerwald NM et al. Maternal age-related differential global expression profiles observed in human oocytes. Reprod Biomed Online. 2007;14(6):700–8.
26. Sanger F, Coulson AR. A rapid method for determining sequences in DNA by primed synthesis with DNA polymerase. J Mol Biol. 1975;94(3):441–8.
27. Cohen AS et al. High-performance capillary electrophoretic separation of bases, nucleosides, and oligonucleotides: retention manipulation via micellar solutions and metal additives. Anal Chem. 1987;59(7): 1021–7.
28. Rusk N. Torrents of sequence. Nat Methods. 2011; 8(1):44.
29. Njoroge SK et al. Integrated microfluidic systems for DNA analysis. Top Curr Chem. 2011;304:203–60.
30. Sieben VJ et al. FISH and chips: chromosomal analysis on microfluidic platforms. IET Nanobiotechnol. 2007;1(3):27–35.
31. Sieben VJ et al. An integrated microfluidic chip for chromosome enumeration using fluorescence in situ hybridization. Lab Chip. 2008;8(12):2151–6.
32. Vedarethinam I et al. Metaphase FISH on a chip: miniaturized microfluidic device for fluorescence in situ hybridization. Sensors (Basel). 2010;10(11):9831–46.
33. Wang X et al. Microfluidic extraction and stretching of chromosomal DNA from single cell nuclei for DNA fluorescence in situ hybridization. Biomed Microdevices. 2012;14(3):443–51.
34. Fan HC, Quake SR. Detection of aneuploidy with digital polymerase chain reaction. Anal Chem. 2007;79(19):7576–9.
35. Lee HJ et al. Electrochemical cell lysis device for DNA extraction. Lab Chip. 2009;10(5):626–33.
36. Vulto P et al. A microfluidic approach for high efficiency extraction of low molecular weight RNA. Lab Chip. 2010;10(5):610–6.
37. Zhang Y et al. An all-in-one microfluidic device for parallel DNA extraction and gene analysis. Biomed Microdevices. 2010;12(6):1043–9.
38. Boles DJ et al. Droplet-based pyrosequencing using digital microfluidics. Anal Chem. 2011;83(22): 8439–47.
39. Pieprzyk M, High H. Fluidigm dynamic arrays provide a platform for single cell gene expression analysis. 2009. Nat. Meth. 6 (iii–iv)
40. Guo G et al. Resolution of cell fate decisions revealed by single-cell gene expression analysis from zygote to blastocyst. Dev Cell. 2010;18(4):675–85.
41. May A et al. Multiplex rt-PCR expression analysis of developmentally important genes in individual mouse preimplantation embryos and blastomeres. Biol Reprod. 2009;80(1):194–202.
42. Morrill BH et al. Use of nanofluidic RT quantitative polymerase chain reaction to study variation in gene expression between single bovine oocyte and blastocyst samples. Reprod Fertil Dev. 2011;24(1): 180–1.
43. Katz-Jaffe MG et al. The role of proteomics in defining the human embryonic secretome. Mol Hum Reprod. 2009;15(5):271–7.
44. Latham KE et al. Analysis of embryonic mouse development: construction of a high-resolution, two-dimensional gel protein database. Appl Theor Electrophor. 1992;2(6):163–70.
45. Shi CZ et al. Protein databases for compacted eight-cell and blastocyst-stage mouse embryos. Mol Reprod Dev. 1994;37(1):34–47.
46. Anderiesz C et al. Effect of recombinant human gonadotrophins on human, bovine and murine oocyte meiosis, fertilization and embryonic development in vitro. Hum Reprod. 2000;15(5):1140–8.
47. Navarrete Santos A et al. Two insulin-responsive glucose transporter isoforms and the insulin receptor are developmentally expressed in rabbit preimplantation embryos. Reproduction. 2004;128(5):503–16.
48. Wang Y et al. Increases in phosphorylation of SAPK/JNK and p38MAPK correlate negatively with mouse embryo development after culture in different media. Fertil Steril. 2005;83 Suppl 1:1144–54.
49. Goldbard SB, Gollnick SO, Warner CM. A highly sensitive method for the detection of cell surface antigens on preimplantation mouse embryos. J Immunol Methods. 1984;68(1–2):137–46.
50. Noci I et al. Embryonic soluble HLA-G as a marker of developmental potential in embryos. Hum Reprod. 2005;20(1):138–46.

51. Mains LM et al. Identification of apolipoprotein A1 in the human embryonic secretome. Fertil Steril. 2011; 96(2):422–7 e2.
52. Katz-Jaffe MG et al. A proteomic analysis of mammalian preimplantation embryonic development. Reproduction. 2005;130(6):899–905.
53. Angelucci S et al. Proteome analysis of human follicular fluid. Biochim Biophys Acta. 2006;1764(11): 1775–85.
54. Katz-Jaffe MG, Schoolcraft WB, Gardner DK. Analysis of protein expression (secretome) by human and mouse preimplantation embryos. Fertil Steril. 2006;86(3):678–85.
55. Beardsley AJ, Li Y, O'Neill C. Characterization of a diverse secretome generated by the mouse preimplantation embryo in vitro. Reprod Biol Endocrinol. 2010;8:71.
56. Cortezzi SS et al. Secretome of the preimplantation human embryo by bottom-up label-free proteomics. Anal Bioanal Chem. 2011;401(4):1331–9.
57. Gao J et al. Integrated microfluidic system enabling protein digestion, peptide separation, and protein identification. Anal Chem. 2001;73(11):2648–55.
58. Herrmann M, Veres T, Tabrizian M. Enzymatically-generated fluorescent detection in micro-channels with internal magnetic mixing for the development of parallel microfluidic ELISA. Lab Chip. 2006;6(4):555–60.
59. Hoegger D et al. Disposable microfluidic ELISA for the rapid determination of folic acid content in food products. Anal Bioanal Chem. 2007;387(1):267–75.
60. Xue Q et al. Multiplexed enzyme assays in capillary electrophoretic single-use microfluidic devices. Electrophoresis. 2001;22(18):4000–7.
61. Chen SH et al. A disposable poly(methylmethacrylate)-based microfluidic module for protein identification by nanoelectrospray ionization-tandem mass spectrometry. Electrophoresis. 2001;22(18):3972–7.
62. Wheeler AR et al. Electrowetting-based microfluidics for analysis of peptides and proteins by matrix-assisted laser desorption/ionization mass spectrometry. Anal Chem. 2004;76(16):4833–8.
63. Young JB, Li L. An impulse-driven liquid-droplet deposition interface for combining LC with MALDI MS and MS/MS. J Am Soc Mass Spectrom. 2006;17(3):325–34.
64. Goluch ED et al. A bio-barcode assay for on-chip attomolar-sensitivity protein detection. Lab Chip. 2006;6(10):1293–9.
65. Jebrail MJ, et al. Digital microfluidics for automated proteomic processing. J Vis Exp. 2009(33).
66. Leese HJ. Metabolic control during preimplantation mammalian development. Hum Reprod Update. 1995;1(1):63–72.
67. Gardner DK. Dissection of culture media for embryos: the most important and less important components and characteristics. Reprod Fertil Dev. 2008;20(1):9–18.
68. Gardner DK et al. Glucose consumption of single post-compaction human embryos is predictive of embryo sex and live birth outcome. Hum Reprod. 2011;26(8):1981–6.
69. Thouas GA, Gardner DK. Metabolomic profiling for selection of the most viable clinical IVF embryo. Curr Women's Health Rev. 2010;6:254–60.
70. Urbanski JP et al. Noninvasive metabolic profiling using microfluidics for analysis of single preimplantation embryos. Anal Chem. 2008;80(17):6500–7.
71. Heo YS et al. Real time culture and analysis of embryo metabolism using a microfluidic device with deformation based actuation. Lab Chip. 2012;12(12):2240–6.
72. Botros L, Sakkas D, Seli E. Metabolomics and its application for non-invasive embryo assessment in IVF. Mol Hum Reprod. 2008;14(12):679–90.
73. Utz M, Landers J. Chemistry. Magnetic resonance and microfluidics. Science. 2010;330(6007):1056–8.
74. Greener J, Abbasi B, Kumacheva E. Attenuated total reflection Fourier transform infrared spectroscopy for on-chip monitoring of solute concentrations. Lab Chip. 2010;10(12):1561–6.
75. D'Alessandro A et al. A mass spectrometry-based targeted metabolomics strategy of human blastocoele fluid: a promising tool in fertility research. Mol Biosyst. 2012;8(4):953–8.
76. Gopichandran N, Leese HJ. Metabolic characterization of the bovine blastocyst, inner cell mass, trophectoderm and blastocoel fluid. Reproduction. 2003; 126(3):299–308.
77. Wei H et al. Cell signaling analysis by mass spectrometry under coculture conditions on an integrated microfluidic device. Anal Chem. 2011;83(24):9306–13.
78. Chen Q et al. Qualitative and quantitative analysis of tumor cell metabolism via stable isotope labeling assisted microfluidic chip electrospray ionization mass spectrometry. Anal Chem. 2012;84(3):1695–701.
79. Lee J, Soper SA, Murray KK. Microfluidics with MALDI analysis for proteomics—a review. Anal Chim Acta. 2009;649(2):180–90.

Index

D.K. Gardner et al. (eds.), *Human Gametes and Preimplantation Embryos: Assessment and Diagnosis*, DOI 10.1007/978-1-4614-6651-2, © Springer Science+Business Media New York 2013

N

O

CPSIA information can be obtained
at www.ICGtesting.com
Printed in the USA
LVHW06*0003221018
594347LV00009B/418/P

9 781461 466505